Applied Speech Technology

Edited by
A. Syrdal
R. Bennett
S. Greenspan

Applied
Speech
Technology

CRC Press
Boca Raton   Ann Arbor   London   Tokyo

Library of Congress Cataloging-in-Publication Data

Syrdal, A. (Ann K.)
    Applied speech technology / A. Syrdal, R. Bennett, S. Greenspan.
      p. cm.
    Includes bibliographical references and index.
    ISBN 0-8493-9456-2
    1. Speech processing systems. I. Bennett. R. (Raymond W.)
  II. Greenspan, S. (Steven L.)   III. Title.
TK7882.S65S97 1994
006.4'54—dc20   94-26882
                                                CIP

No claim to original U.S. Government works
International Standard Book Number 0-8493-9456-2
Library of Congress Card Number 94-26882
Printed in the United States of America 1 2 3 4 5 6 7 8 9 0
Printed on acid-free paper

Table Of Contents

Chapter 1
Speech: Articulatory, Linguistic, Acoustic, and Perceptual Descriptions

Stephen M. Marcus and Ann K. Syrdal
AT&T Bell Laboratories

1. Introduction

Speech has evolved over a period of tens of thousand of years as the primary means of communication between human beings. Since the evolution of speech and of *homo sapiens* have proceeded hand–in–hand, it seems reasonable to assume that human speech production mechanisms, and the resulting acoustic signal, are optimally adapted to human speech perception mechanisms. A deeper understanding of the human communication process may therefore prove very valuable, if not essential, to any who are working on the development and application of speech technology to human–machine interaction *via* speech.

The communication process, seen as a whole, concerns all stages from the origin of a thought in the mind of a speaker to its perception in the mind of the listener. These operations include the selection of a suitable set of words to express the meaning of the speaker's thoughts, the choice of an appropriate word order and grammatical form consistent with this meaning, the expression of each word as speech sounds, and the production of suitable articulatory gestures to give these form as acoustic vibrations in the physical world. The communication process in the listener begins with reception of the acoustic vibrations by the ear, and should ultimately result in the perception of the speaker's intended meaning and thus an insight into his or her thoughts.

The connection between thought and meaning and the selection of words, and the rules and restrictions that govern the order and form of words will not be dealt with here. Although these factors exert an influence throughout the whole process of production and perception, we shall concentrate on the spoken word and its relation to the acoustic signal. After an introductory discussion of the encoded nature of speech, the chapter will describe speech production, the acoustic theory of speech production, linguistic units of speech, acoustic characteristics of speech, auditory perception, and speech perception.

2.   The Encoded Nature of Speech

Several decades ago, two early technical development projects involving speech were initiated but failed because the process of speech communication turned out to be very different from what people assumed it was. Both projects were based on the supposition that speech was composed of a sequence of discrete, distinctive sounds.

In the 1950s, a "reading machine for the blind" was developed in the expectation that by using the auditory modality and sound rather than the tactile modality to perceive raised patterns of dots, faster reading speeds could be achieved for blind users, since reading by braille is significantly slower than reading by sight or listening to a spoken message. The reading machine produced an audibly distinct sound for each alphabetic character in the text to be read. It was initially assumed that any set of highly discriminable sounds would function as efficiently and effectively as speech. Researchers found, however, that reading rates with their device, even with highly trained and motivated users, did not exceed that of Braille or Morse code, and fell far short of the efficiency of speech communication. In fact, the transmission of temporally ordered information in normal speech communication exceeds the temporal resolving power of the ear! This paradox led to the discovery that speech was not a sequential string of discrete sounds, but that the acoustic characteristics of individual speech segments—consonants and vowels—were distributed through the syllable level and even higher (Liberman, 1967). Even though there were no technical failures in the reading machine, it did not work as intended because the process of listening to a series of audibly distinct sounds is different from and much less efficient than what is involved in the perception of speech.

In the early 1960s, there were hopes that an "automatic typewriter" that would produce at least a phonetic version of what was said lay not far in the future. It was supposed that relatively simple decisions could be made to phonetically label each section of the incoming waveform and thus to transcribe the spoken utterance as a sequence of phonemes. Much more is now known about the complex interactions between parts of the acoustic signal that make it impossible to apply any such simple sequential recognition strategy. One such interaction was demonstrated by Pickett and Decker (1960). By inserting a short period of silence (around 100 ms) between the "s" and "l" sounds in the word "*slit*," the modified stimulus is clearly perceived as "*split*." Thus the perception of sounds, and even of a period of silence, depends on the surrounding context in which it occurs.

Although in this case the addition of a period of silence produces the percept of a "p," we cannot simply suppose that a "p–detector" responds to a short period of silence. We would then have difficulty in explaining its fortunate lack of response during other silent intervals. Such context effects are found to occur at all levels in human perception. In the case of speech, the perception of a particular sound depends on the nature of adjacent sounds in the same word, and even on adjacent words in the utterance. It is clear that we cannot build a simple "phonetic typewriter" giving a unique label to each sound without reference to its context.

3. The Production of Speech

Figure 1 shows a schematic diagram of the vocal organs. Speech is generated by the coordinated movements of many anatomical structures. Air pressure built up below the larynx by the efforts of muscles and the lungs provides the energy for the speech signal. The vocal folds within the larynx can be positioned so that air can flow through the glottis (the space between the vocal folds) with or without setting the vocal folds into vibration. During normal speech production, air is forced up from the lungs, and in passing through the glottis and a number of possible narrowings in the vocal tract, either periodic or aperiodic (noise) excitation is produced. The subsequent sections of the vocal tract, including the tongue, jaw, lips, velum, and nasal cavities, act as a set of resonant cavities that modify the spectrum of this excitation before it is emitted from the lips as sound vibrations. While speaking, the articulatory organs are in rapid and almost constant movement, and the sounds produced exhibit many features of a transient nature. Speech perception then requires the integration of these into a continuous stream.

The two broad classes of speech sounds the human vocal tract is capable of producing are vowels and consonants. **Vowels** are produced with a rela-

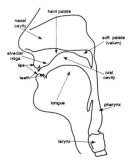

Figure 1. The principal parts of the vocal tract

tively open vocal tract, with little audible obstruction to the passage of air. **Consonants** are produced with a relatively closed vocal tract, resulting in an audible effect on the air flow. There may be a temporary complete closure, as in initial and final sounds in the word "*teak*," or there may be a sufficient closure to produce noticeable turbulence, as in the word "*fish*," or the narrowing may simply result in the sounds of a noticeably lower amplitude and different quality from the vowels, such as "*well*."

To better understand the variety of sounds that may be produced, let us consider the function of the various structures in the vocal tract, beginning at the larynx and working up to the lips.

3.1   The Vocal Folds—Voiced and Voiceless Sounds
The first possible obstruction to the passage of air from the lungs is the **vocal folds** (also called vocal cords)—two small folds of ligament extending from front to back on either side of the larynx. The **larynx** is a stack of cartilages connected by muscles and ligaments that form a series of rings; one of the laryngeal cartilages, the thyroid (or Adam's apple), is easily located because it projects visibly at the front of the neck. The larynx acts as a valve between the lungs and the mouth, and as such it plays an essential role in eating and breathing. Humans have learned to use the laryngeal valve to convert the air stream from the lungs into a sound source for speech. The vocal folds extend from the thyroid cartilage in the front of the larynx to the two arytenoid cartilages at the back. The vocal folds are always held together at the front, but the **glottal opening** can be controlled by moving the arytenoids apart. If the arytenoids and thus the vocal folds are held close together, air pressure builds up behind the vocal folds and eventually blows them apart, releasing the excess pressure, so that the folds return to their closed position. This process repeats, and the repeating cycle causes the vocal folds to vibrate rhythmically, producing a sequence of air puffs heard as a buzzing sound as they open and close. The resulting sound is termed **voiced**. The frequency of vocal fold vibration and of the resulting quasi–periodic sound depends on how fast the folds are blown apart and how quickly they snap back together again. Factors controlling this frequency include the mass, tension and length of the vocal folds, and subglottal pressure; the latter three factors are adjustable by the speaker. The frequency of vibration normally ranges between about 60 Hz and 400 Hz, with an average of around 100 Hz for adult male speakers and 180 Hz for adult female speakers (Peterson and Barney, 1952).

If the vocal folds are somewhat farther apart, turbulence resulting in aperiodic noise will be produced but no periodic vibration. The resulting sound is known as **aspiration**. Aspiration is the sound source for the initial consonant in the word *"house,"* for example, and for all whispered speech.

When the vocal folds are wide open, no sound is produced at the glottis. This occurs during normal breathing and also during the production of some speech sounds, such as all the consonants in the word *"shifts."* The resulting speech sound is then termed **voiceless**. Its characteristic aperiodic turbulence noise source is produced at a narrow constriction higher in the vocal tract. Try producing the sounds "sss..." and "zzz..." or "fff..." and "vvv..." in alternation. The only change between each pair is in the position of the vocal folds (open versus closed) and the voicing of the resultant sound (voiceless versus voiced).

3.2 The Supraglottal Vocal Tract

The quality of the sound produced at the glottis is changed by the configuration of the vocal tract above it. The **pharynx** is the cavity immediately above the larynx (and the esophagus), connecting it with the mouth and nose. The size and shape of the pharynx can be changed either by moving the tongue back or the larynx up, or by contracting the pharyngeal walls. These changes are made routinely during swallowing and also during speech production. The soft palate or **velum** is the muscular, movable portion at the back of the palate, the top structure of the oral cavity. The velum is lowered during normal respiration so that air can flow between the nostrils and the lungs. When it is raised to close against the back of the pharynx, air can only flow through the mouth cavity. This configuration is used for articulating non–nasal (oral) speech sounds. Lowering the velum allows air to flow through the nasal cavities in the production of the nasal consonants, such as those in the words *"name"* and *"Ming,"* and in the nasalization of vowels. The velum is attached to the **hard palate**, which forms the rigid, bony upper roof of the mouth. The juncture of the hard palate and the upper teeth is called the **alveolar ridge**, which is covered by the gums. The tongue and lips are the principle articulators. The powerful muscles surrounding the lips and forming the body of the tongue can, together with the jaw muscles, rapidly change the position of these articulators in relation to the other structures in the vocal tract. The resulting effect on the airflow and the resonances in the vocal tract control the nature and quality of the sound produced.

3.3 American English Consonants

Besides differences in voicing, discussed above, consonants are generally described along two dimensions of their production: their **place of articulation** and **manner of articulation**.

3.3.1   Place of Articulation

The **place of articulation** of a consonant is the point of major closure in the vocal tract during its articulation. The places of articulation of American English consonants are:

(1) **Bilabial**   The main closure or constriction is between the lips, as in the consonants in the words *"wipe"* and *"bomb."*

(2) **Labiodental**   The lower lip approaches or closes against the upper teeth, as in both consonants in the word *"five."*

(3) **Linguadental**   Closure or a major constriction is formed between the tongue tip and the upper teeth, as in initial consonants in the words *"this"* and *"think."*

(4) **Alveolar**   The tongue tip approaches or closes against the alveolar ridge just behind the upper teeth, as in consonants in the words *"tide," "size," "near,"* and *"lull."*

(5) **Palatoalveolar** Closure or major constriction is made between the tongue and the juncture between the alveolar ridge and the hard palate as in the final consonant in the word *"dish,"* the second consonant in *"measure,"* and the initial consonant in *"yell."*

(6) **Velar**   The back of the tongue closes against the soft palate or velum as in the consonants in the words *"king"* and *"gang."*

(7) **Glottal**   A partial closure of the vocal folds, insufficient to result in vibratory activity, but sufficient to produce aspiration noise, as in the initial consonant of the word *"hill."*

3.3.2   Manner of Articulation

Various types of articulatory gesture, or manners of articulation, may be made at the points of closure listed above. Those used in American English are:

1) **Plosives**. These are produced by a complete closure somewhere along the vocal tract, so that air pressure builds up behind the point of closure until the stop is released, resulting in an abrupt burst of energy or "explosion" that characterizes the plosives such as the consonants in the words *"pick," "bid,"* and *"gate."*

2) **Nasals.** Nasals, like plosives, are produced by a complete closure in the oral cavity, but because nasals are also characterized by a lowered (open) velum, the nasal cavities are coupled to the pharynx, allowing airflow through the nasal tract and no pressure build up behind the point of closure. Examples are the final consonants in the words *"same," "sun,"* and *"sing."*

3) **Fricatives**. An extreme narrowing at some point in the vocal tract results in turbulence of the airflow, generating aperiodic hissing noise that primarily excites the oral cavities in front of the constriction, as in the initial consonants of the words *"sea," "zoo," "shoe," "fee," "vee," "hay," "thank,"* and *"they,"* and the second consonant in the word *"measure."*

4) **Affricates**. A complete closure followed by a more gradual release than for a plosive is characterized by some frication. These may be represented as a combination of a stop and a fricative, such as the consonants in *"church"* and *"judge."*

5) **Approximants**. The articulators approach one another, but the constriction formed is not sufficient to produce a turbulent airstream. Two of these sounds, illustrated by the initial consonants of *"wet"* and *"yet,"* are sometimes termed "semivowels" because of their intermediate articulatory status between consonants and vowels. Semivowels are produced by briefly keeping the vocal tract in a vowel–like position and then changing it rapidly to the position required for the following vowel in the syllable. The two other approximants, as in the initial consonants of *"led"* and *"red,"* are often termed "liquids." In the case of the former liquid, the only **lateral** approximant, the airflow is allowed to pass on one or both sides of the tongue. Approximants typically are attached to vowels.

Table I systematically lists the consonants found in American English by place and manner of articulation, and by voicing.

Table I. The consonants of American English listed by place and manner of articulation, and voicing.

Place of Articulation	Manner of Articulation							
	Plosive		Nasal	Fricative		Affricate		Approximant
	Voiced	Unvoiced	Voiced	Voiced	Unvoiced	Voiced	Unvoiced	Voiced
Labial	b	p	m					w[1]
Labiodental				v	f			
Linguadental				ð	θ			
Alveolar	d	t	n	z	s			r,l
Palatoalveolar				ž	š	ǰ	č	j
Velar	g	k	ŋ					
Glottal					h			

3.4 American English Vowels

Vowels are produced with relatively little impediment of the airflow compared with consonants. There are some sixteen vowels in American English. The identity of each vowel is determined, as for the consonants, by the position of the articulators, and in particular the tongue, lips, and lower jaw. The different articulatory positions may be classified as follows:

1) **Tongue height** or **opening** of vocal tract: The terms **high, mid** and **low** refer to the relative height of the tongue at the point of greatest closure. High vowels include those in *"beat"* and *"boot;"* mid vowels, in *"bet"* and *"but;"* and low vowels, *"bat"* and *"bob."* The alternative and equivalent terms **closed, half–open** and **open** refer to the corresponding openness of the vocal tract, the vocal tract being most open when the tongue is lowest.

2) **Horizontal place of articulation: Front, central, back.** The second major parameter is the horizontal location of the point of greatest closure in the mouth. Front vowels include those in the words *"beat," "bit," "bait," "bet,"* and *"bat;"* central vowels, *"but"* and *"bird,"* and back vowels, *"bob," "bought," "boat," "book," and "boot."* Figure 2 shows approximate tongue positions for a number of vowels differing in tongue height and front–back position.

---

1. /w/ is more completely categorized as a voiced labial–velar approximant

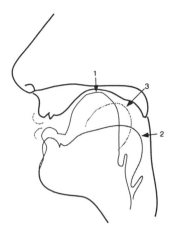

Figure 2. Approximate positions of the vocal organs for the vowels in: (1) *"feed,"* (2) *"fox,"* (3) *"food"*

3) **Lip rounding.** The roundedness of the lips changes the effective length of the vocal tract. This effective length is also influenced by the height of the larynx; lowering of the larynx or rounding the lips both result in an effective increase in vocal tract length. In American English, only back vowels are rounded, as the vowels in the words *"pool," "pull,"* and *"pole."*

4) **Vowel Length.** Vowels also differ in length or temporal duration. In American English, though duration is also subject to many contextual effects, vowels fall into two classes in terms of intrinsic duration — short or long. Short vowels include those in the words *"hit," "head," "hut,"* and *"hood,"* and contrast in duration with spectrally similar long vowels in the words *"heat," "had," "hot,"* and *"who'd,"* respectively.

Other parameters that affect the quality of vowels are diphthongization and nasalization. **Diphthongs** are vowel sounds during which there is a transition from one vowel position to another, although the first part of the diphthong is usually more prominent than the last. American English diphthongs include those in the words *"high," "how," "hay," "hoe,"* and *"boy."* **Nasalized vowels** are produced when the velum is lowered to allow airflow through the nasal cavities. This frequently occurs immediately before the production of a nasal consonant. In English (unlike French), vowel nasalization does not distinguish between words, but it is a feature that varies considerably between speakers.

4. Acoustic Theory of Speech Production

In this section we shall turn from specific details of speech sounds to concentrate on the mechanisms of speech production and the ways they may be represented, modeled and simulated.

The pressure with which air is forced up by the lungs has a primary effect on the intensity of the sounds produced, which can be used to give emphasis to various parts of the utterance. The larynx and the muscular folds of the glottis have the biological function of preventing food from entering the bronchial passageways into the lungs. As we have seen, they also fulfill the important function of giving rise to various types of sound excitation during speech, either of a random (noise) or periodic nature. The spectral characteristics (i.e. the amplitude variation across frequencies) of this excitation are then modified by the resonant and resistive properties of the mouth and nasal cavities, and finally a pressure waveform is emitted from the mouth. While sound is being produced, air is normally flowing out from the lungs, and there is a varying degree of coupling between the cavities above and below the glottis, and in front of and behind any major constriction in the mouth. Sound excitation may be produced not only at the glottis, but also at any such major constriction.

4.1 The Source–Filter Theory

The overall picture of speech production presented above, even without considering the temporal coordination between gestures of various articulators, is a complex one. A valuable simplifying assumption was made by Fant (1960). He suggested that speech could be reasonably approximated by a number of independent elements: an excitation source, an acoustic filter representing the response of the vocal tract, and the transmission characteristic from the mouth into free air. These components of the source–filter model are sketched in Figure 3. The source provides either periodic or noise excitation of rich spectral composition, a composition that is supposedly independent of the subsequent filter. Variations in source repetition frequency result in changes in fundamental pitch. The filter varies with the position of the articulators in the vocal tract. Different filter shapes will characterize different sounds, and very different filter shapes will be found for vowels and consonants. However, it is assumed that the shape of this acoustic filter or vocal tract transfer function does not change as a sound changes in pitch or voicing, as is illustrated in Figure 4. The output characteristic is usually modeled by a simple fixed filter to simulate the low frequency fall–off of the mouth opening. Note that with increasing fundamental frequency the resultant signal becomes less well defined by the more widely spaced harmonics, and this accounts in part for the relatively greater difficulty in adequately analyzing and resynthesizing the voices of women and children compared with that for adult male speakers.

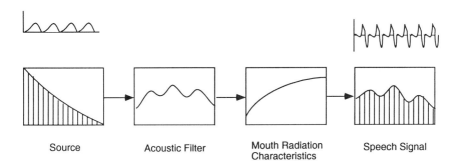

Figure 3. The source–filter model of speech

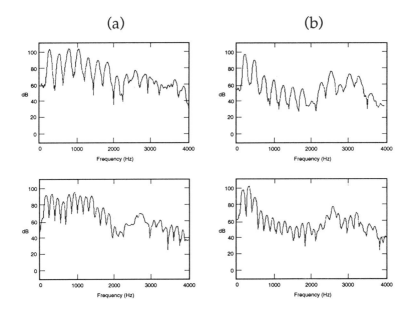

Figure 4. The vowels in (a) "cod" and (b) "key" produced with a higher (top) and a lower (bottom) fundamental frequency

The source–filter model, though a dramatic simplification of physical reality, provides a reasonable approximation to the perceptually relevant characteristics of the speech signal. In order to implement a working model, some further assumptions need to be made concerning the nature of the source and filter. Specific implementations will be described by O'Shaughnessy in Chapter 2, but some general source and filter characteristics will be described here.

4.2   The excitation source
Just as the source-filter theory makes some simplifying assumptions in modeling the filter characteristics, the source is often represented by a very simple excitation function.

A simple train of pulses or a triangular waveform is generally used as the periodic excitation source, and white noise as the noise source. Neither the source waveform nor its spectrum changes with changes in source frequency or amplitude (see section 2.8.6 in O'Shaughnessy's Chapter 2)

More sophisticated systems made possible by digital techniques allow complex source waveforms to be used. At one extreme, the source waveform is chosen such that when it is used to excite the filter, the resulting signal closely approximates the original speech signal. Such systems, though based on the source-filter model, are designed for speech *coding* rather than *modeling* (see section 2.8.7 of O'Shaughnessy's Chapter 2). Others have attempted to more accurately model excitation with parametric models of glottal output, which use various source control parameters that may be adjusted to simulate different speakers or to achieve dynamic changes in the voicing source such as those resulting from changes in modes of vibration or interactions with the vocal tract filter (see for example Klatt & Klatt, 1990).

Some sounds, such as the voiced fricatives beginning the words "*zoo*" and "*veil,*" clearly exhibit both periodic and noise excitation. It is, however, common to limit the source waveform to be either periodic or random noise. In this particular case, voiced fricatives would be generated with periodic excitation, while their unvoiced counterparts, as in "*sue*" and "*fail,*" would be generated with the same subsequent filter, but using noise excitation.

4.3   The Filter: A Formant Representation
One simple form of filter characteristics is expressed in terms of a small number of formants, or vocal tract resonance peaks. In the synthesis of

speech, five formants can be used to produce good quality voiced speech. The two formants highest in frequency, F4 and F5, add little to the intelligibility, but improve the naturalness of the resultant speech. Unvoiced fricatives, where excitation results mainly from turbulence at the point of closure fairly forward in the vocal tract, can be adequately represented by a filter characteristic with a single broad high frequency peak. In analog hardware synthesizers a separate filter is used to produce these sounds, but digital techniques allow a much broader range of individual filter characteristics, and fricatives can be synthesized using the same set as for other sounds.

Each formant peak, and thus its associated filter, varies in frequency, amplitude and bandwidth. A set of formant filters may be connected in parallel, as has been shown in Figure 18 of O'Shaughnessy's Chapter 2. In this case the amplitude of each formant can and must be independently specified. However, the vocal tract is not such an independent system, and in practice a reasonable approximation to empirical filter characteristics can be obtained by a serial configuration, also shown in O'Shaughnessy's Figure 18. Each filter has an asymmetrical shape with a gain of unity for frequencies well below the formant frequency, and a peak at the formant frequency and a high frequency fall–off whose sharpness depends on the formant bandwidth. In this case, the amplitude of each formant is controlled by its own bandwidth and the frequency and bandwidth of each lower frequency peak, and independent specification of amplitude is neither necessary nor possible.

Both serial and parallel configurations require some modification for the adequate production of nasal consonants and nasalized sounds. The configurations shown in O'Shaughnessy's Figure 18 are all–pole filters, involving only spectral peaks. The nasal tract is a damped and lossy cavity, and produces a broad dip in the spectrum around 1.5 kHz. Nasalization may be simulated by introducing zeroes into the filter characteristic, but an alternative is to add an extra 'nasal formant' of low frequency and wide bandwidth. By shifting the spectral balance of the normal part of the synthesizer to higher frequencies and adding these two signals in parallel, an effective dip in the spectrum may be produced. In practice, some synthesizers may have a more or less basic nasal character and produce acceptable speech without such elaborations, just as varying degrees of nasality may characterize different human speakers.

As will be seen in the following chapter, a formant description is only one of many possible representations of the vocal tract transfer function. Since it models the varying resonant peaks, and thus the perceptually most prominent features in the speech signal, a formant representation is a fairly economical one. Unfortunately, although formant synthesizers themselves are relatively straightforward, their parameters are often rather difficult to extract automatically from real speech. However, formant descriptions and synthesis have been of fundamental importance in studying human speech perception and in giving insight into the spectral parameters that cue various phonetic distinctions, and they remain an economical set of parameters for the coding and resynthesis of speech.

4.4 Other Representations of the Acoustic Filter

There are many other descriptions of the acoustic filter that give a good approximation to the observed characteristics of human speech and are useful in modeling and implementing practical systems to decode, recode and synthesize speech. These will be dealt with in detail in the following chapter, but it is useful here to mention the acoustic tube model that attempts to represent the physical vocal tract by a fixed number of tubular sections differing in area. These cross–sectional areas can be readily calculated from the acoustic signal, and bear a close correspondence to a formant description with a number of spectral peaks. Despite the gross differences between such a hard–walled symmetric tube and the soft and irregular cross–section of the vocal tract (see Figure 5), such an approximation can also produce a reasonable representation of the original speech.

4.5 Independence of Source and Filter

The source–filter model has been and is of great theoretical and practical value in studying, analyzing and synthesizing the speech signal. Ultimately, of course, it is only an approximation, and the fine details of the interactions between source and filter characteristics in real speech are being elaborated (e.g. Fant, 1979). These investigations concern the resonant properties of the cavities below the glottis and their coupling with the resonances in the vocal tract that we have considered up to now. This coupling varies with the instantaneous opening of the vocal folds and is thus not independent of the vocal fold excitation function. It also accounts for some of the differences in speech between men and women, since there is more coupling for women speakers or others who tend to have "breathier" voices, for which the vocal folds are open longer or even continuously during a phonatory period, one cycle of vocal fold vibration (Klatt and

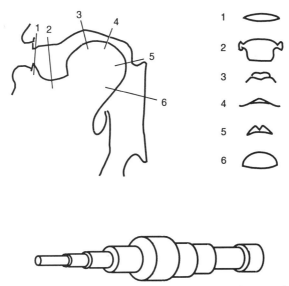

Figure 5. Cross-sections of the human vocal tract (above) estimated from x-rays showing variations from point to point (after Fant, 1968), compared with a symmetric acoustic tube (below)

Klatt, 1990). The larynx itself rises as the pitch of the voice increases, as can be felt by placing a hand on the larynx and singing, or imagining singing, a vowel changing from low to high pitch. As the larynx rises, the vocal tract is effectively shortened and the subglottal cavities lengthened, and once again we see a breakdown of simple independence of source excitation pitch and the resonant characteristics of the vocal tract filter.

Much of this total picture will ultimately have to be modeled in order to synthesize or resynthesize speech that is indistinguishable from that of a human speaker. However, the simplifying assumptions described above remain of great practical value in approximating the perceptually important parameters of speech.

5. Linguistic Units of Speech

Although often related to speech production or acoustics, linguistic descriptions of speech focus on units of speech that function linguistically. That is, rule systems that describe languages define and use linguistic elements that are appropriate for different levels of linguistic analysis. **Phonology** is a branch of linguistics that describes the systems and patterns of sound that occur in a language.

5.1 Phonemes

Phonemes are the smallest segments of sound that can be distinguished by their contrast within words. A phonemic transcription is generally indicated by the use of slashes before and after the phoneme sequence. Thus /b/ and /d/ are different phonemes in American English because *"bark"* and *"dark"* are perceived as different words, and similarly for /i/ and /ɪ/, the sounds distinguishing *"beat"* and *"bit."* Phonemes are abstract units that form the basis for transcribing a language unambiguously such that only the sound variations that make a difference in meaning are recorded. The /k/ portions of *"key"* and *"coo"* are different, the closure for the first being produced further forward in the mouth. However, they never function to distinguish between words in English and are thus the same phoneme. In contrast, in Arabic they are different phonemes, and there are words that differ only in containing one /k/ or the other. There are some 40 phonemes in American English: 24 consonants and 16 vowels. They are listed in Table II. each with its International Phonetic Association (IPA) symbl and an example of its occurrence in a common word.

A phonemic transcription requires a knowledge of the language in order to interpret the sound of each symbol. This contrasts with a **phonetic** transcription that, by means of more detailed and complex symbols, represents each sound in terms of the general articulatory possibilities of the human vocal tract. Phonetic transcriptions are generally indicated by square brackets. They distinguish between the various **allophones** or alternative forms of a phoneme that may be produced depending on context. For example, the phoneme /t/ in American English can be realized as a

Table II. American English Phonemes

IPA symbol	Example	IPA symbol	Example	IPA symbol	Example	IPA symbol	Example
b	bat	ž	measure	i	beat	ɔ	bought
d	dad	f	fun	ɪ	bit	ʊ	book
g	gun	θ	thick	ɛ	bet	u	boot
p	pop	s	sister	æ	bat	eʳ	bait
t	tot	š	ship	ɝ	bird	aʳ	bite
k	kick	h	hay	ʌ	bud	ɔʳ	boy
m	mom	ǰ	judge	ə	about	aʷ	cow
n	none	č	church	ɑ	cot	oʷ	boat
ŋ	sing	w	wine				
v	vine	r	red				
ð	they	l	led				
z	zoo	j	yet				

voiceless aspirated stop with a closure and a release (as in *"top"* and *"attorney,"* phonetically transcribed t̪), as a voiceless unaspirated stop after /s/ (as in *"stop,"* t̪), as a glottal stop (as in *"cotton,"* t̪), as a flap (as in *"writer,"* t̪), as a nasal–released stop (as in *"puritan,"* t̪, as a lateral–released stop (as in *"little,"* t̪), and as an unreleased stop (as in *"white cane"* t̪).

5.2 Distinctive Features

The set of dimensions or properties used by language for phonological contrast represent the distinctive features of sound structure. The goal in defining such dimensions is that all phonemes in the world's languages should be described in terms of a small set of (from about 12 to under 20) distinctive features. For example, the feature Nasal classifies American English phonemes into two categories, those that are [+nasal]—/m n ŋ/—and those that are [−nasal]—all the others. As the above example illustrates, many distinctive features closely resemble the dimensions by which we earlier classified consonant and vowel productions. Other distinctive features may more closely reflect acoustic or perceptual properties or dimensions. There is no single universally accepted set of distinctive features, but the two best known feature systems were developed by Jakobson, Fant and Halle (1963) and by Chomsky and Halle (1968). The Jakobson, Fant and Halle system defined features as binary, and gave priority to the acoustic and perceptual aspects of features. The binary nature of features has been generally accepted by subsequent theorists, but the Chomsky and Halle system and most other recently proposed frameworks have emphasized primarily (though not exclusively) articulatory dimensions. This is because the set of distinctive features can be used to specify sounds that act together in phonological rules, and these regularities in the sound pattern are often more clearly stated in terms of articulation.

Many linguists have maintained that distinctive features rather than phonemes are the basic building blocks of language. One example that is often cited to explain this viewpoint is the formation of plurals in English. Three suffixes are used in English to form the plural of nouns: (1) The suffix is /ɪz/ as in *"nieces,"* *"roses,"* *"peaches,"* *"judges,"* *"bushes,"* *"garages;"* (2) /s/ as in *"lips,"* *"fats,"* *"cakes,"* *"myths,"* *"laughs;"* (3) /z/ as in *"cabs,"* *"lads,"* *"dogs,"* *"games,"* *"cans,"* *"songs,"* *"balls,"* *"cars,"* *"lathes,"* *"caves,"* *"trays,"* *"ties,"* *"toes,"* *"toys,"* *"cows,"* *"bees,"* *"shoes,"* *"furs,"* *"laws."* The description of these rules in terms of the final phoneme of the noun would be: The suffix is (1) /ɪz/ if the noun ends in /s z č ǰ š ž/, otherwise (2) /s/ if the noun ends in /p t k θ f/, otherwise (3) /z/ for all other noun endings. However, the phonemes listed in rules 1 and 2 are similar in terms of distinctive features.

Those in rule 1 are all produced with the blade of the tongue raised to make a constriction, classified as [+coronal], and by high–amplitude, high–frequency noise, classified as [+strident]. The phonemes in rule 2 are all the voiceless English consonants that remain after the [+coronal, +strident] set is removed. Thus, the three ordered rules can be more simply described: The suffix is (1) /ɪz/ if the final phoneme of the noun is [+coronal, +strident], otherwise (2) /s/ if the final phoneme is [–voice], otherwise (3) /z/. Furthermore, the phoneme–based and the feature–based formulation of the rules of English pluralization make different predictions when dealing with nouns with non–English final segments. The phoneme–based rules would incorrectly predict that all such words would be pluralized with /z/, whereas the feature–based rules correctly predict how English speakers pluralize such nouns. An example is the name of the German composer Bach, which English speakers pluralize as /baxs/ as predicted by the feature–based rules, since the German /x/ or ach–laut falls under its rule 2. The predictive success of feature–based descriptions of language has been used to suggest that distinctive features have a psychological reality.

Distinctive features also have been predictive of perceptual confusions commonly made by listeners. The probability of both consonant and vowel confusions can be predicted with reference to distinctive features (Miller and Nicely, 1955; Peterson and Barney, 1952). Miller and Nicely used methods of information theory to analyze consonant intelligibility from confusion matrix data, and were impressed with the independence of distinctive features as separate perceptual channels of information. Wang and Bilger (1973) used multi–dimensional scaling techniques to study consonant confusions in noise, and found that although features were useful for describing patterns of perceptual results and for indicating which acoustic cues were most important in a given context, no set of features consistently accounted for information transmitted better than another. They suggest, on the basis of these results, that articulatory features may not be represented in the underlying perceptual processes. Dubno and Levitt (1981) found that a small set of acoustic variables were good predictors of consonant confusions. Interpretation of consonant errors in terms of features has consistently shown that consonants that are confused have many features in common (Klatt, 1968). Single–feature confusions are by far the most common types of perceptual errrors, and two–feature confusions are much more likely than three–feature confusions, etc. The strength of this regularity, however, breaks down somewhat when synthetic speech (either coded or generated by rule) is considered

(Greenspan, Bennett, and Syrdal, 1989; Greenspan, Bennett, and Syrdal, personal communication; van Santen, personal communication). For example, Greenspan *et al.* (1989) observed that when listeners were asked to identify the initial consonant of consonant–vowel (CV) stimuli, single–feature confusions made up about 75% of the errors for natural speech, but only slightly over 50% of the errors for coded speech, the remainder involving two or more feature errors. This pattern of perceptual confusions for coded or rule–generated synthetic speech probably occurs because the speech signal is subject to several types of acoustic distortions that can affect the perception of speech along several different feature dimensions.

5.3 Morphemes

The morpheme is the minimum meaningful unit into which a word may be divided, and might form important elements in a speech understanding system or a lexicon for speech synthesis by rule. A word may consist of a single morpheme, such as *"dog,"* or it may be built up of one or more root morphemes modified by grammatical prefixes and suffixes. Such a combination may keep a simple relation to the original root form, such as in *"small" "smaller"* or *"mean" "meaningful,"* or some changes in stress and pronunciation may occur, as in *"congress" "congressional"* or *"child" "children."* In other cases the new form may be highly irregular, such as *"is" "was."* Morphemic structure is useful for speech synthesis–by–rule (see Syrdal, Chapter 3), and though the incorporation of such relations into speech recognition systems has not yet occurred, it could be important in future developments.

5.4 Syllabic Structure

The syllable is another constituent of words, a word consisting of one or more syllables. Syllabic structure is important because it constrains possible sequences of phonemes, controls allophonic variation, and can be used to predict stress. There are over four billion arbitrary sequences of from one to six of the 40 phonemes in American English, but only 100,000 possible monosyllablic (one–syllable) words, and 10,000 actual monosyllabic words. Syllabic structure greatly constrains possible phoneme sequences for text–to–speech synthesis as well as candidates in speech recognition. For example, *"atktin"* is not a possible English word because it cannot be broken down into a sequence of well–formed English syllables. Syllabic structure is also important for speech synthesis and recognition because it controls allophonic variation. For example, voiceless stops are unaspirated after /s/ within a syllable (such as *"sprint"*) but not when they belong to two different syllables (such as *"misprint"*). Syllable structure can also be used to predict stress (Liberman, 1975; Liberman and Prince, 1977; Selkirk, 1980; Hayes, 1981). One or more syllables in a given word will be stressed, and this will result in its component sounds being longer, higher amplitude, and articulated with greater clarity.

The syllable has an internal hierarchical structure consisting at the highest level of **onset** (the initial consonant cluster) and **rhyme** (the rest). The rhyme has two components, the **peak**, containing the syllabic nucleus (a vowel in stressed syllables or a vowel or syllabic liquid or nasal in unstressed syllables), and the **coda**, the final consonant cluster. The onset, peak, and coda are considered to be structural units because the tightest phonotactic constraints of syllabic structure obtain within them. For example, in a syllable beginning with two consonants and a vowel, the identity of the vowel does not constrain the identity of the first two consonants (or vice versa) as much as the identity of the first or second consonants constrain each other. For example, in English, if the syllable begins with /p/, the second consonant is constrained to the set of continuants /l r y/ as in *"play,"* *"pray,"* and *"pure."* If the second consonant is /p/, the first consonant is restricted solely to /s/ as in *"spin."* Similarly, tighter phonotactic constraints between peak and coda than between onset and either peak or coda justify the grouping of peak and coda together into a constituent (rhyme). For example, only the subset of English vowels termed "lax" vowels can occur before /ŋ/ in a syllable. **Affixes** may also be added to the end of the syllable, such as /θ z s d t/ in *"twelvth,"* *"themselves,"* *"lifts,"* *"informed,"* and *"marked."* Affix constituents are always [+coronal] and can form strings, as in *"sixths."* They are not considered constituents of the coda because long strings of coronals are not found word–internally.

Another observation about syllabic structure is that syllables constitute peaks of **sonority**. The sonority of a sound is its loudness relative to that of other sounds with the same length, stress, and pitch. In articulatory terms, sonorants are produced with the excitation source at the glottis. Along a continuum of sonority, vowels are the most sonorous speech sounds, followed by semi–vowels, /h/, liquids, nasals, and finally obstruents (stops, affricates, and fricatives), the least sonorous sounds. In distinctive feature terms, obstruents are classified [−sonorant] whereas the others are classified [+sonorant]. The syllabic peak is the constituent of highest sonority in the syllable, and sonority decreases within the syllable proportionally to distance from the peak. In permissible English onset or coda consonant clusters, the segments furthest from the peak (first segments for onsets and last segments for codas) are obstruents, and those closest to the peak are nasals or continuants. For example, the permissible three–consonant onsets in English follow an order of lower to higher sonority; they are /skl skr skw sky spl spr spy str/ as in *"sclerosis," "screw," "squirt," "skew," "splash," "spring," "spurious,"* and *"street,"* respectively. Permissible three–consonant codas follow an order of higher to lower sonority, as for example the ending consonant sounds /nts nst mpt rts rst kst/ in *"intelligence," "against," "exempt," "quartz," "thirst,"* and *"next."*

5.5 Prosodic Structure

Words and their constituents are further organized into **intonation phrases**. Intonation phrases are often, but not necessarily, the same size as syntactic phrases. An intonation phrase has special tonal features at the beginning and the end, and its last syllable is lengthened. Intonation is a major determinant of the patterns of fundamental frequency (F0—pronounced "F zero") observed in speech. It is important for the naturalness and intelligibility of text–to–speech synthesis, and may be used to detect phrases and screen word candidates for speech recognition. In the **declination** effect, the F0 range narrows and declines in frequency over the course of the intonation phrase. There are several approaches to characterizing the continuously varying F0 contour as composed of a sequence of discrete elements, and to implementing the resulting model (Ohman, 1967; Fujisaki and Nagashima, 1969; 't Hart and Cohen, 1973; O'Shaughnessy, 1977; Pierrehumbert, 1981). Pierrehumbert's approach, for example, followed a model of the F0 contour as a series of target values connected by transitional functions. Using Pierrehumbert's terminology, stressed syllables are usually (but not necessarily) marked tonally, with a high, low, or two–target (high–low or low–high) **pitch accent**. The F0 contour "sags" between two high pitch accents that are sufficiently separated in time; otherwise, it is a monotonic curve between two targets.

Descending levels of hierarchically organized constituents of an intonation phrase are word, foot, syllable, and segment. A **metrical foot** is a unit of speech that has one stressed (unreduced) syllable followed by any number of reduced (unstressed) syllables. The inclusion of feet as a level of phonological structure permits formal representation of the stress differences of such word pairs as *"bandanna"-"banana,"* and *"rabbi"-"happy."* This is because the main stressed syllable of a word may be defined as the strongest syllable of the strongest foot. Strong syllables of weaker feet receive what is also termed **secondary stress**. For example, in the word *"constitution,"* the first syllable receives secondary stress, the second syllable is reduced, the

third syllable receives primary stress, and the fourth syllable is reduced. The word is composed of two metrical feet, the second of which is stronger than the first. Besides its possible tonal marking, a stressed syllable is longer in duration, higher in amplitude, and more fully pronounced than an unstressed syllable.

6. Acoustic Characteristics of Speech

6.1 Frequency analysis

The acoustic speech signal is the most easily observed and measured stage of speech communication. Linguists and psycholinguists attempt to characterize the abstract elements and mental activities involved in planning, producing, perceiving, and comprehending speech. Articulatory gestures are often difficult to observe directly. They result in adjustments of the vocal folds, changes in the resonant properties of the oral and pharyngeal cavities, and coupling or decoupling of the nasal cavity, all of which directly affect the resulting speech signal. A representation of the speech signal that is very valuable in revealing significant information about these resonances and how they vary over time is a frequency–time spectrogram. Figure 6 shows an example of such an analysis of a short utterance. The amplitude of different frequency components is indicated by the density of marking.

6.2 Formants

Careful examination of the spectrogram in Figure 6 reveals a number of distinct and semicontinuous bands of energy. These correspond to the main resonances of the vocal tract, termed the formants, and previously discussed as a representation of the vocal tract filter. A full and clear formant pattern will only be seen during sounds in which resonances of the whole vocal tract are involved. When sound excitation is principally produced by a constriction higher in the vocal tract, such as for the burst of plosives and in unvoiced fricatives, primarily the relatively small resonant cavity in front of the constriction is excited and has a high resonant frequency. Figure 7 shows frequency–amplitude sections at the points marked with arrows in Figure 6 and for the vowels the formants are marked and numbered. Each formant may be characterized by a resonant frequency, amplitude and bandwidth. As mentioned in (4.3), generally three to five formants are sufficient to model speech, the lower three characterizing the phonetic quality of the sound itself, while the extra resonances add to the accuracy of the description and to the naturalness of speech resynthesized using such a description. It is possible to synthesize vowels quite

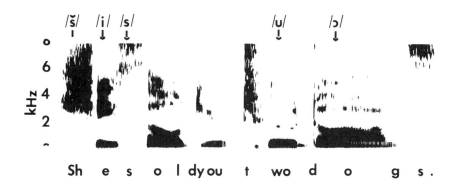

Figure 6. A frequency/time spectrogram for the utterance *"She sold you two dogs."*

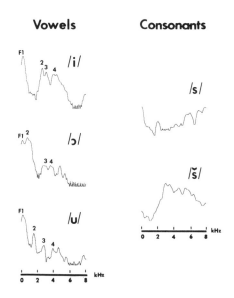

Figure 7. Amplitude/frequency sections at the points marked in Figure 6

successfully (even for a vowel–rich language like Swedish) using two formants, providing that the frequency of the second synthetic formant is set to a value representing the composite perceptual effect of the natural second formant plus higher formants (Carlson, Fant, and Granstrom, 1975).

6.3 Consonants

Speech is produced by rapid movements between the articulatory positions characteristic of each sound. Figure 8 shows stylized spectrograms of the utterances /ba/ and /da/. It can be seen that while the vowel is characterized by the same set of formant positions, the movements from the consonants to the vowel position result in different formant trajectories since the initial consonants begin with different vocal tract configurations. In the case of /ba/there is a large cavity during and immediately after the closure resulting in low formant frequencies and thereafter rising second (F2) and higher (F3 and F4) formants. In the case of /da/ the closure is further back in the mouth and therefore the smaller cavity has a higher resonant frequency and F2 and higher formants fall to their values for the vowel.

It might appear that the difference between /b/ and /d/ is generally indicated by a rising or falling second formant. It can be seen that this is not the case from Figure 9 that shows stylized spectrograms for /di/ and /du/.

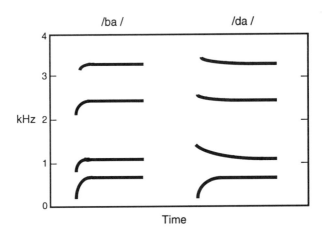

Figure 8. Stylized spectrograms of /ba/ and /da/ show the rising and falling (respectively) F2, F3, and F4 trajectories from consonant to vowel

Here, the initial consonant is the same in both cases. In the case of /du/, F2 again falls, as in the previous example. However, for /di/, F2 rises to its high value for the vowel /i/. In fact we find that the plosive/d/ itself is characterized by an initial F2 of about 1800 Hz, the F2 resonance of this speaker's vocal tract when it is fully closed with the tongue against the alveolar ridge. Since at this point no air can pass, no sound is produced until the tongue has moved away from this position towards the desired vowel. The F2 trajectories in Figure 9 therefore only point toward this initial locus at 1800 Hz.

There are other cues to the nature of stop consonants in addition to such formant movements (see Syrdal, 1983). The release of pressure built up in the closed vocal tract results in a burst of energy whose frequency characteristics give some information about the place of the closure. The timing between this burst and the occurrence of periodic excitation in the speech signal is a major factor in determining whether a plosive will be perceived as voiced or voiceless. The burst of a voiceless plosive is followed by a period of the order of 50 ms during which relative silence precedes vocal fold vibration, whereas voiced plosive bursts are followed immediately (or even preceded) by vocal fold activity. Although formant parameters can be used to synthesize reasonably intelligible and natural speech, a description in terms of a small number of discrete peaks can only approximate the

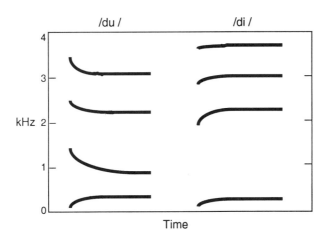

Figure 9. The consonant /d/ may be characterized by rising or falling formant trajectories, depending on the following vowel

spectrum of real speech. The determination and labeling of formant values is performed most reliably by visual inspection of spectrograms with full knowledge of the words and sounds depicted. Resynthesis of speech with these parameters can be used to check the perceptual adequacy of such a description. Some methods of automatic formant extraction are discussed by O'Shaughnessy in Chapter 2.

6.4 Vowels

It would at first appear that the recognition of vowels is somewhat simpler than that of consonants, since the associated formant structure is both clearer and of a less transient nature. Figure 10 shows mean F1 and F2 values for English vowels produced by men, women, and children in /hVd/ context. There is good correspondence between these formant values and the articulatory vowel space described in the previous section. However, the picture is complicated by several factors. As shown in Figure 10, there are large between–speaker differences in the formant structure of vowels (Peterson and Barney, 1952). Men, women, and children have vocal tracts of widely different lengths and shapes (e.g. men's pharyngeal cavities are disproportionately long compared to women's and children's) such that no simple scaling factor can reduce the between–speaker differences. Another complicating factor is dialectical differences, which affect vowels more

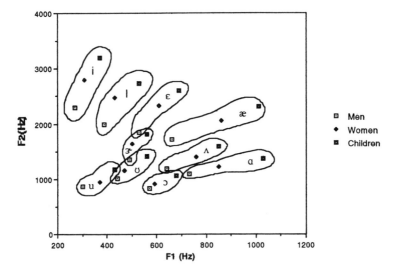

Figure 10. Mean formant frequencies for American English vowels spoken by men, women, and children

than consonants. In addition, the efficient coding and rapid transmission of information in continuous speech results in various phenomena that change the simple picture presented above even within a single speaker.

During normal rapid speech the physical inertia of the articulators does not allow prototypic target articulatory positions to be reached. Instead the articulations for neighboring sounds overlap in time, and these positions are often only approximated. This interaction between adjacent sounds is termed **coarticulation**. Figure 11 illustrates this schematically. The left diagram indicates the formant trajectories in slow speech, while the right diagram shows what might actually be realized in normal or fast speech. The formant positions for the vowel are never reached, and the vowel tends to be reduced in quality, differing vowels becoming more acoustically similar to one another. This phenomenon is termed **vowel reduction** or **neutralization**. Coarticulation and vowel reduction produce a dramatic effect on the acoustic parameters of the sounds actually produced.

7. Auditory Perception

The ear is a remarkably complex device. Through it our perception of sound is characterized by a high frequency resolution and excellent frequency discrimination (tones differing by as little as 0.3% being discriminable), a wide dynamic range of over 120 dB, a fine temporal resolution (able to detect differences as small as 10 μs in the timing of clicks presented to the two ears), and rapid temporal adaptation (faint sounds being audible as

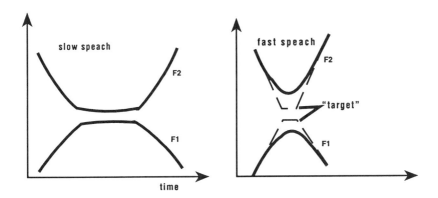

Figure 11. In fast speech articulations do not always reach the target positions they attain in slower speech.

little as 10 ms after the cessation of a moderately loud sound). The lower curve in Figure 12 shows the threshold sensitivity of the ear as a function of frequency. Sound pressure level (SPL) is expressed in dB relative to 20μPa (micropascal).. The solid upper line indicates the threshold above which sounds are experienced as painful. This range almost covers that for which air is a useful medium for sound transmission; at the low end it is some 20–30 dB above the level of noise produced by collisions of air molecules, and at around 160 dB pressure transmission in air itself becomes nonlinear.

7.1 Human audition—Perceptual measures

Figure 12 has shown the absolute range of sound levels and frequencies that may be perceived by an average young adult. There are considerable differences between individuals in sensitivity, but about 90% of the population lies within ± 12 dB of this figure. Very young children are generally 10 dB more sensitive, and above the age of 25 there is a gradually worsening loss of high frequency sensitivity as the hair cells in the cochlea die off (Hincliffe, 1959). Measurements of absolute sensitivity are made using single frequency sinusoidal pure tones presented in isolation.

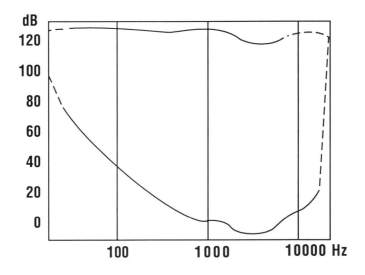

Figure 12. The sensitivity of the ear: Tones are inaudible below the lower line and painful above the upper line.

We live in a world of constant change, and almost constant sound. Such sound is of complex harmonic composition, and we need to examine the relationship between the perception of these complexes and that of pure tones. A first approximation used to experimentally investigate the perception of more complex signals is the perception of one tone in the presence of a second masking tone. For example, a sinusoidal masking tone is presented at 80 dB SPL at 1 kHz and the elevation in threshold level for detecting tones at various other frequencies is measured. This elevation is termed the masking effect of the 1 kHz tone at various frequencies. There are various problems with this approach, such as the presence of audible beats between the two tones, but these may be overcome by techniques of varying sophistication using sharply filtered noise as a masking signal instead. These experiments have led to the auditory perceptual system being characterized by a set of overlapping auditory filters, somewhat analogous to some hardware systems for acoustic signal analysis. It is assumed that tones will be discriminable to the extent that they produce discriminably different activity in different filters, and that they will only mask one another if they fall within the critical frequency band of the same filter. More recent experiments have resulted in a variety of measures, and the resulting critical band scale has been termed the Bark scale (Zwicker, 1961). There are several mathematical approximations of critical bandwidth (Zwicker and Terhardt, 1980; Traunmuller, 1990); these functions are approximately linear up to about 1000 Hz, and approximately logarithmic (about 1/3 octave) thereafter.

7.2 Loudness Estimation
The experiments described above have been concerned with the discriminatory performance of the auditory system—the magnitude and frequency of signals that are just detectable, and the size of just noticeable changes along these dimensions. However, in our everyday experience we are concerned not only with sounds approaching these absolute limits, but also with relative changes in signals lying well within our upper and lower bounds of perception. In such cases we need to know the relation between our subjective experience and the physical characteristics of the signal. Loudness is one such subjective sensation.

The sound pressure level of a pure tone at a particular frequency is easily measured, but this in itself gives little idea of the relative subjective intensity of two tones of differing frequency, or of complex and different harmonic structure. This is of great practical importance, since we often need to equate very different signals, such as speech and music, for subjective loudness, or possibly for annoyance value. A first approach to this problem is to ask listeners to adjust the intensity of a tone of one frequency until it matches that at another frequency. Considerable variability is found between individual adjustments, and data needs to be averaged over a large number of estimates by many listeners in order to provide reliable results. Figure 13 shows a typical set of **equal–loudness contours** for various loudness levels. Each curve indicates the sound pressure level of pure tones at various frequencies that are perceived as subjectively equal in loudness.

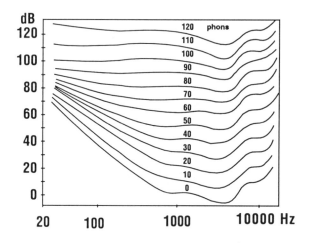

Figure 13. Each line represents a constant subjective loudness (after Fletcher, 1953).

The loudness level of any continuous sound may then be defined in an analogous way. The unit of loudness is the **phon**, and it is measured as the sound pressure level, in dB SPL, of a 1000 Hz tone that is judged as equally loud as the sound. In practice there is an even larger variability in individual judgements of sounds such as automobile engine noise or exhaust fan whine than in the comparison of loudness of pure tones of differing frequency, and a large number of measurements need to be made to obtain useful estimates. Alternative measurements have therefore been developed that in practice allow the perceived loudness of a sound to be predicted from its own spectral composition. Two methods, both of which are international standards, have been developed by Stevens (1956) (ISO

R532 Method A) and Zwicker (1958) (ISO R532 Method B), and rely on complex computations based on the spectral structure of the signal.

In practice, the sound level meter provides a simple but useful method of estimating the approximate loudness of a sound. The pressure detected by a microphone is filtered by an appropriate weighting function to simulate the equal loudness contour of the human ear. The meter is calibrated in dB and adjusted such that a 1000 Hz sinusoid at 40 dB SPL gives a reading of 40 dB. The most frequently used weighting is the 'A-weighting,' approximating the 40 phon equal loudness curve, and the measurements so obtained are termed 'dB (A).' In practice this simple method is of great value since the measuring equipment can be simple, portable and relatively cheap in comparison with the more complex methods mentioned above.

Having determined convenient ways of measuring loudness level, we may estimate the loudness of speech under varying conditions. While a figure of 65 dB SPL at 1 meter is typical, this may vary from 40 dB for a confidential whisper, to 70 dB in a noisy office, to 80 dB for a shout, and to about 90 dB for the loudest shout possible.

7.3 Speech in noise
Of more relevance for the transmission of speech signals is the **dynamic range** of the signal, and the **signal-to-noise ratio** that needs to be maintained for speech to remain intelligible. There is a very wide dynamic range between the loudest vowel segment and the quietest consonant sounds, but in practice a dynamic range of 30 dB may be considered as adequate to retain most of the relevant information. Figure 7 in O'Shaughnessy's Chapter 2 shows the relative frequency distribution of the energy in the speech signal averaged over a long period of time and many speakers of both sexes.

If interfering noise has a relatively flat frequency distribution then a useful 'rule-of-thumb' is that a signal-to-noise ratio above 20 dB will give good communication, down to about +6 dB will result in satisfactory communication, and below 6 dB speech will be no longer intelligible, though it will still be detectable down to about 16 dB. This is of course a continuous process of degradation, and as the signal-to-noise ratio worsens, progressively more speech sounds fall below the noise level. Two important factors that need to be considered in a more detailed analysis are (1) the relative distribution of speech and noise energy with frequency and (2) the contribution of different parts of the spectrum to the intelligibility of speech. Such an analysis, termed the **Articulation Index**, was developed by French and

Steinberg (1949) and refined by Kryter (1962). They divided the frequency range from 200 to 6100 Hz into twenty bands found to be of equal importance for the perception of speech. The relative weighting of these is illustrated in Figure 14. This should be compared and contrasted with O'Shaughnessy's Figure 7 in Chapter 2. Note in particular that the region above 1 kHz, though comprising less than a fifth of the total energy, has the greatest contribution to speech intelligibility. The Articulation Index is based on the relative signal-to-noise ratio measured for each band and thus takes into account both factors mentioned above.

An interesting alternative method is the **Speech Transmission Index** (STI) of Houtgast and Steeneken (1973), since it uses physical measurements that estimate how well the dynamic nature of the speech signal is modified by noise and reverberation. Their computation is based on measurements of the transmission of amplitude modulation of a noise signal through a communications channel or within a particular acoustic environment. Such measurements are made at a range of modulating frequencies, representing those normally found in the envelope of the speech signal, and are then combined. Their method also allows estimated intelligibility to be calculated for complex real or theoretical situations where signal-to-noise and echo characteristics are known.

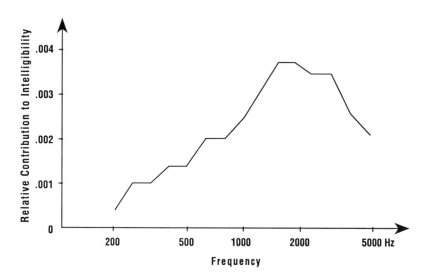

Figure 14. Articulation Index: The relative contribution of different frequency bands to the intelligibility of speech

7.4   Pitch perception

Pitch is also a subjective quality derived in a complex way from the acoustic signal. In the case of a sinusoidal tone, perceived pitch may be assumed (except at frequency extremes) to be equal to the fundamental frequency of the tone. We may then estimate the pitch of other more complex sounds in an analogous way to that used for subjective loudness, adjusting the frequency of a pure tone until it matches that of the complex. In the case of speech, it is found that pitch judgments may be reliably made even when no energy is present at the fundamental frequency. This is commonly the case in speech transmitted over a telephone line or other narrow bandwidth communication channel, where little acoustic energy remains below 300 Hz. Even more dramatically, it is found that a pitch of, say 100 Hz, can be perceived from a few harmonics spaced at 100 Hz intervals and located above 1000 Hz. This phenomenon of **residue** or **periodicity pitch** was first supposed to be due to nonlinearities in the ear and the resultant intermodulation products between the high harmonics in the signal. However, this was questioned by Schouten (1940) and his co-workers, who devised ingenious experiments in which any possible intermodulation products were cancelled out, yet the pitch percept remained. Additionally it was found that if the harmonics were separated by 100 Hz but were not multiples of 100 Hz (e.g. the signals actually used were sinusoids amplitude modulated at 100 Hz), then the perceived pitch differs systematically from 100 Hz. Patterson (1969) showed that the 'missing fundamental' remained perceptible even when noise with a bandwidth of 0 to 600 Hz was added to the signal at a sufficient level to mask any possible distortion products.

Alternative theories suggested that, rather than there being physical energy present at the fundamental frequency, the 'missing fundamental' was detected by finding periodicities in the amplitude-time waveform. However, such a procedure should be highly sensitive to the relative phase of the different frequency components. Although listeners can distinguish subtle differences in the quality of sounds that differ only in the phases of its components, periodicity pitch remains equally discriminable (Patterson, 1973). The ear therefore seems to be relatively insensitive to phase information, and this is exploited by many practical systems of speech coding, where phase information is discarded.

There is no single theory that comprehensively accounts for the apparently simple task of pitch perception, and this is perhaps reflected in the complexity of designing methods of automatic pitch extraction. Two contemporary theoretical approaches are respectively based on a spectral and a temporal analysis of the speech signal. The spectral approach suggests that the pitch extraction is performed by varying the spacing of a "harmonic sieve" until a best match is found with the harmonic composition of the signal (Goldstein, 1973). A mechanism based on the temporal approach would examine temporal periodicities in the output of a set of acoustic filters, perceived pitch being estimated by comparison and combination of these various periodicities.

8. Speech Perception

Speech is a much more complex acoustic signal than is typically used in experiments designed to study auditory psychophysics. In addition, human communication involves the use of speech sounds as a set of categorically distinctive units that convey information very efficiently. Much work in speech perception research has been concerned with investigating the acoustic parameters that influence phonemic labeling of a sound. These experiments have generally taken a pair of sounds that differ along one articulatory dimension, such as voicing(e.g. /d/-/t/), place of articulation(e.g. /d/-/b/), or vowel position (e.g. /ɪ/-/ɛ/), and vary one of the acoustic correlates of this dimension in a number of steps from a clear example of one to a clear example of the other. These variations are generally produced by using a speech synthesizer to simulate and modify a stylized representation of the formant parameters of normal speech. Early work by Liberman and his co-workers (e.g Liberman *et al.*, 1967) suggested that there was a fundamental difference between the perception of consonants and vowels. They found a sudden "categorical" change in perception of variations of the acoustic parameters of consonants in synthetic speech, and a more continuous change in the perception of vowels. The upper panel of Figure 15 schematically illustrates the classification of a series of stimuli varying along a consonant or vowel dimension, and the gradual change from "A" to "B" responses can be seen in both cases. However, the lower panel illustrates discrimination between adjacent pairs of the same stimuli. Discrimination of consonants is considerably better in the region of the boundary between "A" and "B" responses as seen in the upper panel. In contrast, higher overall discriminability but no such peak is found for the vowels. It has been suggested that these effects result from the transient nature of the information relating to consonants compared with the higher amplitude, longer duration vowel information. This lower amplitude transient information decays more rapidly in memory and must be coded almost immediately, in contrast to the louder, relatively steady-state vowel information. In such experiments the sound heard, for consonants, then depends on the category to which the sound is initially assigned (such as "b" or "d"). For vowels the acoustic information itself may still be available as a basis for making a response (Darwin and Baddeley, 1974).

Although coarticulation and vowel reduction complicate the picture, it can be seen that there is a more direct correspondence between a phonemic description and the articulatory gestures than can be found in the resulting

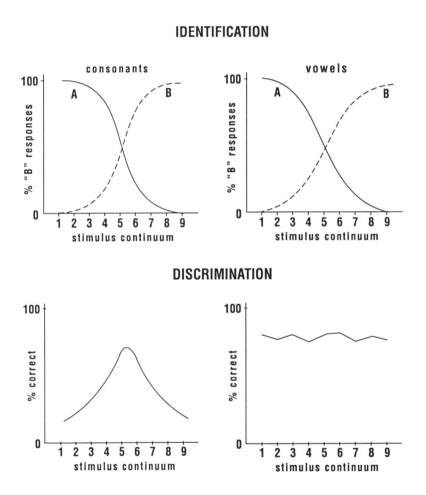

Figure 15. Identification (above) and discrimination (below) functions for speech stimulus continua varying in equal acoustic steps from one consonant or vowel (A) to another (B).

acoustic signal. This observation, together with an emphasis of research on the perception of phonemes rather than of words, led many early workers in the speech field to suggest that the listener perceives speech by reproducing the articulatory gestures of the speaker (Liberman *et al.*, 1967; Liberman and Mattingly, 1985). From inner gestures, which need not result in actual articulation, the listener would know what sounds he or she would have produced, and thus what the speaker had said. There has been much debate about this "motor theory," but in the end the main motivation for formulating it is a good reason for rejecting it—if the relation between acoustics and articulation is so complex, how does the listener come to reproduce the speaker's articulation from the acoustics? If the listener is able to do this, then he or she probably already has enough information to recognize what has been said without resorting to such a device. This is not, of course, to deny the intimate relationship between speech production and perception. We normally grow in our use and understanding of speech by acting both as speakers and listener, and it is through the coordination of these two that we gain our skill.

Many of the theories and experiments in speech perception have centered around the perception of phonemes. More recently the status of phonemes in speech perception has been debated, and there is evidence to suggest that they are neither necessarily perceived nor represented as such by the human listener during normal speech perception (see e.g. Morais *et al.*, 1979; Klatt, 1979; Marcus, 1981). Early work in automatic speech recognition almost always attempted to build phoneme detectors, with varying degrees of limited success. Since then many researchers have worked on systems that directly establish a relationship between the acoustic signal (or some direct parametric representation of it) and the spoken word (e.g. Bahl *et al.*, 1978; see O'Shaughnessy, Chapter 2), rather than using some intermediate stage of representation in terms of phonemes. Since phonemes are abstract units that encompass many allophonic variations, they are not optimal candidates for intermediate units in the process of automatic speech recognition. Use of distinctive features as intermediate units in recognition would appear to be more promising, but few recognition systems have taken this approach.

8.1 Differences between Speakers

Listeners can and do rapidly adjust for a speaker's vocal tract length, as was demonstrated by Ladefoged and Broadbent (1957). They synthesized a word that had formant values intermediate between *"bit"* and *"bet."* They then presented this word to listeners for recognition, preceded by the short initial phrase *please say what this word is*." The initial phrase was synthesized with all the formant values either increased or decreased, corresponding to a larger or shorter vocal tract, relative to the test word. Judgements of the word as "*bit*" or "*bet*" were significantly influenced by this manipulation of perceived vocal tract length, and this occurred even with the much shorter initial phrase "*what's this?*" Some approaches to recognizing speakers from their differences are employed by speaker verification technology, and methods to remove between-speaker differences in order to perform automatic speech recognition are described by O'Shaughnessy in Chapter 2.

There are several models of the perceptual process of speaker normalization. One approach is **extrinsic normalization**, in which the information used to perform the normalization is taken from utterances other than that to be normalized (Gerstman, 1968; Nordstrom and Lindblom, 1975; and Nearey, 1978). Another approach is **intrinsic normalization**, in which the information necessary for normalization is present in the signal to be normalized itself (Syrdal, 1985; Syrdal and Gopal, 1986; Miller, 1989). It is apparent that humans perform both types of normalization. We can usually understand what is being said by a person we have never heard before (as long as we know the language they are speaking), but when we are more accustomed to a person's speaking habits and dialect, we are even more accurate. Experimental results support these observations (Ainsworth, 1975; Nearey, 1989; Mullennix, *et al.*, 1989).

8.2 Continuous Speech

Just as each word is more than a sequence of speech sounds occurring one after another, continuous speech is more than a sequence of concatenated words. The coarticulation effects found between the articulatory gestures within a word are also found between words: the sound that begins one word is affected by the sound that ended the previous word, and vice-versa. In addition to the local effects, the timing and intonation of individual words form a part of a prosodic pattern for the whole utterance. Attempts to generate utterances by concatenating stored waveforms of words spoken in isolation, or in other contexts, demonstrate what happens without correct prosody. The resulting speech is perceived as irregular and disconnected. This effect is, unfortunately, all too common in many applications of voice response technology that use stored speech. In the worst case the sounds may not even appear to belong together in the same utterance (Nooteboom, Brokx & de Rooij, 1976) and the complete sequence may be less intelligible than the individual words spoken in isolation (Stowe & Hampton, 1961). This contrasts with normal connected speech, where words spoken in a meaningful sequence are much more easily recognized than when they are removed from this context and presented in isolation (Miller, Heise & Lichten, 1951).

There are many factors in operation in the perception of continuous speech, and we only have space to deal briefly with a few of them. The context in which a word appears, in terms of its meaning and relationship to adjacent words, has an influence on its probability of being perceived. For example, the word "trees" will be perceived much more easily in the sentence "*Apples grow on trees*" than in a sentence like "*The boy saw some trees.*" Recent perceptual experiments have shown that the effects of grammar and meaning are in operation within a few hundred milliseconds of the beginning of a word (Marslen-Wilson & Welsch, 1978). Since the average duration of a word is some 300–500 ms, this is well before the offset of many words. It therefore appears that speech perception cannot be broken down into stages of recognizing successively larger units. Instead the recognition of the sounds within a word depends on the possible meaningful alternatives for that word.

As noted above, even when words do form meaningful sentences, if the sounds of each word do not form a coherent whole with their neighbors, both the sentence and its component words will be difficult to understand. Such a "coherent whole" consists of the relative timing of each syllable, and the pitch and amplitude with which it is spoken. Speech may be uttered at varying rates, but since some articulatory gestures can be sped up more easily than others, changes in speech rate result in non-linear changes in segment duration. The vowel reduction that accompanies rapid speech has already been mentioned, and changes in speech rate correspond neither temporally nor spectrally to a simple linear transformation of the speech signal. A single parameter of speech rate, in, say, syllables per second, may be of value in examining the overall speech rhythm, but we need also to be aware of the more subtle changes that occur in relative duration.

A characteristic of normal continuous speech is the intonation contour that joins words, spanning whole phrases and sentences. This consists principally of variations in pitch of the speaker's voice, and it may indicate the difference between statements and questions, emphasis of certain words in the utterance, and subtle variations in the speaker's emotional state. It is the intonation contour that gives speech much of its perceptual coherence and naturalness. Figure 16 gives an example of a sentence with its actual measured fundamental frequency (top); the F0 target tones are numbered

T1 through T7 and aligned with syllables and phrase boundaries (%) in the text below. Figure 16 (bottom) shows a stylized pitch contour and its declining baseline and topline within which F0 targets are indicated by decimal numbers representing target values in terms of proportion of F0 range. The adequacy of a stylized pitch contour is tested by resynthesising the sentence with its original pitch and with a stylized contour. Despite the absence of the fine structure of the original contour, listeners judge the stylization as adequately retaining the perceptually relevant information.

9. Summary

This chapter has given a brief outline of the nature of the speech signal. It has been seen that there is not a simple one-to-one relation between the acoustic signal and the sounds perceived. The various articulatory gestures that result in speech have been presented, together with the vowels and consonants found in American English.

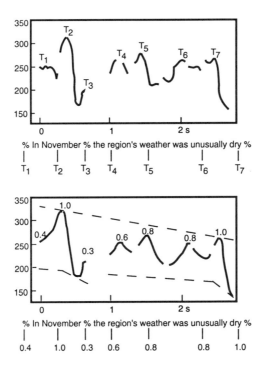

Figure 16. Natural (above) and stylized (below) pitch contours (after Pierrehumbert, 1981).

The acoustic theory of speech production has been introduced, and the source-filter model has been presented as a valuable simplification in representing the acoustic characteristics of speech and speech production. A simple form of the vocal tract filter has been discussed, in terms of either a serial or parallel connection of formant resonances, and the modification of this to include nasal resonances and subglottal aerodynamics briefly mentioned.

Various linguistic units were defined, including phonemes, distinctive features, syllables and their constituents, and intonation phrases. The relation of these linguistic constructs to the description of linguistic rules and to speech production and perception was discussed.

Comparison of the spectral characteristics of even simple utterances and their formant peaks reveals a complex relation between acoustics and articulation, and this is further complicated by coarticulation between adjacent sounds and the vowel reduction that occurs in fast speech as is normally used in fluent conversation.

The section on auditory perception considered perceptual measurements of the characteristics of human audition and the concept of a set of auditory filters each with a particular critical bandwidth. The practical applicability of this both in loudness estimation and speech perception in noise have been mentioned. Finally the perception of pitch has been shown to have a complex relation to the acoustic signal, not simply corresponding to the fundamental frequency of the signal.

The categorical nature of the perception of speech was discussed. Differences between speakers result from differences in the size and shape of their vocal tracts, and differences in the way in which they use them. There is experimental evidence to suggest that listeners can perform between-speaker normalization very rapidly.

In continuous speech various factors operate to give speech its continuity. Meaning and grammatical constraints play an important part even very early in the recognition of each word, while the overall intonation contour of a sentence gives it perceptual coherence and emphasizes important words.

References

Ainsworth, W. (1975). "Intrinsic and extrinsic factors in vowel judgments," in *Auditory Analysis and Perception of Speech*, edited by G. Fant and M. Tatham (Academic, London), pp.103–113.

Bahl, L. R., Bakis, R., Cohen, P. S., Cole, A. G., Jelinek, F., Lewis, B. L., and Mercer, R. L. (1978). "Recognition results with several experimental acoustic processors," IBM Research Report RC7440(#32038),T. J. Watson Research Center, Yorktown Heights.

Carlson, R., Fant, G., and Granstrom, B. (1975). "Two–formant models, pitch and vowel perception," in *Auditory Analysis and Perception of Speech*, edited by G. Fant and M. A. A. Tatham (Academic, London), pp. 55–82.

Chomsky, N., and Halle, M. (1968). *The Sound Pattern of English*. (New York, Harper and Row).

Darwin, C. J. and Baddeley, A. D. (1974). "Acoustic memory and the perception of speech," Cognitive Psychology **6**, 41–60.

Dubno, J. R., and Levitt, H. (1981). "Acoustic factors in consonant confusions," J. Acoust. Soc. Am. **69**, 249–261.

Fant, G. (1960).*Acoustic Theory of Speech Production*, (Mouton, Den Haag).

Fant, G. (1968). "Analysis and synthesis of speech processes," in *Manual of Phonetics*, edited by B. Malmberg (North Holland, Amsterdam), pp. 173–277.

Fant, G. (1979). "Glottal source excitation analysis," Speech Transmission Laboratory Quarterly Progress and Status Report **1**, 83–109.

Fletcher, H. (1953). *Speech and Hearing in Communication*, (van Nostrand, Toronto).

French, N. R., and Steinberg, J. C. (1949). "Factors governing the intelligibility of speech sounds," J. Acoust. Soc. Am. **19**, 90–119.

Fujisaki, H., and Nagashima, S. (1969). "A model for the synthesis of pitch contours of connected speech," Annual Report of the Engineering Research Institute, Tokyo **28**, 53–60.

Gerstman, L. (1968). "Classification of self–normalized vowels," IEEE Trans. Audio Electroacoust. **AU–16**, 78–80.

Goldstein, J. L. (1973). "An optimum processor theory for the central formation of the pitch of complex tones," J. Acoust. Soc. Am. **54**, 373–379.

Greenspan, S. L., Bennett, R. W., and Syrdal, A. K. (1989). "A study of two standard speech intelligibility measures," J. Acoust. Soc. Am. **85**, S43.

`t Hart, J. (1976). "Psychoacoustic backgrounds of pitch contour stylization," I.P.O. Annual Progress Report (Instituut voor Perceptie Onderzoek, Eindhoven, The Netherlands), **11**, 11–19.

`t Hart, J., and Cohen, A. (1973). "Intonation by rule: A perceptual quest," J. Phonetics **1**, 309–327.

`t Hart, J.& Collier, R. (1975). "Integrating different levels of intonation analysis," Journal of Phonetics **3**, 235–255.

Hayes, B. P. (1981). "A metrical theory of stress rules," Chapter 1, Indiana University Linguistics Club.

Hincliffe, R. (1959). "The pattern of the threshold of perception for hearing and other special senses as a function of age," Acustica, **9**, 303–308.

Houtgast, T. & Steeneken, H. J. M. (1973)." The modulation transfer function in room acoustics as a predictor of speech intelligibility," Acustica **28**, 66.

Jakobson, R., Fant, C.G. M., and Halle, M. (1963). *Preliminaries to speech Analysis: The Distinctive Features and their Correlates.* Cambridge, Mass., The MIT Press.

Klatt, D. H. (1968). "Structure of confusions in short–term memory between English consonants," J. Acoust. Soc. Am. **44**, 401–407.

Klatt, D. H. (1979). "Speech Perception: A model of acoustic–phonetic analysis and lexical access," Journal of Phonetics **7**, 279–312.

Klatt, D. H., and Klatt, L. C. (1990). "Analysis, synthesis, and perception of voice quality variations among female and male talkers," J. Acoust. Soc. Am. **87**, 820–857.

Kryter, K. D. (1962). "Methods for the calculation and use of the articulation index," J. Acoust. Soc. Am. **34**, 1689–1697.

Ladefoged, P. (1975).*A Course in Phonetics*, (Harcourt Brace, New York).

Ladefoged, P., and Broadbent, D. E. (1957). "Information conveyed by vowels." Journal of the Acoustic Society of America, **29**, 98–104.

Liberman, A. M., Cooper, F. S., Shankweiler, D. P. and Studdert-Kennedy, M. (1967). "Perception of the speech code," Psychological Review, **74**, 431–461.

Liberman, A. M., and Mattingly, I. G. (1985). "The motor theory of speech perception revised," Cognition **21**, 1–36.

Liberman, M. Y. (1975) "The intonational system of English,"Unpublished doctoral dissertation. Cambridge, Mass.: MIT. Distributed by the Indiana Linguistics Club, 1978.

Liberman, M. Y., and Prince, A. (1977). "On stress and linguistic rhythm," Linguistic Inquiry **8**, 249–336.

Marcus, S. M. (1981). "ERIS–context sensitive coding in speech perception," Journal of Phonetics **9**, 197–220.

Marslen-Wilson W. &Welsch, A. (1978). "Processing interactions and lexical access during word recognition in continuous speech," Cognition **10**, 29–63.

Miller, G. A., Heise, G. A. & Lichten, W. (1951). "The intelligibility of speech as a function of the context of the test materials, "Journal of Experimental Psychology **41**, 329–335.

Miller, G. A. and Nicely, P. E. (1955) "An analysis of perceptual confusions among some English consonants," J. Acoust. Soc. Am. **27**, 338–352.

Miller, J. D. (1989). "Auditory-perceptual interpretation of the vowel," J. Acoust. Soc. Am. **85**, 2124–2134.

Morais, J., Cary, L., Alegria, J. and Bertelson, P. (1979). "Does awareness of speech as a sequence of phonemes arise spontaneously?" Cognition **7**, 323–331.

Mullennix, J., Pisoni, D. , and Martin, C. S. (1989). "Some effects of talker variability on spoken word recognition," J. Acoust. Soc. Am. **85**, 365–378.

Nearey, T. (1978). *Phonetic Feature Systems for Vowels* (Indiana University Linguistics Club, Bloomington, IN).

Nearey, T. (1989). "Static, dynamic, and relational properties in vowel perception," J. Acoust. Soc. Am. **85**, 2088–2113.

Nooteboom, S. G., Brokx, J. P. L. and de Rooij, J. J. (1976). "Contributions of prosody to speech perception," I.P.O. Annual Progress Report (Instituut voor Perceptie Onderzoek, Eindhoven, The Netherlands), **11**, 34–54.

Nordstrom, P.-E., and Lindblom, B. (1975). "A normalization procedure for vowel formant data," *Proceedings of the 8th International Congress of Phonetic Sciences*, Leeds, England.

Ohman, S. (1967). "Word and sentence intonation: A quantitative model," Speech Transmission Laboratory Quarterly Progress and Status Report **2–3**, 20–54.

O'Shaughnessy, D. (1977). "Fundamental frequency by rule for a text–to–speech system," Proc. IEEE Int. Conf. ASSP, 571–574.

Patterson, R. D. (1969). "Noise masking as a change in residue pitch," J. Acoust. Soc. Am. **45**, 1520–1524.

Patterson, R. D. (1973). "The effect of relative phase and the number of components on residue pitch," J. Acoust. Soc. Am. **53**, 1565–1572.

Peterson, G. E. and Barney, H. L. (1952). "Control methods used in a study of vowels." Journal of the Acoustic Society of America **24**, 175–184.

Pickett, J. M. and Decker, L. R. (1960). "Time factors in the perception of a double consonant," Language and Speech **3**, 11–17.

Pierrehumbert, J. (1981). "Synthesizing intonation," J. Acoust. Soc. Am. **70**, 985–995.

Schouten, J. F. (1940). "Five articles on the perception of sound,"Instituut voor Perceptie Onderzoek, Eindhoven, The Netherlands, 1938–1940.

Selkirk, E. (1980) "The role of prosodic categories in English word stress," Linguistic Inquiry **11**, 563–605.

Stevens, S. S. (1956). "Calculations of the loudness of complex noise," J. Acoust. Soc. Am.**28**, 807–832.

Stowe, A. N., and Hampton, D. B. (1979). "Speech synthesis with prerecorded syllables and words," Journal of the Acoustical Society of America **33**, 810–811.

Syrdal, A. K. (1983). "Perception of consonant place of articulation," in *Speech and language: Advances in basic research and practice*, edited by N. Lass (Academic Press, New York) pp. 313–349.

Syrdal, A. K. (1985). "Aspects of a model of the auditory representation of American English vowels," Speech Communication **4**, 121–135.

Syrdal, A. K., and Gopal, H. S. (1986). "A perceptual model of vowel recognition based on the auditory representation of American English vowels," J. Acoust. Soc. Am. **79**, 1086–1100.

Traunmuller, H. (1990). "Analytical expressions of the tonotopic sensory scale," J. Acoust. Soc. Am. **88**, 97–100.

Wang, M. D., and Bilger, Robert C. (1973). "Consonant confusions in noise: A study of perceptual features," J. Acoust. Soc. Am. **54**, 1248–1266.

Wightman, F. L. and Green, D. M. (1974). "The perception of pitch," American Scientist **62**, 208–215.

Zwicker, E. (1958). "Über psychologische und methodische Grundlagen der Lautheit," Acustica **1**, 237–258.

Zwicker, E. (1961). "Subdivision of the audible frequency range into critical bands (Frequenzgruppen)," J. Acoust. Soc. Am. **33**, 248.

Zwicker, E., Flottorp, G.and Stevens, S. S. (1957). "Critical bandwidth in loudness summation," J. Acoust. Soc. Am. **29**, 548–557.

Zwicker, E., and Terhardt, E. (1980). "Analytical expressions for critical–band rate and critical bandwidth as a function of frequency," J. Acoust. Soc. Am. **68**, 1523–1525.

Chapter 2

Speech Technology

Douglas O'Shaughnessy
University of Quebec

1.   Speech Analysis

The previous chapter on speech science examined the production and perception of natural speech and described important aspects of speech for human communication. Applications of speech processing (e,g., coding, synthesis, recognition) exploit these properties (O'Shaughnessy, 1987). To store or recognize speech, reducing redundancy in the speech waveform permits efficient representation of the essential speech aspects in the form of parameters. The relevant parameters for speech recognition must be consistent across speakers, and should yield similar values for the same sounds uttered by various speakers, while exhibiting reliable variation for different sounds. Synthetic speech must replicate perceptually crucial properties of the speech, but may ignore other aspects.

This section briefly examines methods of speech analysis, in both the time and frequency domains. There are tradeoffs when analyzing a time-varying signal such as speech; in examining a window of speech, the choice of duration and shape for the window reflects a compromise in time and frequency resolution. Accurate time resolution helps when segmenting speech signals and determining pitch periods, whereas good frequency resolution helps to identify different sounds. Time analysis is rapid but is limited to simple speech measures, e.g., energy and periodicity, while spectral analysis takes more effort but characterizes sounds more precisely. Phones can be partitioned into manner of articulation classes using simple parameters, but discriminating among vowels (or place of articulation among consonants) requires spectral measures.

An underlying model of speech production involving an excitation source and a vocal tract filter is implicit in many analysis methods. Some techniques try to separate these two aspects of a speech signal. The excitation is often represented in terms of the periodicity and amplitude of the signal, while variations in the speech spectrum are assumed to derive from vocal tract variations.

1.1 Short-Time Speech Analysis

Speech is time varying: some variation is random, but much is under speaker control. For example, a vowel articulated in isolation utilizes a specific vocal tract shape and vibrating vocal cord excitation for a period of time. The resultant speech is only quasi-periodic due to small period-to-period variations in vocal cord vibration and in vocal tract shape. These variations are not important to replicate for speech intelligibility, but probably cause the speech to sound more natural. Aspects of the speech signal directly under speaker control (amplitude, voicing, F0, and shape of the vocal tract) as well as methods to extract related parameters from the speech signal are of primary interest here.

At times, vocal tract shape and excitation may not significantly alter for up to 100 ms. Mostly, however, speech characteristics change more rapidly since phoneme durations average about 80 ms. Indeed, coarticulation and changing F0 can render each pitch period different from its neighbor. It is usually assumed that basic properties of the signal change relatively slowly with time. This allows examination of a *short-time window* of speech to extract relevant parameters presumed to be fixed for the duration of the window. Such parameters are averaged over the time window. Thus, the signal must be divided into successive windows or *analysis frames* so that the parameters can be calculated often enough to follow relevant changes (e.g., those due to different vocal tract configurations). Slowly changing formants in long vowels may allow windows as large as 100 ms without obscuring the desired parameters, but stop releases require windows of about 5-10 ms to avoid averaging spectra of the burst release and an adjacent sound.

Many applications require some averaging to yield an output parameter contour as a function of time that accurately represents some slowly varying aspect of vocal tract movements. Windowing involves multiplying a speech signal $s(n)$ by a (usually finite-duration) window $w(n)$ (Figure 1), which yields a set of speech samples weighted by the shape of the window. The simplest window has a rectangular shape, which just limits the analysis range to N consecutive samples, applying equal weight to all samples. A common alternative is the Hamming window, which has the shape of a raised cosine pulse. Tapering the edges of the window allows periodic shifting of the analysis frame along an input signal without having large effects on the speech parameters due to pitch period boundaries or other sudden changes in the speech signal; it also improves the spectral response of the window.

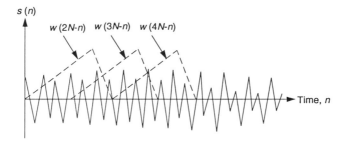

Figure 1: Speech signal $s(n)$ with three superimposed windows, offset from the time origin by $2N$,$3N$,and $4N$ samples.

Due to their slowly varying time waveforms, most windows have frequency responses that resemble lowpass filters. To minimize distortion in the output spectral representation, $W(e^{jw})$, the Fourier transform of the window $w(n)$, should be limited in frequency range: e.g., an ideal lowpass filter (rectangular frequency pulse) strictly limits the frequency range. The output spectrum $X(e^{jw})$ (corresponding to $x(n) = s(n) w(n)$) is a smoothed version of $S(e^{jw})$, where each frequency sample is the average of its neighbors over a range equal to the bandwidth of the lowpass filter. An ideal lowpass filter is not practical because its time signal has infinite duration. Practical finite-duration windows are flawed in not having strictly limited frequency ranges, however, and each sample in the windowed speech spectrum not only is an average of its immediate neighbors but also has contributions from many other frequencies. Virtually all windows limit this undesirable behavior by concentrating most of their frequency response in a *main lobe* centered at zero frequency.

A smoothed output spectrum is often advantageous. Wideband spectrograms and formant detectors need spectral representations that smooth the fine structure of the harmonics while preserving formant structure, which varies more slowly with frequency. For a given window shape, the duration of the window is inversely proportional to its spectral bandwidth. The choice of window duration trades off time and frequency resolution. Traditional *wideband spectrograms* use windows of about 3 ms (good time resolution, capable of examining the decaying amplitude within individual pitch periods), which correspond to a bandwidth of 300 Hz and smooth out harmonic structure (for voices with F0 < 300 Hz). *Narrowband spectrograms*, on the other hand, use a window with 45-Hz bandwidth and a duration of approximately 20 ms. This enables resolution of individual harmonics but smooths time behavior over a few pitch periods. The latter spectral displays are useful for pitch determination, while wideband representations are better for viewing vocal tract parameters, which can change rapidly. If high spectral resolution is desired without using a large number of time samples (e.g., to avoid averaging over events in time), a small number of time samples can be "padded out with zeros" (i.e., M time samples can be augmented by zero-valued samples to a total length of N, which after spectral transformation will yield N frequency samples; if $N \gg M$, much higher frequency resolution is achieved than if M samples are directly transformed).

A good choice for windowing of voiced speech would be a rectangular window having a duration of one pitch period. This would produce an output spectrum very close to that of the vocal tract impulse response, without interference from multiple excitation pulses. Unfortunately, it is often difficult to reliably locate pitch periods, and system complexity increases if window size must change dynamically with F0. Furthermore, since most pitch periods are shorter than the impulse response of the vocal tract, such a window would truncate the impulse response, resulting in spectral degradation, especially for female speech. Using a window of exactly two or three periods alleviates the problem of truncation but includes excitation effects. Most speech analyses use a fixed window size of about 10-25 ms. As the window is shifted without regard for pitch periods (*pitch-asynchronously*), the more periods under the window the less the effects of including/excluding the large-amplitude beginning of any individual period.

1.2   Time-Domain Analysis of Speech Signals
Processing speech in the time domain has the advantages of simplicity, quick calculation, and easy physical interpretation. Several parameters relevant for coding and recognition can be so determined, e.g., energy (or amplitude), voicing, and F0. Energy is commonly used to segment speech; accurate F0 estimation is crucial for many voice coders. Time-domain analysis transforms a speech signal into parameter signals, which usually vary much more slowly than the original signal. This allows more efficient

storage or manipulation of the relevant speech parameters than directly handling the original signal. For example, speech is usually sampled at 6000–10,000 samples/s (to preserve bandwidth to 3-5 kHz), yet sampling a parameter signal at 40-100 samples/s suffices in most cases. Thus, when converting speech into a set of parameters, sampling rates can decrease by two orders of magnitude.

1.2.1 Short-Time Average Zero-Crossing Rate

Normally, to obtain spectral measures from speech requires a frequency transformation of a complex spectral estimation (e.g., linear prediction). A simple measure known as the Zero-Crossing Rate (ZCR) can provide some spectral information at low computational cost. A *zero crossing* occurs in a signal every time the waveform crosses the time axis (changes algebraic sign). For narrow-band signals such as sinusoids, ZCR is an accurate spectral measure. A sinusoid has two zero crossings per period, and thus F0 = ZCR/2 (zero crossings/s).

The ZCR can help determine whether speech is voiced. Most energy in voiced speech is at low frequencies because the spectrum of the glottal excitation decays with frequency at-12 dB/octave. In unvoiced sounds, the broadband noise excitation excites primarily higher frequencies. While no speech sound can be characterized as a narrowband signal, the ZCR correlates well with the frequency of major energy concentration. For vowels and sonorants, the ZCR follows the first formant since it has more energy than other formants. Thus a high ZCR cues unvoiced speech, while a low ZCR corresponds to voiced speech. A reasonable boundary can be found at 2500 crossing/s.

1.2.2 Short-Time Autocorrelation Function

The Fourier transform of a speech signal provides both spectral magnitude and phase. Many applications ignore the phase since it is relatively unimportant perceptually. The time signal corresponding to the inverse Fourier transform of the energy spectrum (the square of the spectral magnitude) is called the *autocorrelation* of the original signal. It preserves information about a signal's harmonic and formant amplitudes as well as its periodicity, while ignoring phase. It has found application in pitch detection, voiced/unvoiced determination, and linear prediction. The autocorrelation function of a signal $s(n)$ is

$$R(k) = \sum_m s(m)s(m-k), \tag{1}$$

which measures the similarity between $s(n)$ and a delayed version of itself as a function of the time delay. The autocorrelation is large if at some delay the two signals have similar waveforms. The range of summation is usually limited (i.e., windowed), and the function can be normalized by dividing by the number of summed samples. For linear prediction, $R(k)$ for k ranging from 0 to 10–16 are typically needed, depending on the signal bandwidth. For F0 determination, $R(k)$ must be evaluated for k near the estimated number of samples in a pitch period; e.g., for k ranging from perhaps 3 ms to 20 ms.

1.3   Frequency-Domain Parameters

The most useful parameters in speech processing are spectral. The vocal tract produces signals that are more consistently analyzed in the frequency, than time, domain. The common model of speech production involving a noisy or periodic waveform exciting a vocal tract filter corresponds well to separate spectral models for the excitation and the vocal tract. Repeated utterances of a sentence often differ considerably in the time domain while remaining quite similar spectrally. The hearing mechanism appears to pay much more attention to spectral aspects of speech than to phase or timing aspects.

One technique of spectral analysis uses a *filter bank* or set of bandpass filters, each analyzing a different range of frequencies of the input speech. Filter banks are more flexible than discrete Fourier transform (DFT) analysis since the bandwidths can be varied to follow the resolving power of the ear rather than being fixed for either wideband or narrowband analysis. Furthermore, many applications require a small set of spectral parameters describing the spectral distribution of energy. The amplitude outputs from a bank of 8–12 bandpass filters typically provide a more compact and efficient spectral representation than a more detailed DFT. A common approach is to space filters following the bark scale, i.e., equally-spaced, fixed bandwidth filters up to 1 kHz, and then to logarithmically increase filter bandwidth.

1.3.1   Short-Time Fourier Analysis

Fourier analysis represents speech in terms of amplitude and phase as a function of frequency. The Fourier transform of speech is the product of the transforms of the glottal (or noise) excitation and the vocal tract response. Since speech $s(n)$ is nonstationary, short-time analysis using a window $w(n)$ is necessary:

$$S_n(e^{jw}) = \sum_{m=-\infty}^{\infty} s(m)e^{-jwm}w(n-m). \tag{2}$$

Assuming $w(n)$ acts as a lowpass filter, the Fourier transform $S_n(e^{jw})$ yields a time signal (a function of n), which reflects the amplitude and phase of $s(n)$ within a bandwidth equivalent to that of the window but centered at w radians. By repeating the calculation of $S_n(e^{jw})$ at different w, a two-dimensional representation of the input speech is obtained: an array of time signals indexed on frequency, each expressing the speech energy in a limited bandwidth about the chosen frequency.

Computationally, the DFT is used instead of the standard Fourier transform so that the frequency variable w only takes on N discrete values (N corresponding to the window duration, or size, of the DFT). Low values for N (i.e., short windows and DFTs using few points) give poor frequency resolution since the window lowpass filter is wide, but they yield good time resolution since the speech properties are averaged only over short time intervals (e.g., in wideband spectrograms, the filter bandwidth is usually 300 Hz). Large N, on the other hand, gives poor time resolution and good frequency resolution (e.g., narrowband spectrograms, with bandwidth of 45 Hz).

1.3.2 Formant Estimation and Tracking

Understanding the time behavior of the first three formants is of crucial importance in many applications. To estimate formant center frequencies and their bandwidths involves searching for peaks in spectral representations (McCandless, 1974, Kopec, 1986). The automatic tracking of formants has been an elusive task, despite the typical spacing of formants every 1 kHz (for a vocal tract 17cm long), the limited range of possible bandwidths (30–500 Hz), and the generally slow formant changes. Acoustic coupling of the oral and nasal cavities during nasals causes abrupt formant movements as well as the introduction of extra formants. Zeros in the glottal source excitation or in the vocal tract response for lateral or nasalized sounds also tend to obscure formants. Many sounds have two formants sufficiently close that they appear as one spectral peak.

1.4 F0 ("Pitch") Estimation

Determining the fundamental frequency (F0) or "pitch" of a signal is a problem in many speech applications. (Although pitch is perceptual and what is being measured here is F0, the estimators are commonly called "pitch detectors.") Many voice coders require accurate F0 estimation to reconstruct speech; in synthesis, natural intonation must be simulated by rule. F0 determination is simple for most speech, but problems arise due to the nonstationary nature of speech, irregularities in vocal cord vibration, the wide range of possible F0 values, interaction of F0 with vocal tract shape, and degraded speech in noisy environments (Hess, 1983). Most pitch detectors operate directly on the speech signal, and also yield a *voicing decision*, in which up to four classes of speech are distinguished: voiced, unvoiced, combined (e.g. /z/), and silence.

F0 can be determined either from time periodicity or from regularly-spaced spectral harmonics. F0 estimators have three components: a preprocessor (to filter and simplify the signal via data reduction), a basic F0 extractor, and a postprocessor (to correct any errors). In the speech signal, time-domain algorithms try finding: the fundamental harmonic, a quasi-periodic time structure, an alteration of high and low amplitudes, or points of discontinuities. Frequency-domain techniques examine the speech signal over a short-term window. Autocorrelation, average magnitude difference, cepstrum, spectral compression, and harmonic matching methods are among the varied spectral approaches. They generally have higher accuracy than time-domain techniques, but require more computation.

1.5   Reduction of Information
Often a major objective of speech analysis is to economically represent information in the signal while retaining parameters sufficient to reconstruct or identify the speech. Coding seeks to reduce the storage or transmission rate of speech while maximizing the quality of reconstructed speech in terms of intelligibility and naturalness. The storage question is secondary for recognition, with accuracy the primary concern. Nonetheless, recognition is faster when the stored data base occupies less memory. In both cases, eliminating redundant information present in the speech signal is important. Whether information is superfluous depends on the application: speaker-dependent aspects of speech are important for talker identification, but are superfluous to identification of the textual message.

It is not always clear which speech aspects can be sacrificed. Acceptable speech can be synthesized with rates under 600 bits/s, which is two orders of magnitude lower than that for the simplest digital representation. However, as bit rate is reduced, small amounts of distortion are gradually introduced into the reconstructed speech. In particular, aspects of the signal relating to the identity of the speaker tend to be removed at low storage rates. Current synthesis models emphasize spectral and timing aspects of speech that preserve intelligibility, sometimes at the expense of naturalness.

2.   Digital Coding of Speech Signals
Digital coding provides efficient, secure storage and transmission of the speech signal. Speech is coded into a bit stream representation, transmitted

over a channel, and then converted back into an audible signal (Figure 2). The decoder is an approximate inverse of the encoder except that some information is lost (e.g., due to the conversion of an analog speech signal into a digital bit stream). Information loss is minimized by an appropriate choice of bit rate and coding scheme. Transmission can be either on-line (*real time*), as in normal telephone conversations, or off-line, as in storing speech for electronic mail (*forwarding*) of voice messages.

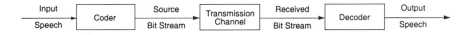

Figure 2: Block diagram of digital speech transmission.

The transmission bit rate is a crucial measure of practicality, because the bandwidth of a transmission channel limits the number of signals that can be carried simultaneously. Coding methods are evaluated in terms of bit rate, costs of transmission and storage, complexity, speed, and output speech quality. Quality normally degrades monotonically (but not necessarily linearly) with decreasing bit rate.

The simplest speech systems are *waveform coders*, which analyze, code, and reconstruct speech sample by sample. Time-domain waveform coders take advantage of signal redundancies, e.g., periodicity and slowly-varying intensity. Spectral-domain waveform coders exploit the nonuniform distribution of speech information across frequencies. More complex systems known as *source coders* or *vocoders* (for *"voice coders"*) assume a speech production model, usually separating speech information into that estimating vocal tract shape and that involving vocal tract excitation. Coding these separately permits a large decrease in bit rate. Vocoders recreate crucial speech aspects that emphasize perceptual quality over waveform accuracy. The vocoder's objective is often to match the original spectral magnitude during successive frames of speech data. Waveform coders typically yield superior output speech quality but operate at bit rates much higher than vocoders. *Signal-to-noise ratio* (SNR) is a very useful measure of speech quality for waveform coders only, since vocoders generate a waveform significantly different from that of the original speech.

2.1 Quantization
All digital speech coders use a form of *pulse-code modulation* (PCM) to convert an analog speech signal into a digital representation, which may be further coded to lower the final bit rate (figs. 3-4). Natural speech waves are

continuous in amplitude and time. Periodically sampling an analog waveform $x_a(t)$ at the Nyquist rate (twice its highest frequency, assuming a lowpass signal) converts it into a discrete-time signal $x(n)$ (where $x(n) = x_a(nT)$ and T is the sampling period). Sampling at the Nyquist rate insures that no information is lost; the original signal can be reconstructed exactly from the analog-coded, discrete-time samples. However, digital applications require number representations with a discrete range, and thus the signal amplitude $x(n)$ at each time instant n must be quantized to be one of L amplitude values (where $B = \log_2 L$ is the number of bits to digitally code each value). The $x(n)$ amplitude is mapped into the nearest discrete value, which minimizes quantization distortion sample by sample. The output value differs from the input by an amount known as the quantization noise e, which is evident in the decoded speech as audible distortion.

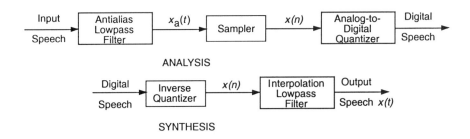

Figure 3:   Block diagram of a pulse-code modulation (PCM) system.

The simplest quantizer has a uniform mapping; a graph of the input-output (x vs. $y = Q(x)$) of a quantizer resembles a staircase due to the finite number of output levels. The *step size* Δ of this staircase represents the spacing between possible output values and is constant in a uniform quantizer but varies with the input x in a nonuniform quantizer. To assign the output levels efficiently, all quantizers assume that the input has a limited range (i.e., $|x| \leq X_{max}$). When the input exceeds these limits occasionally, *clipping* occurs, where the output deviates significantly from the input. Sing $B = \log_2 L$, L is usually chosen to be a power of two to allow an integer number of bits in coding each sample x, with the L output levels symmetrically distributed. The SNR of the average speech energy to the average energy in the quantization error is usually expressed in decibels as $10 \log_{10}$ SNR. For basic PCM, it is $6.02B - 7.27$. Each additional coding bit, which doubles the number of quantizer levels and halves Δ, decreases the noise energy and increases SNR by 6 dB.

Nonuniform quantization can overcome the range problem by making SNR less dependent on signal level. If Δ is not constant but rather proportional to input magnitude, then weaker sounds use a smaller step size than more intense sounds do. For constant percentage of error, the quantization levels should be logarithmically spaced. Compared to uniform PCM, this log PCM process needs about four fewer bits/sample for equivalent quality. Instead of a constant SNR over a wide range of input amplitudes, average SNR is maximized. Statistics of speech amplitudes show roughly Laplacian distributions with decreasing likelihood as amplitude increases. Thus small step sizes are allocated to high-probability, small-input amplitudes.

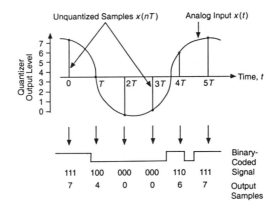

Figure 4: Signals in a PCM system.

Primary concerns in coding speech are bandwidth and perceptual quality. In PCM, individual speech samples are quantized and coded with B bits and then transmitted at the speech sampling rate F_s. Since B is inversely proportional to the noise that degrades the output speech quality, it should be maximized. It is usually also desirable to recover at the output as much as possible of the input speech bandwidth. With F_s samples/s, a bandwidth of up to $F_s/2$ Hz can be represented. A third objective is to minimize transmission rate $I = F_s B$, which corresponds to channel bandwidth reduction in analog speech transmission. Since these three factors conflict, we look for areas of compromise. We assume a speech bandwidth from 0 Hz to almost 4 kHz, with a corresponding $F_s = 8000$ samples/s, typical of many speech coders. This bandwidth choice corresponds roughly to that found in the telephone network (which nonetheless eliminates significant high-frequency energy in sounds like /s/). Basic approaches that code one sample at a time dictate relatively high transmission rates (e.g., 56 kbits/s for log PCM). Many alternative approaches exist; they all assume the same F_s but differ in how the speech samples are coded.

2.2 Speech Redundancies

Speech coders take advantage of redundancies in the speech signal and of perceptual limitations of the ear. Uniform PCM is valid for any bandlimited signal; coders that exploit properties of speech can lower transmission rates. Log PCM takes advantage of the nonuniform distribution of speech amplitudes. Other aspects of speech distinguish it from arbitrary signals. Since natural speech is generated by human vocal tracts, there are distinct limitations on what signals can occur: (1) in general, vocal tract shape and thus speech spectrum change relatively slowly compared to F_s; (2) the vocal cords vibrate rapidly but change rate of vibration (i.e. F0) relatively slowly; (3) successive pitch periods are virtually identical much of the time; (4) the vocal tract spectrum varies slowly with frequency; (5) most speech energy is at low frequency.

Some speech redundancies can be exploited by modeling the speech as periodic or noisy excitation passing through a vocal tract filter. In addition, each sound can be represented with a few parameters, having nonuniform probability distributions.

Concerning audition, vocoders discard phase information since the ear is relatively phase insensitive; other systems code more intense parts of the speech spectrum more accurately than low amplitude frequencies since masking limits the importance of the latter. Below, we show how speech and auditory properties are exploited to lower bit rate while preserving speech quality. The actual information rate of speech in terms of phonemes is very low: assuming about 12 phonemes/s and 5–6 bits/phoneme (since there are 30–40 phonemes in most languages), about 70 bits/s suffice. This calculation ignores other speech information, however, such as intonation, emotions, and speaker identity, which are difficult to quantify.

2.3 Time-Adaptive Waveform Coding

Most speech coders change their characteristics adaptively in time to exploit the tendency for speech traits to vary slowly. In *adaptive-quantizer pulse-code modulation* (APCM), the step size Δ is varied in proportion to the short-time average speech amplitude, which is evaluated over a time window (Figure 5).

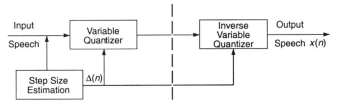

Figure 5: Block diagram representation of adaptive quantization.

For loud sounds, Δ is large, while weaker sounds permit smaller values with little risk of clipping. The choice of window size over which to evaluate the speech energy leads to two classes of APCM coders: *instantaneous* and *syllabic* (Figure 6). Short windows give rapid, "instantaneous" updates and follow amplitude variations within individual pitch periods. Syllabic adaptation, on the other hand, uses longer windows (> 25ms) and follows slower amplitude variations due to changes in the vocal tract.

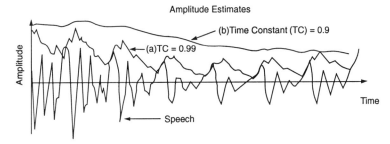

Figure 6: Speech variance estimates in (a) instantaneous, (b) syllabic adaptation. For clarity, values of $\hat{\sigma}_x(n)$ are magnified equally in both plots.

2.4 Exploiting Properties of the Spectral Envelope

The typical short-time speech magnitude spectrum consists of a slowly varying envelope, on which a harmonic line structure is imposed in the case of voiced speech. The envelope shape is primarily due to the poles and zeros of the vocal tract response. In most cases, the center frequencies and bandwidths of the formants describe the envelope well, although zeros have effects in nasals and frication. This section deals with *differential* coders, which exploit the spectral envelope structure.

We have seen that quantization noise is proportional to Δ, which in turn is proportional to the standard deviation of the quantizer input. APCM uses only information about average speech amplitude. Differential PCM (DPCM) achieves more significant gains in SNR by exploiting waveform behavior over intervals of only a few samples. Instead of quantizing speech samples directly, DPCM quantizes the difference between a current sample and a predicted estimate of that sample based on a weighted average of previous samples (Gibson, 1982). The SNR gain from this procedure is due to the high degree of sample-to-sample correlation in voiced speech. Such short-time correlation (over at most 20 samples) corresponds to the spectral envelope; correlation over longer intervals (e.g., periodicity) relates to spectral fine structure and is discussed later.

The average long-term spectrum of speech shows that most energy is below 1 kHz (Figure 7), since most speech is voiced and such energy falls off with frequency because of the dominance of low-frequency energy in glottal waveforms.

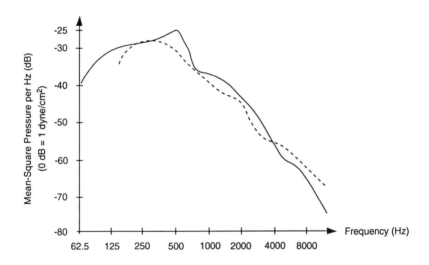

Figure 7   Long-time power density spectrum for continuous speech (solid line is male speech, dashed line is female speech) (Dunn et al., 1940, pp. 278-288).

Nonetheless, F_s cannot be reduced because high frequencies remain very important for intelligibility and naturalness. Thus, voiced speech has a high degree of correlation among adjacent samples. By formulating a prediction estimate and subtracting it from the actual sample, DPCM quantizes a difference value with smaller variance than that of the original speech (Figure 8). Quantization noise is reduced through the use of smaller step sizes, and SNR improves when speech is reconstructed at the decoder with an operation inverting the differentiation. The difference signal is often called a *residual* or *prediction error* since it is the remaining waveform after certain predictable aspects of the speech signal have been extracted.

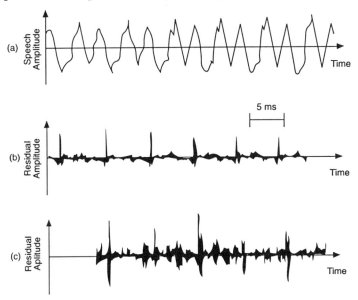

Figure 8 Waveforms of (a) original speech and prediction error after (b) spectrum prediction ($N = 16$) and (c) an additional pitch prediction (of third order). Waveforms (b) and (c) are magnified by $\sqrt{10}$ and 10, respectively.

2.4.1 Differential Pulse Code Modulation (DPCM)

The basic DPCM system forms an estimate $\tilde{x}(n)$ for each speech sample $x(n)$, based on $x(n - k)$, $k = 1,2,3,\ldots,N$, and quantizes the residual $d(n)$ as

$$\hat{d}(n) = Q[d(n)] = Q[x(n) - \tilde{x}(n)] \tag{3}$$

(the ^ notation means "quantized"). At the decoder, $\hat{d}(n)$ passes through an "integrator," yielding the output speech $\hat{x}(n)$. Many DPCM systems do not use such a simple approach because the error at the quantizer output, $e(n) = \hat{d}(n) - d(n)$, is subsequently integrated by the decoder and thus propagates to future samples. In PCM and log PCM, the quantization noise, well modeled as white noise (assuming fine quantization), passes directly through to the output. Integrating the noise instead colors its spectrum, concentrating the distortion at low frequencies. Noise can be spectrally shaped to perceptual advantage, but many applications prefer zero-mean, uncorrelated noise with a flat spectrum. For these reasons, a structure with the predictor P in a closed-loop feedback around the quantizer Q is more common (Figure 9).

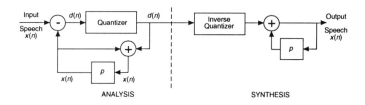

Figure 9: General differential PCM: coder on the left, decoder on the right. P is a linear predictor, and the inverse quantizer simply converts transmitted codes back into a single $\hat{d}(n)$ value.

2.4.2 Linear Prediction
Virtually all DPCM schemes use a *linear predictor* of the form

$$\tilde{x}(n) = \sum_{k=1}^{p} a_k \hat{x}(n-k), \tag{4}$$

where the estimate $\tilde{x}(n)$ is a linear combination of the p previous inputs to the predictor. The reconstructed speech $\hat{x}(n)$ results from passing $\hat{d}(n)$ through a synthesis or reconstruction filter of the form

$$H(e^{jw}) = 1/(1 - P(e^{jw})) = 1/(1 - \sum_{k=1}^{p} a_k e^{-jwk}), \tag{5}$$

where the predictor P is a filter with response $P(e^{jw})$. A good predictor inverse filter $1 - P(e^{jw})$ outputs $\hat{d}(n)$ with a flat error spectrum to achieve minimal quantization error. As a result, $P(e^{jw})$ is chosen so that $H(e^{jw}) \approx X(e^{jw})$. Determination of the optimal values for the filter coefficients a_k yields an $H(e^{jw})$ as close to the speech spectrum as is possible with p coefficients. The usual analysis procedure solves a set of p linear equations (effectively inverting a $p \times p$ correlation matrix). More details on linear prediction will be given in sects. 2.8.1–2.8.2.

2.4.3 Delta Modulation (DM)

An important subclass of DPCM systems is *delta modulation* (DM), which uses 1-bit ($B = 1$) quantization with first-order prediction ($p = 1$ in eq. 5). The main advantages of DM are simplicity and low cost: the quantizer just checks the input sign bit, and each transmitted bit has equal importance, eliminating synchronization problems. To compensate for the otherwise coarse quantization, the sampling rate is several times the Nyquist rate. This oversampling considerably reduces the input variance to the quantizer due to the high sample-to-sample correlation, which yields very small values for $d(n)$. The predictor filter has only one coefficient ($a_1 = a$), which is normally chosen to be just less than 1. A value of exactly 1 would yield a basic differentiator, and the predictor would simply estimate the next input sample to be equal to its last output sample. In DM, the quantized values $\hat{d}(n)$ are $\pm\Delta$, always changing the output by amounts virtually equal to the step size in Figure 10.

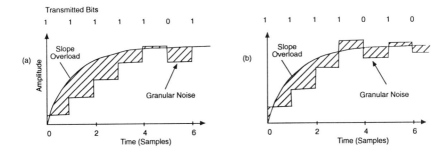

Figure 10 Illustration of slope overload and granular noise with (a) fixed step size (LDM) and (b) adaptive size (ADM).

The choice of Δ is crucial. Since the output magnitude can change only by Δ each sample interval T, the Δ must be large enough to accommodate rapid changes:

$$\frac{\Delta}{T} \geq \max \left| \frac{dx_a(t)}{dt} \right| \approx \max \frac{|x(n) - x(n-1)|}{T} \qquad (6)$$

Otherwise, clipping called *slope overload* results, with the output noise exceeding half the step size. Distortions localized to times of rapid signal change occur, as opposed to noise uniformly distributed throughout the signal as in other PCM schemes. On the other hand, if Δ is chosen too large, the normal *granular* noise becomes excessive since this noise is proportional to step size; e.g., when the speech input is silence, the output still oscillates with amplitude Δ. To improve DM, we can let the step size change dynamically with the input variance; such adaptive DM (ADM) systems are competitive with other waveform coders.

2.4.4   Adaptive Differential Pulse-Code Modulation (ADPCM)

Adaptive differential PCM can refer to DPCM coders that adapt Δ and/or the predictor. Just as PCM and DM benefit from adaptive quantization, SNR can be increased in DPCM if step size may change dynamically. The improvements in SNR are additive: about 6 dB with the differential scheme and another 4–6 dB by adapting the step size. In general ADPCM, both step size and predictor adapt with time, based on either quantizer inputs (feedforward) or outputs (feedback) (Figure 11). The feedforward scheme requires transmission of side information, which is significant for adaptive prediction since *p* coefficients (eq. 5) need transmission. On the other hand, the feedforward scheme allows bit protection against channel errors for the crucial side information, which uses a small percentage of the bit rate.

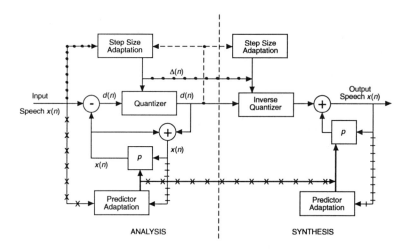

Figure 11:   ADPCM system with both adaptive quantization and adaptive prediction. Paths are marked for the different options: AQF (dots), AQB (dashes), APF (X's), APB (+'s). Paths drawn with heavy lines indicate vector transmission (e.g., several parameters sent in parallel).

With the fixed predictor of DPCM, there is little advantage in a predictor order higher than two or three. When the predictor can adapt to match the short-time characteristics of a dynamic speech signal, prediction gain increases over a wider range of order. SNR improvement saturates much more slowly with increasing order, although the major gains still occur in the first few orders. The closer the reconstruction filter $H(e^{jw})$ can approximate the speech spectrum, the better the coder performance. For a fixed predictor, $H(e^{jw})$ could do no better than to match the long-time speech spectrum. With predictors obtained from windows short enough to consider the speech temporarily stationary, the finer details of individual formants can be modeled in ADPCM. Thus while $p = 1–2$ is sufficient to the model general lowpass characteristic, significant SNR gains can be made up to about $p = 12$ for ADPCM. (Depending on formant separation and bandwidth, typically eight of the filter poles model four formants in 4-kHz bandwidth voiced speech, while additional poles help model the effects of the glottal source and nasality).

2.5 Exploiting the Periodicity of Voiced Speech

To exploit the short-time periodicity of voiced speech, the approach in the previous section could be extended to handle spectral fine structure as well as its envelope. Raising the predictor order p to examine speech over time windows exceeding a pitch period would allow the synthesis spectrum $H(e^{jw})$ to model harmonics. However, p would exceed 100, leading to extremely complicated evaluations of the predictor coefficients plus a complex structure in the predictor filter. This approach is unnecessary since spectral fine structure in voiced speech is highly regular (at least below 3 kHz), with harmonics uniformly spaced at multiples of F0.

The *spectral predictor* of DPCM depends on the speech spectral envelope; to exploit periodicity, we need a pitch predictor. Pitch prediction can be handled well by a filter with only one coefficient, replacing P in eq. 5 with

$$P_d(e^{jw}) = \beta e^{-jwM}, \tag{7}$$

where β is a scaling factor related to the degree of waveform periodicity and M is the estimated period (in samples). This predictor has a time response of a unit sample delayed M samples; so the pitch predictor merely estimates that the previous pitch period repeats itself. Prediction would have no useful effect for unvoiced speech since the fine structure for such speech is flat (the unvoiced excitation being random). Thus $\beta = 0$ for a signal with no detectable period structure and is approximately 1 for steady-state voiced speech. Coders that employ pitch prediction are often called *adaptive predictive coders* (APC) (Figure 12).

2.6 Exploiting Auditory Limitations

In waveform coders, output speech fidelity is usually measured by SNR, with the objective of minimizing output noise energy. Since speech goes to the auditory system, however, it would be better to minimize the subjective loudness of the noise. Auditory masking has strong effects on the perceptibility of one signal (e.g., noise) in the presence of another (speech). Noise is less likely to be heard at frequencies of stronger speech energy, e.g., at harmonics of F0, especially near the intense low-frequency formants.

The general DPCM coder configuration yields white noise of minimal energy in the output speech. While optimal for SNR, the noise is very noticeable during voiced speech at high frequencies, where speech energy is relatively low. If the prediction filter precedes the quantizer, the noise has a spectral pattern identical to that of the input speech, since the white quantization noise is so shaped by the synthesis filter. Perceptually, the speech may improve because the noise is masked to a degree evenly at all frequencies by the speech spectrum. However, the preferred system is a compromise between the two approaches, called *noise feedback coding* (Atal et al., 1979). A noise feedback filter is typically chosen so that the noise follows the speech spectrum, but with a bias toward less noise at low frequencies.

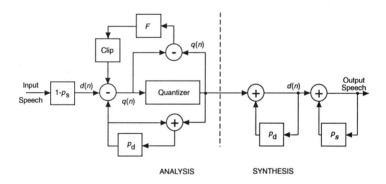

Figure 12: APC system with two stages of prediction: a predictor, P_s, based on the short-time spectral envelope and another, P_d, based on pitch structure. The filter F shapes the quantization noise to have less perceptual effect on the output speech. (After Atal, et al., 1979)

2.7 Spectral (Frequency-Domain) Coders

This section deals with waveform coders that filter the speech into separate frequency bands (called channels or *subbands*) for individual coding.

Within each subband, the filtered speech may be waveform encoded, or relevant measures concerning amplitude and phase may be extracted and coded. The individual coders differ with respect to the number of subbands and the detail with which each subband is coded. Since phase information is always retained, which allows a synchronous comparison between input and output, SNR remains viable.

The short-time Fourier transform $X_n(e^{jw})$ of sect. 1.3 suggests the following spectral coder. Speech is input to a bank of bandpass filters covering the range from 0 to $F_s/2$ Hz, and the output signals are waveform encoded. With proper filter design, no information need be lost in this process, and the speech waveform can be reconstructed by summing the outputs of all channels. Assuming the simplest design, $X_n(e^{jw_k})$ are the time signals in each of N channels centered at frequencies $w_k = \pi(k + 1/2)/N$, where $k = 0,1,2,\ldots,$ $N - 1$. The time window used in defining the frequency transform specifies the shape of the identical, equally-spaced bandpass filters. Since the Fourier transform is invertible, the windowed $x(n)$ can be recovered from $X_n(e^{jw_k})$ (except for the effects of quantization noise). $X_n(e^{jw_k})$ are lowpass signals that may be decimated (following the Nyquist rate) to rates as low as F_s/N samples/s, depending on how closely the window filter approximates an ideal lowpass filter.

Simple filter bank systems are not practical coders. Each decimated channel allows at best a N:1 rate decrease, but there are N channels to code. Thus the total number of samples/s still exceeds the Nyquist rate of the original speech signal. Practical systems require nonuniform channel coding. *Subband coding* divides the spectrum into about 4–8 bands and codes each bandpass signal using APCM (Crochiere, 1977) (Figure 13). Low-frequency channels are transmitted with more bits than higher-frequency bands because the former are more important perceptually. By using individual APCM coders, quantization can be optimized within each band, and the noise in each channel can be isolated from affecting other channels. Bandpass filter design is crucial here. A major potential difficulty with bandpass filtering and subsequent decimation is that of aliasing. Practical filters must have finite-amplitude roll-off with frequencies outside their desired bandwidths, and steeper frequency skirts usually yield more complex filters. Gaps in the output spectrum, due to inadequate filtering, cause perceived reverberation.

2.8 Vocoders
The distinction between waveform coders and vocoders has become blurred in recent years by the design of hybrid systems, which code both temporal

and spectral information. Nonetheless, we distinguish waveform coders that reconstruct speech sample by sample, exploiting redundancies in the time or frequency domain, and vocoders, which exploit speech-specific models. Waveform coders use SNR, while vocoders require subjective evaluation. Vocoders identify certain aspects of the speech spectrum as important to model. The usual parameters of F0, voicing, and formants or broad spectral structure involve the same speech redundancies that waveform coders exploit. However, waveform coders always transmit a residual waveform or spectrum, which represents those aspects of speech that remain poorly understood. Vocoders radically simplify such residuals to reduce bit rates but pay a price in quality. The residual may be of little importance for intelligibility, but vocoders have been unable to attain the naturalness of *toll-quality* speech (quality equivalent to that of analog telephone networks), and usually only approach (lower) *communications quality* in hybrid waveform vocoders which augment the usual vocoder data with residual coding.

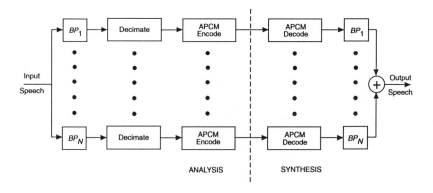

Figure 13: Subband coder with N bands. The decimators have output sampling rates of $2f_i$, where f_i is the high-frequency cutoff for bandpass filter BPi. In many systems, the decimation rate can be as low as twice the bandwidth of BP_i. The decoder in each channel includes the interpolator corresponding to the channel's decimator. (After Flanagan et al. 1979)

Only synthetic-quality speech is possible with basic vocoders due to the loss of phase information. It is usually difficult to compare vocoded speech with waveform-coded speech, since the distortions are different. Waveform coders suffer primarily from additive noise; their noise may be shaped for improved perceptual quality and sometimes takes the form of clicks and pops. Vocoders rarely have such background noise; rather, they suffer from distortions such as whistles, burbles, buzziness, harshness, and muffled quality. The degradations arise from the assumed model of the vocoder.

2.8.1 Linear Predictive (LPC) Vocoders

LPC vocoders typically operate at bit rates under 4.8 kbits/s and yield synthetic-quality speech. Raising the bit rate further yields little quality improvement due to the limitations of the LPC model. The equal spacing of harmonics in voiced speech is exploited by transmitting the spacing (a single F0 value) and requires a binary voicing decision. The addition of a pitch estimator adds complexity, but permits significant reductions in bit rate. Spectral and excitation information is sent at a frame rate selected according to the same criteria for updating side information in waveform coders, usually 30–100 frames/s. Excitation is coded by 5–6 bits for amplitude, 1 bit for a voiced/unvoiced decision and, for voiced frames, about 5–6 bits for F0. The excitation for the synthesis filter is either *pseudo-white noise* (from a random number generator) if the frame is unvoiced or impulses spaced every 1/F0 seconds if voiced. *Variable frame rate* transmission (Viswanathan, et al. 1982) can also reduce bit rate by not sending some frames of data when speech is relatively steady-state: at the receiver, such frames can be replaced by repeating the last frame set, or by waiting for the next one and then interpolating between the two most recently received frames.

LPC provides an accurate and economical representation of speech spectral magnitude that can reduce transmission rates in speech coding, increase accuracy and reduce calculation in speech recognition, and generate efficient speech synthesis (Markel et al., 1976). LPC has been used to estimate F0, vocal tract area functions, and the frequencies and bandwidths of spectral poles and zeros (e.g., formants), but it primarily provides a small set of speech parameters that capture information about the configuration of the vocal tract. This set of LPC coefficients can be directly used in digital filters as multiplier coefficients for synthesis or can be stored as recognition templates. To minimize complexity, the speech signal is usually assumed to come from an all-pole (autoregressive) source; i.e., one assumes that its spectrum has no zeros, despite the presence of zeros due to the glottal source and to nasals and unvoiced sounds.

Following Sect. 2.4.2, each synthetic speech sample $\hat{s}(n)$ is modeled by a linear combination of the p previous output samples and one input sample:

$$\hat{s}(n) = \sum_{k=1}^{p} a_k \hat{s}(n-k) + Gu(n), \tag{8}$$

were G is a gain factor for the input speech. If speech $s(n)$ is filtered by an inverse or *predictor* filter (the inverse of an all-pole $H(e^{jw})$) the output $e(n)$ is the error signal:

$$e(n) = s(n) - \sum_{k=1}^{p} a_k s(n-k), \tag{9}$$

which in voiced speech is normally characterized by sharp peaks separated in time by pitch periods, but also has a significant "noisy" component.

2.8.2   Least-Squares LPC Analysis

Two approaches can be used to obtain a set of LPC coefficients a_k characterizing $H(e^{jw})$. The classical *least-squares* method chooses a_k to minimize the mean energy in $e(n)$ over a speech frame, while the *lattice* approach permits instantaneous updating of the a_k. In the former technique, either the speech or error signal must be windowed to limit the extent of the speech under analysis. In the data windowing or *autocorrelation* method, the speech signal is multiplied by a Hamming or similar time window

$$e(n) = w(n)s(n) \tag{10}$$

so that $x(n)$ has finite duration (N samples, typically corresponding to 20–30 ms). The energy in the residual signal is

$$E = \sum_{n=-\infty}^{\infty} e^2(n) = \sum_{n=-\infty}^{\infty} \left[x(n) - \sum_{k=1}^{p} a_k x(n-k) \right]^2. \tag{11}$$

The values of a_k that minimize E are found by setting $\partial E/\partial a_k = 0$ for $k = 1,2,3,\ldots,p$. This yields p linear equations

$$\sum_{m=-\infty}^{\infty} x(n-i)x(n) = \sum_{k=1}^{p} a_k \sum_{i=-\infty}^{\infty} x(n-i)x(n-k), \text{ for } i = 1,2,3,\ldots,p, \tag{12}$$

in p unknowns a_k. Recognizing the first term as the autocorrelation $R(i)$ of $x(n)$ and taking advantage of the finite duration of $x(n)$, we have

$$R(i) = \sum_{n=i}^{N-1} x(n)x(n-i), \quad \text{for } i = 1,2,3, \ldots ,p, \tag{13}$$

so that eqs. 12 reduce to the Yule-Walker equations,

$$\sum_{k=1}^{p} a_k R(i - k) = R(i), \quad for \ i = 1,2,3, \ldots ,p,$$ (14)

The autocorrelation could be calculated for all integers i, but since $R(i)$ is an even function, it need be determined only for $0 \le i \le p$. There are efficient methods to solve eqs. 14.

In the second least-squares technique, called the *covariance* method, the error $e(n)$ is windowed instead of $s(n)$. A covariance function replaces R, which is quite similar, but differs in the windowing effects. The autocorrelation method uses N windowed speech samples, whereas the covariance method uses the speech samples directly. The autocorrelation approach thus introduces distortion into the spectral estimation procedure since time windowing corresponds to convolving the original short-time $S(e^{jw})$ with the frequency response of the window $W(e^{jw})$. Most windows have lowpass frequency responses; so the windowed speech spectrum is a smoothed version of the original, with the extent and type of smoothing dependent on the window shape and duration. The autocorrelation method is nonetheless popular because it is guaranteed to yield stable synthesis filters and is computationally efficient.

Instead of dividing speech into successive frames of data and obtaining spectral coefficients for each frame, the LPC parameters can be obtained sample by sample. Each new sample updates some intermediate speech measures, from which the LPC parameters are revised. Recalculating and inverting a covariance matrix for each speech sample, as in the block methods, is unnecessary.

2.8.3 Spectral Estimation via LPC

Parseval's theorem for a discrete-time signal (e.g., the error $e(n)$) and its Fourier transform is

$$E = \sum_{n=-\infty}^{\infty} e^2(n) = \frac{1}{2\pi} \int_{w=-\pi}^{\pi} |E(e^{jw})|^2 dw.$$ (15)

Since $e(n)$ can be obtained by passing the speech $s(n)$ through the inverse LPC filter $A(e^{jw}) = G/H(e^{jw})$, the residual is

$$E = \frac{G^2}{2\pi} \int_{w=-\pi}^{\pi} \frac{|S(e^{jw})|^2}{|H(e^{jw})|^2} \, dw. \tag{16}$$

Obtaining the LPC coefficients by minimizing E is equivalent to minimizing the average ratio of the speech spectrum to its LPC approximation. Equal weight is given to all frequencies, but $|H(e^{jw})|$ models the peaks in $|S(e^{jw})|$ better than the valleys (Figure 14). The LPC all-pole spectrum $|H(e^{jw})|$ is limited, by the number of poles used, in the degree of spectral detail it can model in $|S(e^{jw})|$. For a typical 10-pole model, at most five resonances can be represented accurately. The short-time voiced-speech spectrum with rapid frequency variation due to the harmonics as well as the slower variations due to the formant structure cannot be completely modeled. Valleys between formants are less accurately modeled than formant regions, since the error measure emphasizes high-energy frequencies. The choice of the order p for the LPC model is a compromise among spectral accuracy, computation time/memory, and transmission bandwidth. In general, there should be a sufficient number of poles to represent all formants in the signal bandwidth plus an additional 2–4 poles to approximate possible zeros in the spectrum as well as general spectral shaping.

To model the lower-amplitude, higher-frequency formants well, the speech signal is often *pre-emphasized* prior to LPC analysis; i.e., the input to the LPC analyzer is $s(n) - \alpha s(n - 1)$. The degree of pre-emphasis is controlled by a constant α, which determines the cutoff frequency of the single-zero filter through which $s(n)$ effectively passes. This reduces the dynamic range (i.e., "flattens" the speech spectrum) by adding a zero to counteract the spectral falloff due to the glottal source in voiced speech. The pre-emphasis and radiation zeros approximately cancel the falloff and yield formants with similar amplitudes. In LPC vocoders, the final stage of synthesis must contain a *de-emphasis* filter $1/(1 - \alpha e^{jw})$ to cancel the pre-emphasis.

2.8.4 LPC Synthesis

The two basic ways to implement a linear predictor are the *transversal* form (i.e., direct-form digital filter) and the *lattice* form. The lattice method for LPC typically involves both a *forward* and a *backward* prediction (Turner, 1985, pp. 91-134). Block LPC analysis uses only forward prediction (i.e., the estimate $\hat{s}(n)$ is based on p prior samples of $s(n)$), but the estimation can be done similarly from p ensuing samples in a form of backward "prediction"

(Figure 15). The lattice synthesizer has the same form as a vocal tract model, viewed as a lossless asoustic tube of p sections of equal length with uniform cross-sectional area A_m within each section. The reflection coefficients k_m could specify the amount of plane wave reflection at each section boundary:

$$k_m = \frac{A_m - A_{m-1}}{A_m + A_{m-1}}. \tag{17}$$

Efforts to relate the reflection coefficients obtained from speech to corresponding vocal tract areas, however, have met with only limited success because natural vocal tracts have losses and standard models using reflection coefficients must lump all losses at the glottal or labial ends (Wakita, 1979, pp. 281-285).

2.8.5 Window Considerations

Both window size N and order p should be kept small to minimize calculation in LPC analysis. However, since p is specified by the speech bandwidth, only N allows any flexibility to trade off spectral accuracy and computation. Because of windowing distortion, an autocorrelation LPC window must include at least two pitch periods for accurate spectral estimates. In other methods, the lack of signal windowing theoretically allows windows as short as $N = p + 1$. However, the accuracy of the LPC representation increases with the number of samples in the analysis frame.

The LPC model predicts each speech sample based on its p prior samples, following the assumption that an all-pole vocal tract filter describes the signal. It cannot distinguish between vocal tract resonances and excitation effects. Most LPC analysis is done pitch-asynchronously (e.g., on every sample in adaptive lattice techniques or on every N or $N/2$ samples in the block methods), which leads to degraded spectral estimation when pitch epochs are included during an analysis frame. The problem is aggravated when N is small because some analysis frames are dominated by excitation effects. In *pitch-synchronous analysis,* each analysis window is located entirely within a pitch period, which requires an accurate F0 estimator.

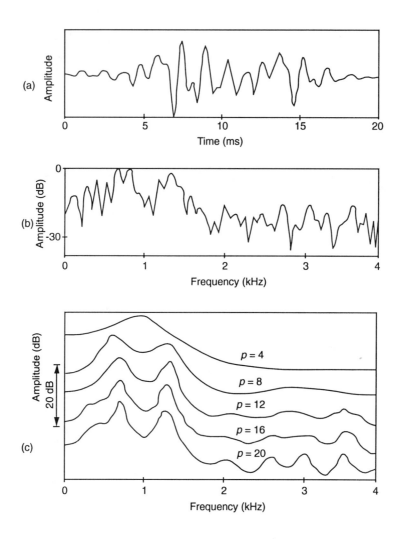

Figure 14: Signals and spectra in LPC for 20 ms of an /α/ vowel at 8000 samples/s: (a) time waveform, (b) speech spectrum, (c) LPC spectra using 4, 8, 12, 16, and 20 poles, respectively.

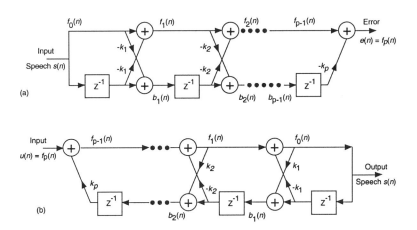

Figure 15: Lattice filters: (a) inverse filter A, which generates both forward and backward error signals at each stage of the lattice; (b) synthesis filter $1/A$. (Boxes labeled z^{-1} represent unit sample delays.)

2.8.6 Excitation for Vocoders

Concerning speech quality, the major problem with most vocoders lies in their simplistic excitation source. Most vocoders code the spectral envelope on one hand and presume that the excitation has a flat spectrum and contains periodicity information. For voiced speech, an excitation of periodically spaced impulses has the desired flat spectral envelope (i.e., equal harmonic amplitudes). However, each harmonic is assigned the same phase of zero at the decoder since no phase information is transmitted. Even if phases appropriate for the formants were to be inserted (and this would require a formant estimator), phase variations due to the glottal source would still be ignored. Only waveform coders retain sufficient phase information (via the transmission of the residual) to capture this important aspect of natural-sounding speech. On the other hand, speech coders that retain phase information operate at rates above 4.8 kbits/s, while most vocoders provide intelligible speech at lower rates.

The standard voiced excitation for vocoders is periodic, often simply one impulse per period, modeling the instant of closure of the vocal cords. The major excitation of the vocal tract in humans occurs at this time, every $1/F0$ seconds. However, this basic model ignores the many other excitations of the vocal tract due to irregularities in vocal cord motion. The vocal cord masses do not close in identical fashion each cycle, and closure may not be complete. Concentrating the excitation energy in one impulse per period leads to a more "peaky" waveform than in natural voiced speech. Some vocoders and synthesizers attempt to distribute the excitation more uniformly by repeating a fixed waveshape every period.

The standard LPC vocoder using a periodic excitation source (most commonly, a single sample per period) for voiced speech yields only *synthetic-quality* speech. The major impediment to toll quality speech lies in the periodic excitation, which adds a "buzzy" or mechanical aspect to the synthetic speech. Part of the problem lies in the binary decision of whether speech during an analysis frame is voiced. The synthesizer chooses either a periodic waveform or white noise to excite the $H(e^{jw})$ filter. Voiced fricatives are thus poorly modeled since they should have a noise excitation with a periodic envelope. More seriously, vowel excitation in natural speech appears to have a noisy component, which is primarily evident above 2–3 kHz.

2.8.7   Multipulse-Excited LPC (MLPC)

In an attempt to enhance speech quality, *multipulse* LPC represents the residual signal with a small number of impulses per speech frame. Decimation factors of about 8:1 are common; e.g., a frame of 64 residual samples is reduced to 8 nonzero samples. In the multipulse residual, the amplitude and position of each sample (or "pulse") are chosen to minimize a perceptually weighted spectral-error criterion (Atal et al., 1982) (Figure 16). The typical multipulse residual resembles a skeleton of the original, in which the major excursions at the start of each pitch period are modeled by several large pulses, and other minor excursions later in the period are modeled by smaller pulses. MLPC is a hybrid coder, combining aspects of waveform coding (for the excitation) and vocoding (for the spectral envelope), and operates in the range of 8–16 kbits/s.

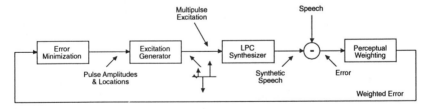

Figure 16   An analysis-by-synthesis procedure for determining locations and amplitudes of pulses in multipulse LPC. (After Atal et al., 1982)

Basic MLPC needs no voicing or F0 detector. The procedure can be implemented iteratively, in an analysis-by-synthesis procedure, starting with a null multipulse residual that excites an LPC synthesizer to yield (null) speech, which is then subtracted from the actual frame of speech to give an error signal. The error here is a form of output quantization noise that is minimized after a perceptual weighting that de-emphasizes the formant regions, since noise at these frequencies is masked by the formant harmonics (similar to APC noise shaping). To obtain higher-quality speech at yet lower bit rates, basic MLPC is often augmented by pitch prediction (as in sect. 2.5), to remove the major pitch epochs in the residual signal.

2.9 Vector Quantization (VQ)

The waveform speech coders described previously have been instantaneous, i.e., the transmitted values $v(n)$ correspond directly with input speech samples. Vocoders consider successive frames of N samples as blocks of data, which yield only a few parameters to transmit (e.g., for 100 speech samples, 10–20 spectral and prosodic parameters). However, these values are often coded independently, taking no account of any redundancies that might exist. Such $v(n)$ values, whether from $e(n)$ in waveform coders or from spectral coefficients in vocoders, are far from random; e.g., humans listening only to $e(n)$ can often understand the speech.

Coders that attempt to remove further redundancy use *vector quantization* (VQ), which considers k samples of $v(n)$ as a block or *vector* and represents them for transmission as a single code, rather than coding k values independently (Gray, 1984). For example, 50 bits might be used in LPC vocoders to send 10 coefficients in scalar quantization, but that same information could be coded with perhaps 10 bits in a VQ scheme. A properly chosen set of 1024 spectra (2^{10} for a 10-bit VQ) should be able to adequately represent all possible speech sounds.

VQ increases complexity in coder analysis. After the normal analysis (yielding k scalar parameters for a frame), the coder must then determine which k-dimensional vector, among a set of M possibilities stored in a *codebook*, corresponds most closely to the set of scalar parameters. A $\log_2 M$-bit code replaces the k parameters. The system's decoder is not more complex, although its memory must be increased to include the codebook. To synthesize the output speech, the decoder uses the parameters listed under the index in the codebook corresponding to the received code.

The key issues in implementing VQ concern the design and search of the codebook. In coding with scalar quantization, distortion arises due to the finite precision for each parameter representation. The distortion in VQ comes from using synthesis parameters from a codebook entry, which differ in general from the parameters determined by the speech analyzer. M should be large enough that each possible input vector corresponds to a codeword whose substitution for the input yields synthetic speech sufficiently close to the original. However, M must be limited for efficient search procedures and because bit rate is proportional to $\log_2 M$.

A distortion measure is needed as a criterion in both the design and operation of the codebook. For coders that use vectors of waveform samples (e.g., k consecutive samples of $e(n)$), the most common measure is a Euclidean distance. Codebook creation usually involves the analysis of a large training sequence, typically of a few minutes, of speech sufficiently varied as to contain examples of all phonemes in many different contexts. An iterative design procedure converges on a locally optimal codebook which minimizes average distortion across the training set.

Compared to scalar coding, the major additional complexity of VQ lies in the search of the codebook for the appropriate codeword to transmit, given a speech vector to code. In a *full codebook search*, the vector for every frame is compared with each of the M codewords, requiring M distance calculations. The SNR performance of VQ increases with increasing dimension k. To code k speech parameters as a block, using $R = \log_2 M$ bits/vector with F_s samples/s and allowing k speech samples/vector, the bit rate is RF_s/k bits/s. Thus, for a constant bit rate, R is directly proportional to k, and the size $M=2^R$ of a VQ codebook rises exponentially with dimension k. Many practical VQ systems rely on fast suboptimal search techniques that reduce search time and sometimes codebook memory, while sacrificing little coder performance.

One major recent application of VQ for speech coding in the 4–9.6 kbits/s range is code-excited linear prediction (CELP), in which short sequences of the LPC residual signal are coded via VQ. It is similar to MLPC in its analysis-by-synthesis procedure and its use of a pitch prediction loop.

2.10   Network Considerations

The choice of bit rates for speech coders has been motivated primarily by the telephone network. Since telephone lines tend to attenuate frequencies above 3200 Hz, 8000 samples/s is considered a standard sampling rate (allowing for imperfect lowpass filtering). Thus, 64-kbits/s toll-quality speech, using 8-bit log PCM, is a benchmark. High-quality coders at 32 kbits/s and 16 kbits/s can double or quadruple the number of voice signals to be sent on a communications link that currently handles one 64-kbits/s signal. Until recently, modem technology could not guarantee digital transmission at rates exceeding 2.4 kbits/s over standard telephone lines. Many low-bit-rate vocoders are designed for standard modem rates at multiples or submultiples of 2.4 kbits/s.

3.   Speech Synthesis

Speech synthesis is the automatic generation of speech waveforms, from either stored speech representations (*voice response*) or from phonetically-based rules (*text-to-speech*). Current speech synthesizers represent tradeoffs among the conflicting demands of maximizing speech quality, and minimizing memory space, algorithmic complexity, and computation time. The memory is often proportional to the vocabulary of the synthesizer, with the simplest speech coding, storage rates near 100 kbits/s result, which are prohibitive except for synthesizers with very small vocabularies. The sacrifices usually made to reduce memory size for large-vocabulary synthesizers involve simplistic modeling of spectral dynamics, vocal tract excitation, and intonation, which yields quality limitations.

3.1   Concatenation of Speech Units

Speech synthesizers can be characterized by the size of the speech units they concatenate to yield the output speech as well as by the method used to code, store, and synthesize the speech. Large speech units (phrases and sentences) can give high-quality output speech but require much memory. Voice response systems handle input of limited vocabulary and syntax, while text-to-speech systems accept all input text. The latter construct speech using small stored speech units and extensive linguistic processing, while the former reproduce speech directly from previously-coded speech.

The simplest synthesis concatenates stored words or phrases. Ideally, each word or phrase should originally be pronounced with timing and intonation appropriate for all sentences in which it could be used. Merely concatenating words originally spoken in isolation usually leads to degraded intelligibility and naturalness. The duration of stored units must be adjusted in concatenation since the durations of units vary in sentential context.

For synthesis of unrestricted text, speech is generated from sequences of basic sounds, which substantially reduces memory requirements since most languages have only 30–40 phonemes. However, the spectral features of these short concatenated sounds (50–200 ms) must be smoothed at their boundaries to avoid jumpy, discontinuous speech. The pronunciation of a phoneme in a word is heavily dependent on its phonetic context (e.g., on neighboring phonemes, intonation, and speaking rate). The smoothing and adjustment process as well as the need to calculate an appropriate intonation for each context results in complex synthesizers with less natural output speech. While commercial synthesizers have been primarily based on word or phone concatenation, intermediate-sized units of stored speech such as syllables (Fujimura et al., 1978) or diphones (Shadle et al., 1979) may be used. *Diphones* are obtained by dividing a speech waveform into phone-sized units, with the cuts in the middle of each phone (to preserve the transition between adjacent phones). When diphones are concatenated in a proper sequence, smooth speech usually results because the merged sounds at the boundaries are spectrally similar.

Smoothing of spectral parameters at the boundaries between units is most important for short units (e.g., phones). Since diphone boundaries interface spectra from similar sections of two realizations of the same phoneme, their smoothing rules are fairly simple. Systems that link phones, however, must use complex smoothing rules to represent coarticulation in the vocal tract. Not enough is understood about coarticulation to establish a complete set of rules to describe how the spectral parameters for each phone are modified by its neighbors. Diphone synthesizers try to circumvent this problem by storing the parameter transitions from one phone to the next since coarticulation primarily influences only the immediately adjacent phones.

High-quality speech requires synthesis using waveform coders and large memories. More efficient but lower-quality systems use vocoders. Vocoder synthesizers are considered *terminal analog synthesizers* because because they model the speech output of the vocal tract without explicitly taking account of articulator movements. A third way to generate speech is *articulatory synthesis*, which represents vocal tract shapes directly, using data from X-ray analysis of speech production (Haggard). Due to the difficulty of obtaining accurate three-dimensional vocal tract representations and of modeling the system with a limited set of parameters, this last method has tended to yield lower-quality speech.

The choice of synthesis method is influenced by the vocabulary size. Because they must model all possible utterances, unlimited text systems are more complex and yield lower-quality speech. Advances in memory technology will increase the vocabulary of low-cost waveform synthesizers; but for greater flexibility, parametric methods are necessary. Parametric synthesis normally produces only synthetic-quality speech because of inadequate modeling of natural speech production. Coding each of about 1200 diphones in English with 2-3 frames of parameters require storage of about 200 kbits. More popular are phoneme synthesizers, which normally store one or two sets of amplitude and spectral parameters for each of the 37 phonemes in as few as 2 kbits.

3.2 Unrestricted Text (Text-to-Speech) Systems

Synthesizers that accept unlimited text need a linguistic processor to convert the text into a form suitable for accessing the stored speech units. The input sentences are translated into a sequence of linguistic codes to fetch the appropriate stored units and intonation parameters are determined to vary F0 and duration properly. The first problem is usually handled by a set of language-dependent rules for converting letters into phonemes (Hunnicutt, 1980). These rules examine the context of each letter; e.g., the letter p is pronounced /p/, except before the letter h (e.g., *telephone*). English needs hundreds of such *letter-to-phoneme* rules to correctly translate 90% of the words in unlimited text situations (Elovitz, et al., 1976). Many common words (e.g., *of, the*) violate basic pronunciation rules; thus, lists of exception words are examined before basic rules are applied.

The pronunciation rules in the MITalk synthesizer (Allen et al., 1979) are preceded by a word decomposition algorithm, which tries to strip prefixes and suffixes from each word. Since there are only a few dozen such affixes in English and they can systematically affect pronunciation (e.g., *algebra* vs. *algebraic*), the decomposition procedure increases the power of the system. MITalk also has a dictionary of morphemes (the basic lexical units that constitute words), which contains not only phoneme pronunciations but also syntactic parts of speech. If this syntactic information is combined with a parser to determine linguistic structures in the input text, intonation can be specified by rule, locating F0 and duration effects to simulate natural intonation. Most synthesizers forgo parsers and large dictionaries as too complex and rely on simplistic intonation rules or leave F0 for the user to specify directly. Poor handling of intonation is a major reason why much unlimited text synthesis sounds unnatural (Akers et al., 1985).

3.3 Formant Synthesis

Most formant synthesizers use a model similar to that shown in Figure 17. The system in Figure 18 shows a specific implementation that forms the basis of most advanced synthesizers, using cascade and parallel structures. The excitation is either a periodic train of impulses, pseudo-random noise, or periodically shaped noise (for voiced fricatives). The vocal tract is usually modelled as a cascade of second-order digital resonators, each representing either a formant or the spectral shape of the excitation source. The cascade filter structure approximates the speech spectrum well for vowels and can be controlled with one amplitude parameter. Advanced synthesizers allow the first four formant frequencies and first three bandwidths to vary as a function of time (variation in higher formants has little perceptual effects. Simpler systems vary only F1-F3, with all bandwidths fixed. Lack of time variation in the bandwidths yields a degradation that is most noticeable in nasal sounds.

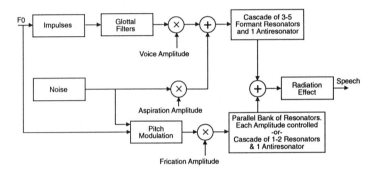

Figure 17:   Simplified block diagram of a formant synthesizer

Synthesis of nasals usually requires one more resonator than for vowels because the acoustic path including the nasal cavity is longer than the oral vocal tract, which increases the number of resonances in the speech bandwidth. To model the spectral zeros that occur in nasals, a second-order antiresonator is often used for the zero with the lowest frequency (higher-frequency zeros have less perceptual importance). For efficient implementation, an extra resonator and antiresonator can be considered as a complex-conjugate pole-zero pair with equal bandwidths, which have canceling effects except when nasals are to be simulated.

A parallel bank of filters may also be used to generate sonorants, but requires calculation of each formant amplitude as well as an extra amplitude multiplication per formant (Holmes, 1983). Special attention must be given to modeling the frequency region below F1 in the all-parallel approach because listeners are sensitive to the large amount of energy present there in natural speech and varying formant positions normally changes the gain below F1 in parallel synthesis. The advantage of an all-parallel method is a simpler synthesizer structure.

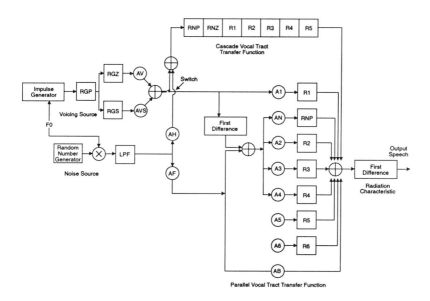

Figure 18: Block diagram of a cascade-parallel formant synthesizer. Digital resonators are indicated by the prefix *R* and amplitude controls by the prefix *A*. Each resonator R_n has associated resonant frequency and bandwidth control parameters. (After Klatt, 1980, pp. 971-995)

To simulate voiced frication, many formant synthesizers excite a parallel set of resonators with a noise source modulated by a waveform with period 1/F0. Typically, F1 has clear harmonic structure in voiced frication, while formants above F2-F3 are fully unvoiced. Providing each formant in a parallel synthesizer with its own control for mixing periodic and noise excitation is one approach. Alternatively in cascade-parallel synthesis, noise can excite a parallel set of resonators while a lowpass-filtered version of the normal glottal signal excites a cascade set of resonators (Klatt, 1980). Whenever formants are added in parallel, they should alternate in sign, i.e., A1 - A2 + A3 - A4..., to account for 180° phase shifts in the vocal tract transfer function at each formant frequency.

3.4 Linear Predictive Coding (LPC) Synthesis

LPC synthesis has a simpler structure than formant synthesis because all spectral properties of speech (except periodicity) are included in the LPC coefficients, which are calculated automatically in the analysis of natural speech. A lattice filter is often used for synthesis because the filter coefficients can be linearly interpolated between frames without yielding an unstable filter. For simplicity, most LPC systems do not allow mixed excitation for voiced fricatives.

The choice between formant and LPC synthesis is governed by tradeoffs. LPC has a simpler and fully automatic analysis procedure. However, our understanding of formant behavior facilitates parameter interpolation at segment boundaries in formant synthesis, whereas interpolation of LPC parameters is usually limited because each coefficient affects a wide range of speech frequencies in a complex fashion. In addition, formant synthesis is more flexible in allowing simple transformations to simulate different voices. The all-pole assumption of standard LPC leads to less accurate spectral estimation for nasal sounds than for other phones, whereas antiresonators in formant synthesis permit direct modeling of the most important spectral zeros in nasals.

3.5   Intonation

Text-to-speech requires determining a natural intonation corresponding to the input text. When the stored synthesis units are large, F0 and intensity are usually stored explicitly (along with the spectral parameters in LPC and formant synthesizers) or implicitly (in residual signals). When concatenating units the size of words or smaller, unnatural speech occurs unless the intonation stored for each unit is adjusted for context. Each language has its own intonation rules, and they can be discovered only by comprehensive analysis of much natural speech.

The domain and method of variation are different for the three prosodics: F0, duration, and intensity. The primary variations in intensity are phoneme-dependent, and so intensity parameters are usually stored as part of the synthesis units. Stressed syllables, however, tend to be more intense, and sentence-final syllables less intense, than average. Thus intensity should be modified at the syllable and sentence level when employing smaller synthesis units. Duration is usually encoded implicitly. In parametric synthesizers, the parameters are evaluated once every frame. For diphone and phone concatenation synthesis, durations must be determined explicitly (from analyses of the input text) since diphones and phones are stored with arbitrary durations.

It is of little use to store F0 for units smaller than a word, since natural F0 patterns are determined primarily at the level of words and phrases: F0 undergoes major changes on the lexically stressed syllables of emphasized words, with F0 rises and falls marking the starts and ends of syntactic phrases, respectively. Even at the word level, substantially different F0 contours can occur depending on the word's position in a sentence. Thus small-vocabulary synthesizers should record each word or phrase in sentence positions appropriate for all possible output contexts. Most F0-by-rule algorithms (Young et al., 1980, O'Shaughnessy, 1977) operate on a sentence-by-sentence basis, assigning a basic falling pattern following the declination effect, with superimposed F0 excursions above the declination line.

4. Speech Recognition

The other aspect of vocal communication between people and computers involves *automatic speech recognition* (ASR), or speech-to-text conversion. Automatic algorithms to perform synthesis and recognition have been less successful for recognition because of asymmetries in producing and interpreting speech. Recognition products often limit the number of speakers they accept as well as the words and syntactic structures that can be used and often require speakers to pause after each word.

To illustrate the difficulty of ASR, consider the problems of *segmentation* and *adaptation*. For both synthesis and recognition, the input is often partitioned for efficient processing, typically into segments of some linguistic relevance. In synthesis, the input text is easily divided into words and letters, whereas the speech signal that serves as input to ASR provides only tentative indications of phonetic segment boundaries. Sudden large changes in speech spectrum or amplitude are often used to estimate segment boundaries, which are nevertheless unreliable due to coarticulation and radically variable phone durations. Boundaries corresponding to words are very difficult to locate except when the speaker pauses. Many commercial recognizers require speakers to pause briefly after each word to facilitate segmentation. Continuous speech recognition allows natural conversational speech (e.g., 150-250 words/min), but is more difficult to recognize. Requiring the speaker to pause for at least 100-250 ms after each word in isolated word recognition (IWR) is unnatural for speakers and slows the rate at which speech can be processed (e.g., to about 20-100 words/min), but it alleviates the problem of isolating words in the input speech signal.

Human listeners adapt to synthetic speech and usually accept it as from a strange dialect. In ASR, however, the computer must adapt to the different voices used as input. It is hard to design a recognition algorithm that can cope with the myriad ways different speakers pronounce the same sentence or indeed to interpret the variations that a single speaker uses in pronouncing the same sentence at different times. Most systems are *speaker-dependent*, requiring speakers to train the system beforehand, by entering their speech patterns into the recognizer memory. Since memory in such systems grows linearly with the number of speakers, less accurate *speaker-independent* recognizers (trained by many speakers) are useful if a large population must be served.

4.1   Performance Evaluation

Most ASR systems quote accuracy or error rates as performance measures. The likelihood of an input being rejected is also important. Evaluation is, however, quite variable across different applications and depends heavily on (a) recording environment; (b) size and confusability of the vocabulary of words the system accepts; (c) whether the system is speaker-trained or speaker-independent; and (d) whether the system accepts isolated words or connected speech. Because performance is so dependent on the choice of vocabulary, several word sets are commonly used to enable comparison of systems. The *digit vocabulary* uses the first ten digits, while the *A-Z vocabulary* has the 26 letters (*ay, bee, cee,..., zee*). The combined 36-word *alphadigit* vocabulary contains some highly confusable subsets, e.g., the *E-set* (B-C-D-E-G-P-T-V-Z-3).

Mean word error rates do not reflect the varying communicative importance of words in an utterance. If ASR replaces typewriters as a means to input text to a computer, then word error rate is a good performance measure. If, however, the objective is to perform some action, then some errors can be tolerated if they do not block understanding. *Speech understanding* systems (Klatt, 1977) measure a recognizer's ability to comprehend the overall speech message. Some systems even operate on a word-spotting principle: the user may say anything, but only stressed words found in the system vocabulary cause action to be taken.

4.2   Basic Pattern Recognition Approach

ASR can be viewed as a pattern recognition task, requiring a mapping between each possible input waveform and its corresponding text. All such tasks involve two phases: *training* and *recognition*. Training establishes a *reference memory* or dictionary of speech patterns, each assigned a text label. The automatic recognition phase tries to assign a label to an unknown input.

Applying pattern recognition methods to ASR involves several steps: normalization, parametrization, feature extraction, a similarity comparison, and a decision (Figure 19). The first three steps concern information reduction, as is done in reducing bit rate for speech coders. Since ASR tries to extract a text message (and not to eventually reproduce the speech), data reduction can eliminate many speech factors that affect naturalness but not intelligibility. Speech coders must preserve both features, but recognizers utilize only aspects that aid in sound discrimination; e.g., low-bit-rate coding in terms of LPC coefficients or formants is practical for ASR because it reduces memory storage while preserving virtually all information dealing with the text message.

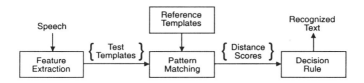

Figure 19: Traditional pattern recognition model for speech recognition.

The initial normalization step attempts to eliminate variability in the input speech signal due to environment. Variability due to the speaker is handled by a later *speaker normalization* step or by incorporating speaker characteristics directly into the memory. The major data reduction occurs in converting the signal into *parameters* and features. Acoustic parameters derive directly from standard speech analysis, while *features* denote the outputs of further reduction.

The focus of recognition is often a comparison between *templates* of parameter (or feature) representations of both an unknown *test* speech signal and a *reference* signal. The reference templates are derived during training. The test template T is usually compared with all reference templates R_i stored in memory, but the memory may be partitioned for a more efficient search. The R_i most closely matching T is usually chosen, yielding an output of text corresponding to that reference. However, if the match is relatively poor or if other R_i provide similar matches, a decision may be postponed and the speaker asked to repeat the utterance.

One can view ASR from either a cognitive or an *information-theoretic* perspective (Levinson, 1985). In the cognitive, or *expert system view*, relationships between speech signals and their corresponding text messages are observed and rules are established to explain the phenomena. For ASR, aspects of human speech production and spectrograms are used to develop techniques to segment and label speech sounds. Capturing all the complex interrelationships of speech redundancies in one comprehensive structural model, however, is very difficult.

The more general information-theoretic approach views speech simply as a signal about which information is derived through statistical analysis. Speech properties are exploited as part of a general framework (often using networks); speech-relevant parameters (e.g., LPC coefficients) are utilized in a statistical model that maximizes the likelihood of choosing the correct symbols (e.g., text) corresponding to an input signal. The models are trained on large amounts of speech and often use general comparison techniques involving templates and standard distance measures. The information-theoretic approach has had more commercial success than the cognitive approach, using either a parametric method (e.g., Markov models) that yields relatively fast recognition or a nonparametric method (e.g., dynamic time warping) which is easy to train but is computationally expensive in the recognition phase.

4.3   Parametric Representation
Most recognizers use a vocoder speech model, which separates excitation and vocal tract response. For a speech frame, excitation is often ignored, while the spectral envelope is represented with about 8–14 coefficients (derived from a Fourier transform, LPC analysis, or bandpass filters). Spectral information is weighted much more heavily than excitation in ASR because amplitude and F0 are more influenced by higher-level linguistic phenomena than by phonemics. Voicing and F0 estimation are also more prone to errors than is estimation of spectral parameters.

4.4   Distance Measures and Decisions
A representation of a speech frame using N parameters can be viewed as an N-dimensional vector (or a point in N-dimensional space). If the parameters are well chosen, in the sense of having similar values for different renditions of the same phonetic segment and distinct values for phonetically different segments, then separate regions can be established in the parameter space for each segment. (As a simple example, the first two formants can partition the vowels along the vowel triangle in two dimensions.) A memory of reference templates, each having an N-dimensional feature vector, is established during training. Generalizing to longer speech segments (words or phrases) requires expanding N to include time variation. In word recognition, templates are M-dimensional vectors, where $M = LN$ and L vectors of dimension N are extracted at uniformly spaced intervals for each word in the system vocabulary.

Given a speech input s, we output the most likely estimated text $\hat{t}$ from among the set of all possible texts t. Using Bayes' rule, we choose $\hat{t}$ so that

$$P(\hat{t} \mid s) = \max_t P(t \mid s) = \max_t \frac{P(t)P(s \mid t)}{P(s)} \; ; \tag{18}$$

i.e., the conditional probability is maximized over all t. Since $P(s)$ does not depend on t, the problem reduces to choosing $\hat{t}$ so that $P(t)P(s \mid t)$ is maximized. Often, either all texts t are equally likely or their *a priori* probabilities are unknown. The problem then reduces to maximizing $P(s \mid t)$.

While recognizers using statistical network descriptions of speech production take this *maximum-likelihood* approach, many other systems (e.g., template-based and acoustic-phonetic systems) follow variations of maximizing likelihood. For template systems, t corresponds to the reference template with the closest match to, or smallest distance from, the test template. Following this *nearest neighbor* (NN) rule, the recognizer calculates distances d_i for $i = 1,2,\ldots,L$ (L = number of templates in the system) and returns index i for d_{min}, the minimum d_i. In systems where there are several stored reference templates for each vocabulary word (corresponding to pronunciations of the word by several speakers, or several repetitions of the word by one speaker), the K-nearest neighbor (KNN) rule may be applied, which finds the nearest K neighbors to the unknown and chooses the word with the maximum number of entries among the K best matches (Gupta et al., 1984).

4.5 Timing Considerations

The discussion of distance measures implicitly assumed a comparison of stationary sounds. However, vocabulary entries usually involve sequences of different acoustic events. Thus, test and reference utterances are subdivided in time, yielding sequences of parameter vectors, e.g., into equal-duration frames of about 10-30 ms. Since reliable segmentation is difficult, ASR often compares templates frame by frame, which leads to alignment problems. Utterances are generally spoken at different speaking rates. To allow frame-by-frame comparison, the interval between frames is normalized so that all templates have a common number of frames.

Accurate time alignment of templates is crucial. Matching templates corresponding to the same word yields a small distance when parallel segments in the two templates are compared. Linear warping is insufficient to align speech events because the effects of speaking-rate change are nonlinear:

vowels and stressed syllables tend to expand and contract more than consonants and unstressed syllables. Thus linear warping of two utterances of the same text often aligns acoustic segments from different phones.

4.6 Segmentation

To simplify the comparison problem, most commercial recognizers offer isolated-word recognition (IWR). Silences between words are sufficient not to be confused with long plosives and allow the recognizer to compare words rather than sentences. Template matching performs poorly on continuous speech because the effects of coarticulation, destressing, and other artifacts of normal speaking are difficult to incorporate into word templates.

Determining time boundaries for acoustic segments in a test utterance is a significant problem for both isolated words and continuous speech. For IWR, accurate location of the endpoints of each word leads to efficient computation and to accurate recognition. Endpoint mistakes cause poor alignment in template comparison and increase the likelihood of rejecting correct reference templates. Weak acoustic segments at misaligned boundaries may be incorrectly matched to background noise.

Most endpoint detectors rely on amplitude functions to separate nonspeech from speech (Lamel et al., 1981, Wilpon et al., 1984). For applications where speech bandwidth exceeds 3 kHz, there is sufficient spectral information at high frequencies to refine energy-determined boundaries with simple spectral measures (Rabiner et al., 1979).

In some applications, it is unnecessary to recognize all words uttered; only a few *keywords* need be recognized. A speaker might be allowed unlimited use of words and phrasing, while the system attempts to recognize only certain words from a limited vocabulary, assuming that the spoken message can be deciphered based on the recognition of these keywords. In general, these systems apply word templates for each keyword to each entire test utterance, shifting the test time axis a few frames at a time (Christiansen et al., 1977).

4.7 Dynamic Time Warping (DTW)

In comparing templates, some recognizers use nonlinear warping one in an attempt to synchronize similar acoustic segments in the test and reference templates. This *dynamic time warping* (DTW) combines alignment and distance computation through a dynamic programming procedure (Itakura, 1975, Sakoe et al., 1978). Deviations from a linear frame-by-frame comparison are allowed if the distance for such a frame pair is small compared with other local comparisons. The underlying assumptions of standard DTW are that (a) global variations in speaking rate for someone uttering the same word on different occasions can be handled by linear time normalization; (b) local rate variations within each utterance are small and can be dealt with using distance penalties known as *local continuity constraints*; (c) each frame of the test utterance contributes equally to recognition; and (d) a single distance measure applied uniformly across all frames is adequate. The first two assumptions appear reasonable, but the latter two are less realistic and have led to refinements of the basic DTW method.

Consider two patterns **R** and **T** (as in sect. 4.2) of R and T frames each. DTW finds a warping function $m = w(n)$, which maps the time axis n of **T** into the time axis m of **R**. Frame by frame, DTW searches for the best frame in **R** against which to compare each test frame. The warping curve derives from the solution of an optimization problem

$$D = \min_{w(n)} \left[\sum_{n=1}^{T} d(T(n), R(w(n))) \right], \tag{19}$$

where each d term is a frame distance between the nth test frame and the $w(n)$th reference frame. D is the minimum distance measure corresponding to the "best path" $w(n)$ through a grid of $T \times R$ points (Figs. 20–21).

Theoretically, TR frame distances must be calculated for each template comparison. In practice, local continuity constraints restrict the search space so that typically only about 30% of the matches are performed. This nonetheless leads to a significant increase in computation. Since DTW calculation usually increases as the square of T (compared to calculation proportional to T for a linear path), computation can become very heavy for long templates involving several words at a time. Commercial recognizers tend to use only 8–16 frames/word to minimize computation.

The main drawbacks to DTW include (a) heavy computational load, (b) failure to adequately exploit temporal information to aid recognition, and (c) treatment of durational variations as noise to be eliminated via time normalization.

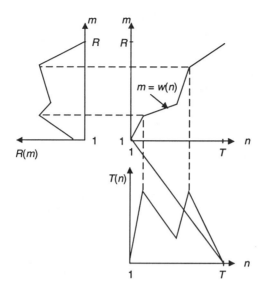

Figure 20: Example of nonlinear time alignment of a test $T(n)$ pattern and reference $R(m)$ pattern. (After Rabiner et al.1978)

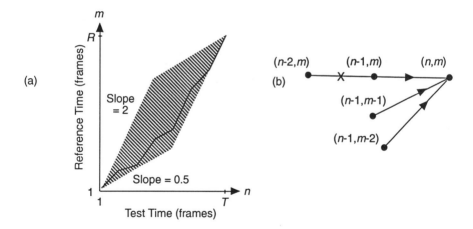

Figure 21: (a) Typical DTW plot, illustrating the optimal warp path $w(n)$ mapping the test time axis n into the reference time axis m. If the template endpoints are forced to match and the warping is restricted to lie within slopes of $^1/_2$ and 2, the shaded area shows the subset of points that is considered. (b) Permitted transitions to the grid point (n,m). Since two horizontal transitions are not allowed, the step marked X is illegal.

Furthermore, the basic form of DTW does not allow distinguishing different parts of an utterance in terms of their information contribution to recognition. For example, in the A–Z vocabulary, consonant identification provides much more information than does vowel identification in determining which of 26 letters was spoken; nonetheless, basic DTW weights all frames of the test template equally, and most frames pertain to vowels since they tend to be longer (Marshall et al., 1983).

4.8 Applying Vector Quantization to ASR

With small vocabularies, the recognizer compares each test template against all reference templates. However, as vocabulary size increases into the thousands of words necessary to handle a general conversation, both memory and the time needed to search it become sufficiently large to warrant more efficient procedures. Vector quantization (VQ), developed primarily to lower the bit rate, provides an alternative to DTW that can reduce computation and indirectly address the temporal problems of DTW. The utility of VQ here lies in the efficiency of using codebook memory for reference templates and codebook searches in place of DTW. In IWR, a separate VQ codebook is usually designed for each vocabulary word, based on a training sequence of several repetitions of the word. Each test template is evaluated by all codebooks, and the word corresponding to the codebook that yields the lowest distance measure is chosen as the recognizer output.

In their simplest form, codebooks have no explicit time information, since the codebook entries are not ordered and can derive from any part of the training words. However, some implicit durational cues are preserved because the codebook entries are chosen to minimize average distance across all training frames, and frames corresponding to longer acoustic segments (e.g., vowels) are more frequent in the training data. Such segments are thus more likely to specify codeword positions than the less frequent consonant frames. Codewords must nonetheless exist for the consonant frames because such frames would otherwise contribute large distances to the codebook. A few codewords often suffice to represent many frames during relatively steady sections of vowels, thus allowing more codewords to represent short, dynamic portions of the words. This relative emphasis that VQ puts on speech transients can be an advantage over DTW for vocabularies of similar words.

4.9 Networks for Speech Recognition

Networks have been used in many ASR systems to represent information about acoustic events in speech (Bahl et al., 1975, Baker, 1975). In continuous speech recognition, knowledge about syntactic and semantic constraints on allowable sequences of words may be efficiently coded in terms of a network whose states are the vocabulary words. Transitions between states are allowed only if the resulting string of words produces a legal sentence following the system's grammar. Networks can be applied to IWR by modeling each word with a set of states linked by likelihood-weighted transitions. The probability of one segment following another weights the transition between the states representing those two sounds. Consider *pass* as a simple example, where states for /p/ closure (silence), /p/ burst, /pæ/ aspiration, /æ/, and /s/ might be selected via coarse segmentation, vector quantization, or some other technique. The transition probabilities between successive stages are normally near unity, but the /p/ burst and/or aspiration may be missing or overlooked in the analysis of some training samples, leading to transitions into the /æ/ state from all three of the earlier states. The transition probabilities typically correspond to the frequency of their occurrence in the training data.

During recognition, the input test utterance is processed by each word network to find the network most likely to have generated the word. Instead of searching a DTW space for a path of minimal distance, each network is searched for the path maximizing the product of all transition probabilities between states corresponding to the test utterance. In practice, log likelihoods are used so that probability values may be summed, instead of multiplied, for faster computation.

The most common network for ASR is the *first-order Markov process* or *chain*, where the likelihood of arriving at a given state depends only on the immediately prior state. To exploit temporal order constraints of speech, only left-to-right transitions are allowed. The networks are sometimes called *hidden Markov models* (HMM) because the models must be inferred through observations of speech outputs, not from any internal representation of speech production. A phone HMM might use three states to represent, in order, an initial transition spectrum from a prior phone, a spectrum from the phone's steady state, and a final transition spectrum to an ensuing phone. To account for variability due to coarticulation, speaking rate, different speakers, etc., each state is represented by a probability density of spectra rather than a fixed spectrum.

4.10 Using Prosodics to Aid Recognition
Despite evidence that F0, duration, and energy convey information in human speech communication, intonation is rarely used in ASR. Other

than including energy as a supplementary parameter to LPC coefficients in template comparisons, most systems assume that spectral cues contain sufficient information for recognition and that prosodic cues are unreliable. Nonetheless, there is clear evidence that performance can be improved by properly exploiting prosodics. Segments of speech corresponding roughly to syllables are more accurately identified if they have the acoustic correlates of stress (longer durations, higher or changing F0, and higher amplitude) (Klatt et al., 1973). If such stressed syllables can be detected, they provide *islands of reliability* in the speech signal, where segmentation and labeling decisions are likely to be more accurate. While most recognizers analyze speech in sequential (left-to-right) order, a hybrid *middle-out* approach can yield superior results at the cost of extra computation: basically proceeding left to right but delaying analysis of unstressed syllables until the next stressed one is found (Klatt, 1977, Waibel, 1986).

Prosodics can also aid in phone identification and in providing syntactic information useful for linguistic postprocessing. The presence and/or identity of consonants is sometimes cued by intonation (Lea, 1980): (a) voiced consonants usually cause a dip in F0 of more than 10%; (b) a 10–20% fall in F0 at the start of a stressed syllable usually indicates the presence of a preceding unvoiced consonant; and (c) relatively long vowels indicate ensuing voiced consonants, etc. Syntactically, an utterance-final F0 rise or a relatively low falloff rate for F0 during the utterance can cue a yes/no question. A syllable identified as stressed is almost always part of a *content word* (e.g., noun, verb, adjective). The primary benefit of intonation, however, appears to lie in identifying major syntactic boundaries: 90% of such boundaries in English are preceded by F0 falls of more than 7% and are followed by rises exceeding 7% (Lea, 1980, pp. 166-205). Parenthetical clauses have even more pronounced (20%) F0 dips.

5.   References

Akers, G., & Lennig, M. (1985). Intonation in text-to-speech synthesis: Evaluation of algorithms. *J. Acoust. Soc. Am.*, *77*, 2157–2165.

Allen, J., Hunnicutt, S., Carlson, R., & Granstrom, B. (1979). MITalk-79: the 1979 MIT text-to-speech system. In J. Wolf & D. Klatt (Eds.), *ASA-50 Speech Communication Papers* (pp. 507–510). New York: Acoustical Society of America.

Atal, B., & Remde, J. (1982). A new model of LPC excitation for producing natural-sounding speech at low bit rates. *Proc. IEEE Int. Conf. ASSP*, 614–617.

Atal, B., & Schroeder, M. (1979). Predictive coding of speech signals and subjective error criteria. *IEEE Trans. ASSP, ASSP-27*, 247–254.

Bahl, L., & Jelinek, F. (1975). Decoding for channels with insertions, deletions, and substitutions with applications to speech recognition. *IEEE Trans. Info. Theory, IT-21*, 404–411.

Baker, J. (1975). The DRAGON system—an overview. *IEEE Trans. ASSP, ASSP-23*, 24–29.

Christiansen, R., & Rushforth, C. (1977). Detecting and locating key words in continuous speech using linear predictive coding. *IEEE Trans. ASSP, ASSP-25*, 361–367.

Crochiere, R. (1977). On the design of sub-band coders for low bit rate speech communication. *Bell Sys. Tech. Journal, 56*, 747–770.

Dunn, H., & White, S. (1940). Statistical measurements on conversational speech. *J. Acoust. Soc. Am., 11*, 278–288.

Elovitz, H. S., Johnson, R., McHugh, A., & Shore, J. E. (1976). Letter-to-Sound Rules for Automatic Translation of English Text to Phonetics. *IEEE Trans. ASSP, ASSP-24*, 446–459.

Flanagan, J., Schroeder, M., Atal, B., Crochiere, R., Jayant, N., & Tribolet, J. (1979). Speech coding. *IEEE Trans. Comm., COM-27*, 710–736.

Fujimura, O., & Lovins, J. (1978). Syllables as concatenative phonetic units. In A. Bell & J. Hooper (Eds.), *Syllables and Segments* (pp. 107–120). Amsterdam: North Holland.

Gibson, J. (1982). Adaptive prediction in speech differential encoding systems. *Proc. IEEE, 68*, 488–525.

Gray, R. (1984). Vector quantization. *IEEE ASSP Magazine, 1*, 4–29.

Gupta, V., Lennin, M., & Mermelstein, P. (1984). Decision rules for speaker-independent isolated word recognition. *Proc. IEEE Int. Conf. ASSP*, 9.2.1–4.

Haggard, M. (1979). Experience and Perspectives in Articulatory Synthesis. In B. Lindblom & S. Ohman (Eds.), *Frontiers of Speech Communication Research* (pp. 259–274). London: Academic.

Hess, W. (1983). *Pitch Determination of Speech Signals: Algorithms and Devices.* Berlin: Springer-Verlag.

Holmes, J. (1983). Formant synthesizers—cascade or parallel? *Speech Comm.*, 2, 251–273.

Hunnicut, S. (1980). Grapheme-to-phoneme rules: A review. *Royal Inst. Tech., Stockholm, STL-QPR*, 2–3, 38–60.

Itakura, F. (1975). Minimum prediction residual principle applied to speech recognition. *IEEE Trans. ASSP, ASSP-23*, 67–72.

Klatt, D. (1977). Review of the ARPA speech understanding project. *J. Acoust. Soc. Am.*, 62, 1345–1366.

Klatt, D. (1980). Software for a cascade/parallel formant synthesizer. *J. Acoust. Soc. Am.*, 67, 971–995.

Klatt, D., & Stevens, K. (1973). On the automatic recognition of continuous speech: Implications from a spectrogram-reading experiment. *IEEE Trans. Audio & Electroac., AU-21*, 210–217.

Kopec, G. (1986). A family of formant trackers based on hidden Markov models. *Proc. IEEE Int. Conf. ASSP*, 1225–1228.

Lamel, L., Rabiner, L., Rosenberg, A., & Wilpon, J. (1981). An improved endpoint detector for isolated word recognition. *IEEE Trans. ASSP, ASSP-29*, 777–785.

Lea, W. (1980). Prosodic aids to speech recognition. In W. Lea (Ed), *Trends in Speech Recognition* (pp. 166–205). Englewood Cliffs, NJ: Prentice-Hall.

Levinson, S. (1985). Structural methods in automatic speech recognition. *Proc. IEEE*, 73, 1625–1650.

McCandless, S. (1974). An algorithm for automatic formant extraction using linear prediction spectra. *IEEE Trans. ASSP, ASSP-22*, 135–141.

Markel, J., & Gray, A. (1976). *Linear Prediction of Speech*. New York: Springer-Verlag.

Marshall, C., & Nye, P. (1983). Stress and vowel duration effects of syllable recognition. *J. Acoust. Soc. Am.*, 74, 433–443.

O'Shaughnessy, D. (1977). Fundamental frequency by rule for a text-to-speech system. *Proc. IEEE Int. Conf. ASSP*, 571–574.

O'Shaughnessy, D. (1987). *Speech Communication: Human and Machine*. Reading, MA: Addison-Wesley.

Rabiner, L., Rosenberg, A., & Levinson, S. (1978). Considerations in dynamic time warping algorithms for discrete word recognition. *IEEE Trans. ASSP, ASSP-26,* 575–582.

Rabiner, L., & Schafer, R. (1979). *Digital Processing of Speech Signals.* Englewood Cliffs, NJ: Prentice-Hall.

Sakoe, H., & Chiba, S. (1978). Dynamic programming algorithm optimization for spoken word recognition. *IEEE Trans. ASSP, ASSP-26,* 43–49.

Shadle, C. & Atal, B. (1979). Speech synthesis by linear interpolation of spectral parameters between dyad boundaries. *J. Acoust. Soc. Am., 66,* 1325–1332.

Turner, J. (1985). Recursive least-squares estimation and lattice filters. In Cowan & Grant (Eds.), *Adaptive Filters* (pp. 91–134). Englewood Cliffs, NJ: Prentice-Hall.

Viswanathan, V., Makhour, J., Schwartz, R., & Huggins, A. (1982). Variable frame rate transmission: A review of methodology and application to narrow-band LPC speech coding. *IEEE Trans. Comm., COM-30,* 674–686.

Waibel, A. (1986). Recognition of lexical stress in a continuous speech understanding system: A pattern recognition approach. *Proc. IEEE Int. Conf. ASSP,* 2287–2290.

Wakita, H. (1979). Estimation of vocal-tract shapes from acoustical analysis of the speech wave: the state of the art. *IEEE Trans. ASSP, ASSP-27,* 281–285.

Wilpon, J., Rabiner, L., & Martin, T. (1984). An improved word-detection algorithm for telephone-quality speech incorporating both syntactic and semantic constraints. *AT&T Bell Labs Tech. J., 63,* 479–497.

Young, S., & Fallside, F. (1980). Synthesis by rule of prosodic features in Word Concatenation Synthesis. *Int. J. Man-Machine Studies, 12,* 241–258.

Chapter 3

Text-to-Speech Systems

Ann K. Syrdal
AT&T Bell Laboratories

1. Introduction

Text-to-speech (TTS) technology, the automatic conversion of stored text to synthetic speech, has progressed due in part to extensive theoretical and empirical contributions from the behavioral sciences. Human factors specialists also play an important role in determining applications appropriate for TTS technology and in further tailoring the technology for a targeted application.

1.1 Applications of TTS

Text-to-speech technology permits communication from computer to human through the natural human communication modality of speech. Terminal-based applications of TTS technology include talking terminals and training devices, proofreading, warning and alarm systems, talking aids for the hearing-impaired and vocally handicapped, and reading aids for the blind. Audiotext services allow users to retrieve information from public or private databases using a telephone as a terminal. The information may include names and addresses from a telephone directory, financial accounts, stock quotations, weather reports, reservations, sales orders and inventory information, or locations of commercial dealers. While some of this information could be provided using stored human speech, TTS systems are appropriate when services access a large or frequently changing database. TTS reduces storage needs from 64 Kb per second for stored telephone bandpass quality speech to a few hundred bits for an equivalent text sentence. Maintaining the database is also simplified, since only the textual data need be updated. Targeting commercial applications of TTS often involves applied research into improving the technology to solve anticipated shortcomings and user interface problems for a specific application.

1.2   Stages of Text-to-Speech Conversion

TTS is probably the speech technology that has involved the most diverse interdisciplinary efforts, and in which behavioral scientists have had the greatest impact thus far. Contributions from the areas of speech production, speech perception, linguistics, and psycholinguistics are incorporated in many of the stages involved in text-to-speech conversion. This chapter will describe the stages of text-to-speech conversion, with a focus on areas in which behavioral scientists have made contributions and on human factors issues and solutions.

The basic steps in the conversion of text to speech are illustrated in Figure 1. These stages include:

- **Text normalization.** input text is normalized in order to distinguish sentence boundaries from abbreviations, expand conventional abbreviations (e.g., St. -> *Saint or Street*), and translate nonalphabetic characters into pronounceable form (e.g., $1234.56 -> *one thousand two hundred thirty four dollars and fifty six cents*).

- **Syntactic parsing.** the syntactic structure of the sentence (e.g. identification of the part of speech of each word — noun, verb, adjective, etc.) is determined by syntactic analysis.

- **Word pronunciation.** with the use of a dictionary and letter-to-sound rules, orthographic characters are mapped into the appropriate strings of phonemes (e.g. the orthographic string gh is translated to the phoneme /f/ in *tough*, to the phoneme /g/ in *ghost*, and is silent in *though*) and their associated lexical stress markers (e.g. record has primary stress on the first syllable if it's a noun, but on the second syllable if it's a verb).

- **Determination of prosody.** Assigning the timing pattern and pitch pattern is necessary for an intelligible and natural-sounding utterance.

- **Speech synthesis.** Phonetic information is transformed into an acoustic structure that results in an audible utterance.

No current text-to-speech system uses an explicit stage of semantic representation, although knowledge about the world may be built into heuristic rules at various stages, such as in the rudimentary sense of probabilities of occurrence. Semantic analysis *per se* plays no role in determining what an abbreviation stands for, how a syntactically ambiguous sentence should be parsed, how a word should be pronounced, or what would be the most appropriate intonation with which to convey the intended meaning of a sentence. In other words, although a TTS system can synthesize any arbitrary utterance in English, it does not "understand" the meaning of what it is saying. Although there are many ways in which a semantic analysis stage would improve TTS conversion, it is beyond the scope of current theory and technology. However, work in text analysis and examination of natural speech databases is beginning to provide discourse information that has been used to construct rules which vary prominence and intonational phrasing in an experimental TTS system (Hirschberg, 1990).

2. Overview of TTS Technology and Behavioral Science Contributions to TTS Technology

2.1 Text normalization

There are many abbreviations, acronyms, nonalphabetic characters, punctuation, and digit strings in unrestricted text. Periods may indicate an abbreviation or the end of a sentence, and must be disambiguated. Many common abbreviations are expanded differently depending on the context. For example, *Dr.* may be expanded as *Doctor* in phrases such as *"Dr. Martin Luther King"* and as *Drive* in phrases such as *"Martin Luther King Dr."*. Other common ambiguous examples are *St.* as an abbreviation for both *Saint* and *Street*, and *N.* as an abbreviation for either *North*, *New*, or the letter *N* when used as an initial. Similarly, common punctuation characters and numbers may be expanded differently, depending upon context: 1/2, for example, may be expanded as *one-half* in some contexts, and as *January second* in others. Such departures from full word equivalents are difficult for TTS systems, which do not have access to semantic information as does the human reader. Syntactic information may be useful in text normalization, but cannot disambiguate all texts. In addition, ASCII text frequently contains embedded escape sequences and other nonalphabetic characters that are not intended to be part of the textual message.

There are two general ways existing TTS systems have dealt with the problems of text normalization. Some systems employ different modes of operation for different types of textual material, which must be determined and set by the user. In some commercial systems the user can set logical switches to determine how various types of nonalphabetic strings are handled. For example, a specialized address normalization mode can be specified by the user whenever a particular field used for addresses is encountered in a database. Another general strategy is to spell out all words that contain nonalphabetic characters, assuming that there is no general solution to the inherent ambiguities of such material. TTS systems may also choose to rely on the host computer to pre-process the material used in its application so that text normalization problems are minimized. In applications in which the input text is from a database with a name field, an address field, and a telephone number field, for example, either the input text could be pre-processed by the host computer to correctly expand abbreviations used in that field and handle other problematic input (which will be more or less successful depending upon the skill of the applications programmers), or the appropriate operational modes of the TTS system could be set in advance by the user for each type of field. Such a solution translates semantic information represented by the different types of database fields to its appropriate text normalization mode, although this translation is performed by the user. A general solution to automatic text normalization is unlikely until TTS systems evolve to handle semantic representation.

2.2   Syntactic Parsing

Syntactic analysis is important for word pronunciation and as one of several components in the determination of prosody. At least a partial syntactic analysis is also important for text normalization. A fairly large class of common English words can be either nouns or verbs (including *record*, *permit*, and *object*) in which the first syllable is stressed for a noun, and the second syllable is stressed for a verb. In order to pronounce these words correctly, the syntactic structure of the input sentence must be determined. Both durational and intonational aspects of prosody are also affected by syntactic structure. Content words (nouns, adjectives, and verbs) generally receive intonational accents, while function words (articles, prepositions, and conjunctions) generally do not. This affects both segment durations and intonation contours. Words such as *like* may be either verbs or prepositions (e.g. *I like green vegetables like spinach.*), and a syntactic analysis is necessary for appropriate prosody. Natural prosodic phrasing depends on locating syntactic phrase boundaries, particularly in sentences with long clauses. Inappropriate prosodic phrasing can result in impaired sentence comprehension (see chapter 6). In text normalization, the correct interpretation or expansion of non-word input may depend upon syntactic context of a standard or specialized type (e.g. the syntax of addresses or telephone numbers).

Syntactic analysis for text-to-speech conversion involves both the generation of possible syntactic parsings for a sentence and the determination of the most probable parsing of the sentence from among the syntactically correct alternatives of a syntactically ambiguous sentence. An example of a syntactically ambiguous sentence is: *Union protests rock cities*, in which either *protests* or *rock* may function as a verb in the sentence. Ideally, syntactic parsing involves not only decisions about syntactic structure, but some knowledge of the world. Since semantic interpretation is not sufficiently developed, knowledge of the world is included in the form of heuristic procedures that utilize probabilities of occurrence. One strategy that was first used successfully in MITalk (an experimental TTS system developed at MIT) involves morphemic decomposition (described in the discussion below on dictionaries) in order to specify information about possible parts of speech of input words for use by the syntactic analyzer. The parser proceded from left to right with the goal of creating the longest possible phrasal constituents, and assigned syntactic categories to sytactically ambiguous words accordingly. This approach would parse correctly our ambiguous sentence, preferring the longer possible noun phrase *Union protests* to the shorter one, *Union*. A simpler strategy adopted by most TTS systems is to use function words to locate phrase boundaries, although this method is insufficient to predict all boundaries. Another simple strategy is to detect verb phrases through a dictionary of unambiguous verbs, although verb phrases that begin with ambiguous verbs are not located. No real-time TTS system has yet incorporated a broad coverage parser, although fuller syntactic information has been provided by experimental interfaces to TTS systems, resulting in more natural-sounding phrasing. Some TTS systems allow the user to add escape sequences to the text to indicate the appropriate part of speech of an input word, which is a useful option for instances of hard-to-resolve syntactic ambiguities.

2.3 Word Pronunciation

The correct pronunciation of words, which involves appropriate phoneme selection and lexical stress assignment, is critical to the intelligibility and acceptability of a text-to-speech system. English orthography is frequently related in a less-than-straightforward way to pronunciation. Pronounciation habits have evolved considerably over time while spelling has remained more stable, and because there are many borrowings from French, Latin, Greek, and other languages. Consequently, letter-to-sound rules cannot yield accurate phonemic transcriptions for a sizable proportion of the words encountered in English text. Many common words are exceptions to the general rules of pronunciation, and their correct pronunciation can only be ensured by including them in an exceptions dictionary. Many of the approaches to word pronunciation used by TTS systems are based on linguistic theory and on psychological studies of strategies humans use to pronounce novel words.

2.3.1   Letter-to-Sound Rules

Letter-to-sound rules predict word pronunciation strictly from orthography. A set of conversion rules is devised assuming there are general correspondences between an alphabetic character or pair of characters in the spelled word and the phonemes in its pronunciation. These correspondences may vary depending upon the neighboring letters in the word, which can be handled by context-sensitive rules (e.g. the well-known "silent e" rule which changes the pronunciation of the preceding vowel from a "short" vowel to a "long" vowel, as in *mad* and *made*). The simplest of these rules are like those frequently taught to young children learning to read. Complex letter-to-sound rule systems contain hundreds of ordered rules (Ainsworth, 1973; McIlroy, 1974; Hunnicutt, 1976; Elovitz, Johnson, McHugh, and Shore, 1976; Carlson and Granstrom, 1976). Attempts have been made to achieve letter-to-sound conversion by using neural nets, statistical learning strategies that try to model some characteristics of a network of neurons, but this approach has been considerably less successful to date than traditional rule sets. Using a self-organizing/connectionist system, Sejnowski and Rosenberg (1987) report letter performance of 80-90%, which corresponds to word accuracy of only 25-50%, assuming 6 letters per word (see Klatt, 1987, for a comparison and discussion of these approaches).

Some of the problems encountered by letter-to-sound rules are that the pronunciation of vowels often depends upon the lexical stress pattern of the word (e.g. *photograph* and *photography*), and that the correct handling of a word depends upon its morphemic structure (e.g. *hothead*, in which the *th* pair does not represent its usual single phoneme). Conversion problems are exacerbated when the pronunciation of proper names is considered, because of the many different languages of origin represented by American surnames. Using American English letter-to-sound rules on non-English surnames often results in very unsatisfactory pronunciations of even common American surnames. Since many applications of TTS involve the pronunciation of proper names, this is a critical problem. Church (1985) developed a two-stage approach to the pronunciation of proper names that first categorizes the probable language family of the name on the basis of the frequency of occurrences of its three-letter sequences in each of many languages. Once the probable language of origin is determined, letter-to-sound and stress rules appropriate for that language are applied.

Stress assignment rules are an important constituent of TTS systems. Incorrect lexical stress assignment is disruptive to the listener because the stress pattern (which affects several acoustic dimensions) is a salient feature in the recognition of a word. Incorrect stress is further disruptive to speech generated by rule because it may cause the mispronunciation of vowels. Stress assignment rules are generally modeled after linguistic theories (Chomsky and Halle, 1968; Halle and Keyser, 1971; Hill and Nessly, 1973; Liberman and Prince, 1977; Hayes, 1980) which predict lexical stress on the basis of general rules that vary considerably in their complexity. Some complex stress rules base stress assignments on the classification of syllables into "heavy" or "light" weight categories depending on vowel length and number of post-vocalic consonants, and on contextual constraints, syntactic category, morphological structure, and etymology (see Church, 1985). Some simpler stress rules base stress assignment on only the number of syllables and basic syllabic structure. Lexical stress prediction is sometimes performed before, and sometimes after, phoneme prediction. Since stress assignment is often important in determining vowel pronunciation, there is an advantage to its being done before the final stage of phoneme prediction. Stress rules may also differ in whether the rules operate backwards or forwards through the letters of the word, although there appears to be an advantage to working backwards because of the many suffixes which determine the stress assignment of preceding syllables.

Letter-to-sound rule systems vary in accuracy. Bernstein and Nessly (1981) evaluated two good 400-rule sets for phonemic accuracy of whole words, using a set of 865 words selected to systematically represent a word frequency range from the 400th most frequent word to the 43, 650th most frequent word in the Brown Corpus (Kucera and Francis, 1967). Both rule sets made phonemic prediction errors in about 25% of the test words. Since about 15% of the words were incorrectly phonemicized by both rule sets, it was proposed that an optimal rule system might achieve 85% phonemic word accuracy. Bernstein and Nessly also estimated that stress assignment was correct in about 75% of the test words for each of two very different algorithms evaluated. Groner, Bernstein, Ingber, Perlman, and Toal (1982) reported 85% accuracy for correct phoneme and stress assignment of whole words using Bernstein's rules without access to an exceptions dictionary. Word accuracy of 85% translates to a phonemic accuracy of over 97%, since there are on average 6 or 7 phonemes in a word, and the probability of correct stress assignment of the segments within a word must be considered also.

2.3.2 Dictionaries

The dictionary approach to word pronunciation is needed for words that don't follow regular rules of English pronunciation or stress assignment. Its disadvantage is that it fails for unknown words, which is why most TTS systems use both a dictionary and letter-to-sound rules. TTS systems use dictionaries of varying sizes, depending on storage constraints and on the accuracy of the letter-to-sound rules used. The dictionary size required to attain a certain level of accuracy depends on letter-to-sound rule performance (Hunnicutt, 1980). If letter-to-sound rules are weak, a larger dictionary is needed to cover its deficiencies. There is a point of diminishing returns in dictionary size, when adding more low-frequency entries will not appreciably improve accuracy. Only about 200 words account for half the words occurring in a typical text, 1,000 words account for almost 70%, but 50,000 words, the size of a typical college dictionary, only account for about 93%. (Hunnicutt, 1980). It is impossible to enumerate all the words that can occur in English, particularly when proper nouns are considered. There have been several attempts to make exception dictionaries more efficient by increasing dictionary coverage with a minimum number of entries. Two such efforts are morphemic decomposition and pronunciation by analogy.

Morphemic decomposition involves dictionary entries of morphemes, the minimal meaningful units of language. Morphemes may be words themselves and are frequently combined to form words, either by adding affixes (e.g. *degradation* -> *de* + *grade* + *ation*) or by combining two free morphemes to create a compound word (e.g. *hothouse* -> *hot* + *house*). The advantages of breaking down a word into its constituent morphemes are broader vocabulary coverage from a set of dictionary entries, and specification of syntactic part of speech information about a word. However, it also requires rules for handling common problems of morphemic decomposition. For example, deletions (*hiking* -> *hike* + *ing*), duplications (*hitting* -> *hit* + *ing*), and modifications (*puppies* -> *puppy* + *s*) of the surface form commonly occur, and must be handled by rules (Lee, 1969). Heuristic rules have also been developed to disambiguate alternative parses of a word (e.g. *scarcity* -> *scarce* + *ity* / *scar* + *city*) depending for example, on frequencies of occurrence of different types of morphemic decomposition (Allen, Hunnicutt, Carlson, and Granstrom, 1979; Coker, 1985; Allen, Hunnicutt, and Klatt, 1987).

Pronunciation by analogy is another approach to increasing the coverage of a limited number of dictionary entries. Pronunciation by analogy was suggested by psychological research showing that humans use analogous known words to pronounce unfamiliar words (Glushko, 1981; Dedina and Nusbaum, 1986). In the analogy approach, the pronunciation of a novel word is predicted by one or more similar words whose pronunciations are known. A major difficulty is devising a similarity metric. One simple solution is to base the degree of similarity on the number of shared letters between the known and unknown words. The frequency of occurrence of analogous known words has also been used in determining the pronunciation of novel words (Dedina and Nusbaum, 1986). Breaking words into substrings larger than characters, such as bigrams and trigrams or syllabic onsets and rhymes, may aid in defining similarity for the purposes of pronunciation by analogy.

Coker, Church, and Liberman (1990) describe how development of morphological and rhyming analogy approaches to dictionary-based word pronunciation in the experimental AT&T Bell Laboratories TTS system have blurred the distinction between traditional letter-to-sound rules and dictionary-based methods. The rhyme analogy method, for example, uses both dictionary look-up to determine the pronunciation of the rhyming portion of the word and letter-to-sound rules to pronounce the novel consonant onset portion of the word. This hybrid approach to word pronunciation provides much greater dictionary coverage than traditional dictionary methods and is far more reliable than traditional letter-to-sound rules.

2.3.3 Subjective Evaluation of Pronunciation Accuracy

Bernstein and Nessly (1981) proposed a metric of Average Words Between Errors (AWBE) as an appropriate measure of people's subjective impression of the pronunciation accuracy of a TTS system. However I am not aware of any research systematically relating this metric to listeners' subjective judgments. Thus, a hypothetical TTS system which achieved 95% accuracy in word pronunciation would translate into an AWBE of 20; i.e. the system would produce a noticeable phoneme or stress error in one word out of 20, on the average. Systems with 93% accuracy and 97% accuracy would result in AWBE measures of about 14 and 33, respectively.

Wisowaty (personal communication) has developed two procedures to evaluate TTS pronunciation of proper names. In one test procedure, naive listeners hear a series of pairings of common American first and last names, and write the name as they hear it. High listener agreement about the correct pronunciation of the common test names can be assumed, so that errors must primarily reflect either errors in TTS-predicted pronunciation (*i.e.* the wrong phoneme or lexical stress was assigned by TTS pronunciation procedures) or poor segmental intelligibility (*i.e.* the correctly assigned phoneme and stress were poorly articulated by the synthesizer). In the second test procedure, naive listeners hear a series of surnames that vary systematically in frequency of occurrence from high- to low-frequency names. Listeners are given a printed list of the names they are presented, and are asked to indicate whether the name they hear is pronounced the same way they would pronounce it, is differently but acceptably pronounced, or is unacceptably pronounced. Wisowaty compared the results of different TTS systems with the results from human speakers. Together, these two evaluations have proved useful in determining the acceptability of TTS name pronunciation.

2.4   Determination of Prosody

Prosody refers to the *way* in which something is said, rather than what words are spoken. Intonation (pitch contours), timing, and intensity are aspects of prosody that affect the sensations of pitch, length, and loudness. Appropriate prosody is very important for a sentence to sound intelligible and natural. Prosody conveys both linguistic information and extra-linguistic information about the speaker's attitude, intentions, and physical and emotional state.

From a linguistic point of view, prosody involves both segmental structure and structural units larger than phonetic segments, termed "suprasegmentals." There are local perturbations of intonation, timing, and intensity due to particular vowels and consonants, and there are more global underlying prosodic patterns that result from the suprasegmental structure of the utterance, *e.g.* morpheme, word, phrase, sentence, and even larger units of discourse such as paragraphs.

The prosodic elements of speech have only recently become a major focus of attention. Previous research focused almost exclusively on the segmental structure of speech because of its principal role in carrying the information conveyed by the speech signal. However, the importance of prosodic structure in both the intelligibility and naturalness of speech became evident with the introduction of speech synthesis-by-rule systems. The poor quality of early rule-generated sentences and phrases highlighted the need for quantitative models of prosodic structure. In addition, the technology for studying the acoustic phenomena associated with prosody became available only relatively recently.

2.4.1 Intonation

In text-to-speech systems, the goal of the intonation component is to generate an appropriate intonation contour for each spoken phrase. An intonation contour is the underlying fundamental frequency (F0) pattern that occurs over time in speech phrases. Physiologically, F0 corresponds to the frequency at which the vocal folds are vibrating. Acoustically, this vocal fold vibration provides the energy source that excites the vocal tract resonances during voiced portions of speech (see Chapter 1). Listeners perceive an intonation contour as a pitch pattern that rises and falls at different points in a phrase. The intonation contour emphasizes certain words more than others, and distinguishes statements (with falling intonation contours) from yes/no questions (with rising intonation contours). It also conveys information about syntactic structure, discourse structure, and the speaker's attitude. Behavioral scientists have been instrumental in basic research demonstrating the importance of intonation in the perception and production of speech, and in developing and evaluating intonation algorithms.

Some of the simpler commercial TTS systems do not tailor an intonation contour to each sentence that is synthesized. They either use a monotone with a falling pitch at the end of the sentence, or they synthesize a sentence like a list of words, treating each word like a declarative sentence in which pitch first rises and then falls at the end of the word. Either of these treatments is highly unnatural and can be tedious and confusing to the listener.

The better TTS systems generate an intonation contour that is tailored for each sentence. Intonation rules used in TTS systems generate overall patterns of pitch contours. F0 typically declines gradually over the course of a phrase, although there are several local peaks and valleys superimposed on the general pattern of F0 declination. Intonation contours are frequently used to distinguish between different types of sentences. A final rising intonation contour is generated for yes/no questions (*e.g.* "*Do you want to play a game?*"). A final falling contour is generated for statements (*e.g.* "*I like to play chess.*") and for questions that cannot be answered by yes or no (e.g. "*What game do you want to play?*"). A continuation falling-rising contour is generated between two clauses within a sentence (*"I like to play chess, but he prefers checkers."*).

The intonation pattern generated also depends in part upon the syntactic function of words used in the sentence. Typically, content words like nouns, verbs, and adjectives are assigned stress that is associated with rising (or sometimes with falling) pitch accents. These accents account for many of the local peaks and valleys in an F0 contour. Function words like articles and prepositions are typically unstressed, and do not receive pitch accents. For example, in the following sentence the upper-case content words are accented, and the lower-case words are not: "The OLD MAN SAT in a ROCKER." Some intonation algorithms employ a detailed part-of-speech hierarchy to determine pitch accent levels; for example, nouns are given higher prominence than verbs. Other algorithms employ simpler heuristics to assign alternately higher or lower prominence to content words regardless of grammatical category. Algorithms also vary in their placement of pitch accents in time. Generally, the accent peak is placed within the accented vowel, but the exact placement varies among algorithms and may vary within an intonation algorithm depending on phonetic and phonological context.

Phonetic structure influences fundamental frequency by causing local segmental perturbations. For example, in acoustic measurements of human speech, F0 is typically higher near voiceless consonants (e.g. [p],[t],[k]) than near voiced consonants (e.g. [b],[d],[g]), and F0 is typically higher for "high" vowels such as [i] and [u] than for "low" vowels such as [ae] and [a], although the strength of this effect depends upon phonological context. Such effects have been modeled in "micromelody" intonation rules for TTS synthesis, but most TTS systems do not use such detailed algorithms. There is, however, perceptual evidence that segmental effects can enhance the intelligibility and naturalness of synthetic speech (see Silverman, 1987).

Units larger than a phrase or sentence also influence intonation. Semantic factors and the structure of discourse affect intonation in systematic ways. When new information is introduced, it tends to receive intonational emphasis, but in repeated occurrences, the effects on F0 are reduced. This effect is exemplified in the following sentences, in which the upper-case words are accented, and the lower-case words are de-accented: "At the TOP of the MENU are TWO BUTTONS. The LEFT button is USER-DEFINED." The structure of discourse (longer passages of connected speech involving several sentences) affects intonation as well. Speakers tend to raise their F0 range at the beginning of a paragraph, and to lower F0 range near the paragraph end. Discourse-level intonational variations are used by speakers and listeners to organize discourse into paragraph units that each focus on a topic. Discourse-level changes in intonational range should not be neglected because they can affect the comprehension and interpretation of spoken messages (Silverman, 1987).

Intonation is also commonly used by speakers to indicate their attitude about what is being said. For example, a rise-fall-rise F0 pattern is typically interpreted as expressing a discrepancy between what is being said and beliefs about the current reality. Most speakers would use a rise-fall-rise intonation contour when saying "Evelyn knows the answer," when they intend to convey that Evelyn, in contrast to the listener or another person being discussed, does know the answer. The message implied by the rise-fall-rise intonation in the previous sentence is "so why don't you?". Inappropriate TTS intonation can unintentionally convey rudeness to listeners. For example, a standard neutral declarative intonation pattern for the phrase "Good-bye" in a TTS-synthesized announcement can sound very abrupt and rude. For reasons such as this, it is advantageous for a TTS system to have a flexible, user-modifiable intonation system. Since the author's intentions are often ambiguous (even to the human reader, who has access to sophisticated semantic interpretation), the appropriate goal of TTS automated intonation is an intentionally neutral, syntactico-semantically informed intonation.

There are several types of quantitative intonation models used in text-to-speech synthesis. They differ in naturalness and flexibility, as well as in ease of implementation and in underlying phonological theories on which they are based. A discussion of implementation and theoretical linguistic issues involving intonation models is beyond the scope of the present chapter. Issues of naturalness and flexibility, however, will be briefly discussed.

A diagnostic evaluation of the naturalness of a TTS intonation algorithm is ideally performed in a series of perceptual experiments, each one testing a specific effect or aspect of the algorithm, while keeping all other parameters equal. For examples of these kinds of evaluations, see Silverman (1987). Perceptual preference judgments comparing one entire intonation system to another should be conducted within the framework of a single TTS system that is identical in all other respects. For an example of this type of evaluation, see Akers and Lennig (1985). Either of these types of evaluations can be quite difficult in practice, however, because many intonation algorithms are proprietary. Furthermore, they frequently cannot be easily moved from one TTS system to another for evaluation purposes, because different intonation algorithms require different levels or types of input from other components of the TTS system. A perceptual comparison of intonation as used by TTS systems that differ by more than their intonation algorithms is so confounded by uncontrolled variables that no valid conclusions about intonation *per se* can be reached. However since intonation interacts with other aspects of prosody, as will be discussed below, there may be some advantages to comparing entire prosodic systems.

2.4.2   Segmental Durations

Speech timing is an important aspect of prosody, and affects both intelligibility and naturalness. Text-to-speech systems typically use duration rules to determine a target duration for each phonetic segment in an utterance. There are basically four types of effects that duration rules model: the inherent durations of various phonemes, the effects of syntactic, phonological, and phonetic contexts on durations, non-linguistic factors such as speaking rate that affect segment duration, and the interactions of these factors. Duration rules may vary in complexity from system to system. For example, the simplest systems may use only inherent durations to determine segment target durations, without modeling even major contextual effects.

There are very large differences in the inherent durations of different phonetic segments. For example, Klatt (1979) lists the inherent duration of a flapped /t/ (as in *butter*) as 20 ms, and the inherent duration of the diphthong /ɔ' / (as in *boy*) as 280 ms, a 14-fold increase. Vowels in general have longer inherent durations than consonants (see Chapter 1), and there is a great deal of systematic variation within each of these categories as well. For instance, tense vowels (as in beet) and diphthongs (as in *bait*) have longer inherent durations than lax vowels (as in *bit* and *bet*), and open vowels (as in *bat*) have longer inherent durations than closed vowels (as in *boot*).

There are numerous contextual effects on segment durations. Syntactic boundaries (*e.g.* the ends of sentences, phrases, and clauses), phonological markers (*e.g.* stress and accent assignment and phonological phrasing), and phonetic context (e.g. preceding and following segments) all have substantial influences on segment durations. It is well known, for example, that segments immediately preceding a phrase boundary are lengthened, that stressed vowels are lengthened, and that vowels preceding a voiced stop are lengthened. There are many other such contextual effects that have been reported in acoustic-phonetic studies of natural speech.

Speaking rate has the obvious effect of shortening segment durations for faster rates, and lengthening durations for slower rates. However, there are spectral as well as temporal effects of speaking rate (Lindblom, 1963; Gopal and Syrdal, 1988), that some segments are affected by rate much more than others (Picheny, 1981; Picheny et al., 1986; Uchanski, 1988), phonological modifications may co-occur with changes in speaking rate, and the occurrence, location, and duration of pauses in connected speech are strongly affected by speaking rate (Goldman-Eisler, 1968).

Rule systems that model the numerous effects on duration must also model their interactions. Duration rules generally use either additive, multiplicative, or incompressible (a combination of multiplicative and additive rules developed by Klatt, 1979) models of the interaction of factors affecting duration. Which model best fits observed speech data is a current topic of research interest. The implementation of efficient duration rule algorithms is also a practical problem for developers of real-time text-to-speech systems.

Several evaluations of text-to-speech duration rule systems have been reported. Carlson, Granstrom, and Klatt (1979) performed a quantitative study of the importance of different specifications of durational structure on both naturalness and intelligibility within the context of one TTS system. Their results indicated, among other things, that accurate vowel duration is more important than accurate consonant duration, that phrase-final lengthening is important for both naturalness and intelligibility, and that durations generated by complex duration rules were both significantly more intelligible and more natural sounding than those generated by simple rules. The results strongly confirmed the importance of segment duration to sentence perception. Syrdal (1989) compared listener preference for durations generated for an experimental AT&T Bell Laboratories' TTS system by two complex sets of duration rules, one modeling interactions as primarily additive, the other modeling interactions as primarily incompressible. Results indicated that the incompressible rules were preferred to the additive rules, and that they also more closely approximated durations measured in natural speech. Furthermore, listeners also slightly preferred the incompressible rule-generated durations over durations obtained from natural speech. Interestingly, "goodness of fit" measures (i.e. comparisons of rule-generated durations with durations obtained from natural speech) did not reliably predict perceptual preference or judgments of naturalness obtained from listeners in either of the two studies. This may be due in part to interactions between duration and other aspects of the TTS systems, such as intonation and other acoustic characteristics of the segments. The fact that physical distance was not a reliable predictor of perceptual distance in either study, however, underscores the importance of perceptual testing in evaluating text-to-speech algorithms and systems.

2.4.3   Intensity

Intensity is the least important of the components of prosody, and is not modeled per se in most text-to-speech systems. Although intensity was initially believed to be a primary acoustic cue to the perception of stress, perceptual and acoustic studies have consistently shown that it is secondary to duration and F0 (Fry, 1955; Fry, 1958; Lehiste and Peterson, 1959). Intensity increases with F0, vowel height, laryngeal state, and other factors associated with stress. Intensity typically becomes weaker near the end of an utterance, but again this appears to be a secondary effect of changing voice source characteristics. The dynamic changes in voice source that occur within an utterance are a current topic of research, and it is anticipated that such effects eventually will be modeled in text-to-speech systems. These additional prosodic rules should further improve the naturalness of speech synthesized by rule.

2.5   Speech Synthesis

Synthesis involves the transformation of the linguistic message from a visual modality (phonetic symbols) to an auditory modality (an acoustic signal). Text-to-speech systems achieve this phonetic to acoustic conversion in several ways.

Formant-based synthesis uses heuristic acoustic-domain rules to control a formant synthesizer. The rule-generated acoustic parameters are updated every 5 to 10 ms, and include formant frequencies and bandwidths, fundamental frequency, source specification and parameters, etc. Research in acoustic phonetics and speech perception has identified perceptually salient acoustic features that are reliably associated with specific phonetic segments. These findings are useful for all types of TTS systems, but particularly for formant-based synthesis, because of its knowledge-based approach. Advantages of formant-based synthesis are its flexibility, its ability to generate smooth transitions between segments, and its relatively small storage requirements. The major disadvantage is the difficulty of specifying sufficiently detailed rules to synthesize acoustically rich and redundant, robust segments, especially consonants. Many experimental and commercially available TTS systems, including MITalk, Klattalk, DECtalk[1], CallText 5050[2], Infovox[3], Votrax[4] and others use formant-based synthesis.

Concatenative synthesis uses an inventory of pieces of natural speech as building blocks from which any arbitrary utterance may be constructed. The size of these inventory units is limited by various constraints. Whole words as units are impractical because there are too many English words to store and access readily, and coarticulation and phonetic recoding at word boundaries could not be provided for, resulting in highly unnatural connected speech. The syllable is another impractical option; there are over 10,000 different syllables in English — fewer than the number of words, but still too large an inventory for TTS purposes — and there is the problem of syllable boundary coarticulation. At the other end of the spectrum of possible units is the phoneme itself, of which there are only about 40 in English. While the size of a phoneme inventory would be easily manageable, the large coarticulatory effects between adjacent phonemes make the phoneme an unsatisfactory concatenative inventory unit. There are two types of inventory units, larger than phonemes but smaller than syllables, that have been used successfully for concatenative synthesis, the diphone and the demi-syllable.

Peterson, Wang, and Sivertsen (1958) originally proposed the diphone as the appropriate minimal unit for concatenative synthesis. The diphone is the acoustic piece of speech from the middle of one phoneme to the middle of the next phoneme. The middle of a phoneme tends to be acoustically more stable and less affected by coarticulation than other regions within a phoneme, which often involve rapid acoustic transitions from one phoneme to the next. A minimum inventory of about 1,000 diphones is required to synthesize arbitrary English text, since not all of the 1,600 possible different combinations actually occur (see Chapter 1). Because concatenative synthesis preserves the richness and fine acoustic detail of natural speech in its acoustic inventory elements, diphone synthesis is generally highly intelligible. This advantage is particularly notable in the synthesis of consonants. One disadvantage of diphone synthesis is that coarticulation is only provided with the immediately preceding and following phonemes,

---

[1] DECtalk is a product of Digital Equipment Corporation.
[2] CallText 5050 is a product of Speech Plus
[3] Infovox is a product of Infovox
[4] Votrax is a product of Votrax

whereas some phonemes, such as /r/ and /l/, can strongly affect the articulation of several preceding phonemes. Another disadvantage is that transitions between diphones may not be sufficiently smooth, and perceptually disruptive discontinuities can be introduced in the middle of a phoneme when they are concatenated. Examples of TTS systems that use diphone concatenative synthesis are an experimental AT&T Bell Laboratories system (Olive, 1977; Olive and Liberman, 1985), an early version of which is demonstrated at the Epcot Center of Walt Disney World, and an experimental multilingual TTS system developed at IPO (Institute for Perception Research) in the Netherlands (Elsendoorn, 1984; van Rijnsoever, 1988). The IPO system uses a relatively large inventory of stressed and unstressed variants of diphones for each language.

The demi-syllable is an alternative unit for concatenative synthesis suggested and developed by Fujimura & Lovins (1978). A demi-syllable is half a syllable; that is, either a syllable-initial consonant or consonant cluster plus the first half of the vowel, or the second half of the vowel plus the syllable-final consonant or consonant cluster. The number of demi-syllables in English is comparable to the number of diphones, approximately 1,000. Although demi-syllables allow for considerable coarticulation within a syllable, they have difficulty handling between-syllable coarticulatory effects, as discussed above for syllable concatenative units. An example of a current demi-syllable concatenative synthesis TTS system is Bellcore's system, Orator (see the July, 1990 issue of *Scientific American* pp. 92–93).

A concatenative synthesis system that uses variable-phone units has been recently developed at AT&T Bell Laboratories by Olive (1990). In this TTS system a majority of the acoustic inventory elements are diphones, but many longer multi-phone elements are used for commonly occurring and highly coarticulated sequences. The resulting synthesis is consistently judged more natural-sounding than strictly diphone concatenative synthesis.

Concatenative synthesis methods use various representations of the small units of speech that are concatenated together to form connected speech. For example, multipulse linear prediction analysis and synthesis techniques (see Chapter 2) were used to create the diphone inventory for the original version of an experimental AT&T diphone concatenation TTS system (Atal and Remde, 1982). In a recent hybrid version of the system, formant tracking is applied to voiced regions, which are synthesized by cascade formant synthesis, and unvoiced regions are synthesized with LPC techniques (Olive, 1989). Waveform synthesis is a relatively new technique that uses a time domain representation of the signal for concatenative synthesis. Several experimental systems using waveform synthesis are currently being developed in Europe (Moulines, et al., 1990). Whatever representation of the constituent speech units is used, rules must be provided for stretching or compressing them to achieve the target durations determined by duration rules and for smoothing the transitions between concatenated diphones. In addition, an F0 contour is imposed on the concatenated units, according to the system's intonation rules.

Articulatory synthesis is another synthesis method being developed for experimental TTS systems. Articulatory synthesis represents phonemes as articulatory targets, and employs rules that model how articulators move in time and space to generate connected speech. It is hoped that the articulatory approach will lead to simpler, more elegant rules that more closely model the way people actually speak. A lack of complete, detailed articulatory data from studies of human speakers, however, has made optimization of articulatory TTS systems difficult. An example of an articulatory TTS system is an experimental system developed at AT&T Bell Laboratories (Coker, 1968; Coker et al., 1973; Coker, 1976). A number of experimental articulatory synthesis programs that are not part of a TTS system have also been developed; one such system was developed at Haskins Laboratories (Rubin et al., 1981). Articulatory control parameters rather than text input or acoustic parameters control these synthesizers.

Evaluations of TTS synthesis algorithms involve tests of both speech intelligibility and speech quality (see the Schmidt-Nielsen chapter). Without careful attention to faithful modeling of acoustic details, TTS systems using formant-based synthesis tend to have problems with intelligibility. They can also lack the natural richness of human speech, and can tend towards a more mechanical, "thin" quality, although recent improvements on more realistic voice source models should improve the quality of formant synthesis (and possibly of other synthesis methods) considerably. Concatenative synthesis using linear predictive analysis and synthesis can have a buzzy quality that is characteristic of much LPC encoded speech. Concatenative synthesis methods also can introduce disruptive acoustic discontinuities when two diphones or demi-syllables are concatenated and the transition between them is abrupt; these discontinuities usually adversely affect speech quality more than intelligibility. Careful LPC-based concatenative synthesis can be highly intelligible—equivalent to or exceeding that of LPC-encoded human speech (Pols and Olive, 1983).

Synthesis methods that work adequately for the synthesis of a male voice may not be adequate for the synthesis of a female voice. Because of the higher fundamental frequencies of female (and children's) voices, it is harder to estimate formant frequencies. Female voice quality is often characterized by increased breathiness, due to voicing source differences between females and males. Vowels spoken by women do not conform as well to an all-pole model assumed by LPC methods; there is appreciable sub-glottal coupling, which introduces additional extraneous peaks and dips in the spectrum, and there are also source/tract interactions. Only a few TTS systems provide a female voice, and its intelligibility and quality are generally judged inferior to the system's male voice (Logan et al., 1989). Female voices are more adversely affected by telephone bandpass filtering than are male voices. In DRT intelligibility evaluations (see Chapter 5) of telephone bandpass filtered human speech, we typically observe about 33% more errors on average for female speakers than for male speakers. Issues involved in how to adequately model the female voice are active research topics (see Klatt and Klatt, 1990).

3.   TTS Evaluations

The preceding sections on the stages involved in text-to-speech synthesis, although focused on describing the technology, have also discussed evaluations of each of these stages of processing. Stage-specific evaluations are useful primarily in the development of the technology. They should provide diagnostic information with which to improve a component of text-to-speech conversion.

Overall evaluations of TTS systems generally involve testing the intelligibility, subjective speech quality, and comprehension of synthetic speech output. These topics are covered in chapters 5 and 6 of this book, and will not be discussed in detail here. However, it should be noted that speech synthesized by rule presents more problems for intelligibility and quality evaluations than does encoded human speech, because of all the dimensions along which it can differ from human speech. For example, with encoded speech, intonation and timing are provided by human speech input and are likely to be quite faithfully maintained, but natural prosody cannot always be expected in rule-generated TTS output. In addition, TTS intelligibility cannot be adequately evaluated by a test of initial consonants of monosyllabic words, as some intelligibility tests used frequently for encoded speech attempt to do. Results of overall evaluations may be diagnostic, but often they are simply used to determine a unidimensional score against which other systems' scores can be compared. Unidimensional scores, while less useful to researchers and developers, are often valued by those responsible for selecting one system over another.

Evaluations may also be developed to test the suitability of TTS systems for specific applications. Application-specific evaluations are potentially very useful. If well-designed, they provide the best means for determining the selection of a system, because they test those aspects of the system that are most relevant for its intended use in a task situation similar to that of the actual application. In other words, good application-specific evaluations are highly predictive of performance in the intended application.

There are various considerations that are important for the design of a good application-specific evaluation. First, duplicating the type of environment to be encountered in the actual application is very important (e.g. will the system be accessed through the telephone or by a terminal, is the environment likely to be noisy or quiet, private or public, etc.). Second, the evaluation should include TTS synthesis of the same type of text (e.g. names, addresses, product names, news articles, user-entered electronic mail or TDD (Telecommunications Device for the Deaf) conversations, etc.) in the same format that will be generated in the intended application. In addition, it is important that the evaluation simulate as closely as possible the level of experience and motivation as well as the demographic similarity of the likely users of the intended application. Marketing information should be of considerable assistance in this regard. Another factor that can be important in the design of application-specific evaluations is the nature of the existing service or system (if any) that is being replaced by TTS. This affects user experience, expectations, and motivation, and may have a large impact on the use and acceptance of TTS-generated speech.

For example, in an AT&T marketing trial of an automated mail-order telephone service which used recorded voice prompts for unchanging announcements (greetings, instructions) and TTS output for messages that varied for each user (verification of credit card, name and address information, customer order verification, inventory status), many users expressed more trust in the accuracy of the computer-generated TTS information than they did in human sales representatives whom they felt from past experience were more prone to error or laziness. Most users had no problems understanding and accepting synthetic speech (some surprisingly did not even notice the difference in voice quality between the recorded announcements and TTS messages), and those who were initially unaccepting of synthetic speech reported that if its use resulted in increased access (24-

hour order service) and lower product costs, they were willing to accept an automated service with TTS messages.

4.   Human Factors Issues in Tailoring TTS Technology for Specific Applications

Human factors specialists can and do play an important role in improving the user acceptability of text-to-speech technology as a user interface. This can be done through identifying appropriate and useful applications of TTS and by identifying deficiencies and supplementing the technology in order to overcome them. For example, market research may show that the TTS synthesis of proper names and addresses is needed for most TTS applications, and behavioral evaluations may indicate that current algorithms do not do a sufficiently good job in pronouncing them to be successful in the intended application. Applied behavioral research can then help to develop methods to improve proper name pronunciation. Other examples might involve the text normalization and intonation of addresses, determining the most appropriate speaking rates for various types of applications, or the most preferred voice or voice quality for an application.

4.1   Wording and Tuning TTS Announcements

The wording and structuring of voice prompts is a common human factors project. It is also a problem that is crucial for the acceptability of any voice interface, particularly a TTS interface. A standard announcement or voice prompt offers an opportunity to show text-to-speech synthesis at its best. Since the speaker's intention and the meaning of the message are known by the designer in advance, emphasis and intonation can be carefully tuned to convey the information optimally and to sound as natural as possible. Many TTS systems provide for the inclusion of additional control text or escape sequences that override defaults generated by rule, and are able to provide for carefully tailored announcements. Unfortunately, these options are often not taken advantage of by TTS service designers, who may have little training in speech or TTS technology. However, it is a challenge to TTS researchers and developers to construct and provide adequate instructions and examples for less experienced designers to follow in developing TTS announcements.

For all voice interfaces, but especially for TTS-generated announcements, it is important to follow general strategies for announcement structure and wording that place a minimal cognitive load on the listener. That is, the listener's perceptual and cognitive abilities and memory should be minimally taxed by hearing and comprehending the voice announcement. This is especially true for TTS announcements, because research (discussed in the Ralston, Pisoni, and Mullennix chapter on perception and comprehension) indicates that synthetic speech may require more attention from the listener to process than human speech does. An example of a strategy in structuring voice prompts that minimizes the cognitive load to the listener is, when listing a series of listener-selectable options, to first state the function of the option, and to then state the operation the listener is to perform to select this option. In this way, the listener must simply listen for the desired function, and then listen to and follow the subsequent instructions. An example of this structure is: "To listen to your message, press star 5; for help at any time, press star 4; to quit at any time, just hang up." If the order is reversed so that the operation precedes the function (as unfortunately often happens in poorly designed announcements), the listener must temporarily hold the operation information in memory until the function of the option is explained, and then the listener can determine whether to follow it or forget it and listen to the next operation. An example of a poorly designed prompt is: "Press star 5 to listen to your message; press star 4 for help at any time; just hang up to quit at any time."

5.   Summary and Conclusions

Text-to-speech technology allows computer-to-human communication through the natural human communication modality of audible speech. TTS is particularly useful in applications that provide access to large and frequently changing databases, for which stored human speech would be impossible or impractical. The development of TTS technology has been a multi-disciplinary effort, in which behavioral scientists have played many important roles. The basic stages of conversion of text to speech include text normalization, syntactic analysis, word pronunciation, determination of prosody, and speech synthesis. Text normalization involves locating sentence boundaries, expanding abbreviations, and translating nonalphabetic characters to a pronounceable form. Syntactic analysis classifies each word into its part of speech, and is important for word pronunciation and the determination of prosody. A dictionary and letter-to-sound rules are used to map orthographic characters into strings of phonemes and to assign lexical stress. The determination of prosody involves assigning a pitch pattern and a timing pattern to an utterance, stages which are important for both intelligibility and naturalness. The final stage of speech synthesis transforms phonetic symbols to an audible acoustic speech signal. Synthesis methods used for TTS include formant-based synthesis, several concatenative synthesis methods, and articulatory synthesis. A variety of evaluations are useful diagnostically during the development of a TTS system, and are also helpful in comparing and selecting systems for specific applications. Human factors input can improve the acceptability of TTS synthesis as a user interface by tailoring the technology for various applications and by carefully designing the wording and structure of voice prompts.

6. References

Ainsworth, W. A. (1973). A system for converting English text into speech. *IEEE Trans. Audio Electroacoust.*, **AU-21**, 288–290.

Akers, G. and Lennig, M. (1985). Intonation in text-to-speech synthesis: Evaluation of algorithms. *J. Acoust. Soc. Amer.*, **77**, 2157–2165.

Allen, J., Hunnicutt, S., and Klatt, D. H. (1987). *From Text to Speech: The MITalk System.* Cambridge Univ. Press: Cambridge, UK.

Allen, J., Hunnicutt, S., Carlson, R., and Granstrom, B. (1979). MITalk-79: The MIT text-to-speech system. *J. Acoust. Soc. Am.* Suppl. 1 **65,** S130.

Atal, B. S., and Remde, J. R. (1982). A new model of LPC excitation for producing natural-sounding speech at low bit rates. Proc. Int. Conf. Acoust., Speech Signal Process. **ICASSP–82**, 614–617.

Bernstein, J., and Nessly, L. (1981). Performance comparison of component algorithms for the phonemicization of orthography. *Proc. 19th Annu. Assoc. Comp. Ling.*, 19–22.

Carlson, R., and Granstrom, B. (1976). A text-to-speech system based entirely on rules. *Proc. Int. Conf. Acoust. Speech Signal Process.* **ICASSP–76**, 686–688.

Carlson, R., Granstrom, B., and Klatt, D. H. (1979). Some notes on the perception of temporal patterns in speech. In B. Lindblom and S. Ohman (Eds.), *Frontiers of Speech Communication Research,* Academic Press: London, New York and San Francisco, 233–243.

Chomsky, N., and Halle, M. (1968). *Sound pattern of English,* Harper and Row: New York.

Church, K. W. (1985). Stress assignment in letter-to-sound rules for speech synthesis. *Proc. 23rd Meeting Assoc. Comp. Ling.*, 246–253.

Coker, C. H. (1968). Speech synthesis with a parametric articulatory model. In J. L. Flanagan and L. R. Rabiner (Eds.), *Speech Synthesis*, Dowden, Hutchinson and Ross: Stroudsburg, PA, 135–139.

Coker, C. H. (1976). A model of articulatory dynamics and control. *Proc. IEEE* **64**, 452–459.

Coker, C. H. (1985). A dictionary—intensive letter-to-sound program. *J. Acoust. Soc. Am.* Suppl. 1 **78**, S7.

Coker, C. H., Church, K. W., and Liberman, M. Y. (1990). Morphology and Rhyming: Two powerful alternatives to letter-to-sound rules for speech synthesis, *Proceedings of the European Speech Communications Association (ESCA)*, September, 1990.

Coker, C. H., Umeda, N., and Browman, C. P. (1973). Automatic synthesis from ordinary English text. *IEEE Trans. Audio Electroacoust.*, **AU–21**, 293–297.

Dedina, M. J., and Nusbaum, H. C. (1986). Pronounce: A program for pronunciation by analogy. *Speech Research Laboratory Progress Report 12*, Indiana University, Bloomington, IN, 335–348.

Elovitz, H., Johnson, R., McHugh, A., and Shore, J. (1976). Letter-to-sound rules for automatic translation of English text to phonetics. *IEEE Trans. Acoust. Speech Signal Process.*, **ASSP–24**, 446–459.

Elsendoorn, B. A. G. (1984). Heading for a diphone speech synthesis system for Dutch. *IPO Annual Progress Report* **19**, 32–35.

Fry, D. B. (1955). Duration and intensity as physical correlates of linguistic stress. *J. Acoust. Soc. Amer.*, **27**, 765–768.

Fry, D. B. (1958). Experiments in the perception of stress, *Lang. Speech* **1**, 126–152.

Fujimura, O., and Lovins, J. (1978). "Syllables as concatenative phonetic elements," in A. Bell and J. B. Hooper (Eds.), *Syllables and Segments*, North-Holland: New York, 107–120.

Glushko, R. J. (1981). Principles for pronouncing print: The psychology of phonography. In A. M. Lesgold and C. A. Perfetti (Eds.), *Interactive processes in reading*, Erlbaum: Hillsdale, NJ.

Goldman-Eisler, F., (1968). *Psycholinguistics: Experiments in spontaneous speech*, Academic Press: New York.

Gopal, H. S., and Syrdal, A. K. (1988). Effects of speaking rate on temporal and spectral characteristics of American English vowels. *Speech Communication Group Working Papers, Volume VI*, Research Laboratory of Electronics, M. I. T., 162–180.

Groner, G.F., Bernstein, J., Ingber, E., Pearlman, J., and Toal, T. (1982). A real-time text-to-speech converter. *Speech Technol.* **1**, 73–76.

Halle, M., and Keyser, S. J. (1971). *English stress: Its form, its growth and its role in verse*. Harper and Row: New York.

Hayes, B. P. (1980). *A metrical theory of stress rules*. Ph.D. thesis, MIT, Cambridge, MA.

Hill, K., and Nessly, L. (1973). Review of the sound pattern of English, *Linguistics* **106**, 57–101.

Hunnicutt, S. (1976). Phonological rules for a text-to-speech system. *Am. J. Comp. Ling*. Microfiche 57, 1–72.

Hirschberg, J. (1990). Accent and discourse content: Assigning pitch accent to synthetic speech. *7th National Conference of the American Association for Artificial Intelligence*, Boston, MA, July 29–August 3, 1990, 952–957.

Hunnicutt, S. (1980). Grapheme-to-phoneme rules, A review. *Speech Transmission Laboratory, Royal Institute of Technology, Stockholm, Sweden*, **QPSR 2–3**, 38–60.

Klatt, D. H. (1979). Synthesis by rule of segmental durations in English sentences. In B. Lindblom and S. Ohman (Eds.), *Frontiers of Speech Communication Research*, Academic Press: London, New York and San Francisco.

Klatt, D. H. (1987). Review of text-to-speech conversion for English. *J. Acoust. Soc. Amer*., **82**(3), 737–793.

Klatt, D. H., and Klatt, L. C. (1990). Analysis, synthesis, and perception of voice quality variations among female and male talkers. *J. Acoust. Soc. Amer*., **87**, 820–857.

Kucera, H., and Francis, W. N. (1967). *Computational analysis of present day American English*. Brown Univ. Press: Providence, RI.

Lee, F. F. (1969). Reading machine: From text to speech. *IEEE Trans. Audio Electroacoust*. **AU–17**, 275–282.

Lehiste, I. and Peterson, G. E. (1959). Vowel amplitude and phonemic stress in American English. *J. Acoust. Soc. Amer*., **31**, 428–435.

Liberman, M., and Prince, A. (1977). On stress and linguistic rhythm, *Linguistic Inquiry* 8, 249–336.

Lindblom, B. (1963). Spectrographic study of vowel reduction. *J. Acoust. Soc. Amer.*, 35, 1773–1781.

Logan, J. S., Greene, B. G. and Pisoni, D. B. (1989). Segmental intelligibility of synthetic speech produced by rule. *J. Acoust. Soc. Amer.*, 86, 566–581.

McIlroy, M. D. (1974). Synthetic speech by rule. Unpublished Technical Memo, Bell Laboratories, Murray Hill, NJ.

Moulines, E., Emerard, F., Larreur, D., Le Saint Milon, J. L., Le Faucheur, L., Marty, F., Charpentier, F., and Sorin, C. (1990). A real-time French text-to-speech system generating high-quality synthetic speech, *Proc. Int. Conf. Acoust. Speech Signal Process.* **ICASSP–90**, 309–312.

Olive, J. P. (1977). Rule synthesis of speech from diadic units. *Proc. Int. Conf. Acoust. Speech Signal Process.* **ICASSP–77**, 568–570.

Olive, J. P. (1989). Mixed spectral representation — Formants and LPC coefficients. *J. Acoust. Soc. Am. Suppl. 1* 85, S59.

Olive, J. P. (1990). A new algorithm for a concatenative speech sythesis system using an augmented acoustic inventory of speech sounds. *Proceedings of the European Speech Communications Association Workshop on Speech Synthesis*, Autrans, France, 25–29.

Olive, J. P., and Liberman, M. Y. (1985). Text-to-speech—An overview. *J. Acoust. Soc. Am. Suppl. 1* 78, S6.

Peterson, G., Wang, W., and Sivertsen, E. (1958). Segmentation techniques in speech synthesis. *J. Acoust. Soc. Amer.*, 30, 739–742.

Picheny, M. A. (1981). *Speaking Clearly for the Hard of Hearing*, Ph.D. thesis, MIT, Cambridge, MA.

Picheny, M. A., Durlach, N. I., and Braida, L. D., (1986). Speaking clearly for the hard of hearing II: Acoustic characteristics of clear and conversational speech. *J. of Speech and Hearing Research*, 29(4), 434–446.

Pols, L. C. W., and Olive, J. P. (1983). Intelligibility of consonants in CVC utterances produced by diadic rule synthesis. *Speech Commun.* 2, 3–13.

Rubin, P., Baer, T., and Mermelstein, P. (1981). An articulatory sythesizer for perceptual research. *J. Acoust. Soc. Amer.*, 70, 321–328.

Sejnowski, T., and Rosenberg, C. (1987). Parallel networks that learn to pronounce English text, *Complex Systems*, **1**, 144–168.

Silverman, K. E. A. (1987). *The structure and processing of fundamental frequency contours*. Ph.D. thesis, Cambridge University, Cambridge, UK.

Syrdal, A. K. (1989). Improved duration rules for text-to-speech synthesis. *J. Acoust. Soc. Am. Suppl. 1*, **85**, S43.

Uchanski, R. M. (1988). *Spectral and temporal contributions to speech clarity for hearing impaired listeners*, Ph.D. thesis, MIT, Cambridge, MA.

van Rijnsoever, P. A. (1988). A multilingual text-to-speech system. *IPO Annual Progress Report* **23**, 34–40.

Chapter 4

Using Speech Recognition Systems: Issues in Cognitive Engineering

Howard C. Nusbaum, Jenny DeGroot, and Lisa Lee
The University of Chicago

1. Abstract

A number of fundamental human factors issues arise when considering the design and use of speech recognition systems. Some human factors problems are determined specifically by characteristics of the user, such as individual differences between talkers that affect the success of recognition performance. Other issues are more general, and relate more directly to the design of the user/system interface, such as the type of feedback presented to the user. Still others stem from properties of the environment and context in which speech recognition is used. While many of these issues will be the same for small and large vocabulary recognition systems, discrete and continuous speech recognition systems, and talker-dependent and talker-independent systems, their relative importance and the way these issues are resolved will be very different. We will outline some of these basic differences and discuss some new human factors issues that may arise with the next generation of speech recognition systems.

2. Acknowledgments

Preparation of this chapter was supported, in part, by a grant from NIDCD, DC00601 to the University of Chicago. The second author was supported, in part, by an NSF Graduate Fellowship.

3. Introduction

Speech is the most common mode of communication between people. We issue commands, requests, and assertions by directly speaking to another person, and although speech communication is not a perfect process, we understand each other with a very high success rate. Language encodes an idea, or "message", into an utterance in a number of partially redundant representations. Thus, there are two aspects of spoken language use that are probably critical to its effectiveness as the normal means of communication among people. First, the redundant representation of a message in an utterance provides a very robust method of transmitting information. We have extensive knowledge of linguistic structure and of the methods and styles of communication, extensive knowledge about the world and concepts we discuss in general, and immediate knowledge about the situation in which communication is taking place. All of this knowledge allows us to recognize and understand an utterance using both its pattern properties (acoustic characteristics) and inferences about what the utterance might possibly mean. Moreover, a series of utterances is not treated as a sequence of dissociated patterns or meanings. In spoken discourse each utterance provides some information that can constrain the interpretation of previous and subsequent speech (Halliday & Hasan, 1976).

For example, in the speech signal itself a number of different acoustic cues may each provide information about the identity of a consonant or vowel sound; simultaneously, knowledge about grammar, words, and sentences, and knowledge about the world all contribute to spoken language understanding. This redundancy in the representation of speech helps us to understand what other people say. For example, if part of a word is obscured by noise or through misarticulation, knowledge of the whole word, of the sentence in which it occurs, or of the situational context can be used to "fill in the blank" (see Samuel, 1986) or correct the perceptual error (e.g., Cole & Jakimik, 1980; Cole & Rudnicky, 1983).

Second, spoken language is used interactively by the speaker and listener. In many cases, the success of speech communication depends on the ability of speakers and listeners to exchange roles rapidly and frequently to provide feedback to each other. Communication depends on people's ability to make requests and to summarize and restate previous utterances. This type of interaction allows a listener to request clarification, elaboration, and expansion, and it allows a speaker to fulfill those requests, which can be done by providing information directly as well as by directing the listener's attention to parts of an utterance. When a communication channel is noisy (e.g., speech over a telephone or at a crowded party) or distorted, more interaction may occur. Speakers may change the way they speak, increasing pitch, amplitude, and duration because they understand that noise affects the perception of their speech (Dreher & O'Neill, 1957; Pisoni et al., 1985; Summers et al., 1988). Listeners may become more active in requesting information. In conversation, speakers may change their selection of words, syntax (sentence structure and word order), and overall style of interaction as they cooperate to maximize communication. In addition, when an utterance is not understood completely or correctly, there are a number of conventions for error correction and recovery that can be used to assist comprehension. For example, if we misunderstand a word, we can directly request that the speaker clarify some part of an utterance.

By comparison, speaking to machines is a much less satisfactory communication process. Speech recognition algorithms do not exploit the redundant sources of information in spoken language. Even the best commercially available speech recognition devices rely primarily on "bottom-up" pattern recognition. In bottom-up (or data-driven) pattern recognition, the pattern structure or properties of a particular input signal are compared to the patterns within a set of known signals. Recognition occurs when the input pattern is sufficiently similar to a known pattern. This contrasts with the kind of recognition that humans use, which includes "top-down" (or conceptually driven) processing. In top-down processing, sophisticated knowledge about the likelihood of signals and the relations among signals and other sources of information can be used to infer the identity of an input signal. For example, in top-down processing, inferences could be made about what might be a plausible utterance given a particular linguistic context or communicative situation.

Commercially available recognition systems use only the crudest and most simplistic acoustic representation of speech and do not employ any inferential processes at all (see Moore, 1986, for a discussion of template and hidden Markov model recognition systems). As a result, the recognition performance of these systems is far worse than speech perception by humans (e.g., see Nusbaum & Pisoni, 1987). Even in research laboratories, where speech understanding systems apply some minimal linguistic and contextual knowledge to exploit some (but by no means much) of the information encoded in an utterance, recognition performance is still not up to human standards (see Klatt, 1977, for a review).

Furthermore, none of these systems exploits the kinds of communicative interactions that permit and facilitate the process of error recovery in communication between people. For example, if there are two known words whose patterns are equally similar to an input word, recognition systems do not have any inherent method of resolving this confusion by requesting clarification from the talker. Even in the most advanced speech recognition systems and speech understanding systems that make use of linguistic knowledge or contextual expectation, there are no inherent strategies for error recovery based on exploiting communicative interactions. In some cases, when a spoken word is very unlikely in a particular context, linguistic or contextual expectations may actually be sufficiently strong to override bottom-up pattern recognition in favor of a more contextually appropriate word. In doing so, without asking for clarification, a system can reject the correct word and make a "perceptual" error. Unlike humans, these systems have no means of detecting or correcting these errors. Therefore, speaking to a computer is generally much less successful and satisfying than speaking with a human. Speaking to a computer could even be frustrating, if recognition performance is sufficiently poor and feedback to the user is sufficiently uninformative.

Besides the amount of miscommunication that can occur when computers are given the task of recognizing speech, there are other problems that confront someone who is talking to a computer. Clearly, talking to a machine using current speech technology is not as simple and natural as talking with a person. Speaking to humans subjectively seems to be a relatively effortless task; but speaking to a computer may be very demanding. For most recognition systems, talkers must carefully choose each word from a restricted set of alternatives, and they must speak clearly and regularly, pausing between words. Choosing words from a restricted vocabulary and speaking in a precise fashion may require a great deal of effort and attention. This may cause problems, because the ability of humans to carry out simultaneous tasks is limited by the basic structure of our cognitive and perceptual systems (Nusbaum & Schwab, 1986). The more a particular task requires attention, the more we are limited in performing other tasks that demand "cognitive resources" such as working memory (see Baddeley, 1986; Shiffrin, 1976). If speaking to a computer requires a lot of attention, it could degrade the talker's ability to remember important information, solve a problem, or perform some other task (see Wickens, 1980). Furthermore, our cognitive limitations become most apparent when we try to combine language-oriented tasks, like speaking, writing, and listening (Brooks, 1968; Wickens, 1980). Thus, for example, it might be especially difficult to compose a memo while talking to a recognizer, because both are linguistic activities.

The constant effort of speaking in an unnatural way to a computer could very well hinder some aspects of the talker's job performance. But there may be other unfavorable effects as well. The interaction between human and machine is seldom an intelligent dialogue; the unfamiliar nature of feedback about errors and error correction strategies may be frustrating to the user. For example, some recognition errors may require repeating the same utterance over and over ad nauseum (in worst cases) until the computer successfully recognizes what is said (or the talker quits trying). Thus, speech recognition systems may not only increase cognitive load but may also increase fatigue and stress.

In general, as the tasks involving speech recognition become more complex, we expect to see reductions in overall task performance. If the accuracy of a particular recognition algorithm is low for a specific vocabulary or talker, this should cause even greater degradation of task performance. Moreover, the complexity of the operator's task may interact with the form of the user-system interface, the accuracy of the recognition device, and the individual user's ability to deal with increased frustration, stress, and cognitive load. Indeed, it is likely that with increased cognitive load, fatigue, and stress, the talker will produce speech differently (Summers et al., 1989), thereby reducing recognition performance and task performance. This could then further amplify stress, fatigue, and load effects.

There should be little doubt, then, that the use of speech recognition systems in a variety of applications—data entry, command and control, and information retrieval—may produce human factors problems that might not arise with the use of other interface technologies, such as keyboard or joystick input. These problems can be approached from a cognitive engineering perspective (see Norman, 1984). Rather than address the issues surrounding the use of speech technology as more technologically advanced, but similar to the issues surrounding the use of knobs and dials, it is important to understand that new interface technologies such as speech recognition systems are themselves information processing systems. In the past, human factors analyses of a particular device or service required understanding issues such as response compatibility in controls and legibility of displays. The psychological research most relevant to these issues comes largely from the fields of motor control and sensory psychophysics. However, speech technology does not just provide a more advanced control and display system. Speech technology directly engages the cognitive system of the operator by involving psycholinguistic, inferential, attentional, and learning mechanisms. This requires a more sophisticated approach to understanding the use of speech technology—an approach informed by basic and applied research in cognitive psychology.

Unfortunately, there has been very little work directed at understanding the use of speech technology as a problem of applied cognitive psychology. Research has investigated a few basic human factors problems that are involved in the use of commercially available, isolated utterance, small vocabulary speech recognition devices for database retrieval, command and control, and personnel training applications (see Simpson et al., 1987). However, there has been very little research directed at the issues surrounding the use of large vocabulary recognition systems (although see Gould et al., 1984) or the next generation of recognition systems still under development. In other words, it is difficult to anticipate the types of problems that will arise in using the next generation of speech recognition systems, which will be designed to accept continuous speech input (i.e., without pauses between words), with large vocabularies, and with more natural sentence structure. Indeed, although vocabulary size has been cited as a significant limiting factor on the usability of speech recognition devices (National Research Council [NRC], 1984), it does not seem reasonable to assume that simply increasing vocabulary size alone will greatly enhance the performance or effectiveness of the technology. Increasing vocabulary size will probably introduce reductions in recognition performance for many reasons (e.g., reaching limits of recognition algorithms and increased confusability of vocabulary items) and will introduce new human factors issues in providing information to the user. Thus, changing one aspect of the limitations on recognition technology will not automatically increase the utility of the technology, because there will be concomitant effects on the user interface. Rather, it is important to consider in detail the nature of the new limitations on speech technology and tailor the user interface to surmount those limitations and address new problems when possible. In addition, improvements in technology such as increasing vocabulary size will make possible new applications, such as dictation, and these applications will raise new human factors problems that must be addressed systematically but cannot be entirely anticipated.

Therefore, our purpose in the present chapter is not to propose specific solutions to particular human factors problems posed by speech recognition technology, but rather to describe the kinds of problems that are likely to arise and to advocate a more general approach to developing solutions since the solutions will change with the technology. There is a need for more research that investigates the causes of these human factors problems, and we argue that solutions will come from theoretically motivated, empirical investigations of the use of this technology. At present, there is simply too little information available about the human factors issues that must be addressed in developing and using the next generation of speech recognition systems. However, it is clear that three aspects of the use of speech recognition systems must be understood: (1) the design and functions of the speech recognition system (consisting of hardware and software), (2) the limitations and capabilities of the human operator, and (3) the environment and context within which recognition takes place (including the selection of the task or application). Each of these areas must be understood, because they will interact to determine the overall effectiveness and performance of a speech recognition system for a particular task or application and because together they will constrain the choices that must be made in designing a user interface to the technology.

4. The Recognition System

For our purposes, a recognition system can be defined to consist of the hardware and software that instantiate the algorithms for training the system (storing examples of the specific utterances that it will have to recognize) and for recognition itself, along with any software for user interaction with the recognizer's functions (e.g., changing the type of error feedback, if a system permits it). There are four basic components to be considered in understanding the operation of a speech recognition system. First, in order to know what a talker has said, the recognition system must have some way of encoding, learning, and representing a set of utterances (i.e., the known vocabulary) that it will recognize. Second, during recognition, there must be some type of pattern-matching algorithm that compares a representation of a particular input utterance with the representations in the known vocabulary. Third, given the comparison of some input with the vocabulary, there must be an algorithm that decides which utterance in the vocabulary was produced. Finally, there must be some kind of user interface to the functions and operation of the recognition system.

4.1 Characteristics of Speech Recognition Systems

Given this basic description of a speech recognition system, we can outline some of the differences among systems. First, speech recognition systems can be speaker-dependent or speaker-independent. Speaker-dependent systems can recognize a particular person's utterances only if that person has previously stored examples of his or her speech in the system. Speaker-independent systems do not have this limitation they can recognize speech across talkers without prior experience with the talker's speech.

Another difference among systems is whether they accept discrete, connected, or continuous speech input. Systems that recognize discrete, or isolated-word, input require a brief pause after every word or may allow only one word as input. Systems that recognize connected speech input accept a sequence of concatenated citation-form words. Systems that recognize continuous speech should accept fluent speech produced as if directed at a human listener.

A third characteristic difference among speech recognition systems is the size of the vocabulary. Some systems can recognize only a small set of words, perhaps even as few as the ten digits and a few words such as yes and no (currently this kind of restricted vocabulary is the only kind found in speaker-independent devices, since this is the only way to achieve reasonable performance; an example is the Conversant Systems recognition system, discussed in Schinke, 1986). Other systems can recognize much larger sets of words, even into the tens of thousands. Some recognition systems permit syntaxing or vocabulary switching so that different vocabularies are available contingent on the outcome of recognizing an utterance. For example, recognizing the word defect could switch in a vocabulary of codes for part defects whereas recognizing the utterance part number could switch in a digit vocabulary. Partitioning a large vocabulary into smaller, context-dependent subsets reduces confusability of vocabulary items.

Finally, systems can differ in the way they represent the acoustic properties of utterances, the way sets of utterances are combined to form vocabularies, and the way they determine which vocabulary item was actually spoken (the recognition algorithm). Choices among the features and capabilities of different recognition systems usually represent a tradeoff among speaker dependency, style of speech input accepted, and vocabulary size. These properties interact with the recognition algorithm and the representations of utterances and vocabularies, to affect system performance.

Recognition systems all form some internal representation of an utterance through an encoding process. Some recognition devices use a time-domain representation of the signal (e.g., the Dragon System, described in Baker, 1975), but most represent the spectro-temporal properties of an utterance (e.g., the Interstate and Votan systems). In other words, most systems represent the pattern of information within an utterance by encoding the way the distribution of acoustic energy across frequencies changes over time. Extracting spectro-temporal information is computationally costly since the time-varying waveform (the speech soundwave itself) must be converted by filtering or by carrying out fast Fourier transforms (see

Ramirez, 1985, for background on FFTs). Thus a system that uses spectro-temporal patterns will either be computationally slower than a system that encodes only the time-domain properties of the speech waveform or will require specialized hardware.

4.2 Training a Recognition System

Recognition systems also store a recognition vocabulary, which is typically a representation of the information present in several different tokens (instances) of each vocabulary item. Recognition systems differ in the way this vocabulary is formed. They may use training algorithms that maintain different tokens as separate patterns or may combine pattern information from different tokens based on statistical analyses. The most common commercially available recognition systems start out as a *tabula rasa*: They do not have any a priori representation of the set of utterances they can recognize. On one hand, this is a kind of advantage since the vocabulary can be tailored to suit a particular application. When a speech recognition interface to an application must be defined in a limited vocabulary of 200 words, it is important to have flexibility in constructing the application vocabulary. For example, the vocabulary for using a word processor (including utterances such as "italicize text" or "format paragraph") would be quite different from the vocabulary for a database application (such as "define field" or "find record").

On the other hand, the reason that these systems start without a predefined vocabulary is that the most common commercial word recognition systems employ speaker-dependent recognition algorithms. This means that the recognition device does not just need a list of utterances that constitute the task vocabulary; it needs a representation of the acoustic patterns of those utterances produced by a particular person. Speaker-dependent recognition systems must be trained on the utterances of the specific talker who will use the recognition system. The acoustic patterns of speech differ between talkers such that two talkers may produce the same intended utterance with different acoustic properties and different utterances with the same properties (Peterson & Barney, 1952). In order to recognize accurately a talker's speech, a speaker-dependent recognition system must be trained to know how that talker says each word.

Training consists, typically, of the talker reading the vocabulary items one at a time while the recognition device stores an acoustic representation of each utterance. Initial enrollment of a vocabulary occurs when the first token of each item is produced, analyzed, and stored as an acoustic pattern associated with some type of system response or orthographic string (i.e., the spelling of a word or phrase). Many systems have the ability to use more than one token of each vocabulary item and thus permit the talker to update the vocabulary with subsequent repetitions of each item. This allows a recognition device to have a better (richer) representation of the possible acoustic patterns that may exemplify an utterance.

When training a system, it is important to keep in mind that talkers seldom say the same thing twice with precisely the same acoustic pattern (e.g., Peterson & Barney, 1952). For example, changes in speaking rate will change the acoustic pattern of an utterance (Miller, 1981). In addition, when the linguistic context for an utterance changes, the acoustic properties of that utterance change as well (Liberman et al., 1967). Thus even when training a recognizer on a list of vocabulary items, it is important to sample vocabulary items in the context of a range of different words and with different intervals between words (to allow for variation in speaking rates). Simply saying the same item repeatedly and then saying the next item afterwards will restrict the amount of variation in utterances, and thus fail to represent the range of acoustic variability that may occur when the recognition device is actually used in an application. It is much better to randomize (Simpson et al., 1987) or systematically sample vocabulary items in different contexts. Internally, these samples could be stored as a list of different forms of the same word, or the statistical properties of the set of tokens corresponding to a single vocabulary item could be used as a representation of the ensemble. In fact, these statistical properties could be (but seldom, if ever, are) used to adaptively check the similarity of the training tokens of each vocabulary item, in order to make sure an optimal sampling is obtained. Furthermore, the training tokens of a given word could be (but seldom, if ever, are) compared to the representation of the entire vocabulary, to determine whether the system is performing a suffi-ciently detailed acoustic analysis. If there is insufficient resolution in the analysis, then the training tokens of similar-sounding words may not be distinctive enough.

Another training issue is that there are substantial acoustic differences between spontaneous speech and speech that is produced by reading aloud (Mehta & Cutler, 1988; Remez et al., 1987). It is generally true, for many reasons, that training conditions should match the conditions under which the recognizer will be used. This ensures that the distribution of acoustic properties of speech produced during training will be maximally similar to the distribution of properties of speech produced when the recognizer is used. Thus, if vocabulary items are to be read aloud from a screen during normal operation, training should be carried out the same way. Utterances that are spoken spontaneously during training will probably be somewhat different acoustically from utterances read aloud during actual use of the recognition system, making it harder for the recognizer to match an input utterance to a stored vocabulary item.

Training constitutes a major difference between speaker-dependent and speaker-independent recognition systems. As noted earlier, speaker-independent systems do not require training. Speaker-independent systems are designed to recognize utterances from many different talkers, without training on any particular talker's speech, since they start out with a representation of speech from a large sample of talkers for a predefined vocabulary (e.g., Schinke, 1986; Wilpon, 1985). These systems are appropriate for applications in which training is not possible, typically because the individual talkers are not known in advance or because each talker may use the system only once or infrequently. Certain types of customer services provide examples: Even if a business knows which employees will talk to the recognizer, it cannot always identify a priori all its customers. An example of a speaker-independent system is the Conversant Systems recognition device (Schinke, 1986), which can recognize digit sequences (such as, "Five, three, six") regardless of the talker. One of its possible uses is recognizing bank account numbers spoken over the phone by customers to retrieve current balance information. A bank cannot train its recognizer on speech from all its customers, and these customers may not access their accounts by phone sufficiently often to make the inconvenience of a training session worthwhile. Using a speaker-independent recognition system with a restricted vocabulary for limited customer interactions with the service addresses this problem.

Speaker-independent recognition systems require a representation of the vocabulary in a form that will be sufficient to match almost any talker's speech. One way to accomplish this is to construct a vocabulary that represents each item as the statistical average of speech produced by a large number of talkers. However, there are potential problems with this approach. In one case, a speaker-independent recognition system developed on a database of New Jersey speech performed terribly in Louisiana (Wilpon, 1985). On one hand, if talkers are sufficiently homogeneous in dialect (and thus more similar in the phonological characteristics of their speech), it seems feasible to develop a statistical representation of that dialect. But what happens when speech is taken from a sufficiently variable sample of talkers, changing the phonetics and phonology of the speech (Oshika et al.,

1975)? As the disparity among tokens increases, not only will the patterns that constitute a single item become as different as the patterns corresponding to different vocabulary items, but different vocabulary items may now become more similar. For example, in some dialects, the pronunciation of pen is identical to pin, while in others pen is closer to pan. If a sample of speech includes tokens from these different dialects, there will be two results: great variation within the set of pen tokens, and increased overlap of the pen set with the sets of pin and pan tokens.

One way to limit the amount of overlap between word types is to limit the vocabulary size. This is why the only truly speaker-independent recognition systems have very small vocabularies, such as the ten digits. Thus, vocabulary size is an important practical and theoretical distinction among speech recognition systems and may be constrained by other properties of a recognition device or application.

4.3 Speech Input

For related reasons, the nature of the speech input that can be accepted for recognition constitutes another important distinction among speech recognition systems. Discrete input consists of words produced carefully as isolated, citation-form utterances which display much less acoustic variability than words produced in the context of other words. Citation-form words are well-defined and much more similar from token to token than are words in conversational speech.

Connected speech input does not have the pauses between words that discrete input requires, but it still requires the operator to speak carefully so that words are phonologically intact and largely unmodified by the phonological influences of neighboring words. In connected speech, speakers try to produce words as a concatenated sequence of citation-form utterances, hopefully minimizing the phonological and coarticulatory influence of adjacent utterances while still producing an unbroken stream of speech. Of course, it is impossible to eliminate the coarticulatory effects and phonological influence of neighboring words, but with careful articulation these effects can be reduced.

Finally, continuous speech input is much closer to natural, fluent speech. Talkers produce speech as a more acoustically integrated utterance rather than as a list of discrete words. Thus the articulation of one word may restructure pronunciation of adjacent words: Sounds may be elided, combined, or modified through a combination of phonological and phonetic effects. In fluent, continuous speech, the phonological pattern of sounds in words may change from context to context, and the acoustic-phonetic properties of particular sound segments will also change (see Oshika et al., 1975).

In recognizing words produced in isolation as discrete input, a recognition algorithm uses a simple energy detector to determine when a word starts and when it ends. The energy between these points is then coded into the acoustic form used for pattern matching to the stored recognition vocabulary. However, in continuous or connected speech input, a recognition device must segment the continuous acoustic structure of an utterance into its constituent word-length patterns before comparing these patterns to the stored vocabulary representations. Segmentation requires recognizing the beginning and ending of a word. However, this cannot be carried out successfully based on an energy detector alone, because in natural speech there are usually no silences between words. Indeed, there is no simple, single acoustic property that marks the beginning or ending of a word in fluent or connected speech. Thus, for a system to recognize individual words from continuous speech, it must either use more subtle and complex acoustic cues to the word boundaries (Nakatani & Dukes, 1977), or identify boundaries via its stored knowledge of phonology, the lexicon, or syntax.

The simplest approach to segmentation (but apparently the one used by human listeners; see Greenspan et al., 1988) is for segmentation to be a consequence of recognition rather than its precursor. If a recognition device begins processing acoustic information at the start of an utterance, once the first word in the utterance is recognized, the beginning of the next word is directly located. Recognition of the second word can begin, using the acoustic information following the first word. However, this approach may not be very robust: Incorrect recognition of the first word may impair recognition of subsequent words by imposing an incorrect segmentation and mistakenly locating the word boundary inside either the first or second word. Recognition of the second word starting at this point will most certainly fail.

Segmentation can also be approached as a separate recognition problem from recognizing words. A recognition device can attempt to recognize word boundaries from some of their acoustic or linguistic properties (e.g., Nakatani & Dukes, 1977; Lamel, 1983). Connected or continuous speech may be recognized best by speaker-dependent systems, because the subtle acoustic cues to word boundaries may differ across talkers. Similarly, connected or continuous speech is currently better recognized by small vocabulary systems, because smaller vocabularies require less lexical and syntactic knowledge than large vocabularies within which many more interactions are possible (see Chen, 1986, for an implementation with connected digits). Thus vocabulary size, speaker independence, and fluency of input may trade off against each other in determining optimal recognition performance, depending on the needs of the application.

4.4 Contributions from Speech Perception Research

Vocabulary size, speaker independence, and fluency of input are much less limiting for human listeners than they are for recognition systems. Human listeners are quite good at recognizing continuous speech from multiple talkers using large vocabularies. Speech recognition technology will certainly benefit from research on how humans perform these tasks, since humans are the only effective and robust examples of speech recognition devices.

On one hand, a functionalist perspective might state that we do not need to understand the human's perceptual system to model the functioning of that system. Certainly, airplanes do not flap their wings. But the principles of aerodynamics that govern bird flight also govern the flight of planes. We understand much less about the principles that govern human speech perception currently than was understood about aerodynamics when the first successful plane was flown. Even if we do not implement human speech perception algorithms as the internal structure of recognition devices, understanding the operation of human speech perception may suggest ways of improving computer speech recognition systems.

For example, consider the problem of recognizing speech produced by different talkers. At present, some speaker-independent systems are restricted to tiny vocabularies (on the order of less than 20 words) because small vocabularies can be constructed to maximize the acoustic-phonetic differences between words, even when produced by a broad range of talkers. Also, acoustic data must be collected from a very large group of talkers in order to capture the most general acoustic characterization of the vocabulary across talkers. Since the amount of data is a function of the vocabulary size and the set of talkers, given the large number of talkers that are needed even small vocabularies represent a huge data analysis problem.

Computer recognition systems may therefore benefit from a better understanding of how people recognize speech produced by different talkers. The prototypical idea of speaker-independence is that a recognition system should recognize speech produced by any talker, without any prior experience with that talker's speech. However, it is interesting to consider that even human listeners are probably not speaker-independent recognition systems in the way that engineers seek to develop speaker-independence for computers. For example, word recognition is faster and more accurate for speech produced by a single talker than it is for speech produced by several talkers (Mullennix et al., 1989; Nusbaum & Morin, 1989). Thus, speech recognition performance in humans is affected by talker variability.

Talkers differ in head-size, vocal tract length and shape, and the ways in which they articulate utterances. These differences affect the acoustic properties of speech such that listeners may need this information to recognize correctly a particular talker's speech. For example, Peterson and Barney (1952) demonstrated quite clearly that two vowels produced by different talkers may have similar acoustic patterns and the same vowel produced by different talkers may have very different acoustic patterns. In order to resolve the many-to-many relationships between the acoustic patterns of speech and the linguistic interpretation of those patterns, listeners need to use information about the vocal characteristics of talkers.

Joos (1948) suggested that perhaps listeners normalize differences between talkers by calibrating their perceptual system on an initial greeting such as, "Hi. How are you?" In other words, he proposed that the necessary information about the talker's vocal characteristics can be extracted from such stereotypical greetings, for which the phonetic structure would be specified a priori. In fact, this approach is entirely possible. Gerstman (1968) has shown that if listeners can recognize correctly a talker's point vowels (i.e., the vowels in heat, hot, and hoot, which are the extremes of the American English vowel space—the acoustic range of vowels), all of the acoustic patterns for that talker's other vowels can be inferred correctly. Moreover, Ladefoged and Broadbent (1957) demonstrated that listeners perceive target words such as bit and bet differently when the same word is heard presented in context sentences synthesized to represent different talkers. Thus, listeners modify recognition based on the vocal characteristics of a talker conveyed by a context sentence. Listeners seem to use a context utterance to form a representation of the talker's vowel space that is used to guide recognition of subsequent utterances.

Nusbaum and Morin (1989) have provided further support for the conclusion that listeners use context to map out the talker's vowel space. In addition, however, they have shown that listeners seem to use another mechanism for recognizing speech when a prior context is not available. Listeners appear to use a more computationally intensive process for recognizing speech when they first encounter a talker or when they encounter multiple talkers in succession. Moreover, this second mechanism seems to operate based on cues that Syrdal and Gopal (1986) suggested should be relevant for normalizing talker differences (Morin & Nusbaum, 1989).

These findings on how humans recognize speech from multiple talkers point to a way for computer systems to achieve the same goal. Most generally, these results suggest that recognition systems should employ several different approaches to talker normalization. The effectiveness and robustness of human speech perception may be less a function of having a single, highly optimized algorithm than having available a set of different algorithms each of which may operate most effectively under different conditions. Moreover, research on speech perception suggests that the engineer's idealization of recognition performance may not be achievable even by the most effective recognition system available—the human listener. An unrealistic goal for developing a recognition device may mislead engineers from seeking more pragmatic solutions to recognition problems.

More specifically, in the present case, the results from speech research suggest that listeners do not operate in accordance with the prototypical concept of perfect speaker-independence. On one hand, performance is much better than chance when speakers vary, but on the other hand it is still worse than when the speaker is constant. Furthermore, the research on human listeners suggests that it may be better to employ two different kinds of mechanisms rather than a single normalization algorithm. One algorithm should be designed to develop a representation of talker-specific information based on a "calibration utterance" or set of utterances that is spoken in lieu of training (cf. Gerstman, 1968). Indeed, this kind of speaker-specific "tuning" is employed in the IBM Tangora system. A set of sentences spoken by the operator is processed to modify the recognition model to incorporate speaker-specific information. This is the only source of talker-specific information for the recognition model and thus represents the only normalization process. It is interesting that the calibration utterances were chosen randomly rather than designed specifically to reveal, through their linguistic properties, the acoustic properties that are most diagnostic of a talker's vocal characteristics. It is possible that this speaker-tuning process could be made more effective by a more analytic selection of utterances or by modifying the process to adaptively select for a talker a set of diagnostic utterances contingent on the analysis of an initial token.

A second normalization algorithm should be capable of performing recognition even without prior experience with a particular talker's speech (cf. Syrdal & Gopal, 1986). Although this algorithm may be less accurate in recognition performance, it could operate in circumstances where the previous algorithm could not, such as when talkers change quickly (e.g., when several different speakers are issuing commands). By combining these algorithms, a recognition system could adapt to a talker over time, using vocal characteristics extracted from each token to improve the recognition of subsequent tokens. This is somewhat similar to the adaptive recognition function in the Dragon System recognizer, which can update its recognition model using speaker-specific information computed during recognition processing, without requiring a new, separate training session (Baker, 1975).

Addressing the issue of recognizing speech from multiple talkers is only one specific case for which basic research on human speech perception could affect the development of recognition technology. Every aspect of the recognition process, from the encoding and representation of speech signals to the matching of an input utterance to the stored vocabulary to the decision regarding which item in the vocabulary was spoken, may be affected by research on human speech perception. For example, the acoustic properties of an input utterance are encoded by a recognition system into a simple temporal or spectral representation which is very impoverished compared to our knowledge about the auditory representation of speech in the peripheral nervous system. For years it has been accepted that human listeners encode speech into a neurogram (like a spectrogram; see Licklider, 1952) as the first stage of auditory processing in speech perception. However, while complex spectro-temporal properties appear to form the primary representation of speech for the human auditory system, the precise form of this representation is still a debated research question (see Carlson & Granstrom, 1982). There have been several recent attempts to create more neurophysiologically plausible models of auditory coding for speech recognition systems (Lyon, 1982; Seneff, 1986) and these approaches may improve recognition performance in computers (see Searle et al., 1979). Indeed, Cohen (1989) has shown that an auditory front end can improve an existing speech recognition device based on a statistical pattern matching model, although the generality of improvement provided by neurophysiologically plausible auditory coding has been questioned for other pattern-matching approaches (Blomberg et al., 1986). Moreover, there is clearly a great deal of important information in the temporal structure of speech (see Scott, 1980) that is not currently exploited in speech recognition systems.

With additional knowledge about the use of temporal structure in human speech perception, this information could be brought to bear on pattern recognition by computers. In fact, although speech recognition devices only represent an utterance as a single, simplified acoustic pattern, human listeners undoubtedly represent and maintain several different, partially redundant, complex spectro-temporal representations in different parts of the auditory system, each slightly more appropriate for different types of perceptual decisions.

Similarly, while current speech recognition systems employ only one strategy for segmenting fluent speech into word-length sections of waveform for subsequent pattern matching, human listeners may employ several different strategies simultaneously. Whereas a recognition system may either model the acoustic cues to word boundaries explicitly or carry out segmentation as a consequence of sequential recognition, humans may flexibly select among these and other strategies to determine the optimal approach for any particular utterance. Speech perception research has shown that there are some acoustic-phonetic cues that listeners may to use to locate word boundaries in natural fluent speech (Nakatani & Dukes, 1977). In addition, listeners appear to use stress patterns and contrasts between strong and weak syllables as information about the presence of a word boundary (Cutler & Norris, 1988; Taft, 1983). For some utterances, human listeners may also perform "segmentation by recognition" (Henly & Nusbaum, 1991), in which recognition of a word locates the boundaries of its neighboring words within an utterance. In addition, unlike computer recognition systems, which are rigid, human listeners can learn to adopt new segmentation strategies with moderate amounts of experience and feedback about performance (Greenspan et al., 1988).

Similarly, humans are much more flexible about recognition processing than are computers. Recognition devices represent all utterances using the same type of acoustic analysis, compare input speech with vocabulary items with a single pattern matching algorithm, and decide which item matches best with a single decision metric. Humans can employ a number of different sources of information during recognition and can trade these off against each other in various ways. Foss and Blank (1980) argued that listeners can recognize phonemes using acoustic-phonetic information from the speech signal in a bottom-up pattern matching mechanism as well as make top-down inferences about the presence of phonemes based on knowledge of lexical structure. Recently, Nusbaum and DeGroot (1990) have provided evidence supporting this idea that listeners are flexible in the process by which they recognize the sound patterns of speech. This same kind of flexibility also shows up when listeners recognize spoken words. Word recognition seems to trade off bottom-up processing of acoustic-phonetic information against inferences made on the basis of linguistic context (Cole & Jakimik, 1980; Grosjean, 1980; Marslen-Wilson & Welsh, 1978).

There are two general conclusions that can be drawn from these examples of research on human speech perception. First, although there may be some surface similarities between particular algorithms and some aspect of processing carried out by listeners, there are numerous differences. A better understanding of the representations and processes that mediate human speech perception will probably have a significant impact on the development of more effective speech recognition systems. Indeed, since most recognition systems were constructed without exploiting any current knowledge about speech perception, it is entirely possible that applying what little we know about the perceptual processing of speech to recognition systems could improve recognition performance.

Second, by comparison to humans, speech recognition devices employ extremely simple strategies. Recognition devices use a single representation of speech and a single approach to segmentation and pattern comparison. Human listeners are both flexible and adaptive. Speech perception may involve a number of different, redundant representations and processes, allowing the listener to select the best approach for any specific set of conditions. In addition, as speech perceivers, we can learn from experience and adopt new strategies for recognition. In fact, flexibility and adaptability may be the hallmarks of human cognitive processing compared to artificial intelligence. It is very likely that these abilities are central to explaining superior human performance in tasks for which computers are currently adequate. Certainly in any human-computer interaction, the human will be the more flexible and adaptable participant.

There are really two conclusions to be drawn from this simplistic comparison of human and computer processing of speech, one for the engineer concerned with developing more effective speech recognition devices and one for the engineer concerned with incorporating speech recognition into a particular application. In terms of designing a speech recognition system, it is clear that there is a great deal of basic information about human speech perception that could be exploited in improving computer speech recognition. In terms of the most effective use of speech recognition systems in applications, it is important to exploit the flexibility and adaptability of the human operator as much as possible. In order to do this effectively, it is necessary to consider carefully the interface between the operator and the speech recognition system.

4.5 The User Interface

There are actually two user interfaces that must be considered: The recognizer interface involves the operator's interactions with the speech recognizer— how people speak to it, what they say, how feedback is presented to them. The application interface consists of the transmission of information between the operator and the target application, such as a database management system or word processing system, through the speech recognition system. In this section, our primary concern is with the information and control provided by the recognizer interface. The term "user interface" will generally refer to the recognizer interface throughout this chapter, unless specifically qualified.

According to Norman (1983), a user interface not only provides communication and control for a system, but also conveys a system image. The system image can be thought of as a kind of depiction of the operation of the system itself. The system image is essentially the set of displays and controls that are provided to the user, along with the coordination among these during the use of the system. Since the user interface is the main point of contact between an operator and a system, it is through this interface that the user forms a mental model of the operation of the system. In essence, this mental model is the way the user thinks about the system, including the beliefs, inferences, and expectations that arise from experience with a particular system image. The mental model of a system allows the user to interact with, interpret, understand, and predict the behavior of the system, serving as a mental guide for the user's behavior. In a well-designed interface, the system image reflects the operating principles of the system, directing the user toward appropriate, productive interactions with the system.

In considering the development of a user interface for speech recognition systems, although there is often discussion of the type of feedback that should be provided to the user (e.g., Van Peursem, 1985), there has been very little discussion about the nature of the system image conveyed to users. This is an important consideration, because the system image is the basis for the mental model formed by the user, and the mental model determines the manner in which speech is produced, that is, the speaking behavior of the talker. It is easy to imagine that before using a computer speech recognition system, an operator has a mental model of speech recognition that is at odds with reality. This model is probably based largely on human-to-human communication and could lead the operator to interact with a recognition device in ways that are not effective. Consider one example of the error recovery strategies used in human-to-human communication when communication fails: In talking to a non-native listener (e.g., a native German speaker presented with English), it is fairly common for a talker to repeat an utterance more loudly even though the original utterance was quite audible. The "system image" presented by the non-native listener (i.e., the listener's behavioral response to an utterance that is not understood) seems to accord well with a listener who has a hearing impairment rather than someone who doesn't know the language; consequently, this is the mental model the speaker forms of the listener. Thus, the speaker's response to the feedback is guided by the wrong mental model. While speaking loudly is effective as an error correction strategy for a listener with a hearing impairment, an improved signal-to-noise ratio does not improve recognition for someone who speaks a different language.

Similarly, this mental model would not be a good one for guiding speaking behavior when interacting with a recognition device, even though it is probably the default one, given a failure to recognize an utterance. In designing a user interface, it is important to provide feedback and displays that are not just informative about the present state of the recognition system, but are also informative about its overall operation. It is also important for the talker to receive information that allows the construction of a more appropriate mental model of a computer speech recognition system. Telling the operator not to shout and to speak more carefully or to speak as they did during training would provide better guidance than just giving a beep signal to indicate a recognition failure. In any case, information provided by the user interface should allow the operator to infer a mental model that would direct appropriate speaking behavior and successful error correction strategies.

To date, the role of the system image for a speech recognition device has not been explored systematically. As a result, there are few empirical results that could guide the development of an effective system image. Although the recognition systems are governed by relatively simple operating principles, especially those with small vocabularies, overlooking the role of the system image in conveying those principles to the user ignores a potentially important method of increasing the effective use of speech recognition technology. Moreover, as the complexity of recognition systems increases, efficient use of these devices will depend on interfaces that modulate the user's expectations about how to speak, about recognition performance, and about how to control the recognizer's functions.

Recently, Zoltan-Ford (1984) demonstrated how the system image of speech technology can influence the speaking behavior of users. Subjects spoke freely with unconstrained syntax and vocabulary to a computer simulation of a recognition system, which responded using a limited vocabulary and syntax. Without explicit instruction, the subjects learned the syntactic and lexical constraints provided by the simulation, and adopted them in their own speech to the computer. Thus, it is apparent that the user does indeed form a mental model about speech technology through relatively subtle interactions with the user interface. Furthermore, by projecting the appropriate system image, it is possible to modify a user's speaking behavior (and thus the acoustic-phonetic properties of the user's speech) to conform to the requirements of a recognition system, thereby improving performance. This might occur by the same process that allows us to alter the complexity of our speech depending on which human listeners we are addressing. Perhaps talkers are guided by a general communicative principle of observing their listeners' responses to determine how complex the utterances should be; this is why speech to young children (sometimes called "motherese") is different from speech to professional colleagues. The same strategy might generate a "userese" style of speech, appropriate to the capabilities of current speech recognition systems (Biermann et al., 1985; Haggard, 1983).

Although we have been focusing on the global effects of the user interface on the operator, in terms of inducing a mental model of the recognition system, the user interface also has more immediate, local effects on the operator's behavior. To some extent, we can think of the interaction between the user and the speech recognition device as a kind of dialogue. However, the interaction between the user and the device is typically not as flexible as the give-and-take of information between two people engaged in a normal communicative interaction such as a conversation. Nevertheless, the recognition system does provide some feedback—responses to the user's input—that guides the user's subsequent actions. For example, the system provides feedback when it tells the user what word it has recognized or requests clarification of a word it could not recognize. The operator's response to this information will be governed by a combination of the immediate demands of the situation (e.g., fix the error) and the mental model that suggests strategies for generating responses (e.g., speak more clearly).

Although there has been some research about the type of feedback needed to improve the effectiveness of recognition technology by influencing the user's responses (e.g., Schurick et al., 1985), it is unlikely that the results of this research will be appropriate for the next generation of speech recognition systems, which will process connected or continuous speech with large vocabularies. For example, Schurick et al. found that word-by-word visual feedback, confirming each recognized word, was helpful in a small vocabulary data entry task. But it is unclear whether word-by-word visual feedback in a large vocabulary task like dictation will speed up the process or slow it down. Like modality, the amount of feedback can also be varied. Mountford, North, Metz, and Warner (1982) provided users with varying amounts of feedback in an aircraft navigation data entry task; for example, in "verbose" mode, feedback followed each entry, while in "succinct" mode there was no feedback after entries. Users preferred the succinct mode, even though they felt it required more attention, because the verbose style made the transactions too lengthy. Another aspect of feedback is its timing. For nonspeech computer interactions, it has been found that users' tolerance for delays can vary, depending on the feedback they are waiting for, such as a "ready" signal or an error message; in fact, in some circumstances, error messages can be annoying if they are too fast (see Rosenthal, 1979, for a review). Simpson et al. (1987) recommend selecting a feedback modality and amount that are "appropriate" for the application at hand. They do not give guidelines on how to determine the appropriate verbosity and modality, but basic and applied research can address this question. It is possible that feedback from speech recognizers will be easiest for users to assimilate if its modality, verbosity, and timing are similar to the feedback that humans give each other during a conversation.

When one person talks to another, communication errors are inevitable. When speaking to a speech recognition system, recognition errors are much more frequent and error recovery is more difficult than it is with humans. Sometimes a recognition device makes a substitution error; that is, it matches the user's utterance to the wrong vocabulary item. For example, the user says, "eight," but the machine identifies the word as "date." In other errors, the system might "recognize" nonspeech, such as a cough or background noise, as a vocabulary item. When either of these happen, the system will proceed as if there were no error; it is unaware that it has made a mistake. The human operator must realize that an error has occurred and step in to set it straight. Thus, every user interface must have a mechanism that allows the user to detect and correct substitution errors (Simpson et al., 1987). This has implications for the style of feedback a system provides. First, the user has to receive enough feedback, in an appropriate modality, to be able to see that an error has occurred, either directly by noting the state of the recognition system or indirectly by determining that an inappropriate action was taken by the recognizer or the application. Second, the timing of the feedback should allow the user to correct the error before it causes any trouble, but perhaps, depending on the task, after reaching a convenient stopping point, like the end of a sentence during dictation.

Besides substitution errors, a different type of error also occurs when a person talks to a speech recognition system: the system sometimes fails to recognize any word at all. There are several varieties of this problem. In some cases, the operator says a word, but the system does not detect any speech. As with substitution errors, the system does not "know" it has made this error; the user is responsible for detecting the error from the overall behavior of the system. When the system is providing the user with word-by-word feedback, the user can readily identify the problem and simply repeat the word, perhaps speaking more loudly or adjusting the microphone. When a different feedback style is used, it should allow the operator to see that a word was missed earlier, and to insert the word (i.e., correct the error).

In another type of error, the system detects an utterance, but cannot identify it. The utterance might be too different from any vocabulary item for it to be recognized, or it might be similar to more than one vocabulary item, and the system cannot choose among the alternatives. The recognition device, rather than the operator, is the one that detects these errors. Its threshold for error detection, however, is determined by humans, and should be adjusted to meet task needs.

For example, a system can be set so that it requires a very close match between the input and a stored vocabulary item, or it can be set to match the input word to the most similar vocabulary item, even if they are rather different acoustically. Similarly, if the input is similar to two different vocabulary items, the system can simply select the closest matching item, or it can signal an error if the second-best candidate is too similar to the input. In one way, this is similar to what a human listener does. Human listeners do not understand every word they hear; when they are not confident that they have understood what a speaker said, they ask for clarification (Van Peursem, 1982). A speech recognition system does the same thing, but the user or software developers should determine its "confidence" in accordance with the needs of the task.

When the recognition system detects an error, it must present an error message, to notify the user that an utterance was not recognized and request a clarification. There are numerous types of error messages. To begin with, the message can be presented visually or auditorily. If auditory, the signal can take the form of synthetic speech ("Please repeat") or nonspeech, such as a beep. A beep can be accompanied by a visual signal, such as a blinking cursor at the error location on a screen (Morland, 1983). The request for a correction from the user can take a variety of forms, as well. If the system has narrowed its answer down to two word candidates, it can present the candidates as choices for the user ("Which did you say: five or nine?"). A few investigators have made recommendations about the types of error messages that promote efficient error correction (Van Peursem, 1982). For example, Schmandt, Arons, and Simmons (1985) suggest that queries about an unrecognized word should be structured to elicit one-word answers from the talker, rather than sentences like, "I said X."

This type of error correction strategy may be effective for restricted vocabulary tasks such as data entry, but it is likely to be less effective for large vocabulary dictation tasks for which people have grown accustomed to other types of correction queries. Indeed, when human secretaries miss a word while taking dictation, they often repeat the whole phrase to ask for clarification of a single word (e.g., "...revise our policies and what?"), rather than simply asking, "What did you say?" The person giving dictation responds using the same phrase ("...our policies and procedures."). These interactions appear to be an easy and "natural" way to correct errors during dictation (see Levelt & Kelter, 1982, for a study of this phenomenon in answering questions). Yet such interactions are very different from the single-word correction methods of small vocabulary systems. In order to select the most efficient error correction methods, the user's natural speaking style must be weighed against ease of recognition; then, as Schmandt et al. (1985) suggest, the error message can be designed to elicit the appropriate type of response from the user.

Given that a user interface has been developed to provide basic information about the state of a recognizer and to convey an appropriate system image, how closely should the interface be integrated with the recognizer itself? In most cases, not very closely. Norman (1983) has suggested that in any domain it is important to separate the user interface or system image from the rest of a system. The separate interface module makes it much easier to modify and improve the interface independent of the main functions of the system. In the case of a speech recognition device, this means keeping the information display and control functions that the operator sees (e.g., asking for clarification, confirming the recognized word) separate from the implementation of the recognition algorithm itself. On the other hand, it is most efficient to handle the application interface differently: It is important for the developers of an application (e.g., a word processor) to build the interface with the recognizer into the application. Since it is unlikely that the applications developers will be familiar with the requirements of a speech interface, they should also receive guidance on how speech can be integrated into an application, along with examples of error correction procedures and feedback to the user. It is also important to note that just as the user interface to the recognition system will provide the basis for a mental model of the operation of the recognition device, and the application interface will provide the basis for a mental model of the operation of the application itself, the interactions between the recognizer interface and the application interface will provide the basis for forming a mental model of the operation of speech recognition within the application.

The user interface with both the recognition device and the application governs the user's behavior in two ways. At the global level, the system image conveyed by the interface allows the operator to construct a mental model that specifies the strategies appropriate for using the system. At the local level, specific information about the current state of the system allows the operator to select the most appropriate action from among those strategies in response to any particular situation. To the extent that the operator infers an accurate mental model and feedback is informative about the state of the system, the operator will be able to respond optimally to the demands of any particular task using the recognition device. Given the optimal user interface, then, the success of a speech recognition device for a particular application will be limited only by the accuracy of the basic pattern recognition system itself, and by the appropriateness of using speech recognition for controlling the application. Conversely, if a recognition device is extremely accurate, the success of system use will be limited primarily by the adequacy of the user interface and, again, by the appropriateness of speech input for the application. However, since it is unlikely that either the user interface or the recognition algorithm will be optimally designed, the limitations of both will interact to degrade overall system performance. Lower recognition accuracy will require more accurate and diagnostic error detection to facilitate error correction—in other words, more interactions between the user and the system, and more opportunities for any flaws in the user interface to have a detrimental effect. Thus, in order to understand how successful using a particular speech recognition device will be for any application, it is important to measure the recognition performance of the speech recognition system.

4.6 Performance Assessment

The success of implementing a speech recognition system as part of an application depends to a large degree on the recognition performance of the system. If a recognition system has a very high error rate, it may be preferable to use an interface technology other than speech recognition, unless there is no other recourse (e.g., both the operator's hands are occupied as part of the application). When selecting among several vendors' products, it is important to consider the performance of the recognition device along with its cost and features. Basic information regarding the performance of a speech recognition system is important for assessing the suitability of the system for a particular application and for making price/performance comparisons between systems. Moreover, recognition performance represents a significant human factors issue in the implementation of this technology, perhaps more so than for other types of technologies such as keyboards or mice. As noted earlier, as recognition performance decreases, an operator will depend more on the user interface for providing diagnostic information about problems and for suggesting ways of solving those problems. Furthermore, decreases in recognition accuracy may increase the difficulty of controlling the application, thereby causing other types of human factors problems. However, since performance assessment has not been critical to other interface technologies (such as keyboards), it has not generally been viewed as part of the human factors of speech recognition systems.

Recognition performance is an important human factors issue that must be investigated as part of the process of incorporating a recognition device into an application and as part of the development of the user interface. However, very little research investigating the performance of speech recognition systems has been carried out systematically, that is, under carefully controlled and matched conditions (although see Doddington & Schalk, 1981; Baker, 1982). For example, some vendors of recognition systems have cited performance of their technology at 98-99% accuracy, without specifying the conditions under which testing was carried out. Without knowing something about the structure of the testing vocabulary, how many talkers and tokens of speech were used, how training was carried out, or what signal-to-noise ratio or microphone was used, it is not possible to determine what 99% correct recognition means, or how it compares to some other performance measure.

A systematic approach to performance testing of speech recognition systems is important for several reasons. First, routine performance testing is necessary for improving existing recognition systems and developing new and more robust recognition algorithms. Without measuring recognition performance under controlled conditions, it is almost impossible to determine whether changes in a recognition algorithm have resulted in reliable improvements in recognition performance. Also, detailed analyses of a recognizer's performance can provide diagnostic information about the specific problems inherent in a particular recognition algorithm and can suggest how an algorithm can be improved to optimize performance.

Second, performance testing provides data on speech recognition systems that may be important for determining how appropriate a particular recognition system is for a specific application. For example, if a particular application requires highly accurate recognition, there must be a procedure for determining which systems offer high enough accuracy. For some applications, the operator has little choice about using the recognition device and so will simply be forced to accept high error rates, especially if there is no alternative technology or interface. On the other hand, customers of a service (e.g., database access or bank balance querying) might well turn to a competitive service using a different technology if recognition accuracy is low.

Finally, performance testing can serve an important function for advancing basic research on speech recognition. Detailed analyses of the data collected in performance tests can provide fundamental knowledge about individual differences in speech production, the effects of noise on speech production, the role of lexical stress in distinguishing vocabulary items, and a number of other basic issues in speech research. Although recognition systems have not played a large role in basic speech research in the past, their potential contribution may be substantial (see Yuchtman & Nusbaum, 1986; Yuchtman, Nusbaum, & Davis, 1986). Thus, performance testing of recognition systems is important to a number of issues surrounding the development, application, and advancement of recognition technology, as well as the advancement of basic speech research.

No single test procedure can completely address all the possible issues related to the assessment of recognition performance. For example, performance testing carried out with input utterances from a stored, standard database of speech will not produce precisely the same effects as testing carried out within an applications environment with "real users". (For our purposes we can define real users as subjects sampled from the population that will actually use the application, as opposed to talkers who were hired just to produce speech.) These different test procedures address different aspects of performance. A standard test, using a standard and publicly available database of speech, permits applications-independent comparisons of different recognition devices across testing sessions and testing laboratories—a kind of benchmark test. In contrast, a test carried out with real users will assess how a particular user population (perhaps with very specific characteristics) will interact with a recognition system when performing a specific task. Although it is likely that the general pattern of test results for a number of recognition systems on one type of test would be related to results on the other type, there may be important differences. Certainly the latter type of test will provide information that is much more specific and appropriate to designing a user interface, whereas the first type of test may be more useful in developing and improving recognition algorithms.

Unfortunately, of the few systematic performance assessment programs carried out with recognition systems, none have been reported comparing a wide range of recognition devices across several application-specific tests together with application-independent benchmarks. If such data were available, we could empirically determine the relationship between different types of tests, and use that information to attempt to generalize from one set of results to predict relative performance across applications. In the absence of such data, however, we can try to anticipate the factors that should be most significant in determining performance, and assess the relative impact of these factors on recognition performance for several systems. Even in the absence of application-specific tests, data such as these should provide a rough guide to the relative performance of different recognition devices.

Minimally, then, without the definition provided by a specific application, the most general kind of performance testing should be carried out. Optimally, the performance testing protocol should be clearly specified so that the testing methodology can be replicated over time in other locations. The development of an explicit and coherent testing procedure permits a direct comparison of performance data collected in different laboratories. Furthermore, using a standard, readily available database of speech that is in the public domain provides another level of comparability among test results from different laboratories.

In addition, performance testing should be carried out automatically, under computer control. In general, when performance assessment is carried out informally, a few (friendly) users are given access to a recognition system and allowed to play with it. Under these conditions, speech varies from test to test, and users may select for themselves how much training to provide and how to score recognition results. As a result these data are the least useful for comparison purposes because of the uncontrolled nature of the assessment procedure. However, even when a standard database of speech is used and a specified testing protocol is followed, it is still possible to introduce variability into results by carrying out the testing under direct human supervision. The timing and presentation of the speech may vary when a human operator starts the speech signal (from either a tape recording or digital playback), and scoring may depend on the operator's interpretation of the recognizer's response to the speech. Nusbaum and Pisoni (1987) advocated carrying out testing under computer control to eliminate as much operator-introduced variability and measurement error as possible and described a system that was implemented for this purpose.

Using a computer-controlled testing system, with a standard database of speech, Nusbaum and Pisoni (1987) tested six speaker-dependent speech recognition devices. They used a database of speech collected by Doddington and Schalk (1981) and distributed by the National Bureau of Standards. The speech was produced by eight male and eight female talkers and consists of two vocabularies. The TI-20 vocabulary contains the ten digits and ten control words: YES, NO, GO, START, STOP, ENTER, ERASE, RUBOUT, REPEAT, and HELP. The TI-Alphabet vocabulary contains the names of the 26 letters of the alphabet. For each vocabulary item, each talker produced 10 tokens for training purposes and another 16 tokens for recognition testing.

The words in the TI-20 vocabulary are highly discriminable, with the majority of confusions occurring between GO and NO. By comparison, the alphabet is a much more difficult vocabulary because it contains several confusable subsets of letters, such as {B, C, D, E, G, P, T, V, Z} and {A, J, K}. By testing performance using a relatively discriminable vocabulary and a relatively difficult vocabulary, recognition accuracy is measured at two extremes on the performance curve for a specific device. Thus, it may be possible to predict the relative performance of recognition systems on an application vocabulary by interpolation. If the rank ordering of performance by a variety of recognition devices is similar for both very difficult and highly discriminable vocabularies, then the same rank ordering might be obtained for most vocabularies in between these extremes. In other words, if the same recognizers consistently perform well on a range of vocabularies, and other recognizers perform poorly on these vocabularies, the same relative performance rank-ordering of these recognizers might be obtained for almost any vocabulary.

There are other reasons to measure performance on different vocabularies. The TI-20 vocabulary is a good choice because it has been used for other tests and therefore can serve as a standard benchmark of performance. Unfortunately, however, the TI-20 database has been circulating in the public domain for a number of years, and it is possible that recognition systems were "tuned" specifically for this database. It is likely that systems have been developed, tested, and improved using this database to assess performance in the vendors' own laboratories. As a consequence, performance on this database might simply be better because algorithms were tested and improved using these speech samples and this vocabulary. By comparison, the TI-Alphabet database was not distributed in the public domain long enough to have been used in the development of the systems tested by Nusbaum and Pisoni (1987). As a result, it is unlikely that those systems were optimized for performance on these speech samples.

Another reason for testing performance on different databases of speech is to determine how recognition performance depends on the acoustic-phonetic structure of the vocabulary. Changes in vocabulary size and confusability are likely to have very large effects on recognition performance. By measuring performance with more than one vocabulary, it is possible to investigate the relative influence of different vocabularies on the performance of a number of different recognition systems and to carry out appropriate comparisons of the performance of the same recognizers under different conditions.

Nusbaum and Pisoni (1987) noted several ways in which a particular recognition algorithm might perform better under certain conditions. For example, they measured recognition performance on several different tests, each based on a different number of training tokens: one, three, or five. Training on one token is, in some respects, biased against recognition systems that are based on statistical modeling principles (such as hidden Markov models) compared to template-based systems (Pallett, 1985). On the other hand, for a particular recognition device, baseline performance data after training on a single token, in comparison to training with several tokens, will indicate the relative importance of training on more speech samples. Furthermore, performance after training with one token may indicate what could be expected in performance if users are unwilling to go through complex training protocols and engage in only minimal vocabulary enrollment. In terms of human factors problems, it is entirely possible, under some working conditions, that operators will seek to minimize the demands of their workload by reducing the amount of training.

In general, the results of the comparison reported by Nusbaum and Pisoni (1987) were somewhat surprising. Although there were some performance differences among the recognition systems with minimal training, these differences were greatly reduced when the devices were trained according to the vendors' specifications. Moreover, there was a fairly complex relationship among algorithm type, vocabulary difficulty, and the effect of amount of training. For the TI-20 vocabulary, which is simple and relatively discriminable, training on three tokens of speech produced the largest improvement for all recognition devices. Training on more tokens of speech did not produce reliable performance improvements for most of the recognition devices, including those based on statistical modeling techniques, such as the Dragon system. Even providing as many as ten training tokens for the systems that employed statistical modeling did not reduce substitution errors compared to training with three tokens of speech. However, on the TI-Alphabet, a much more difficult vocabulary, the performance of almost all the recognition systems improved reliably when the number of training tokens was increased above three. In addition, the systems that employed statistical modeling made reliably more effective use of ten tokens of speech—which exceeded the training ability for template-based systems. These results indicate that increased training is more beneficial to recognition performance with more difficult vocabularies. Thus, for difficult and confusable vocabularies, there may be a performance advantage for statistical algorithms, which can take advantage of more training tokens. For more discriminable vocabularies, however, it is important to note that performance differences among recognition systems were slight when the devices were trained according to the vendors' instructions.

In general, examining recognition performance as a function of training may provide some indication of the optimal amount of training required for a particular recognizer and vocabulary. An asymptote in recognition performance as a function of training indicates the minimum amount of training required to obtain the highest level of recognition performance. Moreover, performance curves may also indicate the relationship between increased training and increased performance. Since training the recognition devices requires time and effort, for some applications it may be important to assess the costs of increased training against the benefits in recognition performance. The data reported by Nusbaum and Pisoni (1987) suggest that in some cases the cost of additional training may not be justified in terms of the size of the improved recognition accuracy that results.

Although it is reasonable that users will prefer a system with high recognition accuracy, it is not clear to what extent users would accept reduced recognition accuracy for other features of a system. For example, different recognition systems differ substantially in their speed of recognition (Nusbaum & Pisoni, 1987). For some applications, users might accept lower accuracy with a very fast system response time. In other applications, users might accept lower accuracy in a system that allows them to dictate connected speech, even if accuracy is lower than in a recognition system that requires isolated word input. A measure of overall performance must acknowledge a variety of factors such as these (Simpson et al., 1987). Furthermore, these tradeoffs can be addressed only in the context of a particular application. Often, for example, people dictate drafts of documents, which will be proofread. In such cases, recognition errors are not costly; they are likely to be detected during proofreading (Mangione, 1985).

Similarly, it is also possible that listeners will accept different levels of accuracy for different types of errors. Imagine that the recognition algorithm of one device biases it to make errors that are spectrally based whereas another device tends to make errors that are based on temporal properties of utterances. Spectrally based errors might result in confusions among certain vowels that are similar in frequency patterns, such as /o/ and /u/, or among stop consonants differing in place of articulation, such as /p/, /t/ , and /k/. Temporally based errors might result in confusions of segments of that differ in duration, such as /b/ and /w/, or /t/ and /s/. It is entirely possible that although one recognizer has a nominally lower error rate on a standard performance testing database, the nature of the errors made by that device for some specific application would actually produce worse performance on the vocabulary specific to the application. As recognition algorithms become more complex and sophisticated, it is possible that the nature and distribution of errors will differ among recognition systems. Thus, in the future, it will not be sufficient to report the overall accuracy of a recognition device; it will be necessary to diagnose its error patterns.

Ohala (1982) has suggested that diagnostic vocabularies could be used for this purpose. Words differ from one another on a number of dimensions (e.g., stress pattern, word length, phonotactic properties), and recognition devices may differ in the ways they process and recognize these dimensions. It should be possible to construct vocabularies that represent a wide range of variation along these different dimensions. These vocabularies could then be used for performance assessment. An examination of the pattern of errors across these dimensions should make it possible to diagnose the "recognition deficiencies" of a particular system. By analyzing a proposed application vocabulary along the same dimensions as the diagnostic vocabulary, it should be possible to predict which application utterances would be most confusable for a specific recognition device based on the pattern of errors on the diagnostic vocabulary.

As recognition systems become more sophisticated and complex, the problems of assessing recognition performance will also increase. Similarly, all the human factors issues surrounding the use of these recognition systems will change and become more complicated. For example, while we have attempted to spell out some guidelines for performance testing with the current generation of recognition systems, we can only begin to imagine the performance assessment issues that will arise in the future. Simply classifying recognition errors for systems that accept fluent speech input will be a much more difficult task. For the current generation of systems, the possible errors are quite limited: A recognition device can fail to respond to an utterance or it can substitute a different vocabulary item. However, when the number of responses can vary as well (i.e., the number of responses may be different from the number of words in the input utterance) and recognition errors can be compounded by segmentation errors (i.e., misplacing a word boundary), scoring recognition accuracy and characterizing recognition performance will be much more difficult. Similarly, as we consider increasing vocabulary size dramatically and shifting from speech recognition to language understanding with concomitant increases in linguistic knowledge, the human factors issues will become considerably more complex and we can point to the need for more research in this area.

4.7 The Next Generation of Recognition Systems

Vocabulary size is one of the first attributes of recognition systems that is viewed as a limitation and therefore desirable to change. As vocabulary size increases, there will be problems in determining how to train a speaker-dependent system. For example, there may be 5000 or more words in an isolated utterance recognition system, or hundreds of thousands of possible sentences in a connected speech recognition system, and it is not practical to train a device on all the utterances that it must recognize. As a consequence, it will be important to combine talker tuning of a recognition system (in which a talker provides a few key utterances prior to using the system) and talker adaptation (in which the stored representations of vocabulary items are changed on the fly following each recognition pass) in order to achieve acceptable performance. As noted earlier, these approaches seem much closer to the way human listeners take into account information specific to a particular talker. However, these approaches raise the problem of developing tuning vocabularies, sets of training utterances that inform the recognition system about the speech of the particular talker it must recognize, and training protocols, methods for collecting the training utterances that ensure that talkers speak the same way during training as they will when actually using the system. Unfortunately, there has been little or no systematic research on this problem or on other human factors problems that stem from the size of the vocabulary in the next generation of recognition systems.

In fact, there has been only one well-documented investigation of some of the issues that may arise with large vocabulary recognition systems. Gould et al. (1984) measured users' speed of composing and proofing letters in a dictation task, using a simulation of a recognition system with several different vocabulary sizes. They found that, for users who were experienced at dictating letters, speed of dictation with connected speech input was independent of vocabulary size, but speed of dictation with isolated words was greatly affected by vocabulary size. For these experienced subjects, dictation performance became slower for isolated word input as the vocabulary size decreased, that is, as the set of recognizable words became more restricted. In general, for vocabularies of 5000 or 1000 words, Gould et al. found that connected speech produced better performance by the users experienced in dictating letters. The results of this study have implications for the design of recognizers to be used for dictation tasks. However, it is reasonable to suspect that a different pattern of results might be obtained for other applications. For example, in command and control applications such as directing a manufacturing process, or information request applications such as a database query, discrete speech may be as easy or easier to produce than continuous speech. In these situations, a user will have to construct a command sequence or perhaps a string of key words using relatively artificial (and much less familiar) rules of word order. This process may require sufficient thought that the user's speaking rate could slow substantially, resulting in short pauses between words. In any case, it is clear from this study that the type of speech input and vocabulary size are two issues that must be investigated more thoroughly.

Another issue of some importance for dictation tasks is the presence and weighting of a language model in a recognition system. A language model is a set of principles describing language use. When processing dictation or any spoken discourse, recognition systems can exploit more information than is contained in the signal alone. As Newell (1975) has suggested, in fluent speech the acoustic pattern may actually underdetermine the linguistic content of an utterance. Speech perception may be a combination of pattern recognition and sophisticated guessing based on some linguistic and contextual knowledge; such knowledge might be summarized in a language model. To a great degree, speech understanding systems such as Harpy and Hearsay (see Klatt, 1977) exploited linguistic and contextual knowledge to aid in the recognition process; however, these systems did not organize such information into a model. The next generation of speech recognition systems, reflected currently in commercial prototype systems such as Tangora (Jelinek, 1986) use similar linguistic information but instantiated in a different form: The Tangora system uses a language model as part of its recognition algorithm. Millions of words of office correspondence were analyzed to find all possible three-word sequences, and the probability of occurrence of every possible sequence. These probabilities were encoded into a hidden Markov model (a summary of transition probabilities), which is the particular language model Tangora uses for recognition. Since the ordering of words in text is constrained by a combination of syntax, semantics, and pragmatics, this three-word language model represents a statistical approximation to the operation of all of these knowledge sources together. The language model makes the recognition of some word sequences much less likely than others, because the occurrence of these sequences has been found to be unlikely. Thus the language model, when appropriate to a particular domain of discourse, can serve to constrain the set of possible word choices during recognition.

On one hand, a language model that is built to constrain word recognition can improve performance in a dictation system as long as the speech input conforms to the expectations of the model. On the other hand, a highly weighted language model that is built on a particular database of text could actually introduce errors in recognition if the user's syntax and vocabulary were inconsistent with the model. It is important to investigate whether users can learn to accommodate tacit feedback from a language model or whether language models must be made to adapt to the talker over time.

Syntax subsetting of a vocabulary, or "syntaxing," is a related technique for improving recognition accuracy available in current recognition systems. In a system with this feature, the vocabulary used in an application is divided into subsets (e.g., see Coler et al., 1978). Each subset is activated only by certain vocabulary items. For example, a recognizer for a file management system might recognize the command open. After that vocabulary item has been recognized, the recognizer would deactivate all words except those that can logically follow the open command. For example, file, record, and directory might be included in the recognizable subset, while save, zero, and the word open itself might be excluded. This type of sequential information is not an attempt to capture the knowledge of sentence structure that the term "syntax" refers to in linguistics. Rather, syntaxing is simply a technique for improving recognizer performance by reducing the number of word candidates that a recognizer must consider at any point. The recognizer can settle on a match faster when it has fewer vocabulary items to evaluate. Furthermore, its matches are more likely to be accurate, because fewer incorrect alternatives are available. Of course, the user is responsible for remembering what words are allowable at any time during the interaction. A word from the wrong subset will not be recognized, no matter how clearly it is pronounced (Bristow, 1984).

It is interesting that there has been so little research on the human factors issues that surround the use of syntaxing in speech recognition. This could reflect the fact that syntaxing is not used to full advantage in current recognition systems. But it is possible that research carried out on the problems and benefits of incorporating syntaxing into a recognition system would predict some of the human factors issues that will arise in conjunction with the more sophisticated language models incorporated by the next generation of recognition systems.

Finally, it will be important to consider how the user will change modes of operation in more sophisticated recognition systems. In current recognition devices, there are few options for a user to choose. In future recognition devices, there may be several modes of operation that will be integral to the user interface. For example, in their simulation of a dictation application, Gould et al. (1984) provided several modes of operation to the user, including a dictation mode (the default), a spell mode, a number mode, and a formatting and punctuating mode. They provided clear keywords to enter and exit these different states. This is an important human factors issue, since many errors in text editing occur because users become confused about the current mode of a system. A user who enters text when the system is expecting commands could actuate a sequence of unintended commands that could actually destroy data.

Norman (1982) has made four general suggestions about the design of a user interface for any complex information processing system. First, feedback to the user should provide clear information about the current state of the system. Second, different types of functions should be invoked using discriminable (acoustically different) commands; this might help the user keep track (in memory) of the different commands, as well as minimize substitution errors by the recognizer. Third, the user should be able to undo almost all actions. Finally, it is important for commands to be as consistent as possible across the different modes of a system. For example, the delete function in a recognizer that takes dictation should be activated in the same way in dictation, spell, and number modes, to help the user remember the commands.

In general, few if any of these human factors issues have been investigated systematically for the operation of the next generation of speech recognition systems. As the capabilities of recognition systems improve to better approximate the spoken language abilities of humans, we will see entirely new human factors problems. At the simplest level, users' expectations regarding system capabilities will be raised substantially, perhaps leading to problems based on treating recognition systems more like human listeners when this is inappropriate. At the same time, improved capabilities will permit new domains of applications to exploit speech recognition technology. The human factors problems inherent in dictation tasks are not the same as those in simple command and control tasks. As task complexity increases, the demands on the cognitive abilities of the user will also increase. Thus it is important to realize that the human factors issues regarding the operation, performance, and user interface of the recognition system cannot be completely understood without considering the limitations and capabilities of the human operator.

5. The Human Operator

The effectiveness of any recognition system depends on the human who provides the speech input and makes use of the technology. In turn, the effectiveness of the human operator depends on limitations on several aspects of the human cognitive system. First, the operator's knowledge forms a basic constraint on performance. For example, a user who understands the technical principles of a speech recognition device will probably interact with a recognition system very differently from a user who has no understanding of the technology at all. For example, understanding how a recognition system operates would lead a user to speak as consistently as possible. Explicit knowledge about the operating principles of a recognition system would also constrain users' interpretations of recognizer errors and guide their actions. Similarly, knowledge about the properties of speech and speech production could affect user behavior. Also, users with a very deep understanding of the application that employs the recognition device may behave quite differently from users with no background knowledge.

Second, experience using a recognition device probably affects user behavior as well. Understanding the operating principles of a device is not a direct substitute for the experience of talking to a particular recognizer and learning how to relate speaking to recognition performance. In much the same way, understanding the general principles of database access or some telecommunications service will affect behavior somewhat differently from the specific experience of using that service. Most simply stated, the user's knowledge can provide a framework for developing an accurate and appropriate mental model of a recognition device or application. Without that framework, experience with the user interface will be the complete source of information for forming a mental model. In the absence of a priori knowledge about the workings of recognition systems, experience with a poorly designed system image may lead the user to form an incorrect mental model of the particular recognition device or application being used. It is also easy to see how users with background knowledge but without the requisite experience may have a framework for guiding general interactions with a recognition system and application, but will lack the specifics until they have some actual experience with the system. One way to think about this is to imagine how someone would play tennis after reading a book about tennis playing with no experience using a tennis racquet. Then consider how different things would be if someone tried to learn to play tennis with no prior knowledge about the rules or goals of the game.

Third, the human information-processing system is basically a limited capacity system. Cognitive capacity can be thought of as the mental "resources" that humans have in limited supply and must allocate judiciously to each of the cognitive processes being performed at the same time (Norman & Bobrow, 1975). For example, short-term memory is a mental resource that may affect performance in information processing tasks by providing a limited cognitive "workspace" (Baddeley, 1986; Shiffrin, 1976). Other mental resources may be specific to different modalities or cognitive subsystems, such as psycholinguistic processes or spatial processes (Navon & Gopher, 1979; Wickens, 1980). Any particular task, such as data entry or dictation or part quality inspection, may require several different cognitive processes, such as memory encoding and retrieval, speech production and perception, or visual pattern recognition. Any two cognitive processes may involve some central cognitive resources, such as short-term memory, and may also share some modality-specific resources, such as those that may be involved in word recognition. To the extent that the knowledge, sensory inputs, and response outputs are shared by "simultaneously operating" cognitive processes, performance interactions can be expected between these processes (see Navon & Gopher, 1979). In many cases, these interactions could take the form of interference, in which one process retards, inhibits, or degrades performance of another process. A classic example of this type of interaction is Stroop interference, in which subjects are slower to name the color of ink used to print a word when the word spells a color name that differs from the ink color (Stroop, 1935). For this particular example, it has been shown that the interference comes largely from the response generation process in which the color-naming response competes with a well-learned process of reading the word (Egeth & Blecker, 1969).

Indeed, modality-specific interference can be very striking. When subjects are asked to combine two linguistic tasks or two spatial tasks, performance is considerably worse than when a spatial and linguistic task are combined (Brooks, 1968). Wickens (1980) has demonstrated that modality-specific interference can be due to shared input modalities and/or response modalities. Specifically, Wickens showed that use of a speech recognition device was impaired more than keyboard input when stimulus information was presented using synthetic speech as opposed to a visual display. Although it is important to note that perception of synthetic speech requires more capacity than perception of natural speech (Luce et al., 1983) and may also require more capacity than recognizing digits on a visual display system, it is the modality-specific interactions that are of greatest relevance. Presenting operators with speech rather than visual displays is more likely to cause performance problems for the use of a speech recognition system than for the use of a keyboard. Conversely, operators' speech perception may well be adversely affected by the demands of speaking to a speech recognition system. These interactions could be due to the combined demands placed on limited resources commonly used in speech perception and production, or they could be due to changes in the way humans strategically approach perception and responding within a single modality. In either case, it is important to recognize the existence of such interactions when implementing a speech-based interface for any particular application.

It is also important to understand that as the capacity demands made by one process (e.g., speech perception) increase, there will be an impact on other processes (e.g., speech production). Since perception of synthetic speech requires more capacity than perception of natural speech, using synthetic speech to provide the operator with information may have a greater impact on the use of a recognition system. Indeed, there is reason to believe that the intelligibility and capacity demands of synthetic speech are related (see Nusbaum & Pisoni, 1985), so that the quality of synthetic speech in a user interface may affect the use of a speech recognition system. As speech perception requires more effort and attention, speech production may be impaired. Thus, using lower quality synthetic speech may degrade recognition performance by affecting the resources available to the operator for speech production. This suggests that if a speech recognition device is to be used with synthetic speech feedback and displays, the highest quality speech output system should be employed, all other factors being equal. Thus, if a relatively small or fixed set of voice messages is required for the user interface, high quality coded speech may be more effective and have less of an impact on recognition performance than a low cost text-to-speech system.

In general, then, capacity limitations can affect how well a user interacts with a speech recognition system. This is true even when the amount of modality-specific interference is reduced as much as possible. For example, a speech recognition system may require the user to issue verbal commands to the system while simultaneously reading feedback on the computer screen and typing on the keyboard. Although the three processes of speaking, reading, and typing share some central cognitive resources (related to linguistic processes), the amount of modality-specific interaction is reduced for the stimulus input and response outputs. Nevertheless, the user must allocate some cognitive capacity to each of the processes. If there are too many processes or if each demands too much central cognitive capacity, the user will not be able to allocate sufficient resources to each task, and performance of one or more tasks will suffer. Thus, even if the only use of speech within an application is the user's speech to the recognizer, other perceptual and cognitive processes may have an impact on speech production. To understand and predict the performance of a speech recognition system as it will actually be used in a particular application, it is therefore important to understand the total cognitive demands on the human operator. There is clearly a need for understanding the effects of these cognitive demands on the acoustic-phonetic structure of speech (NRC, 1984).

One recent study addressed this topic and found that cognitive demands indeed affect how people produce speech (Summers et al., 1989). Summers et al. analyzed the speech of people who were required to speak while performing a cognitively demanding perceptuo-motor tracking task. In this tracking task, subjects kept a pointer on a video screen from hitting the sides of the display by manipulating a joystick. Subjects also performed a speech task, in which they said phrases that were presented on the video screen. Subjects performed the speech task alone (the control condition) and in conjunction with the tracking task (the high cognitive load condition). Comparisons of the speech produced under these two conditions indicate that when under cognitive load, talkers tend to speak more loudly and with greater variability in amplitude. Increases in amplitude were generally greater at the higher frequencies of the speech signal than at the lower frequencies. In addition, talkers tended to speak more quickly and with less variation in pitch when under cognitive load. Formant frequencies of speakers' productions (another aspect of the spectro-temporal information measured), however, did not vary with workload.

These results indicate that cognitive load affects speech production. Of all the effects observed, the most relevant for predicting the performance of speech recognition devices is the increased variability of the acoustic properties of speech. As the acoustic structure of speech varies more from token to token, it is more difficult for a recognition device to represent vocabulary items and perform reliable pattern matching. Some of the effects of cognitive load on the performance of a recognition system can be reduced if training is carried out under the same conditions as will hold during the routine use of the recognizer. If users are under the same capacity demands while training the device as they are during the actual use of the application, then these capacity demands should affect the acoustic properties of the training utterances the same way they affect the utterances produced while actually using the application. This will ensure that the range and values of the acoustic properties included in the stored representation of vocabulary in the recognition device will be similar to the properties of the utterances produced when the recognition device is used in the context of the application. However, the increased variability in acoustic properties will most likely still reduce recognition performance. In order to understand better the effects of cognitive load on recognition performance, much more research is needed to discover how the changes in speech production resulting from increased cognitive load affect the performance of speech recognition devices.

Of course, the interaction between effort and speech recognition performance is a two-way street. As mentioned above, high cognitive workload changes some of the acoustic-phonetic properties of speech, and these changes in the acoustic structure of speech could affect recognition performance. Simultaneously, the use of a recognition system itself may increase the operator's effort. First, talking to a recognition device is not like talking to another human. The entire "style" of speaking is different, requiring the talker to pay constant attention to the act of speaking in an unfamiliar way, with artificially limited vocabulary and syntax.

In general, the goal of speaking to a computer is to be as acoustically consistent as possible and to provide as much redundant acoustic information as possible by speaking in citation forms. While there are many goals that govern normal conversation, these goals are not set at the level of acoustic criteria but instead in terms of linguistic and cognitive strategies (see Hobbs & Evans, 1980). Therefore, most users of recognition systems have not had much practice speaking in a style appropriate for computer speech recognition. Indeed, subjectively it seems more difficult to produce isolated words than to produce connected speech and more difficult to produce connected speech than to produce fluent continuous speech. No data have been reported on the effort required to dictate passages of text with isolated word input. Although Gould et al. (1984) reported data on the performance of talkers in a dictation task using isolated utterances as input, they did not report the effects of this requirement on the cognitive capacity of the talker, compared to the cognitive effects of fluent, continuous speech production. It is possible that dictating discrete words requires a great deal of attention and effort, so that speech production performance may degrade over time at a faster rate than it would for continuous speech input.

Similarly, the restriction of dictating with a limited vocabulary of 1000 to 5000 words or a constrained language model may require more effort than dictating from an unrestricted vocabulary (as large as 10,000 or even 100,000 words; see Seashore, 1933; Hartman, 1946) or using unconstrained word order.

If it is indeed the case that using a recognition system demands cognitive resources, we should expect these attentional demands to affect the performance of other tasks. For example, Mountford et al. (1982) had commercial pilots use speech input to perform a navigation task in a flight simulator. Some pilots requested notepads for written notes during the task, suggesting that using a speech recognition system placed significant demands on short-term memory. Navigation is a complex cognitive task and it is not surprising that the cognitive demands of using a speech recognition system are observed under these conditions. It is especially interesting, however, that the pilots found it difficult to keep track of the speech recognizer's mode, the navigation system's mode, or the airplane's status, during navigation. Since much of this information is normally maintained in a pilot's memory, the additional demands of using a recognition system seems to have had a significant impact on cognitive capacity. It should be clear that writing on notepads to provide an "externalized" expansion of memory capacity would nullify one of the major benefits of cockpit voice recognition—keeping the pilot's eyes and hands free for flight control.

From this study, we can make two suggestions for reducing the increased capacity demands of using a recognition system. First, the recognizer, in conjunction with the application itself (e.g., navigation), must provide feedback to let the user know the status of the task; this will reduce the memory demands of the application. In many cases, if this feedback is immediate, it prevents possible confusion for the operator (Simpson et al., 1987) and reduces the operator's need to maintain information in short-term memory. To the extent that the user must integrate several pieces of information, presented over a span of time, in order to understand the state of a system or task, memory demands will be greater. The goal of immediate feedback should be to elicit an immediate response from the operator, rather than presenting some information that the operator will need to remember for a later point in time. However, it is important to remember that, as noted earlier, immediate feedback and the requirements of an immediate response may be disruptive for some tasks. The format and frequency of feedback should depend on the complexity of a specific task.

The second suggestion is that memory demands can be reduced to the extent that information is cognitively "transparent." If an operator must integrate several sources of information and come to a conclusion or make some kind of inference, cognitive load will be higher than if the system presents the inference or conclusion directly. For example, it is generally true that more cognitive capacity will be required if a user must remember the current state of a system in order to interpret information provided by the system. Indeed, all user interfaces can benefit from the observation that in any human-machine interaction, the best memory aid is understanding (Norman, 1981). A system, including the system of switching between modes (such as the "command" and "number" modes that a navigation system might use or the "dictation" and "spell" modes that a recognizer itself might use), should be designed in a logical and consistent way. If users can easily understand the system, be it a recognition system or an application, it will be easier for them to interpret information and to remember how to provide input.

Factors such as effort (associated with the difficulty or complexity of a particular task), stress, and fatigue can clearly affect the performance that may be achieved with a recognition system. Thus, the overall effectiveness of recognition technology depends on a thorough understanding of the limitations of the human operator. However, at the same time it is also important to remember that the human operator is much more flexible and accommodating than a speech recognition system. Humans are able to quickly adopt new strategies for interacting with the technology if they are given appropriate and informative feedback and training. The human information processing system is adaptable and can respond to the requirements and make up for the limitations of technology when the technology is inflexible. Despite the limitations on cognitive capacity that constrain performance, there are also important capabilities that the human can use to cope with and overcome limitations inherent in technology. A pertinent example is Zoltan-Ford's (1984) finding that people change their vocabulary and sentence structure to match a simulated system image.

Thus, if attentional limitations are found to affect users' performance with speech recognition systems, these effects may be reduced through appropriate training and experience. Recent studies have found that human listeners can be trained to improve their ability to recognize computer-generated speech (Greenspan et al., 1988; Schwab et al., 1985). Significantly, as their ability improves, the listening task begins to require less attention (Lee & Nusbaum, 1989). This demonstrates that the human listener is flexible enough to adopt new perceptual strategies to improve recognition performance with synthetic speech. It seems quite reasonable to predict that attentional demands may be similarly reduced for interacting with speech recognition systems by giving the user appropriate training and experience. It is possible that this training may be used to modify a talker's speech to improve recognition performance. Thus, even if a particular operator does not use a speech recognition device effectively when first introduced to the technology, it may be possible to improve performance through a systematic program of training.

Just as a single talker's performance with a recognition device may differ as a function of training, knowledge, experience, and the cognitive demands of a task, talkers may differ in their use of speech recognition devices. Although there has been a great deal of research on individual differences in cognitive functioning and abilities (e.g., Crowder, 1976; Posner, 1978), there has been very little research on the way talkers differ in using speech recognition systems. We can make a few inferences at the most general level, though. First, since there are individual differences in cognitive capacity (Davies et al., 1984), these differences could affect the use of recognition devices in that talkers could vary in their sensitivity to the cognitive demands of any task. Second, talkers differ in intelligibility, although there is not a lot of research in this area. However, in a seminal study on measuring the intelligibility of natural speech (House et al., 1965), there was a difference in the intelligibility of the talkers who provided the speech stimuli. Certainly talkers differ in the acoustic properties of their speech (Peterson & Barney, 1952), and these differences could affect the processing of speech by computers. Third, talkers may differ in their mental models of speech recognition systems, either because of different kinds of knowledge about speech or speech recognition or because of different amounts of experience with the technology. This might lead to different strategies for interacting with recognition systems or different degrees of motivation for using speech technology.

There has been some initial consideration of very gross differences in the ability of people to use speech recognition systems. Doddington and Schalk (1981) suggested that people could be classified as either "sheep" (successful users) or "goats" (unsuccessful users). Of the possible accounts of this distinction among users, there are three explanations that have been discussed informally. First, sheep may be highly motivated to use the technology while goats are not. It is not clear precisely how a lack of motivation affects performance, but it is easy to generate several possible results, such as mumbling, not responding to feedback, or not paying attention to the state of the system; any of these might result in poorer system performance. This might be thought of as the "Luddite" explanation in the sense that such users might show resistance to any kind of new technology. The explanation is not specific to speech production in any way, and in fact goats of this type should produce speech that is acoustically equivalent to the speech produced by sheep. A second explanation is that sheep and goats may differ in the acoustic-phonetic structure of their speech such that the utterances produced by goats are simply less discriminable from each other than those of sheep. According to this explanation, under the appropriate testing conditions, it should be possible to show that even for human listeners, speech produced by goats would be less intelligible than speech produced by sheep. This hypothesis suggests that acoustic measurements of the speech produced by goats and sheep should show different patterns such that acoustic-phonetic cues are more distinctive for sheep than for goats. Finally, goats may be less consistent in their productions so that the utterances used to train the recognizer are very different from each other and from utterances provided as input when the recognition device is used in an application. This explanation implies that acoustic measurements of speech produced by goats should show more variability than speech produced by sheep, even if the mean values of those properties do not differ between these groups. It has been suggested that 25% of any population of users is likely to have this type of inconsistent speech pattern (Simpson et al., 1987).

Of course, it is also possible that there is more than one explanation for differences in performance between sheep and goats. Indeed, Nusbaum and Pisoni (1987) reported some data that suggest that none of the above explanations is entirely correct. During their tests of the performance of several speech recognition systems on a pre-recorded database of speech from 16 talkers, they discovered a talker that might be classified as a goat. When trained on five tokens of this talker's speech using the TI-Alphabet vocabulary, 85% of the Votan's responses were substitution errors whereas the average substitution error rate for the entire group of talkers for this vocabulary was close to 20%. Moreover, this was the only talker for whom the error rates were even over 30%. Since performance on this talker's speech was so poor compared to the other talkers in the database, at first glance it would seem that this talker has the requisite characteristics of a goat. In fact, this is generally how goats have been identified in the past: For one particular recognition device, using a specific vocabulary after a set training protocol, recognition performance for one talker's speech is much worse than recognition performance for other talkers.

A closer examination of the entire set of data argued against this interpretation, however. First, for a different vocabulary, the TI-20, the Votan's performance on the "goat's" speech was the same as performance on the other talkers' speech. Certainly, motivation would not differ across vocabularies, and thus we can rule out low motivation as an explanation of performance. Second, an examination of recognition performance on the goat's speech across different training protocols with the Votan recognition system provided some interesting information. Recognition performance decreased with increasing amounts of training. This would seem to rule out as an explanation the relative intelligibility of the goat's speech, since acoustic-phonetic distinctiveness of the testing tokens for the alphabet is not affected by the number of training items presented to the recognizer. On the other hand, this is exactly the pattern of results that would be expected if this goat was more variable in speech production than were the sheep.

Unfortunately, there were two more findings that argue against the variability hypothesis. The goat was a goat only for the Votan. Performance on this talker's speech was indistinguishable from performance on other talkers' speech for all the other recognition systems. Also, when Nusbaum and Pisoni bypassed the built-in training mechanism of the Votan and used their own training mechanism, performance on the goat's speech became equivalent to performance on the other talkers' speech. This demonstrates that it is not the inherent variability of the training tokens that affected performance and it was not the specific acoustic-phonetic properties of the speech per se. Rather these findings suggest that some deficiency in the training algorithm was responsible for one talker appearing to be a goat.

Since the goat was a goat only for a specific combination of vocabulary, training protocol, training algorithm, and recognition system, it appears that none of the explanations alone is sufficient. In fact, the issue of goats and sheep may be less a function of the talker and more a function of the recognition technology itself. The definition of a goat may depend on interactions among characteristics of the talker, the training algorithm, the recognition algorithm, and the specific vocabulary used for recognition. It is much too simplistic to consider being a goat as entirely a property of the talker. From the perspective of human factors, there may be more solutions to recognition problems than simply blaming the talker. In cases where it is not feasible to replace the operator, it may be the case that performance problems with a particular recognition device can be alleviated by changing the application vocabulary in some way, modifying the training algorithm, changing the training protocol, or adopting a different recognition device.

From this example study, it should be apparent that we need much more research on the way talkers produce speech to recognition systems. It is important to the success of implementing a recognition device that we understand how the limitations and abilities of the human operator affect the performance of a recognition system. Speech is a product of a complex motor skill controlled by and embedded in complex cognitive and linguistic systems. There are many ways in which the interactions among these mechanisms can be affected, and understanding these interactions is necessary for designing a user interface and optimizing the use of this technology. Moreover, just as the limitations and abilities of the human operator are fundamental to determining the performance of a recognition system, the context in which recognition takes place is important to determining how the operator is affected by cognitive and sensory-motor limitations and can exploit cognitive and sensory-motor abilities.

6. The Recognition Environment and Context

Speech recognition takes place within the context of a physical environment and an application environment. The physical environment includes the ambient noise background, including the user's speech to people nearby (Simpson et al., 1987) and speech directed at the user (and therefore at the recognizer), as well as nonacoustic characteristics of the recognition setting, such as temperature, or the vibration and acceleration of a vehicle. These physical characteristics can affect recognition performance either by changing the way the talker produces speech or by affecting the input or operation of the recognition system. In particular, the effects of high levels of background noise on recognition performance are well known (NRC, 1984). However, recent research has demonstrated that the acoustic-phonetic properties of speech are modified for speech produced in noise, compared to speech produced in quiet (Pisoni et al., 1985). This is important because it has generally been assumed that the effects of the noise environment are principally on the signal characteristics of the speech input to the recognition system. If noise affects only the signal input, these effects could be eliminated by the appropriate acoustic filtering. By contrast, if noise affects the way the talker produces speech, the types of solutions to the performance problems introduced by noise will be quite different.

Pisoni et al. (1985) demonstrated a number of effects of noise on speech production, even beyond the relatively well-documented Lombard effect of increased duration, pitch, and amplitude (e.g., see Lane & Tranel, 1971). When a person produces speech while listening to noise, high frequencies in the speech signal are amplified, and lower frequencies are attenuated— in other words, there is a change in the tilt of the power spectrum for certain segments. In addition, the formant frequencies (spectral patterns) characteristic of a given vowel are different, depending on whether it is produced in noise or in quiet. These changes can greatly reduce recognition performance. If a recognition system is trained in a quiet environment, the acoustic patterns of a talker's speech will have a set of acoustic-phonetic characteristics that are spectrally quite different from the same utterances produced in a background of noise. Thus the encoded forms of speech produced in noise during actual use will not match the training patterns from a quiet environment. To avoid this problem, new recognition systems will have to adapt to changes in a talker's speech that might occur as a consequence of a wide range of environmental factors or perhaps even model the effects of certain environmental factors on the acoustic properties of speech. For the present, the best rule of thumb is to train a recognition system under the same set of conditions that will hold during actual use of the system. This will ensure that the environmental factors operating on the talker will be held constant.

Beyond the human factors problems engendered by conditions of the physical environment, it is also important to understand the effects of the application environment on the performance of speech recognition systems. The application environment consists of the tasks and applications for which speech recognition is being used. Over the history of commercial speech recognition systems, one of the most significant human factors problems has been finding applications for which speech recognition will be an effective interface technology. In the most general terms, speech recognition should be employed when it can provide a more effective or efficient replacement for an existing interface technology, when it is the only possible interface technology, or when it makes certain applications economically feasible or available to a wider population (e.g., visually disabled people).

The most commonly suggested applications for the current generation of speech recognition systems are those in which a keyboard is unavailable, or impractical for entering data or commands, either because the operator's hands or eyes are busy, or because the operator needs to walk around, such as while taking inventory in a warehouse (in the latter case, a wireless microphone can allow speech input; Lea, 1980). As a general rule, this is probably not a bad guide for small vocabulary recognition systems (e.g.,

Simpson et al., 1987). For example, speech input may allow a pilot to display information on a screen in the cockpit without letting go of manual flight controls to press a keypad. Similarly, a clerk taking inventory in a warehouse, a quality control inspector, or even a pathologist may record data by voice without having to look away from the items being counted or inspected. Telecommunications services can be provided over the telephone when there is no keyboard available: Speech recognition can eliminate the need to type in complex codes on the limited keypad of a touchtone phone and can even provide services to a rotary dial phone that were previously available only to a touchtone phone. In all of these application environments, small vocabulary speech input provides some definite advantages over the traditional, manual mode of input to a computer.

However, the need for a new input or control channel may not be the most important criterion when selecting applications for the next generation of large vocabulary speech recognition systems, which may accept connected or continuous speech input. Instead of changing the mode of communicating with a machine, these more powerful recognizers may be most useful for tasks that already use speech, but that currently rely on a human listener. These are cases in which a human currently provides an interface to some kind of computer or machine. Perhaps the most prototypical example is dictation, in which text is spoken to a secretary for transcription. The secretary serves as a highly intelligent interface to a word processor. However, there are other examples as well, such as information retrieval, in which queries might be made by phone to a human operator. Any request over a telephone that is currently handled by a human operator such as requesting a service (e.g., calling a taxi, ordering a pizza, inquiring about a bank account) is a potential target for implementing a speech recognition system. If speech recognition can be used efficiently in tasks like these, it can benefit both the talkers and the service providers. The customer or talker can dictate a letter or retrieve information at short notice, even if support personnel are not available, and the costs associated with providing some services may be decreased by reducing the need for costly human labor. Meanwhile, secretaries and reference librarians will be free to work on projects other than dictation and information lookup. Humans can be freed to perform tasks that require more intelligence than serving as a passive interface for speech to a computer system or machine.

Among these types of tasks, then, which ones are the best applications for the next generation of speech recognition systems? There are currently no strong criteria for answering this question. Most suggested criteria are based simply on physical demands of the application, as if they were criteria for small vocabulary recognition. In order to select the best applications for large vocabulary speech recognition, however, research is needed on the relationship between the cognitive representations inherent in different application environments, the goals and needs of the user for those applications, and the functions that might be provided by a large vocabulary recognition system. It seems reasonable that computer speech recognition is likely to be most appropriate whenever speech is used for communication among humans—in other words, when communication is carried out by expressing propositions. Making requests, providing declarations and assertions, and issuing imperatives are all standard linguistic behaviors that could be spoken to an intelligent computer as well as to a human listener. A rule of thumb is that this includes most interactions that people can conduct easily by telephone: obtaining flight schedules, querying medical records, performing banking transactions.

On the other hand, it is probably difficult for most people to describe graphic information verbally. Consequently, graphic information display or manipulation will probably be a poor candidate for speech input to a computer, just as it is for speech to a human: architectural plans and magazine layouts are usually displayed, not described verbally to people. Thus, the selection of a task for large vocabulary computer speech recognition can be guided by the cognitive representations most generally used for that task when it is performed without computer speech recognition. Of course, instead of applying recognition to various tasks based on this type of intuition, the possible criteria for task selection should be investigated systematically. It is important to analyze the requirements of a candidate task to determine how speech recognition could possibly provide a useful and effective interface and then to implement a recognition system in a prototype application to validate this analysis. It is entirely possible that an analysis of a task may not take into account the way the limited performance of a particular recognition system constrains the kinds of interactions that could take place with an application.

To be effective in a particular application environment, speech recognition systems must be designed so that, regardless of whether a human or a machine is listening, there is little difference in difficulty for the user. This is necessary because extra demands on the user may cause fatigue or stress and a corresponding change in the speech produced, which could result in degraded recognition performance. Computers are inferior to human listeners, both in pattern matching (determining what word was uttered, based on the acoustic signal) and in linguistic processing (e.g., determining the meaning of a sentence after its individual words have been identified). Therefore, some technological advances will be necessary in order to achieve a state in which talking to a machine is as easy as talking to a person. For example, database queries are generally made by constructing artificial sentences from a database query language. Speech recognition could substitute for typing in these queries and allow them to be made over a telephone. However, even with a discrete input recognition system, database queries might be made more easily if some rudimentary linguistic abilities were present. On one hand, this can be achieved by severely limiting the user's syntax (sentence structure)—for example, allowing a user to say, "I want some recent articles by Smith" but not, "Are there any recent articles by Smith?" It might, however, take a great deal of effort for users to restrict themselves to a limited set of sentence structures. To avoid such a requirement, the system must have more flexible linguistic capabilities—semantic capabilities, to allow access to word meanings, and syntactic capabilities, to understand different sentence structures (Hayes-Roth, 1980). To ensure that appropriate linguistic knowledge is included in a system, this knowledge should be developed from samples of utterances directed at the application (Hayes-Roth, 1980). Linguistic processing capabilities will also make it more feasible for untrained users, such as clients who call a service office, to talk to a computer instead of a human.

Although a database query is quite different from dictating a letter, there will be some considerations in common, such as the need for sophisticated linguistic abilities. Dictation may place even greater demands on a recognition system beyond word recognition and sentence processing. A database query will generally consist of just a few sentences and so could be produced as sequences of discrete words. Dictating letters generally produces many more sentences and dictating isolated words might fatigue a talker faster than dictating connected speech; recognition performance might decline as a consequence. A recognizer would therefore have to recognize words in connected speech in order to allow maximum efficiency in a dictation system.

Even after addressing the foregoing concerns, there are no guidelines on precisely how to integrate recognition functions into an application. With large vocabulary recognition systems, there may be a temptation to place all the functions of the application under the control of the recognizer. However, this may not be the best approach for all applications. For example, in a dictation task, speech may provide the best means of entering the original text into the system, but it may be more efficient to edit the text using a keyboard and a mouse.

Finally, the utility of a speech recognizer for any application may be limited by the users' view of whether it is a valid application of speech technology, and their readiness to modify their behavior to make it work (Haggard, 1983; Van Peursem 1985). Therefore, speech recognition should facilitate the task in some way that is readily apparent to the user. In some cases, the benefits to the operators themselves are not direct, such as with the use of small vocabulary recognition systems for voice data entry tasks. In this application, a significant advantage is the immediate entry of data into a computer system for other employees to access and analyze or the immediate availability of data for managers; the operators use voice data entry only because they are required to do so.

In the case of an application like dictation, the users themselves must be motivated to change from a human listener to a machine. In this case, the potential operators may be executives, who can choose whether or not to use a computer for their dictation. Some managers might perform dictation only occasionally, and might therefore be unwilling to invest much effort in preparation for computer speech recognition, such as learning to speak in discrete words or training the system on the characteristics of their own speech (Mangione, 1985); they might choose not to use a dictation system that requires such preparation. Alternatively, they might use the system incorrectly, leading to high error rates and frustration with the technology.

Customers and clients of a service make up another group that must be positively motivated to use speech recognition effectively. Wilpon (1985) reported that AT&T customers calling a particular service were presented with a recorded message instructing them to say their phone number with a pause after each digit. Instead of talking, many customers simply hung up. With additional encouragement or motivation, these customers might have spoken to the recognizer. For example, the recorded instructions might have included a promise of faster or less expensive service as a result of the new system. Also, customers should be informed in advance that the computer will repeat their phone number for confirmation; such reassurance could help motivate them to try the new technology.

It is important to remember that speech recognition is an interface technology and not an application itself. While that may seem to be an obvious statement, the complexity of implementing speech recognition systems often focuses so much effort on the speech technology that the relationship between the recognition system and the application is ignored. Sometimes there is an interest in implementing speech recognition technology for a particular application because the abstract idea of talking to an application seems so appealing. The reality of current recognition technology is far from the ideal of talking to another person; the performance could potentially reduce the desirability of an application or service. The decision to implement a speech recognition interface for a particular application requires a consideration of the capabilities and limitations of the human operator, the capabilities and limitations of the available recognition technology, and the suitability of the application and physical environment for speech recognition. Since these factors all interact in complicated ways, there can be no simple set of guidelines for the selection and implementation of a recognition system or for the design of the user interface.

7. Conclusions and Implications

When first confronted with the problem of implementing a speech recognition system as the interface to a particular application, there are a number of questions that must be addressed: (1) Is speech recognition an appropriate interface technology for this application? (2) Which aspects of the application will benefit most from a speech interface and which will be more effectively handled using other types of interfaces? (3) What kind of interface should be provided to the speech recognition system itself, separate from the interface provided by the recognition system to the application? (4) Which particular recognition device would be best for this application? (5) Which aspects of the recognition system should be under control of the operator and which should be under control of the application or service? (6) How should the application vocabulary (and syntax if any) be defined for this application? (7) What training protocol should be used for a speaker-dependent recognition system? (8) How can operators (or customers, for that matter) be trained to make most effective use of the recognition system interfaced to the application?

None of these questions is simple, and some of them implicitly entail other questions as well. However, the development of an effective speech recognition interface for an application depends on the answers to these questions. Unfortunately, there are no simple criteria or guidelines to provide answers for most situations. The answers to these questions depend on understanding how the limitations and abilities of the human operator interact with the limitations and functions of a recognition system, through some system image, in the context of a particular physical environment and application. It may seem that there should be some simple rules of thumb that should apply regardless of the specific considerations of these interactions. Our view is that while it may be possible to specify some heuristics to guide the implementation of a speech recognition system, these may only apply in very simple situations, and should not be treated as general rules.

In recent years, there has been some research directed at investigating the human factors problems in using speech recognition systems from the perspective of providing general guidelines (e.g., Simpson et al., 1987; Van Peursem, 1985). However, this research has focused primarily on small vocabulary systems and the applications that are appropriate for this more limited technology. Increasing the capabilities of recognition systems will also increase their complexity. As we noted earlier, the next generation of speech recognition systems will be used in very different applications and will place different demands on the human operator. In order to understand better how to use these systems effectively, it is important to investigate more thoroughly a number of human factors issues, taking into account the full range of complex interactions that may occur between the characteristics of the recognition system and its user interface, the characteristics of the human operator, and the recognition environment.

There have been some attempts to specify guidelines for the use of recognition, based on the limited research that has been carried out on speaker-dependent, small vocabulary recognition devices. However, even a cursory examination of these indicates the difficulties involved in making useful recommendations. For example, Van Peursem (1985) has suggested five general implementation guidelines. Three of these can be thought of as directed at inducing a positive attitude in the user and are not specific to speech recognition technology per se. These three guidelines could be summarized as making users happy by providing for their needs and expectations and letting users feel in control of the system by giving them control but not overwhelming them with demands. The remaining two guidelines similarly have nothing specific to do with speech recognition. In these guidelines, Van Peursem suggests giving clear feedback and guidance that eliminates the need for a manual.

On one hand, it is a laudable goal to give the user a positive attitude about the technology and to make feedback and online help clear and informative. In fact, these are important goals for any user interface. But they do not directly address the questions that need to be answered in implementing a speech recognition system in an application. Moreover, while the general strategy of user interface development outlined by Van Peursem might well make the naive operator's very first encounters with a recognition system more enjoyable, it is far from clear whether that will improve productivity, the effectiveness of the recognition system, or even operator satisfaction in the long run. One way of characterizing Van Peursem's suggestions is that they seem to derive from the perspective of the user as someone who must be appeased by the interface, rather than as an adaptive intelligent agent operating the system. For some user populations and applications, it may very well be important to "pander" to the user in some ways. It is unlikely that this will be the most effective approach for all applications and user populations. As we noted earlier, research has demonstrated that people can quickly alter their speech production and perception to meet new demands—even without explicit instructions on how to change (Greenspan et al., 1988; Lee & Nusbaum, 1989; Zoltan-Ford, 1984). Given such adaptability, it might be more efficient and effective to design user interfaces with this perceptuo-motor and cognitive flexibility in mind, than to try to match the interface to a supposedly inflexible and untrainable operator. For some populations, it may be much more effective to provide a system image that is intended to induce an optimal mental model of the recognition system, rather than focusing primarily on inducing a positive attitude.

Simpson et al. (1987) have also offered some considerations for implementing a speech recognition system. They classify these considerations into the categories of Task Selection, Message Design, Performance Measurement, User Training, Recognizer Enrollment, and System Design. While these considerations come closer to addressing the questions we posed, they do not do so systematically. Some of the considerations are very specific to a certain kind of technology such as a speaker-dependent recognition device, whereas others are much more general. Still other recommendations may conflict with each other. For example, in the category of Performance Measurement, Simpson et al. provide a formula for computing message recognition accuracy assuming independent recognition of the words within each message; they note that this does not take into account the effects of syntax, without providing an alternative method. In contrast, under Message Design, they strongly argue for the use of syntax in subsetting vocabularies, thereby invalidating the formula provided for computing accuracy. Also under Message Design, they suggest that it is important to avoid acoustically similar vocabulary items, but they also suggest that users be allowed to select their own vocabulary. This potential for conflicts among a single set of recommendations for implementing a speech recognition system illustrates that it is almost impossible to make specific recommendations that are appropriate for all different recognition technologies, for all types of applications, and for all user populations.

Of course, it is important to point out that as separate recommendations, taken individually for a specific recognition system, user population, and application, the considerations suggested by Simpson et al. should be quite useful. However, it will be difficult to treat these or any other existing guidelines as a coherent and integrated set of answers to the implementation questions we posed at the start of this section. Moreover, in order to use these considerations effectively, it is important to know which type of recognition technology, which user populations, and which types of applications are most likely to benefit from them. It may require as much expertise to determine when to follow these recommendations as it does to formulate them.

Guidelines to the implementation of a speech recognition system are likely to be either too general to provide any concrete assistance or too specific to be broadly applicable. Rather than advocate any particular "cookbook" approach, our view is that there is insufficient knowledge currently to make suggestions regarding all possible combinations of speech technology, user populations, and applications. For a few relatively simple cases, based on previous experience, some suggestions already exist (e.g., Simpson et al., 1987). But for the increasing number of more complex situations and for the future, we suggest an empirical approach cast within a particular theoretical framework.

To develop the most effective implementation of a speech recognition system, there is no substitute for understanding the operation of the recognition system, the characteristics of the user population, and the demands and requirements of the application. Each of the questions that we posed in the beginning of this section can be addressed by carrying out small controlled studies and by analytic consideration. The theoretical framework is relatively general: It seems reasonable to view spoken interactions between a computer and human as a degraded or impoverished form of human-to-human communication. Taking this as a model or theoretical ideal provides a general set of guidelines for implementing a speech recognition system that can be summarized quite simply. Try to make the interaction between human and computer as close as possible to the types of interactions that occur in person-to-person conversation. Thus the user interface should be as adaptive and interactive as possible. Information should be exchanged between human and computer and not just displayed. The computer should have a repertoire of responses rather than a single fixed response to any situation, to allow elaboration and guide the human operator's behavior. To the extent that the computer models human interaction—even if it fails to achieve recognition and comprehension performance comparable to the human—the human operator will be able to make use of a well established mental model for guiding behavior. For example, Schmandt et al. (1985) have demonstrated that the performance of relatively low-cost speech recognition and synthesis systems can be substantially enhanced by exploiting the properties of human communicative interactions. Given the extremely non-interactive nature of most speech recognition systems, it seems that at least as a working model, human communication may provide a good starting point.

Empirical studies can be used to compare different recognition systems. Of course the cost and the features and functions of different recognition devices can be compared directly. But these comparisons may be a bit misleading. For example, the cost of a recognition device may be small compared to the cost of training a human operator to use a particular device. Similarly, the functions of two recognizers can be compared in terms of the vendors' specifications. However, some functions may not operate as effectively as advertised, and some may be difficult to implement because of programming considerations. Therefore it is important to carry out performance evaluation tests that exercise the functions of different recognition systems and permit an assessment of the ease of use of the systems. Other studies should be carried out to test user interfaces and to examine performance within the context of a simulation of the application, if not the application itself. In carrying out these studies it is important to employ operators drawn from the user population and to interview them extensively to determine how well they understood the recognition system and application and how useful they found the implementation. Although it is often impractical to carry out fully controlled experiments, a great deal can be learned even from a few typical users.

Without explicit criteria to guide the implementation of a speech recognition system, and without extensive prior research, it is necessary to learn from empirical investigation the answers to the questions we have posed. In all cases, it is important to remember that a successful implementation of a speech recognition system will depend on understanding the operation of three systematic constraints: (1) the characteristics of the recognition system, including the user interface; (2) the limitations and abilities of the human operator; and (3) the requirements and demands of the recognition environment and context. These three general constraints interact to determine the overall performance of a particular recognition system, and there can be little doubt that as the complexity of recognition systems increases, so will the importance of understanding the human factors problems inherent in each constraint.

8. References

Baddeley, A. (1986). *Working Memory*. New York: Oxford.

Baker, J. (1975). The Dragon System—An overview. *IEEE Transactions on Acoustics, Speech, and Signal Processing*, **23**, 24–29.

Baker, J. M. (1982). The performing arts—how to measure up. In D. S. Pallett (Ed.), *Proceedings of the Workshop on Standardization for Speech I/O Technology*. Gaithersburg, MD: National Bureau of Standards.

Biermann, A. W., Rodman, R. D., Rubin, D. C., & Heidlage, J. F. (1985). Natural language with discrete speech as a mode for human-to-machine communication. *Communications of the ACM*, **28**, 628–636.

Blomberg, M., Carlson, R., Elenius, K., & Granstrom, B. (1986). Auditory models as front ends in speech recognition systems. In J. S. Perkell & D. H. Klatt (Eds.), *Invariance and variability in speech processes* (pp. 108–114). Hillsdale, NJ: Erlbaum.

Bristow, G. (1984). *Electronic speech synthesis: Techniques, technology and applications*. New York: McGraw-Hill.

Brooks, L. R. (1968). Spatial and verbal components of the act of recall. *Canadian Journal of Psychology*, **22**, 349–368.

Carlson, R, & Granstrom, B. (Eds.). (1982). *The representation of speech in the peripheral auditory system*. Amsterdam: Elsevier.

Chen, F. R. (1986, April). Lexical access and verification in a broad phonetic approach to continuous digit recognition. Paper presented at IEEE International Conference on Acoustics, Speech, and Signal Processing, Tokyo, Japan.

Cohen, J. R. (1989). Application of an auditory model to speech recognition. *Journal of the Acoustical Society of America*, **85**, 2623–2629.

Cole, R. A., & Jakimik, J. (1980). A model of speech perception. In R. A. Cole (Ed.), *Perception and production of fluent speech* (pp. 133–163). Hillsdale, NJ: Erlbaum.

Cole, R. A., & Rudnicky, A. I. (1983). What's new in speech perception? The research and ideas of William Chandler Bagley, 1874–1946. *Psychological Review*, 90, 94–101.

Coler, C. R., Huff, E. M., Plummer, R. P., & Hitchcock, M. H. (1978). Automatic speech recognition research at NASA-Ames Research Center. In R. Breaux, M. Curran, & E. Huff (Eds.), *Proceedings of the Workshop on Voice Technology for Interactive Real-Time Command/Control Systems Application* (pp. 143–170). Moffett Field, CA: NASA Ames Research Center.

Crowder, R. G. (1976). *Principles of learning and memory.* Hillsdale, NJ: Erlbaum.

Cutler, A., & Norris, D. (1988). The role of strong syllables in segmentation for lexical access. *Journal of Experimental Psychology: Human Perception and Performance*, 14, 113–121.

Davies, D. R., Jones, D. M., & Taylor, A. (1984). Selective–and sustained–attention tasks: Individual and group differences. In R. Parasuraman & D. R. Davies (Eds.), *Varieties of attention* (pp. 395–447). Orlando, FL: Academic.

Doddington, G. R., & Schalk, T. B. (1981). Speech recognition: Turning theory to practice. *IEEE Spectrum*, 18, 26–32.

Dreher, J., & O'Neill, J. J. (1957). Effects of ambient noise on speaker intelligibility for words and phrases. *Journal of the Acoustical Society of America*, 29, 1320–1323.

Egeth, H. E., & Blecker, D. L. (1969). Verbal interference in a perceptual comparison task. *Perception & Psychophysics*, 6, 355–356.

Foss, D. J., & Blank, M. A. (1980). Identifying the speech codes. *Cognitive Psychology*, 12, 1–31.

Gerstman, L. J. (1968). Classification of self-normalized vowels. *IEEE Transactions on Audio and Electroacoustics*, AU–16, 78–80.

Gould, J. D., Conti, J., & Hovanyecz, T. (1984). Composing letters with a listening typewriter. *Communications of the ACM*, 26, 295–308.

Greenspan, S.L., Nusbaum, H. C., & Pisoni, D. B. (1988). Perceptual learning of synthetic speech produced by rule. *Journal of Experimental Psychology: Learning, Memory, and Cognition*, **14**, 421–433.

Grosjean, F. (1980). Spoken word recognition processes and the gating paradigm. *Perception & Psychophysics*, **28**, 267–283.

Haggard, M. P. (1983, August). The human impact of speech technology. Presidential Address to Psychology Section, British Association.

Halliday, M. A. K. & Hasan, R. (1976). *Cohesion in English*. London: Longman.

Hartman, G. W. (1946). Further evidence on the unexpected large size of recognition vocabularies among college students. *Journal of Educational Psychology*, **37**, 436–439.

Hayes-Roth, F. (1980). Syntax, semantics, and pragmatics in speech understanding systems. In W. A. Lea (Ed.), *Trends in speech recognition* (pp. 206–233). Englewood Cliffs, NJ: Prentice-Hall.

Henly, A. & Nusbaum, H. C. (1991). The role of lexical status in the segmentation of fluent speech. *Journal of the Acoustical Society of America*, 2011, 9SP8 (Abstract).

Hobbs, J. R., & Evans, D. A. (1980). Conversation as planned behavior. *Cognitive Science*, **4**, 349–377.

House, A. S., Williams, C. E., Hecker, M. H. L., & Kryter, K. (1965). Articulation–testing methods: Consonantal differentiation with a closed-response set. *Journal of the Acoustical Society of America*, **37**, 158–166.

Jelinek, F. (1986). Continuous speech recognition—An IBM research project. Paper presented at the Voice Input/Output Applications Show and Conference, New York.

Joos, M. A. (1948). Acoustic phonetics. *Language*, **24**(Suppl. 2), 1–136.

Klatt, D. H. (1977). Review of the ARPA speech understanding project. *Journal of the Acoustical Society of America*, **62**, 1345–1366.

Ladefoged, P., & Broadbent, D. E. (1957). Information conveyed by vowels. *Journal of the Acoustical Society of America*, **29**, 98–104.

Lamel, L. F. (1983). The use of phonotactic constraints to determine word boundaries. *Journal of the Acoustical Society of America*, 74, 515 (Abstract).

Lane, H. L., & Tranel, B. (1971). The Lombard sign and the role of hearing in speech. *Journal of Speech and Hearing Research,* **14,** 677–709.

Lea, W. A. (1980). Speech recognition: What is needed now? In W. A. Lea (Ed.), *Trends in speech recognition* (pp. 562–569). Englewood Cliffs, NJ: Prentice–Hall.

Lee, L. & Nusbaum, H. C. (1989). The effects of perceptual learning on capacity demands for recognizing synthetic speech. *Journal of the Acoustical Society of America,* **85,** S125 (Abstract).

Levelt, W. J. M., & Kelter, S. (1982). Surface form and memory in question answering. *Cognitive Psychology,* **14,** 78–106.

Liberman, A. M., Cooper, F. S., Shankweiler, D. P., & Studdert-Kennedy, M. (1967). Perception of the speech code. *Psychological Review,* **74,** 431–461.

Licklider, J. C. R. (1952). On the process of speech perception. *Journal of the Acoustical Society of America,* **24,** 590–594.

Luce, P. A., Feustel, T. C., & Pisoni, D. B. (1983). Capacity demands in short-term memory for synthetic and natural word lists. *Human Factors,* **25,** 17–32.

Lyon, R. F. (1982). A computational model of filtering, detection, and compression in the cochlea. *Proceedings of the IEEE International Congress on Acoustics, Speech, and Signal Processing,* **82,** Paris, France.

Mangione, P. A. (1985). Speech recognition and office automation. *Proceedings of the Voice I/O Systems Applications Conference* (pp. 59–67). Sunnyvale, CA: AVIOS.

Marslen-Wilson, W. D., & Welsh, A. (1978). Processing interactions and lexical access during word recognition in continuous speech. *Cognitive Psychology,* **10,** 29–63.

Mehta, G. & Cutler, A. (1988). Detection of target phonemes in spontaneous and read speech. *Language and Speech,* **31,** 135–156.

Miller, J. L. (1981). Effects of speaking rate on segmental distinctions. In P. D. Eimas & J. L. Miller (Eds.), *Perspectives on the study of speech* (pp. 39–74). Hillsdale, NJ: Erlbaum.

Moore, R. (1986). Computational Techniques. In G. Bristow (Ed.) *Electronic speech recognition: Techniques, technology, and applications* (pp. 130–157). New York: McGraw–Hill.

Morin, T. M., & Nusbaum, H. C. (1989, November). Cues to perceptual normalization of talker differences. *Journal of the Acoustical Society of America,* **86,** S100 (Abstact).

Morland, D. V. (1983). Human factors guidelines for terminal interface design. *Communications of the ACM,* **26,** 484–494.

Mountford, S. J., North, R. A., Metz, S. V., & Warner, N. (1982). Methodology for exploring voice–interactive avionics tasks: Optimizing interactive dialogues. *Proceedings of the Human Factors Society 26th Annual Meeting,* 207–211.

Mullennix, J. W., Pisoni, D. B., & Martin, C. S. (1989). Some effects of talker variability on spoken word recognition. *Journal of the Acoustical Society of America,* **85,** 365–378

Nakatani, L. H., & Dukes, K. D. (1977). Locus of segmental cues for word juncture. *Journal of the Acoustical Society of America,* **62,** 714–719.

National Research Council (1984). *Automated speech recognition in severe environments,* Committee on Computerized Speech Recognition Technologies, Washington, D. C.

Navon, D., & Gopher, D. (1979). On the economy of the human–processing system. *Psychological Review,* **86,** 214–255.

Newell, A. (1975). A tutorial on speech understanding systems. In D. R. Reddy (Ed.), *Speech recognition: Invited papers presented at the 1974 IEEE Symposium* (pp. 3–54). New York: Academic Press.

Norman, D. A. (1981). The trouble with UNIX. *Datamation,* **27**(12), 139–150.

Norman, D. A. (1982, March). Steps toward a cognitive engineering: Design rules based on analyses of human error. In *Proceedings of the Conference on Human Factors in Computer Systems,* Gaithersburg, MD.

Norman, D. A. (1983). Design principles for human–computer interfaces. In *Proceedings of the CHI 1983 Conference on Human Factors in Computer Systems* (pp. 1–10). Amsterdam: North–Holland.

Norman, D. A. (1984). Design rules based on analyses of human error. *Communications of the ACM,* **26,** 254–258.

Norman, D. A., & Bobrow, D. J. (1975). On data–limited and resource–limited processes. *Cognitive Psychology,* **7,** 44–64.

Nusbaum, H. C., & DeGroot, J. (1990). In M. S. Ziolkowski, M. Noske, & K. Deaton (Eds.), *Papers from the parasession on the syllable in phonetics and phonology.* Chicago: Chicago Linguistic Society.

Nusbaum, H. C., & Morin, T. M. (1989). Perceptual normalization of talker differences. *Journal of the Acoustical Society of America, 85,* S125 (Abstact).

Nusbaum, H. C., & Pisoni, D. B. (1985). Constraints on the perception of synthetic speech generated by rule. *Behavior Research Methods, Instruments, & Computers, 17,* 235–242.

Nusbaum, H. C., & Pisoni, D. B. (1987). Automatic measurement of speech recognition performance: A comparison of six speaker-dependent recognition devices. *Computer Speech and Language, 2,* 87–108.

Nusbaum, H. C., & Schwab, E. C. (1986). The role of attention and active processing in speech perception. In E. C. Schwab & H. C. Nusbaum, (Eds.), *Pattern recognition by humans and machines: Vol. 1. Speech perception* (pp. 113–157). New York: Academic Press.

Ohala, J. J. (1982). Calibrated vocabularies. In D. S. Pallett (Ed.), *Proceedings of the Workshop on Standardization for Speech I/O Technology* (pp. 79–85). Gaithersburg, MD: National Bureau of Standards.

Oshika, B. T., Zue, V. W., Weeks, R. V., Neu, H., & Aurbach, J. (1975). The role of phonological rules in speech understanding research. *IEEE Transactions on Acoustics, Speech, and Signal Processing,* **ASSP–23,** 104–112.

Pallett, D. S. (1985). Performance assessment of automatic speech recognizers. *Journal of Research of the National Bureau of Standards, 90,* 371–387.

Peterson, G. E., & Barney, H. L. (1952). Control methods used in a study of the vowels. *Journal of the Acoustical Society of America, 24,* 175–184.

Pisoni, D. B., Bernacki, R. H., Nusbaum, H. C., & Yuchtman, Y. (1985). Some acoustic-phonetic correlates of speech produced in noise. In *Proceedings of ICASSP 85.* New York: IEEE Press.

Posner, M. I. (1978). *Chronometric explorations of mind: The third Paul M. Fitts lectures.* Hillsdale, NJ: Erlbaum.

Ramirez, R. W. (1985). *The FFT: Fundamentals and concepts.* Englewood Cliffs, NJ: Prentice-Hall.

Remez, R. E., Bressel, R. S., Rubin, P. E., & Ren, N. (1987). Perceptual differentiation of spontaneous and read utterances after resynthesis with monotone fundamental frequency. *Journal of the Acoustical Society of America*, 81, S2 (Abstract).

Rosenthal, R. I. (1979). The design of technological displays (Tutorial Paper). In P. A. Kolers, M. E. Wrolstad, & H. Bouma (Eds.), *Processing of visible language: Vol. 1.* (pp. 451–472). New York: Plenum.

Samuel, A. G. (1986). The role of the lexicon in speech perception. In E. C. Schwab & H. C. Nusbaum (Eds.), *Pattern recognition by humans and machines: Vol. 1. Speech perception* (pp. 89–111). New York: Academic Press.

Schinke, D. (1986). Speaker independent recognition applied to telephone access information systems. *The Official Proceedings of Speech Tech '86: Voice Input/Output Applications Show and Conference*, 1(3), 52–53.

Schmandt, C., Arons, B., & Simmons, C. (1985). Voice interaction in an integrated office and telecommunications environment. *Proceedings of the Voice I/O Systems Applications Conference* (pp. 51–57). Sunnyvale, CA: AVIOS.

Schurick, J. M., Williges, B. H., & Maynard, J. F. (1985). User feedback requirements with automatic speech recognition. *Ergonomics*, 28, 1543–1555.

Schwab, E. C., Nusbaum, H. C., & Pisoni, D. B. (1985). Some effects of training on the perception of synthetic speech. *Human Factors*, 27, 395–408.

Scott, B. L. (1980). Speech as patterns in time. In R. A. Cole (Ed.), *Perception and production of fluent speech* (pp. 51–71). Hillsdale, NJ: Erlbaum.

Searle, C. L., Jacobson, J. Z., & Rayment, S. G. (1979). Stop consonant discrimination based on human audition. *Journal of the Acoustical Society of America*, 65, 799–809.

Seashore, R. H. (1933). Measurement and analysis of extent of vocabulary. *Psychological Bulletin*, 30, 709–710.

Seneff, S. (1986). A synchrony model for auditory processing of speech. In J. S. Perkell & D. H. Klatt (Eds.), *Invariance and variability in speech processes* (pp. 115–122). Hillsdale, NJ: Erlbaum.

Shiffrin, R. M. (1976). Capacity limitations in information processing, attention, and memory. In W. K. Estes (Ed.), *Handbook of learning and cognitive processes: Vol. 4* (pp. 177–236). Hillsdale, NJ: Erlbaum.

Simpson, C. A., McCauley, M. E., Roland, E. F., Ruth, J. C., & Williges, B. H. (1987). System design for speech recognition and generation. *Human Factors*, **27**, 115–141.

Stroop, J. R. (1935). Studies of interference in serial verbal reactions. *Journal of Experimental Psychology*, **18**, 643–662.

Summers, W. V., Pisoni, D. B., & Bernacki, R. H. (1989). Effects of cognitive workload on speech production: Acoustic analyses. *Research on Speech Perception* (Progress Report No. 15). Bloomington, IN: Indiana University, Speech Research Laboratory.

Summers, W. V., Pisoni, D. B., Bernacki, R. H., Pedlow, R. I., & Stokes, M. A. (1988). Effects of noise on speech production: Acoustic and perceptual analyses. *Journal of the Acoustical Society of America*, **84**, 917–928.

Syrdal, A. K., & Gopal, H. S. (1986). A perceptual model of vowel recognition based on the auditory representation of American English vowels. *Journal of the Acoustical Society of America*, **79**, 1086–1100.

Taft, L. (1983, December). Prosodic constraints in lexical segmentation. Paper presented at the Meeting of the Linguistic Society of America.

Van Peursem, R. S. (1982). Speech recognition performance: A function of the application. In D. S. Pallett (Ed.), *Proceedings of the Workshop on Standardization for Speech I/O Technology* (pp. 43–46). Gaithersburg, MD: National Bureau of Standards.

Van Peursem, R. S. (1985). Do's and don'ts of interactive voice dialog design. *The Official Proceedings of Speech Tech '85: Voice Input/Output Applications Show and Conference*, **1**(2), 48–56.

Wickens, C. D. (1980). The structure of attentional resources. In R. S. Nickerson (Ed.), *Attention and Performance VIII* (pp. 239–257). Hillsdale, NJ: Erlbaum.

Wilpon, J. G. (1985). A study on the ability to automatically recognize telephone–quality speech from large customer populations. *AT & T Technical Journal*, **64**, 423–451.

Yuchtman, M., & Nusbaum, H. C. (1986). Using template pattern structure information to improve recognition performance. *Proceedings of the Voice I/ O Systems Applications Conference* (pp. 375–392). Sunnyvale, CA: AVIOS.

Yuchtman, M., Nusbaum, H. C., & Davis, C. N. (1986). Multidimensional scaling of confusions produced by speech recognition systems. *Journal of the Acoustical Society of America*, **79**, S95–S96.

Zoltan-Ford, E. (1984). Reducing variability in natural language interactions with computers. In *Proceedings of the Human Factors Society 28th Annual Meeting* (Vol. 2), Santa Monica, CA: Human Factors Society.

Chapter 5

Intelligibility and Acceptability Testing for Speech Technology

Astrid Schmidt-Nielsen
Naval Research Laboratory

1.   Abstract

The evaluation of speech intelligibility and acceptability is an important aspect of the use, development, and selection of voice communication devices—telephone systems, digital voice systems, speech synthesis by rule, speech in noise and the effects of noise stripping. Standard test procedures can provide highly reliable measures of speech intelligibility, and subjective acceptability tests can be used to evaluate voice quality. These tests are often highly correlated with other measures of communication performance and can be used to predict performance in many situations. However, when the speech signal is severely degraded or highly processed, a more complete evaluation of speech quality is needed, one that takes into account the many different sources of information that contribute to how we understand speech.

2.   Introduction

The need for evaluation occurs at many stages of speech technology development—during development to determine whether improvement has occurred, in manufacturing to determine if specifications are met, and in selection to compare and choose among competing equipment or techniques. In order to evaluate the performance of a speech communication, processing, or synthesis system, some form of intelligibility or acceptability testing involving human listeners is usually conducted. The tests that are used can vary considerably in sophistication and reliability. In intelligibility testing, one or more listeners perform a task in which they listen to the transmitted or synthesized speech and report what they hear.

Depending on the specific test, the listener's task may be to write down a sentence, word or sound to select the response that most closely matches what was heard from two or more alternatives. In contrast to measures of speech intelligibility, which can be objectively scored, evaluations of speech acceptability are based on subjective listener judgements. Subjects listen to speech samples and rate the quality of speech using either a numerical scale or verbal labels (which can later be converted to numbers).

The problem of conducting intelligibility and acceptability tests to evaluate voice communication systems is especially difficult because the listeners and speakers that are used to evaluate the speech can vary considerably from person to person and from study to study, whereas the performance of the equipment itself is highly stable from one time to another and among different units of the same model. This chapter discusses intelligibility and acceptability test methods. The use of physical measures of the speech signal as possible indices of speech intelligibility or acceptability is also briefly considered. An overview of the testing process and a discussion of the factors that contribute to speech intelligibility and acceptability precede a review of intelligibility and acceptability test methods. Finally, experimental relations among different tests and considerations in selecting test methods will be discussed, and some general recommendations will be made.

The general concept of intelligibility refers to how well the speech can be comprehended or understood. Speech that is more intelligible is easier to understand. This leads more or less directly to the notion of measuring intelligibility by counting the number of words or speech sounds that are correctly understood, but in real life factors other than the fidelity of the acoustic signal also contribute to how well the speech is understood (e.g., listener expectations, subject matter, etc.). It is important to remember that the score obtained on an intelligibility test is only a predictor or estimate of what we really want to know and is not an end in itself. The goal of testing is not merely to obtain high scores but to develop usable systems.

Intelligibility testing is a compromise that requires trade-offs among conflicting goals and sometimes incompatible test requirements. One of the most important goals is to determine the usability of a communication system for the given application. Potential users of the equipment want to know how well the system will perform in operational environments with realistic vocabularies. It is also highly desirable to be able to compare the results of different test conditions with one another. Decision makers who use scores for selection prefer to deal with exact numbers; they want to know that the score is 92 and do not want to be told the next time that the score may be 87 even if the system would still have the same rank ordering as before. For the purpose of writing procurement or manufacturing specifications, a specific criterion is needed—i.e., that the score meets or exceeds the specified value. Practical considerations of time, cost, and human resources are also important in determining the kind of testing that can be carried out. Realistic field tests are time consuming and expensive, and it is often difficult to quantify the results. Field tests are also highly specific to a particular situation and do not generalize well to other situations, nor do they allow for meaningful comparisons of test scores with the results of tests made under other conditions. The result is that intelligibility testing usually involves relatively simple listening tasks; this allows tests to be given and scored quickly and inexpensively so that the test does not end up evaluating extraneous factors rather than the performance of the speech system. These intelligibility test tasks differ from the tasks involved in the actual use of a system, which might involve, for example, specialized vocabulary and grammar, rapid responses in emergencies, or fatigue through extended use. Unfortunately, the test materials that give the most repeatable results, like rhyme tests or nonsense syllable tests, are often the least realistic, while the most realistic speech materials, sentences or conversations, tend to produce the least repeatable results. If the correlations among tests using different types of speech materials were entirely consistent, it would be possible to predict performance with more realistic vocabularies and speech materials from rhyme test scores. However, as will be seen later in this chapter, generalizing from one type of test to another is questionable, especially when comparing very different speech systems or degradations.

In selecting and using speech intelligibility and acceptability tests and interpreting the test scores, it is important to understand how the test tasks relate to actual tasks in order to make intelligent decisions about when and how test results can be extrapolated to performance in the real world. The most obvious consequences of poor speech intelligibility are mistakes in understanding the spoken message—misperceptions, confusions among words, or words that are missed altogether—and this of course is the reason for intelligibility tests. Poor speech quality can have consequences, even when all of the words are correctly understood. When more effort is required to understand speech, it may be harder to integrate and store the information in memory (Luce et al., 1983), and in high workload or multiple task situations, the added effort of listening to degraded speech can lead to poorer performance on concurrent tasks (Schmidt-Nielsen et al., 1990).

Many of these effects are difficult to track or quantify because the human being is an extremely flexible information processor who develops new strategies or uses more effort to compensate for deficiencies in the system and thus manages to perform the required task in spite of poor speech quality. The long term effects of listening to degraded speech over extended periods of time, such as fatigue and stress, are even more difficult to document, but are probably nonetheless real. Standard intelligibility tests can provide standard and repeatable scores that make it possible to compare results across different conditions, but it is often useful to supplement standard test results with tests and experiments to evaluate other aspects of system performance.

3.   Overview of the Testing Process

The basic elements of a voice transmission system are shown in Figure 1, and these are also the principle elements involved in the testing of voice systems. For simplicity, a number of links have been left out of this simplified system, for example an input device such as a microphone and an output device such as a loudspeaker or headphones. Each of the elements in the diagram may be subject to considerable elaboration, and the elements need not all be present for any given test situation. The testing of speech synthesizers, for example, includes only the right half of the diagram, and the transmission channel may be omitted in some tests.

Characteristics of each of the elements depicted in Figure 1 will affect the outcome of the testing process and can also interact with the other elements in determining the final score. Some of these (e.g., background noise) may be of specific interest to the evaluation process and may be systematically varied in a test series. Others (e.g., listener differences) may only contribute random variability to the test scores and should be carefully controlled. In deciding how to conduct a series of tests, the tester should have a clear idea of which aspects are of interest to the evaluation process and which ones need to be controlled.

3.1   The Speaker
Different speakers have different voice characteristics that affect the performance and intelligibility of the voice system. It is well recognized that some voices, especially female voices, can cause problems for narrowband digital voice systems, such as linear predictive coding (LPC) algorithms. A speaker whose voice performs well in one environment may not be best for another.

3.2 The Speaker Environment

Voice communication systems are often used in environments where background noise is present. This may vary from relatively benign environments like an office to severe environments such as a helicopter or tank. Even though people generally tend to speak more loudly when there is background noise, some voices are considerably more intelligible in noise than others. The background noise environment not only affects the voice characteristics of the speaker, causing changes in amplitude, pitch, duration, and formant frequencies (e.g., Summers et al., 1988), but when the noise enters the microphone, the performance of the voice system may also be degraded. Some communication systems degrade when there is background noise while others are quite robust. Systems designed primarily to handle speech may be particularly susceptible to degradation from nonspeech sounds.

3.3 The Voice Processor

Digital voice transmission systems, wideband and narrowband, consist of a speech analyzer at the input, which analyzes and codes the speech signal and a synthesizer at the output to reconstruct the speech signal and transform it back to analog voice output. Noise reduction by various techniques is a form of speech processing that may be used either at the input of a communication device before the speech is coded and transmitted or at the output after noisy speech is received. Speech synthesis for computer voice output uses rules or stored segments to generate the voice instead of the human speaker.

3.4 The Transmission Channel

When a communication system is tested in back-to-back mode, with the output of the analysis portion going directly into the synthesis portion, the only degradation is due to the voice processor itself, yielding the best performance that can be expected. In actual use, the transmission channel for voice communication systems is another possible source of degradation. Telephone links may suffer from echo or crosstalk. Radio transmissions may be subject to various forms of interference, natural or human made. Digital voice processors are susceptible to bit errors, random or burst, from various sources of interference. Digital voice transmissions may sometimes involve tandems, i.e., more than one digital processing link, with the speech being converted back to analog from transmission through the next link. Combinations of degradations may interact with one another to cause even more severe degradation.

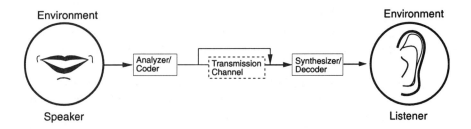

Figure 1   Simplified diagram of the elements needed in a communication system and for intelligibility testing.

3.5   The Listener
Listeners vary in their ability to make speech discriminations. When listeners with normal hearing are used, listener variability is generally smaller than speaker variability for most intelligibility tests (Voiers, 1982). Listener variability tends to be greater than speaker variability for acceptability tests (Voiers, personal communication). With more complex speech tasks, involving sentence or dialogue comprehension, other skills of the listener, such as the attention span or language ability, can also affect the results.

3.6   The Listening Environment
Like the speaking environment, the listening environment may have more or less severe background noise, which can affect speech intelligibility. However, the listener can often compensate by increasing the volume of the speech.

Tape recording is frequently used at various stages of the testing process for standardization and control of the test materials as well as for portability and reproducibility. The speakers used in an intelligibility test may be recorded reading the test materials and the recorded materials processed through the voice equipment. The output can also be recorded for later use in testing and played back to the listeners. Background noises of various types may be recorded and the levels noted so they can later be played back at the same levels to simulate different speaking or listening environments.

4.   Factors that Influence Speech Intelligibility and Acceptability

When speech is used for communication, information that can be used to decode and understand the speech sounds is available on many different levels. Human listeners are versatile and efficient processors of information with remarkable capabilities for understanding even a degraded speech signal. They will use every available source of information to perform the speech task. Several types of information are available to the listener in a typical communication situation. There is the acoustic-phonetic information in the speech signal itself as well as the contextual information from the surrounding circumstances. The information carried by the speech signal includes segmental information (the acoustic-phonetic cues for consonant and vowel identity) and suprasegmental or prosodic information (the intonation, timing, and intensity cues that carry information about word stress and word and sentence structure.) Words spoken in isolation carry more acoustic detail relating to phonetic structure of the word while prosody and context assume greater importance in understanding connected speech. The words in spoken sentences are highly intelligible within the sentence context, but individual words extracted from such speech are poorly recognized (Pollack and Pickett, 1964). Contextual information include the grammatical and semantic constraints imposed by sentence structure as well as specific situational knowledge and general knowledge which influence the listener's expectations. If there is little information available from the context, as for example in trying to identify nonsense syllables, the listener must rely almost exclusively on acoustic-phonetic information in the signal for correct identification, and conversely, the more information there is in the context, the less accurate acoustic information the listener needs to correctly identify the speech. Different types of tests present different levels of information to the listener and measure different aspects of the comprehension process. In this section we will consider some of the types of information that people may use in the communication process, how the distortion of this information by a voice processing system might affect the intelligibility or judged acceptability of a system, and the extent to which it is measured by existing tests.

4.1   Segmental Information

The acoustic-phonetic information that allows us to identify individual speech sounds needs to be correctly transmitted for the speech to be intelligible. In analysis-synthesis voice transmission systems, especially low data rate systems, the acoustic cues needed to correctly identify the speech sounds are not always correctly reproduced, and this reduces intelligibility. Speech synthesis by rule does not always produce the correct sounds either, and the effects of coarticulation (the influence of adjacent speech sounds on one another) may not be correctly reproduced in some contexts, so that phoneme intelligibility may vary considerably depending on word position, surrounding phonemes, etc. Intelligibility tests explicitly test phoneme intelligibility, but the standard tests include discriminations only in initial and final positions in single syllable words.

4.2   Suprasegmental Information

Prosodic information—variations in pitch, intensity, and timing across segments—conveys information about stress levels and word and sentence structure, as well as more subtle nuances of meaning and emotion. In spoken English, the intonation is often the only cue that distinguishes a statement from a question. (Compare "He did?" with rising intonation and "He did." with falling intonation.) Some low data rate digital voice transmission systems may have problems with pitch and intensity, especially if there are rapid changes, but for most voice transmission systems pitch and intensity changes as well as segmental timing tend to be reasonably accurately reproduced, so testing prosody explicitly is not usually necessary. In speech synthesis by rule, intonation and timing rules that follow the constraints of the spoken language must be explicitly built into the system, and the effect of prosody on intelligibility and naturalness needs to be evaluated. The extent to which prosodic information is correctly conveyed is usually not explicitly tested in intelligibility tests, although tests using sentences or paragraphs may implicitly test the goodness of the prosody. Incorrect or distorted prosody will also tend to lower scores on voice acceptability tests.

4.3   Nonspeech Sounds

Other sounds—laughter, sighs, throat clearings, breath noises—also occur in voice communications and can provide information about the speaker's state or intentions. For naturalness, a voice transmission system should be able to transmit these sounds in a reasonably faithful manner. Low data rate voice algorithms that are optimized for speech may produce some rather odd effects when they encounter nonspeech sounds (Kemp et al., 1989). Voice tests seldom, if ever, include such sounds, although they can influence acceptance of the system in actual use.

4.4   Contextual Information

Context from several sources can help the listener to understand the spoken message. Grammatical constraints, realized in the sentence structure, provide one kind of context that helps us to know what kinds of words to expect next. In addition to the obvious constraints of English grammar military communication has its own special structures which constrain the word order and type of words that are used to convey a message. Context is also provided by semantic constraints, that is, the meaning of the words in a sentence or paragraph provide clues and create expectations about what will be said next. The comparison of everyday sentences with semantically anomalous but grammatically correct sentences can be used to evaluate some of the effects of context.

When a voice system is used in the real world, situational knowledge is an important contextual factor. This can be anything from knowing the topic of a conversation to knowing what to expect at any given time in a fairly constrained scenario like air traffic control or ordering in a fast food restaurant. An important effect of context is that it limits the number of alternatives that can occur at any given time in the message. As the size of the response set decreases, intelligibility scores will be higher and will decrease more slowly with increased noise levels (Miller, Heise, and Lichten, 1951; related research is reviewed in Ralston, et al., Chapter 6).

4.5 Speaker Recognition

Although speaker identity is not directly related to intelligibility, speaker recognition can be an important aspect of user acceptance and deserves at least to be mentioned. Testing for speaker recognition can be very difficult and will not be discussed in this chapter.

5. Overview of Speech Evaluation Techniques

Intelligibility tests evaluate the number of words or speech sounds that can be correctly identified in a controlled situation. The responses can be objectively[1] scored as a percentage of correct responses. Acceptability or quality[2] tests evaluate the acceptability of the system based on listener judgements of subjective voice quality. In an attempt to avoid some of the problems of using human listeners, various physical measures of the speech signal have also been used with variable success to predict speech intelligibility or acceptability.

---

[1] The terms objective measures and subjective measures have been used in different ways in various contexts. As used in this chapter, objective refers to any measure that can be objectively scored, as for example the percentage of correct responses or the number of requests for repeats, while subjective refers to expressions of opinion (which may be assigned numeric values). Some authors have used the term subjective tests for all tests using human listeners, regardless of the basis for scoring, and the term objective has been used to describe aspects of the speech signal that can be physically measured. I prefer to call the latter physical measures and to retain the distinction between objective and subjective aspects of listener behavior.

[2] Acceptability and quality have been both used to refer to subjective judgement tests. The term acceptability is probably more accurate (Voiers et al., 1990), but the term quality is also in widespread use for such tests. In order not to create confusion as to whether these are separate types of tests, both terms are used in this chapter.

5.1   Intelligibility Test Methods

The basic methods of intelligibility testing for voice communication systems have been in existence for a long time. As early as 1910, Campbell used consonant-vowel (CV) syllables to test telephone transmissions. The classic paper by Fletcher and Steinberg (1929) describes test methods and results using a variety of speech materials, including consonant-vowel-consonant (CVC) nonsense syllables, multi-syllable utterances, and English words, and it also included sentence comprehension based on questions like *Explain why a corked bottle floats*. However, the 1960 standard for monosyllabic intelligibility (ANSI, 1960) contains the following statement:[3]

"At present it is not possible to compare with precision two systems or conditions by testing one system or condition in one laboratory and the other system or condition in another laboratory."

Much subsequent research has been aimed at developing highly controlled and repeatable methodologies to reduce test-to-test variability, allowing for more accurate replicability and comparison of tests conducted at different times and places. In addition to the phonetically balanced (PB) monosyllabic word test specified in the 1960 standard, the current standard on speech intelligibility (ANSI, 1989) includes two rhyme tests, the Diagnostic Rhyme Test (DRT) and the Modified Rhyme Test (MRT). (The DRT and the MRT are independent tests; the MRT is a modification of an earlier test (Fairbanks, 1958).)

This section gives an overview of intelligibility test methods with examples of different test types. This review is not intended to be exhaustive or to cover all possible tests or types of tests that have been used to evaluate speech intelligibility. Rather, selected commonly used or promising test methods are described with a discussion of some of their major advantages and disadvantages. An excellent summary of a large number of different intelligibility tests can be found in Webster (1972), and Kryter (1972) also discusses various aspects of intelligibility testing for speech communication. The three tests included in the ANSI (1989) standard will be discussed first. These tests have been thoroughly validated and have been used extensively for testing voice systems, and there is a large body of literature using these tests. The standard describes methods for conducting intelligibility tests, including the selection and training of the speakers and the

---

[3] The American National Standards Institute periodically studies and recommends standard methods for measuring the intelligibility of speech. (ed.)

listeners, how to conduct the test sessions, and analysis of the results. The guidelines presented in the standard are applicable to other monosyllable and rhyme test materials as well as those described in the standard.

5.1.1   Standard Tests

The PB words, the DRT, and the MRT are all tests of phoneme intelligibility. In a phoneme intelligibility test, scores are based on the number of phonemes correctly identified by the listeners. Most frequently, single syllable words or nonsense syllables are used, and they may be spoken either as isolated utterances or in a carrier phrase, for example, "You will write the word _____ now." A phoneme test can be either open response, where the listener writes the word or syllable that was heard on the answer sheet, or closed response, where the listener is given two or more choices in a multiple-choice format and selects the word that is closest to the one heard. A detailed discussion of the controls that need to be exercised over the test procedures, listener and speaker selection, recording and reproduction equipment, levels, etc., can be found in the ANSI (1989) standard.

5.1.1.1   PB Words

The PB word test is an open response test consisting of 1000 monosyllabic CVC words grouped into 20 lists of 50 words each, usually presented in a carrier phrase. Several variants of this type of test have been developed that are used for testing the hearing impaired. The Harvard phonetically balanced (PB) word test (Egan, 1948) was until recently the only standard method for testing voice systems (ANSI, 1960), although closed response rhyme tests are now more common. Correctly training the speakers and listeners for this test is a cumbersome and expensive procedure often taking several weeks, and even then the listeners' scores continue to improve gradually with repeated testing, so that it is difficult to compare scores obtained at different times or in different laboratories.

5.1.1.2   Diagnostic Rhyme Test

The Diagnostic Rhyme Test (DRT) (Voiers, 1977, 1983) is a two-alternative closed response test that consists of 96 rhyming word pairs, in which the initial consonants differ only by a single distinctive feature (e.g., moot-boot differ only in the feature nasality). The features are derived from the Jacobson, Fant and Halle (1952) distinctive feature system. The words are presented without a carrier phrase, so more words can be presented in the same time than for tests using a carrier phrase. In addition to an overall intelligibility score, the DRT provides diagnostic feature scores on six phonemic features (voicing, nasality, sibilation, sustention, graveness, and compactness) A correction for guessing is used in scoring the DRT. Standard input tapes using the same six speakers in quiet and in a variety of military background noises (helicopter, jeep, tank, etc.) can be used. A test session usually uses ten listeners, and the two who are the most inconsistent are eliminated, leaving eight listeners for the final scores.

5.1.1.3   Modified Rhyme Test

The Modified Rhyme Test (MRT) (House et al., 1965) is a closed response test that consists of 300 words presented as six lists of 50 words each and uses a six-alternative format (e.g., rust, just, dust, must, gust, bust). A carrier sentence is usually used. Some of the alternatives differ from the target word by only a single distinctive feature and some differ by more than one feature. Both syllable initial and syllable final consonants are tested. A correction for guessing is not usually used in scoring.

5.1.1.4   Other Rhyme Tests

Rhyme tests have also been developed for other languages. Spelling modifications have been made to ensure that DRT pairs rhyme for British pronunciation (Pratt et al., 1987). There is a six-alternative test similar to the MRT for German, and diagnostic rhyme tests for French and Dutch have been developed following the same principles as the DRT (Peckels and Rossi, 1971; Steeneken, 1982). A PB monosyllabic word test also exists for Dutch (Houtgast and Steeneken, 1971). Finally, a "rhyme" test for vowels also exists (Clarke, 1965), which may be helpful in evaluating speech synthesizers.

5.1.1.5   Comparison of Tests

Both the DRT and the MRT have been extensively used to evaluate military and commercial voice systems. This means that there is a large amount of historical data against which to evaluate the results of any new tests. Scores on the DRT and MRT tend to be very highly correlated with one another over a wide variety of speech degradations (e.g., Voiers, 1983), so given the score on one of the tests, it is possible to predict the other and to make comparisons between the two. The DRT has the advantage of providing diagnostic feature scores, and the MRT has the advantage of testing final as well as initial consonants. A diagnostic counterpart of the DRT, the Diagnostic Alliteration Test (DAT) (Voiers, 1981), has been developed for final consonants and is highly correlated with the DRT and MRT. Scores on the MRT tend to be lower for final consonants than for initial consonants, and scores on the DAT also are consistently lower than equivalent DRT scores (Voiers, 1981).

Closed response tests, such as rhyme tests, are easier to administer and score, and they produce more consistent results with less variability than open response tests. Test procedures for closed response tests can be standardized to the point where scores of the same system obtained at different times can be highly repeatable. The Department of Defense (DoD) Digital Voice Processor Consortium, an inter-agency consortium to coordinate secure voice research, has conducted numerous tests of processors and modems over the years using the DRT. When voice systems were tested more than once, scores were usually within one or two percentage points of one another, with the exception of extremely low scores, which have greater variability. The average standard error for over 100 DRT scores listed in Sandy (1987) was 0.84. Closed response tests are also ideally suited for computerized data collection and scoring. The amount of practice needed to obtain stable performance is relatively small, and proper randomization procedures can be used effectively to prevent continued improvement due to guessing.

Open response tests have the advantage that the listeners can indicate the sounds they actually heard and are not limited to the choices provided by the test developer. Another possible advantage is that scores on open response tests are usually lower, so with very good systems there is less possibility of "ceiling effects" (scores that are so near the maximum that differences in performance are indistinguishable). These advantages are offset by the greater variability in scores for open response tests, which means that there is less possibility for discriminating among closely competing systems. More listeners can be used to compensate for this effect. A more serious drawback is that practice and learning effects are also greater for open response tests, where the same pool of words is used repeatedly in different randomizations. Considerable practice is needed before performance becomes reasonably stable, and gradual continued improvement occurs even after extensive practice. This effect makes it very difficult to make accurate comparisons of results obtained at different times or in different laboratories. Open response tests are also relatively expensive to administer and score because the written responses must be tallied by hand.

5.1.2   Sentence Tests: Harvard and Haskins Sentences

Tests that use complete sentences evaluate a number of speech cues not included in simple phoneme tests. Words in sentences tend to be less carefully articulated than words spoken in isolation, but sentences are often more intelligible because of grammatical and semantic constraints. Sentence structure also affects suprasegmental cues—pitch, intensity, and segmental duration. Sentence intelligibility is usually scored on the basis of the number of key words in the sentence that are correctly transcribed.

The Harvard Sentences (Egan, 1948) consist of sets of phonetically balanced, meaningful but not highly predictable sentences (e.g., *The birch canoe slid on the smooth planks*.) Transcription accuracy is usually scored on the basis of five key content words in each sentence.

The Haskins Sentences consist of sets of grammatically correct but semantically anomalous sentences (e.g., *The old corn cost the blood*), (Nye and Gaitenby, 1973). The content words in each sentence are scored. These sentences serve to evaluate sentence comprehension with grammatical constraints but without semantic constraints to aid in word recognition. The Haskins and Harvard sentences are often used in the same experiment to separate the effects of grammatical and semantic constraints.

Like open response tests, sentence tests are cumbersome to administer and score. Sentence tests are by nature very difficult to adapt for use as a repeatable standardized intelligibility test in that they cannot be used repeatedly with the same listeners because once a sentence has been heard and understood, it is known to the listener. This means that a sustained testing program would require either an enormous supply of listeners or an inexhaustible source of sentences that have been equated for difficulty. However, sentence tests can be useful for one-time comparisons in a controlled experiment when it is important to evaluate the intelligibility of connected speech, as for example with text-to-speech synthesis.

5.1.3   Other Speech Materials

A variety of other speech materials (e.g., polysyllabic words, paragraphs) and methods (memory, comprehension, reaction time) have been used to evaluate the effects of speech systems on performance. Many of these methods cannot be adapted for the repeated testing required for an extended testing program and are more suitable for limited experimental comparisons where only the speech systems tested at the same time can be meaningfully compared. Other types of material, for example consonants in other than initial and final positions (consonant clusters, intervocalic consonants), can be used to provide additional information in evaluating certain types of systems, e.g., synthesizers. Schmidt-Nielsen (1983) found that for LPC processed speech, the confusions for intervocalic consonants were different from the confusions for initial consonants as tested by the DRT. To be a useful evaluation tool, any test using a different type of speech materials would have to be extensively tested and validated and the procedures standardized to assure that reliable results can be obtained that will be comparable across a variety of situations.

Experiments also have been conducted testing specialized vocabularies such as military phrases (e.g., Webster, 1972). The intelligibility of the International Civil Aviation Organization (ICAO) spelling alphabet and digits has been compared with DRT intelligibility for a number of digital and analog conditions (Schmidt-Nielsen, 1987a, 1987b). The spelling alphabet uses a small, highly distinctive vocabulary, so it is subject to ceiling effects for most ordinary voice systems, but it can be useful for evaluating the usability of very degraded systems where the DRT or other standard intelligibility scores are so low as to be considered unacceptable for normal use. The spelling alphabet is suitable for generating multiple randomizations and for standardizing procedures for repeated use. It can be readily adapted for machine scoring, as the letter or number responses can be typed on an ordinary keyboard. A randomization procedure has been developed that tests all of the letter names and digits while including some repetitions so that listeners will not develop expectations about the remaining words, and tape recordings have been made using four of the speakers who have been used for DRT recordings.

5.2   Acceptability Test Methods

Acceptability or quality tests deal with subjective opinions of how the speech sounds. It is important to evaluate acceptability in addition to intelligibility because some degradations may affect one more than the other. While subjective quality is often highly correlated with intelligibility, there are situations in which intelligibility may be high but speech quality is degraded. For example, a high pitched whine in the background may not reduce intelligibility noticeably but could be so annoying as to make the speech almost intolerable to listen to, and certain degradations like peak clipping may have a relatively small effect on intelligibility but can still make the speech sound unpleasant (e.g., Licklider and Pollack, 1948). There can also be circumstances in which speech quality is improved but speech intelligibility is still poor. Noise removal techniques, for example, can improve acceptability scores (Kang, 1989) but often tend to lead to lower segmental intelligibility scores (Sandy and Parker, 1984).

The two most commonly used procedures for quality tests are paired comparisons and rating scales, or category judgements. Paired comparisons may be made among a set of voice systems of interest, pairing each system with every other system, or the system(s) of interest may be compared with a set of standard reference systems consisting of controlled noise levels or other distortions. The listener hears a sentence for each of two speech conditions and selects the one that is preferred. All pairs should be presented twice so that each system is presented both in first and second place. For ratings, listeners hear one or more sentences and are asked to rate the quality or acceptability of the speech on some form of rating scale. The listeners may be instructed either to assign labels—category judgements— (e.g., excellent, good, fair, poor, bad), which can later be converted into numerical scores, or they may assign numerical values directly. Reference systems are usually included in the test to make comparisons with previous results easier.

The IEEE Recommended Practice for Speech Quality Measurements (1969) outlined three quality measurement techniques—the isopreference method, the relative preference method, and the category judgement method. The former two are paired comparison methods. The isopreference method developed by Munson and Karlin (1962) uses isopreference contours based on speech level and noise level. The relative preference method (Hecker and Williams, 1966) compares the test system to five reference systems consisting of different degradations. More recently, subjective quality has been referenced to varying amounts of multiplicative white noise, and the quality of the speech transmission device or distortion is given in terms of subjective speech-to-noise ratio (Nakatsui and Mermelstein, 1982). The selection of a single reference dimension such as subjective speech-to-noise levels allows for standardization of comparisons, but it is not clear that it is possible to make valid comparisons among widely different distortions (as in different kinds of digital voice algorithms) along a single dimension. The use of several different reference distortions raises the problem of selecting the appropriate distortions and also increases the number of paired comparisons that must be made. The use of paired comparisons tends to be very inefficient for comparing more than a very few systems, both in terms of listening time and in terms of the time needed to generate the test materials. If large numbers of reference systems are used, or if many different voice systems are to be compared directly with one another or with all of the reference systems, the number of pairs to be compared becomes very large.

The use of ratings or category judgements instead of paired comparisons greatly simplifies the data collection since each system being tested need be rated only once for each speaker. Experimental evidence (e.g., Voiers, 1977b) as well as many informal experiences in different speech laboratories indicate that the rank orderings assigned by the use of rating scales and by paired comparisons are very highly correlated.

The most serious problem with using rating tests (and to some extent also paired comparisons) for speech quality is listener variability. Listeners can vary widely in their preferences, and in how they use the scales, in the extent to which they spread their responses over the entire scale or use only a portion of the scale. A variety of control procedures, such as listener training, listener normalization, etc., can be used to provide greater repeatability and stability of scores. Speaker variability can be controlled by using the same speakers in all tests, but caution should be used in comparing data for different speaker sets.

5.2.1   Diagnostic Acceptability Measure (DAM)

The Diagnostic Acceptability Measure (Voiers, 1977b; Voiers et al., 1990) is the quality test that has been taken the farthest toward standardizing test procedures developing techniques for reducing variability, and compensating for differences between individuals and for changes over time. Voiers et al. (1990) list the measures used to control systematic and random error in the tests: 1) Direct and indirect estimates of acceptability, 2) Separate evaluation of signal and background quality, 3) Explicitly identified anchors to give the listeners a frame of reference, 4) Probes to detect shifts in listener adaptation level, 5) Listener screening procedures, 6) Listener training procedures, 7) Listener calibration procedures, 8) Listener monitoring procedures.

The DAM uses standard input tapes consisting of 12 sentences for each of six speakers, three males and three females; listening crews include at least 12 listeners. There are 21 rating scales: ten signal quality scales, eight background quality scales, and three scales evaluating overall speech characteristics. The rating scales are negatively oriented and evaluate the detectability of the effect in question on a 10-point scale that ranges from undetectable to overwhelming. The category labels (e.g., barely detectable, very conspicuous, etc.) for the ratings were experimentally selected from a large set of possible labels to be as perceptually equidistant as possible. Potential listeners are screened for normal hearing, for their ability to discriminate different features of the speech signal, and for their consistency in using the rating scales. Upon selection and periodically thereafter all listeners are calibrated against a large set of speech systems for which normative historical data has been obtained. This yields a set of constants and coefficients based on each individual listener's mean and standard deviation that can be used to transform that listener's scores to those of a theoretical "normative listener." These transformations are applied to future data obtained for that listener and are periodically updated. Anchors and probes are also built into each listening session, and additional adjustments are made based on probe performance for individuals who may be having a particularly lenient or strict day. The scales used on the DAM were derived from factor analysis. An overall composite acceptability score is arrived at by a complex set of combining equations. The diagnostic scales and the summary scores on the DAM have been validated against an extensive set of systematic speech degradations (Voiers, et al., 1990).

Over the years, the DoD Digital Voice Processor Consortium has conducted a large number of DAM tests, including many repetitions. In most cases, scores have been within one or two points of one another. On one occasion there was a difference of as much as five points after several years, but a source of bias was later identified in this case. The recently revised DAM II introduced some modifications to the way the questions are presented to the listener that should result in even better repeatability than with the previous version. Data collected over a period of two and a half years (Voiers, et al., 1990) indicate that the standard deviation for inter-run variation of DAM scores was 1.01 points for unadjusted scores and 0.59 for probe adjusted scores.

5.2.2   Mean Opinion Score (MOS)

Mean Opinion Score refers to a general procedure that has been widely used for evaluating telephone systems (CCITT, 1984a) and can have many variations. The speech material, typically sentences, is played through the voice systems of interest and presented to listeners for scoring. The listener assigns scores on a five point scale defined by category labels such as excellent, good, fair, poor, and bad. Sentences spoken by several different speakers may be used, often two males and two females. Large numbers of naive listeners rather than small numbers of trained listeners are generally used. A modification of the absolute category rating procedure, the Degradation MOS (DMOS) (CCITT, 1984b), uses a five point degradation or annoyance scale and includes a high quality reference system in order to obtain greater sensitivity than the usual MOS procedure, especially for high quality systems (Pascal and Combescure, 1988). Instead of calibrating the listeners, scores are referenced to the modulated noise reference unit (MNRU) (CCITT, 1984c). Reference systems that are degraded by modulated noise at various speech-to-noise levels are included in tests of voice systems, and the scores for each system are referenced to equivalent Q-levels or modulated signal-to-noise levels. At least five reference systems at different signal-to-noise levels should be included. Goodman and Nash (1982) conducted tests of a number of communication and reference circuits using the same general procedure in seven different countries. They reported that average MOS scores differed considerably from country to country but that much of this variability was due to an additive scale shift. The average standard deviation for U.S. listeners was 0.75 on a scale of 1 to 5. There were 31 listeners, so the standard error in this case would be about 0.14.

5.2.3   Phoneme Specific Sentences

A set of phoneme specific sentences was developed by Huggins and Nickerson (1985) for subjective evaluations of speech coders. Different sets of sentences contain consonants belonging only to certain phonetic categories or combinations of categories. For example, the content words in the sentence *Nanny may know the meaning* has only nasal consonants and vowels. They had the listeners first rank the speech conditions for each sentence and later provide degradation ratings for the same materials. Different sentence types were sensitive to different aspects of degradation due to LPC processing. This type of test could provide a form of diagnosticity that is different from that provided by the DAM and perhaps more similar to that provided by the DRT. No listener calibration or standardization procedures were used.

5.3   Communicability Tests

Communicability tests are a variant of quality tests using two-way conversations. Standard quality and intelligibility tests using prerecorded materials are essentially one-way in that the speaker does not have the opportunity to modify his manner of speaking to fit the situation. In ordinary two-way conversations, there is feedback between the speaker and listener, and the person can speak more loudly or enunciate more clearly if necessary. Communicability tests use a two way communication task followed by a rating questionnaire, and result in subjective opinion scores.

Communicability tests are cumbersome to administer in that all of the voice systems to be tested need to be assembled and set up in the same location. So far, communicability tests have not been standardized for individual listener differences, so the scores are relative within a single test series and are not comparable across different tests. This means that all of the voice systems to be compared must be tested at the same time. Communicability tests are useful primarily for determining whether system deficiencies are compensable or non-compensable (Voiers & Clark, 1978). For example, a noisy connection can be overcome by speaking more loudly, but other degradations, such as the garbling caused by high bit errors in a digital transmission, may be more difficult to overcome.

5.3.1   Free Conversation Test

Conversational methods have been widely used in Britain to evaluate telecommunication systems (e.g., Richards & Swaffield, 1958; Richards, 1973). A task or problem to solve is given to each of two participants, who discuss the problem in a natural manner over the voice system to be evaluated and then rate the quality of the communication link after they are finished. Scores are Mean Opinion Scores based on a five point rating scale of effort. In one version (Butler & Kiddle, 1969), each participant is given one of two pictures taken a short time apart, and they discuss the pictures until they can agree on which came first. Reference systems are generally included for comparison, but listener calibration procedures for communicability tests are not well developed. The test materials are not reusable in that once a given problem has been solved, the answer is known to the participants. The problems given to the participants with the Free Conversation Test also tend to vary in difficulty, and the time to reach a solution may vary from problem to problem.

5.3.2   Diagnostic Communicability Test

This test (Voiers & Clark, 1978) uses five participants and a stock trading game. The stocks assigned to each person vary from game to game; therefore the test materials are reusable and are also consistent in difficulty. There are 15 rating scales including both signal and background diagnostic scales. To implement this test, a five-way communication setup would be needed for the systems to be tested.

5.3.3   NRL Communicability Test

The NRL Communicability test (Schmidt-Nielsen & Everett, 1982) is a reusable variation of the Free Conversation method. The test uses an abbreviated version of the pencil and paper "battleship" game. Each player places two "ships" on a five-by-five grid, and the players take turns shooting at each other specifying cells in the grid, e.g., "alfa four" or "charlie three". The game can be used repeatedly with the same participants because the players place their own "ships" at the beginning of each game. The speech content is relatively uniform from game to game because the vocabulary used in playing the game is quite limited. There is some variability in game duration, but the time per move can be determined; however, Schmidt-Nielsen (1985) found that measures of speaker behavior such as time per move, changes in vocabulary, or requests for repeats were less reliable measures of performance than were the subjective ratings. Scores obtained on the NRL test are relative and are not repeatable from one occasion to another, so reference systems should be included for comparison, and it is best to test all of the systems that need to be compared with one another at the same time.

5.4 Physical Measures of the Speech Signal

It is appealing to try to use physically measurable characteristics of the speech signal to evaluate intelligibility or voice quality because of the accuracy and repeatability of physical measurements compared with tests involving human listeners. Physical measures are also considerably cheaper and less time consuming than listener tests. Such measures can be useful for limited applications but should not be considered as substitutes for listener tests.

5.4.1 Articulation Index (AI)

The Articulation Index (French and Steinberg, 1947) is computed as the average of the estimated articulation, based on speech to noise levels, in each of 20 contiguous frequency bands that contribute equally to speech intelligibility. The approximate relations of AI to the intelligibility of various types of speech materials including PB word sets of different sizes, nonsense syllables, rhyme tests, and sentences are given in Kryter (1972, p. 175). These are valid only for male speakers (Kryter, p. 190). Plots of AI and PB word intelligibility for wideband and especially for narrowband noise (Kryter, p. 191, 192) show considerable scatter of the scores around the prediction curves, indicating that there can be considerable discrepancy between listener results and AI.

5.4.2 Speech Transmission Index (STI)

The Speech Transmission Index (Steeneken and Houtgast, 1980) is an improvement of the AI in that it takes into account distortion from adjacent bands. The STI uses an artificial test signal and measures the effective signal to noise ratio in seven octave bands calculated from the modulation index of each band. The STI has been implemented in measuring devices— STIDAS and RASTI (rapid STI). The STI has been shown to be very effective for noise and for auditorium measurements. Steeneken and Houtgast (1980) found a high correlation between STI and PB monosyllable intelligibility for Dutch for a variety of speech degradations and even for some wideband voice coders, and Anderson and Kalb (1987) also found a high correlation between STI and PB words for English. However, Schmidt-Nielsen (1987c) notes that the prediction errors (5.6%) associated with these correlations were too large for comparisons among systems with similar scores to be useful.

5.4.3   Combined measures

As part of an ongoing program to develop predictors for speech acceptability, Barnwell and his colleagues (e.g., Quackenbush, Barnwell, and Clements, 1988; Barnwell, 1990) have tested a large number of objective measures of the speech signal as possible predictors of subjective speech quality. The test conditions covered a large number of different distortions including a variety of coding algorithms and a set of controlled distortions that include several levels of each of a variety of different distortions, such as additive noise, bandpass filtering, interruption, clipping, and voice coders. Subjective quality scores for each of the distortions were obtained using the Diagnostic Acceptability Measure, and regression techniques were used to evaluate many possible objective physical measures, including signal to noise measures of various kinds, a number of different distance measures, and others. No single measure performed very well in predicting acceptability over the entire database, although some were found to be very good for the subsets of the database. Composite measures performed better than simple measures but even the best (based on 34 regression coefficients) had a correlation coefficient of only 0.84 and a standard error of estimate of 4.6. Segmental signal-to-noise ratio was an important attribute, and frequent variant segmental signal to noise ratio was an excellent predictor for the subset of waveform coders, with a correlation of 0.93 and a standard error of estimate of 3.3 for this subset.

Physical measures of the speech signal can be a convenient method for estimating the effects of simple distortions such as noise, but it is important to realize the limitations of such measures for more complex distortions. They should not be used in making comparisons among different types of distortions of different classes of speech processing techniques. They are also not appropriate for evaluating non-waveform coders such as linear predictive coders (LPC). Listener tests are essential in evaluating the effects of voice processor improvements because coder distortions can interact in complex ways with perceptual processes.

6.   Relations Among Different Tests

Tests are often highly correlated with one another because many of the degradations that occur due to digital processing, background noise or channel degradations affect many characteristics of the speech signal globally. There are also a number of degradations that affect some characteristics of the speech more than others, and in these cases one would expect tests that evaluate different characteristics to give divergent results. This section reviews some of the interrelations, similarities as well as discrepancies, that have been found for different types of speech materials and evaluation methods.

There is a large body of research to suggest that although the difficulty of task may vary, measures of speech intelligibility are often highly intercorrelated. Fletcher and Steinberg (1929) showed systematic relations between intelligibility scores for various speech units—phonemes, syllables, sentences—for a variety of telephone circuit conditions. Miller, Heise, and Lichten (1951) demonstrated a systematic effect of the size of the response set on the percentage of correct responses under varying degrees of noise degradation. Correlations have also been found between rhyme tests and other types of speech materials (Kryter & Whitman, 1965), including military vocabularies (Montague, 1960; Webster, 1972). A considerable number of the comparisons of different types of speech materials have involved systematically degrading the speech signal along a simple dimension using different levels of the same type of degradation, often noise or bandpass limiting. With systematic degradations along a single dimension, one would expect tests using different speech materials to be highly correlated even though they might differ in difficulty. A high degree of cross predictability between the DRT and the MRT has been demonstrated using a variety of different degradations (Voiers, 1983), but it should be noted that the speech materials for these two tests are very similar.

A discrepancy between the DRT and MRT has been noted in testing speech synthesizers. Pratt and Newton (1988) tested several speech synthesis systems using the DRT, the MRT and another test, the Four Alternative Auditory Feature Test (FAAF). They obtained different rank orderings of the synthesizers with the DRT than with the other two tests, which gave results comparable to one another. It can be speculated that the discrepancy may be attributable to the fact that the DRT tests only initial consonants, while the MRT and FAAF test both initial and final consonants. Logan, Pisoni & Greene (1985) found different groupings of synthesizers for final consonants than for initial consonants on the MRT. Unlike analysis-synthesis systems, syntheses-by-rule systems do not necessarily yield similar performance on initial and final consonants (but final consonants are less intelligible than initial consonants, even for analysis-synthesis systems).

A number of researchers have found that different degradations can affect different kinds of speech materials in different ways. Hirsch, Reynolds, and Joseph (1954) compared nonsense syllables and one-, two-, and multi-syllable words for different noise levels and for high- and low-pass filtering. The relations among the different types of speech materials were not the same for the different degradations. Williams and Hecker (1968) used four different test methods (PB words, the Fairbanks Rhyme Test, the Modified Rhyme Test, and lists of Harvard Sentences) to evaluate several different types of speech distortion—additive noise, peak clipping, and a channel vocoder at different error rates. They also found that the relationships among test scores and the rank orderings for the different speech distortions were not the same across speech materials, and they concluded that results for a given test were highly dependent on the nature of the distortion. Greenspan, Bennett, and Syrdal (1989) found very similar DRT scores for unprocessed speech and for two digital voice coders, but acceptability as measured by the DAM was considerably lower for both coders than for the unprocessed speech. When they used an open response cv intelligibility test and naive listeners, both coders scored well below the unprocessed speech, and one of the coders had a lower score than the other. Tests with a large number of response alternatives are generally more difficult than tests with a small number of alternatives and may be less subject to ceiling effects for high intelligibility voice systems. Furthermore, there were significantly more multiple-feature confusion for the coded speech than for the unprocessed speech for which errors were primarily single-feature confusions.

Schmidt-Nielsen (1987a, 1987b) conducted several tests comparing DRT intelligibility to the intelligibility of the International Civil Aviation Association (ICAO) spelling alphabet ("alfa", "bravo", "charlie", etc.) and the digits "zero" to "niner". Digital voice test conditions included LPC algorithms with different levels of random bit errors and an 800 bit/sec pattern matching algorithm. Analog conditions used speech transmitted over AM radio with noise jamming. These included continuous jamming conditions of various degrees of severity and several interrupted jamming conditions. Within the LPC conditions, scores on both tests decreased as the bit error rate increased, and there was a consistent relationship between the two sets of scores. Both DRT and spelling alphabet scores also decreased with increased severity of the radio jamming conditions, but the relationship between the two sets was less consistent, especially for the interrupted conditions. The relationship between the DRT scores and spelling alphabet scores was quite different for digital than for analog speech degradations. LPC conditions with low DRT scores showed very poor spelling alphabet recognition, but the noise degraded radio jamming conditions with similarly low DRT scores showed much higher spelling alphabet recognition. A DRT score near 50 corresponded to spelling alphabet intelligibility of just over 50% for LPC with bit errors but to spelling alphabet intelligibility of about 80% for noise jamming. This result makes sense in terms of the way different degradations affect the speech materials on the two tests. DRT scores would be expected to be more vulnerable to noise degradation than are spelling alphabet scores. The DRT is based on consonant discriminations, and consonants have less acoustic energy than vowels and can be expected to degrade considerably in noise. The spelling alphabet was developed specifically to be robust in noise, so the letter names differ from one another in their main vowels as well as in the number and pattern of the syllables. LPC, in contrast, is an analysis-synthesis system, and errors in the bit stream will cause the wrong signal to be reconstructed at the receiver, which affects the entire speech signal, so that the vowel and prosody cues that help the spelling alphabet in the noise context are not as well preserved under the digital degradations.

It is not unusual to encounter speech systems for which the intelligibility is good but for which the voice quality is degraded in some dimension. However, when intelligibility is poor, judged voice quality usually goes down as well. An exception to this seems to occur when noise reduction techniques are used to remove or ameliorate background noise. The results of a National Research Council panel on noise removal (1989) indicate that noise reduction may lead to a subjective impression of improvement, but that there seems to be no evidence for any overall improvement in intelligibility as measured by standard phoneme intelligibility tests such as the DRT. Test of a noise reduction preprocessor by the DoD Digital Voice Processor Consortium (Sandy and Parker, 1984) using military background noises (helicopter, tank, etc.) indicated that intelligibility as measured by the DRT did not improve. In several cases DRT scores were actually lower with noise reduction than without, while only one noise (helicopter) showed any improvement. In contrast, Kang and Fransen (1989) tested the same noise condition using the DAM and found dramatic improvements in quality using a spectral subtraction technique for noise suppression. Speech samples with background noise were processed through a 2400 bit LPC voice processor with and without the noise processor as the front end. There was improvement in all cases, with an average gain of 6 points, and a maximum gain of 13 points in the DAM Score.

The purpose of testing is ultimately to determine the adequacy of the speech system for use in a real environment, although selection among several candidates for an application may also require the ability to make fine discriminations among closely competing systems. In actual use, the factors discussed in an earlier section that can affect intelligibility and acceptability interact in complex ways to determine how well the speech is understood and whether users will find the system acceptable. In testing, the demands that are made on the listener may vary with the type of task and the test materials that are used. The kind of information that is available to the listener in order to determine the correct response varies with the type of speech materials that are used. With rhyme tests the listeners must rely almost entirely on segmental information for their responses, whereas with meaningful sentences, they have access to context from other words in the sentence and to information about grammatical structure from suprasegmental cues. The way in which the degradation interacts with the relevant speech cues should be considered in selecting test methods.

7.   Selecting Test Methods

Speech system evaluation is conducted in a variety of contexts with different goals and requirements, depending on the purpose of the test, the type of speech system to be evaluated, and the kind of comparisons that need to be made.

7.1   Reasons for Testing

Some important reasons for speech evaluation tests might include developmental testing, diagnostic evaluation of defects, comparison and selection, operational usability evaluation, and the development of procurement specifications. Selection and specification testing rely heavily on standard test methods and highly controlled procedures that produce reliable numerical scores, whereas developmental and usability tests more often include nonstandard materials and evaluation experiments that cannot be generalized beyond the immediate context.

During the development of new voice systems or voice processing techniques, testing needs to be carried out regularly to monitor progress, to determine the weaknesses of the system, and to evaluate improvements. At times a very specific test may be needed to evaluate a particular aspect of the system that needed improvement, while at other times a wide variety of tests may be desirable to determine strengths and weaknesses and to guide future efforts. Much of this testing is highly informal, often consisting simply of listening to the output or perhaps asking one or two colleagues for an opinion. Periodically, more formal tests need to be carried out to monitor progress and to guard against the listener becoming so accustomed to the system that its defects are no longer noticed. Caution should be exercised in relying too heavily on a single standard intelligibility test when developing and refining new techniques. It is possible to "tune" the system too much to the particular features of a given test to the detriment of overall performance. A discrepancy between subjective quality evaluations and intelligibility scores can be an indication that this is happening.

The most common application of standard intelligibility and quality tests is for decision making or selection purposes. This may involve the selection of the best system for a particular application from several competing candidates or comparing a newly developed or improved system with existing systems. Controlled test procedures that eliminate variability in the test results due to irrelevant factors are required in order to make fair comparisons. It is highly desirable to simulate conditions that may occur in use such as environmental background noise or channel degradations.

Tests of user acceptance of telephone devices may include user opinions of test sentences or conversations based on ratings or customer interviews. Operational evaluation of military voice systems usually involves field tests in which the developers of the systems are not involved. When tests are conducted in operational environments, it is often difficult to get the users to conduct controlled conversations or to be analytic about the quality of the voice system; if the user does not like it or if some part of the system fails to operate properly when needed, the system is unacceptable, even if the reason for the failure is unrelated to the quality of the voice transmission. Laboratory tests may be conducted for the purpose of predicting the usability of a device in a given environment. Estimates of user acceptance may also be developed from experiments establishing correlations of standard tests with field tests or user evaluations.

When establishing specifications of minimally acceptable intelligibility levels for procurement contracts, very exact test procedures are needed. If the specification establishes a target intelligibility score that must be met or exceeded, the test must be capable of producing scores that are repeatable from one occasion to the next with very little variability. With tests that produce good discriminations but have less numeric stability, an alternative is to specify that the test score must be within a specified number of points of the score of a reference or standard system to be tested at the same time.

7.2   Type of Voice Application and Comparisons to be Made

The type of speech system to be evaluated and the nature of the degradation of the speech signal should be considered in relation to its effect on the factors that influence speech intelligibility and acceptability. The way in which the test materials and tasks affect and interact with the relevant types of speech information (segmental cues, prosody, context, etc.) can then be used to select the tests that will be the most informative. If background noise or poor channel conditions are likely to be present in the intended application, they should be included in the test program, and the robustness of the competing systems under these conditions would be an important consideration in the selection process.

For voice communication systems that start with human speech at the input and reproduce a more or less faithful version of the same speech as output at the receiving end, a consonant test is a reasonably accurate predictor of intelligibility because if consonant sounds are reproduced correctly, chances are that other segmental information will also be right. Existing wideband algorithms for digital telephone transmission generally have very good to excellent intelligibility. Sometimes the intelligibility may be high enough to produce ceiling effects on standard rhyme tests, giving little discrimination among the scores for competing methods. Where intelligibility is so high as to be considered good enough for normal communications, minor differences may be unimportant, and the quality of the voice system becomes the overwhelming consideration. For most narrowband systems, there is likely to be some loss in speech intelligibility and quality, so ceiling effects are less of a problem. Although some modern narrowband systems approach wideband systems in intelligibility, very low data rate systems can have substantially reduced intelligibility. Some military applications include adverse conditions where intelligibility may fall into ranges that would be unacceptable for normal communications but may still be quite usable for the restricted and distinctive vocabularies used in many military communications.

No single test is equally sensitive to small differences across the entire range of intelligibility. Different speech materials and test formats vary in the difficulty of the acoustic discriminations needed for the responses. In general, we would expect a difficult test to be more sensitive to small amounts of degradation, but when the speech quality is very poor the test would lose sensitivity because of floor effects. A test with easier discriminations or more context would discriminate well among poor speech conditions but would be subject to ceiling effects for less degraded speech.

Both intelligibility and quality tests are important for evaluating voice transmission systems. The choice between the DRT and the MRT will depend to some extent on the historical background. If the MRT has been used extensively in the past in a given context, it may be convenient to continue to use it even though the DRT provides more detailed diagnostic information. The DoD Digital Voice Processor Consortium has used the DRT since the early 1970's and has accumulated a large historical database of DRT scores for wideband and narrowband digital voice systems for military applications (e.g., Sandy and Parker, 1984; Sandy, 1987). The MOS has been widely used in telephone applications, but the DAM produces highly repeatable results, offers diagnostic scales, and has been extensively used to evaluate digital voice systems for military applications (Sandy and Parker, 1984; Sandy, 1987). A disadvantage of the DAM is that the details of the scoring procedure are at present proprietary to a single company that provides testing services. Many of the advantages of the DAM could be reproduced by using appropriate diagnostic scales and rigorous listener calibration and monitoring procedures with other materials. Communicability tests can provide two-way conversations under controlled conditions at considerably less expense than field tests. For systems or conditions where intelligibility and quality can be expected to be very poor it may be useful to conduct supplementary tests. Research at NRL with the ICAO spelling alphabet indicates that a test using this limited and distinctive vocabulary can be useful for evaluating usability when DRT scores fall into the unacceptable range.

For other applications, such as synthesis-by-rule systems, it is necessary to consider other phoneme categories and word positions. Rhyme tests can give an indication of synthesizer performance (Pratt, 1987), but the speech materials on such tests are too limited for a complete evaluation of synthesis systems. The MRT tests both initial and final consonants, but a combination of the DRT for initial consonants and the DAT for final consonants would give more diagnostic information about specific weaknesses. It is important also to include tests of consonants in other positions, such as word medial position or consonant clusters, as well as vowels in different consonant contexts and at different stress levels. Intonation and timing rules that follow the constraints of the spoken language must also be explicitly built into the system, and the effects of prosody on intelligibility and naturalness need to be evaluated. Tests using sentence materials can be used to evaluate multiple phonemic contexts as well as the effects of prosody on intelligibility and quality. The Harvard sentences and Haskins sentences may be useful, but they do not provide the possibility of repeated use necessary for making accurate comparisons of different synthesis systems. A subjective acceptability test that provides numeric stability and diagnostic scales is also very useful in evaluating the naturalness of speech synthesizers.

In general, the more highly processed the speech signal (i.e., synthesis, very low data rate speech algorithms, noise removal techniques), the more important it is to include tests that evaluate several different speech processing methods or different types of speech degradations.

8.   General Recommendations

1. Whenever possible, use standard test materials. It is highly desirable to use standard evaluation methods so that comparisons can be meaningfully made among different types of voice systems and among tests conducted at different times and in different places. If standard tests are inappropriate for the application or if additional tests are needed, consideration should be given to high reliability and to selecting test materials that have been used by other researchers and for which historical data are available.

2. Reference conditions are essential. Except when using rhyme tests like the DRT and MRT with standard speakers and scored by laboratories with trained and screened listening crews, it is necessary to include reference systems, such as high quality unprocessed speech and several known degradations for which previous historical data are available, in order to provide a context for interpreting the scores. This is especially important if nonstandard speech materials, unknown speakers, or untrained listeners are used.

3. Use multiple speakers. Given that speaker differences can be quite large, at least six to twelve speakers should be used for most intelligibility tests. A larger number of speakers may be needed for sentence materials than for rhyme test materials. Both male and female speakers should be used unless the application is known to be restricted to only one sex.

4. Use a sufficient number of listeners. The IEEE Recommended Practice for Speech Quality Measurements (1969) recommends 6-10 trained listeners or at least 50 untrained listeners. These numbers, or a few more listeners, are also reasonable for intelligibility tests. The DRT procedure starts with 10 listeners and eliminates the two that are the most inconsistent over an entire session, so that there are actually 8 listeners for each score.

5. Exercise the system. For communication systems, test different environmental conditions that may occur in use—e.g., background noise, channel degradations. For synthesizers, include a variety of speech materials to evaluate prosody. In general, the more highly processed the speech is, the more important it is to evaluate several different types of speech materials covering different types of speech cues that contribute to intelligibility.

6. When comparing very different processing methods or speech degradations, use several different types of tests and speech materials. When comparing similar processing methods or degradations, a more limited set of speech materials may be used, but it may be useful to include a variety of environmental conditions.

7. Meticulous care should be exercised in the selection, setup, and maintenance of all recording and playback equipment, the storage and copying of tapes, etc. Seemingly minor deficiencies like dirty tape heads or a bad connector can significantly reduce speech quality and render the outcome of an entire test series invalid.

8. When comparing scores, the proper statistical procedures should be used. There have been references to the measurement error inherent in using human listeners throughout this chapter, and proper statistical methods are needed to make the correct comparisons among the different systems that have been tested. These might include, for example, analysis of variance and multiple comparison tests. When in doubt, consult someone with a broad knowledge of behavioral statistics.

9.   Acknowledgments

I would like to thank my colleagues and friends, and also the editors of this book, who have read and commented on an earlier version of this chapter. I am especially grateful to Thomas H. Crystal, John D. Tardelli, and William D. Voiers for their thoughtful reading and helpful suggestions.

10.   References

American National Standards Institute. (1960). *American standard method for measurement of monosyllabic word intelligibility* (ANSI S3.2-1960). New York: American Standards Association.

American National Standards Institute. (1989). *Method for measuring the intelligibility of speech over communication systems* (ANSI S3.2-1989 — A revision of ANSI S3.2-1960). New York: American Standards Association.

Anderson, B. W. & Kalb, J. T. (1987). English verification of the STI method for estimating speech intelligibility of a communications channel. *Journal of the Acoustical Society of America*, 81, 1982–1985.

Barnwell, T.P. (1990). A new objective speech quality measure for speech coding systems. *Journal of the Acoustical Society of America*, 87, S13.

Butler, L.W., & Kiddle, L. (1969). *The rating of delta sigma modulating systems with constant errors and tandem links in a free conversation test using the reference speech link* (Report No. 69014). Signals Research and Development Establishment, Ministry of Technology, Christchurch, Hants.

Campbell, G.A. (1910, cited in Fletcher & Steinberg, 1929) Telephonic intelligibility *Phil. Mag.* Jan., 1910.

CCITT (1984a). Absolute category rating (ACR) method for subjective testing of digital processors, Red Book, Volume V, (Annex A to Suppl. 14).

CCITT (1984b). Subjective performance assessment of digital encoders using the degradation category rating (DCR) procedure, Red Book, Volume V, (Annex to Suppl. 14).

CCITT (1984c). Recommendation P.70 (Subjective voice-ear measurements—modulated noise reference unit), Red Book, Volume V, 111–114.

Clarke, F.R. (1965). *Technique for evaluation of speech systems* (Contract DA 28-043 AMC-00227(E)). Final report of Stanford Research Institute Project 5090 on U.S. Army Electronics Laboratory.

Egan, J.P. (1948). Articulation testing. *Laryngoscope*, 58, 995–991.

Fairbanks, G. (1958). Test of phonemic differentiation: The rhyme test. *Journal of the Acoustical Society of America*, 30, 596–600.

Fletcher, H. & Steinberg, J.C. (1929). Articulation testing methods. *Bell System Technical Journal*, 8, 806–854.

French, N.R., & Steinberg, J.C. (1947). Factors governing the intelligibility of speech sounds. *Journal of the Acoustical Society of America*, 19, 90–119.

Goodman, D.J., & Nash, R.D. (1982). Subjective quality of the same speech transmission conditions in seven different countries. *IEEE Trans. Commun.* COM-30, 642–654.

Greenspan, S.L., Bennett, R.W., & Syrdal, A. .K. (1989). A study of two standard intelligibility measures. *Journal of the Acoustical Society of America*, 85, S43 (Abstract).

Hecker, M.H., & C.E. Williams. (1966). Choice of reference conditions for speech preference tests. *Journal of the Acoustical Society of America*, 39 (5, Pt.1), 946–952.

Hirsch, I.J., Reynolds, G., & Joseph, M. (1954). Intelligibility of different speech materials. *Journal of the Acoustical Society of America*, 26 (4), 530–538.

House, A.S., Williams, C.E., Hecker, M.H.L. & Kryter, K.D. (1965). Articulation Testing Methods: Consonantal differentiation with a closed response set. *Journal of the Acoustical Society of America, 37*, 158–166.

Houtgast, T. & Steeneken, H.J.M. (1971). Evaluation of speech transmission channels using artificial signals. *Acoustica, 25,* 355–367.

Huggins, A.W.F. & Nickerson, R.S. (1985). Speech quality evaluation using "phonemic-specific" sentences. *Journal of the Acoustical Society of America,* 77, 1896–1906.

IEEE Subcommittee on Subjective Measurements (1969). IEEE recommended practice for speech quality measurements. *IEEE Transactions on Audio and Electroacoustics, 17,* 227–246.

Jacobson, R., Fant, C.G.M., & Halle, M. (1952). *Preliminaries to Speech Analysis: the Distinctive Features and their Correlates,* Tech. Rep. No. 13. Acoustics Laboratory, MIT.

Kang, G.S. & Fransen, L.J. (1989). Quality improvement of LPC-processed noisy speech by using spectral subtraction. *IEEE Transactions on Acoustics, Speech, and Signal Processing,* ASSP-37, 939–942.

Kemp, D.P., Sueda, R.A., & Tremain, T.E. (1989). An evaluation of 4800 BPS voice coders. *IEEE ICASSP-89.*

Kryter, K.D. (1972). Speech communication. In Van Cott, H.P. & Kincade, R.G.(Eds.), *Human Engineering Guide to Equipment Design.* Washington, DC: U.S. Government Printing Office.

Kryter, K.D. & Whitman, E.C. (1965). Some comparisons between rhyme and PB word intelligibility tests. *Journal of the Acoustical Society of America,* 37, 1146.

Licklider, J.C., & Pollack, I. (1948). Effects of differentiation, integration, and infinite peak clipping upon the intelligibility of speech. *Journal of the Acoustical Society of America, 20,* 42–51.

Logan, J.S. Pisoni, D.B. & Greene, B.G. (1985). Measuring the segmental intelligibility of synthetic speech: Results from eight text-to-speech systems. *Research of Speech Perception Progress Report No. 11.* Bloomington, IN: Indiana University.

Luce, P.A., Feustel, T.C. & Pisoni, D.B. (1983). Capacity demands in short-term memory for synthetic and natural speech. *Human Factors*, 25, 17–32.

Miller, G.., Heise, G.A., & Lichten, W. (1951). The intelligibility of speech as a function of the context of the test materials. *Journal of Experimental Psychology*, 41, 329– 355.

Montague, W.E. (1960). *A comparison of five intelligibility tests for voice communication systems*. (Report No. 977). San Diego, California: U.S. Navy Electronics Laboratory.

Munson, W.A., & Karlin, J.EE. (1962). Isopreference method for evaluating speech transmission circuits. *Journal of the Acoustical Society of America*, 34, 762–774.

Nakatsui, M. & Mermelstein, P. (1982). Subjective speech-to-noise ratio as a measure of speech quality for digital waveform coders. *Journal of the Acoustical Society of America*, 72, 1136–1144.

National Research Council Panel on Noise Removal. (1989). *Removal of noise from noise-degraded speech signals*. Panel on removal of noise from a speech/noise signal. Washington, DC: National Academy Press.

Nye, P.W., & Gaitenby, J. (1973). Consonant intelligibility in synthetic speech and in a natural control (Modified Rhyme Test Results). *Haskins Laboratories Status Report on Speech Research*, SR-33, 77–91.

Pascal, D., & Combescure, P. (1988). Evaluation de la qualite de la transmission vocale Evaluation of the quality of voice transmission . *L'Echo des RECHERCHES*, 132 (2), 31–40.

Peckels, J.P. & Rossi, M. (1971). (Cited in Voiers, 1983). Le test de diagnostic per paires minmales adaptation au francais du Diagnostic Rhyme Test de W.D. Voiers. *Journee d'Etudes sur la Parole*, Groupement des Acousticiens de Langue Francais, April, 1971.

Pollack, I., & Pickett, J.M. (1964). Intelligibility of excerpt from fluent speech: Auditory vs. structural context. *Journal of Verbal Learning and Behavior*, 3, 79–84.

Pratt, R.L. (1987). Qualifying the performance of text-to-speech synthesizers. *Speech Technology*, March/April, 54–64.

Pratt, R.L., Flindell, I. H., Belyavin, A.J. (1987). *Assessing the intelligibility and acceptability of voice communication systems* (Report No. 87003). Malvern, Worcestershire: Royal Signals and Radar Establishment.

Pratt, R.L. & Newton, J.P. (1988). Quantifying text-to-speech sythesizer performance: An investigation of the consistency of three speech intelligibility tests. *Proceedings of Speech 1988, 7th FASE Symposium*, Edinburgh.

Quackenbush, S.R., Barnwell, .P., & Clements, M.A. (1988). *Objective Measures of Speech Quality*. Englewood Cliffs, Prentice Hall.

Richards, D.L. (1973). General background. *Telecommunications By Speech* London: Butterworth & Co. (Publishers) Ltd. (pp.1–27).

Richards, D.L., & Swaffield, J. (1958). Assessment of speech communication links. *The Institution of Electrical Engineers*, paper no. 2605 R, 77–92.

Sandy, G.F. (1987). *Digital Voice Processor Consortium Report on Performance of 16 kbps Voice Processors MTR-87W161*. McLean, VA, Mitre Corp.

Sandy, G.F., & Parker. (1984). *Digital Voice Processor Consortium Final Report MTR-84W00053*. McLean, VA, Mitre Corp.

Schmidt-Nielsen, A. (1983). Intelligibility of VCV segments excised from connected speech. *Journal of the Acoustical Society of America*, 74, 726–738.

Schmidt-Nielsen, A. (1985). Problems in Evaluating the Real-World Usability of Digital Voice Systems. *Behavior Research Methods, Instruments, and Computers*, 17, 226–234.

Schmidt-Nielsen, A. (1987a). Evaluating degraded speech: Intelligibility tests are not all alike. *Official Proceedings of Military Speech Tech 1987* (pp 118–121). New York: Media Dimensions, Inc.

Schmidt-Nielsen, A. (1987b). The effect of narrowband digital processing and bit error rate on the intelligibility of ICAO spelling alphabet words. *IEEE Transactions on Acoustics, Speech, and Signal Processing*, ASSP-35, 1101–1115 (1987).

Schmidt-Nielsen, A. (1987c). Comments on the Use of Physical Measures to Assess Speech Intelligibility. *Journal of the Acoustical Society of America*, 81, 1985–1987.

Schmidt-Nielsen, A. & Everett, S.S. (1982). A conversational test for comparing voice systems using working two-way communication links. *IEEE Transactions on Acoustics, Speech, and Signal Processing*, ASSP-30, 853–863.

Schmidt-Nielsen, A., Kallman, H.J., and Meijer, C. (1990). Dual Task Performance using Degraded Speech in a Sentence Verification Task. *Bulletin of the Psychonomic Society*, 28, 7–10.

Steeneken, H.J.M. (1982). (Cited in Voiers, 1983). *Ontwikkeling en Toetsing van een Nederlandstalige Diagnistische Rijmtest voor het Testen van Spraak-Kommunikatiekanalen.* Report No. IZF, 1982–13. Institut voor Zintuigfysiologie TNO Soesterberg.

Steeneken, H.J.M., and Houtgast, T. (1980). A physical method for measuring speech-transmission quality. *Journal of the Acoustical Society of America,* 67, 318–326.

Summers, W.V., Pisoni, D.B., Bernacki, R.H., Pedlow, R.I., & Stokes, M.A. (1988). Effects of noise on speech production: Acoustical and perceptual analyses. *Journal of the Acoustical Society of America,* 84, 917–928.

Voiers, W.D. (1977a). Diagnostic Evaluation of Speech Intelligibility. In M.E. Hawley, (Ed.), *Speech Intelligibility and Speaker Recognition.* Stroudsburg, PA.: Dowden, Hutchinson, and Ross.

Voiers, W.D. (1977b). Diagnostic Acceptability Measure for speech communication systems, ICASSP-77, *IEEE International Conference on Acoustics, Speech, Signal Processing,* New York.

Voiers, W.D., & Clark, M.H. (1978). *Exploratory research on the feasibility of a practical and realistic test of speech communicability* (Final Rep. on Contract No. N0039-77-C-0111, Dept. of the Navy, Navy Electronics Systems Command, Washington, D.C.). Austin, TX: Dynastat, Inc.

Voiers, W.D. (1981, October). Uses, limitations, and interrelations of present-day intelligibility tests. *Proceedings of the National Electronics Conference,* Vol.35, Chicago, Illinois.

Voiers, W.D. (1982). Some thoughts on the standardization of psychological measures of speech intelligibility and quality. *Proceedings of the Workshop on Standardization for Speech I/O Technology,* National Bureau of Standards, Gaithersburg, Md, March 18–19, 1982.

Voiers, W.D. (1983). Evaluating processed speech using the Diagnostic Rhyme Test. *Speech Technology.* Jan/Feb., 0–9.

Voiers, W.D., Panzer, I.L., & Sharpley, A.D. (1990). *Validation of the diagnostic acceptability measure (DAM II-B)* (Contract No. MD904-87-C-6026 for National Security Agency Ft. Meade, MD). Austin, TX: Dynastat, Inc.

Webster, J.C. (1972). Compendium of speech testing material and typical noise spectra for use in evaluating communications equipment. (Technical Document 191). San Diego, CA: Naval Electronics Laboratory Center, Human Factors Technology Division.

Williams, C.E. & Hecker, M.H. (1968). Relation between intelligibility scores for four test methods and three types of speech distortion. *Journal of the Acoustical Society of America*, 44, 1002–1006.

Chapter 6

Perception and Comprehension of Speech[1]

James V. Ralston, David B. Pisoni and John W. Mullennix
Indiana University[2]

1. Introduction

Most perceptual evaluations of coded speech to date have utilized restricted sets of stimuli presented in isolation for identification and discrimination judgments (see Logan et al., 1989 and Schmidt-Nielson, this volume). However, because comprehension of speech engages mechanisms beyond those mediating phonemic and lexical recognition, it is likely that the processes involved in comprehension of fluent connected speech cannot be adequately assessed from intelligibility measures alone. Unfortunately, there have been very few studies assessing comprehension of passages of fluent connected speech reported in the literature. In this chapter, we first discuss several preliminaries related to assessing the comprehension of speech, including the nature of voice output devices, behavioral evaluations of segmental intelligibility, the process and measurement of comprehension, and the role of attention. Next, we review and evaluate the existing body of research devoted specifically to assessing the comprehension of speech, including recent findings from our own laboratory on the comprehension of synthetic speech produced by rule. Finally, we discuss the major issues that need to be addressed in the future.

---

[1] This is a draft of a chapter to appear in R. Bennett, A. Syrdal, and S. Greenspan (Eds.), *Behavioral Aspects of Speech Technology: Theory and Applications.* New York: Elsevier. This research was supported, in part, by NSF Research Grant IRI-86-17847.

[2] This chapter was completed while all the authors were at Indiana University. Currently, J.V. Ralston works at Ithaca College, Ithaca, NY; J.W. Mullennix works at Wayne State University, Detroit, MI; and D.B. Pisoni remains at Indiana University.

1.1   Voice Output Devices

Although our primary interest in this chapter is with rule-based speech synthesis systems, particularly text-to-speech (TTS) systems, most of what we say pertains as well to other forms of coded speech. However, due to a general lack of comprehension research on coded speech other than TTS, we will primarily describe studies using TTS stimulus materials.

Most consumers are familiar with systems using stored speech—that is, naturally produced speech waveforms that have been digitally recorded and processed, so they can be played back to listeners at a later time. The chief advantages of stored speech are its high intelligibility and natural sounding speech quality. However, digitally-stored waveforms require large amounts of storage capacity that depend on such factors as sampling rate, amplitude resolution, size of the message set, and length of the utterances. Therefore, digitally encoded speech is more appropriate for applications that require relatively short utterances in a fixed repertoire, such as menus, warning messages, and command systems. Some coding methods (e.g., LPC, CVSD, TDHS) reduce storage requirements, but the storage constraints may still be fairly substantial with long messages or a large corpus of utterances. If the output system is designed for the production of a large or variable set of messages, stored speech may become unwieldy and infeasible (Allen et al., 1987; Klatt, 1987). In the case of unlimited and unrestricted voice output, the use of stored speech simply becomes impractical. In addition, if one desires to alter the content of the stored messages, the entire recording process must be repeated for each new message. To overcome these problems, it has become common to use synthetic speech produced automatically by rule using a TTS system (Allen et al., 1987; Klatt, 1987).

TTS systems are devices that take input text, typically ASCII characters, and transform it into a speech waveform (see Klatt, 1987). In more sophisticated TTS systems such as DECtalk[2], several linguistic rule-based modules are used to process the phonemic, morphologic, lexical and syntactic aspects of the input string to derive a representation that can be used to produce the final speech waveform (see Syrdal, Chapter 3). Although less natural sounding and somewhat less intelligible than natural speech, these systems can produce an unlimited number of messages without recording or storage constraints. Thus, text-to-speech systems are by their design much

---

[2] DECtalk is a product of Digital Equipment Corporation.

more flexible than waveform coding systems and are ideally suited for applications such as reading machines, computer-assisted learning devices, data-base query systems, and audiotext, all of which must produce unrestricted connected discourse (Allen, 1981).

1.2 Behavioral Evaluation

Because of the large number of different TTS systems currently available, it is important to have some basis to objectively evaluate and compare speech quality using reliable experimental techniques. The most valid method is assessment of human preference and performance in situations resembling actual applications environments. However, this is often not feasible and laboratory studies have had to serve as the benchmark for assessing and comparing different systems. Five major factors have been shown to influence listeners' performance in laboratory situations (Pisoni et al., 1985). These are: (1) the quality of the speech signal, (2) the size and complexity of the message set, (3) short-term memory (STM) capacity of the listener, (4) the complexity of the listening task or other concurrent tasks, and (5) the listener's previous experience with the system.

Generally, performance is enhanced with higher-quality synthetic speech signals that are closely modeled after natural speech. However, many current speech synthesizers produce impoverished and inappropriate acoustic cues to signal phonetic distinctions (see Syrdal, this volume). The size of the message set affects listener expectations and indirectly affects performance. Research has shown that listeners display higher levels of performance with signals drawn from smaller message sets. STM is one of the most important structural limitations on human performance. STM functions as a general purpose mental workspace with limited processing resources (Baddeley & Hitch, 1974; Kahneman, 1973). Consequently, individuals have a limited ability to encode and process the multitude of sensory inputs impinging on the senses at any given time. The proportion of this limited capacity that different mental tasks require has been shown to be related to the number and complexity of their component subprocesses (Wickens, 1987). Finally, the experience of a listener with a given task can have profound effects on performance with even poor quality synthetic speech (Greenspan et al., 1988; Schwab et al., 1985). Perceptual learning allows the listener to develop processing strategies that optimize performance in a given task. The role of each of these factors in the comprehension of synthetic speech will be addressed in the sections below.

1.3   Intelligibility

As a first approximation, intelligibility is often assumed to reflect speech quality. Speech intelligibility measures listeners' ability to recognize different phonemes or words when they are presented in isolation. As such, speech intelligibility provides an index of the lower bounds of perceptual performance for a given transmission device when no higher-level linguistic context is provided (Schmidt-Nielson, Chapter 5). Standardized guidelines have been developed to measure speech intelligibility (ANSI, 1969). Although efforts are underway, no standards have been developed to date to measure intelligibility or comprehension of synthetic speech. Several recent studies have compared the segmental intelligibility of synthetic and natural speech (Hoover et al., 1987; Logan et al., 1989; Nusbaum et al., 1984; Nye & Gaitenby, 1973; Pisoni & Hunnicutt, 1980). A popular intelligibility test is the Modified Rhyme Test (MRT), in which a list of 300 monosyllabic CVC words are presented to naive listeners in a forced-choice format (House et al., 1965). Subjects respond by choosing one of six alternative words on each trial. Overall, these studies have found lower intelligibility and different patterns of perceptual errors for synthetic speech compared to natural speech.

In one study carried out in our laboratory, Logan et al. (1989) obtained MRT scores for synthetic speech produced by ten TTS systems. The results of this study are presented in Figure 1 along with control data from an adult male talker. Performance for different synthesizers varied widely from nearly perfect scores for natural speech to about 90-95% correct for "high-end" synthesizers and 60-70% correct for "low-end" synthesizers. Although some of the segmental confusions for synthetic speech were similar to those observed for natural speech, there were more errors overall for fricative and nasal phonemes. For some systems, the errors appeared to be quite unique to the particular synthesis techniques used.

The same systems and the natural control stimuli were also tested using an open response format test. The original forced-choice form of the MRT provides a closed set of six alternative responses (House et al., 1965). Subjects in the open response condition were required to write their responses to each word on blank lines in a test booklet. Figure 2 shows error data for open and closed formats for the same systems. Error rates for the open response condition were roughly double those observed for the closed response condition across all systems. In addition, for the same stimuli the increase in errors from closed to open response set was larger for synthesizers with the greatest closed response errors. The only change was in the response format. In the closed MRT, the listeners had to select one response from six available alternatives. In the open MRT, the response set was all the words a listener knew.

A closer analysis of the pattern of errors indicated a greater diversity of errors in the open response condition. However, the rank order of the errors was the same for the two response conditions. These results are important because they illustrate the effect of message set size on listener performance. Although the stimuli were the same in both conditions, from the listener's perspective the potential set of stimuli on each trial was much larger in the open response condition. These findings with synthetic speech produced by rule replicate earlier results (Pollack & Decker, 1958).

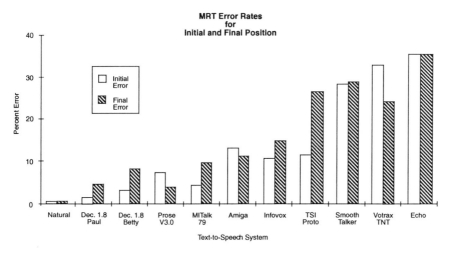

Figure 1 Error rates (in percent) for several TTS systems tested with a closed-format MRT. Open bars represent error rates for syllable-initial contrasts and striped bars represent error rates for syllable-final contrasts (from Logan et al., 1989)

From an applications perspective, it is of paramount importance to recognize that by increasing stimulus context or message redundancy, one effectively reduces the size of the message set and consequently enhances listener performance. This has been demonstrated in classic studies by Miller and his associates, who had subjects transcribe words presented in isolation, or embedded in random word strings or more meaningful sentences (Miller & Isard, 1963; Miller et al., 1951). Transcription scores were always higher when stimulus materials formed coherent, meaningful

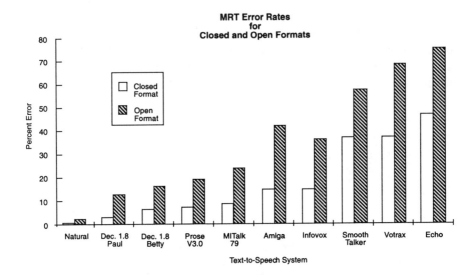

Figure 2   Error rates (in percent) for several TTS systems tested with both closed- and open-format MRT. Open bars represent error rates for the closed-response format and striped bars represent error rates for the open-response format (from Logan et al., 1989)

sentences. The implications for speech applications are straightforward: the greater the redundancy of a message, the greater the probability is that the message will be correctly received and decoded.

Although differences in the detailed time course of synthesis are generally believed to account for most performance differences among synthesis systems, the suprasegmental structure of an utterance (i.e., duration, stress pattern and intonation contour) also influences speech intelligibility. Suprasegmental effects operate at two levels. First, inappropriate suprasegmental information often affects some phonetic judgments (Haggard et al., 1970). Second, suprasegmental information provides syntactic and semantic cues to clausal structure and directs attention to certain portions of the speech signal, particularly stressed syllables (Cutler, 1976; Shields et al., 1974; Wingfield & Klein, 1971). "Low-end" synthesizers typically concatenate phonemes without smoothing, and often do not automatically encode suprasegmental information. For example, the durations of words produced in sentential context by the Votrax Type-N-Talk synthesizer are identical to those produced in isolation (Greenspan et al., 1988). On the other hand, systems such as Prose 2000[3], Infovox[4], and DECtalk encode substantial prosodic information that is governed by a large number of complex linguistic rules that consider morphemic, lexical, and syntactic structure of an input text (Klatt, 1987). Thus, differences in intelligibility between various TTS devices are due not only to differences in segmental cues to phonemes but also to differences in suprasegmental information as well.

1.4 Comprehension

Relatively few studies have examined the comprehension of synthetic speech, particularly long passages of fluent connected speech. Whereas intelligibility measures assess the perception of individual spoken segments or words, comprehension measures assess a listener's "understanding" of the spoken message, not just the recognition of specific words in the sentence. At present, there are no standardized methods for measuring the comprehension of synthetic speech. Webster's New World Dictionary (2nd Ed.) defines comprehension as "the act of grasping with the mind, the capacity for understanding ideas or facts, or the knowledge that results from these processes". Psycholinguists have described comprehension as

---

[3] Prose 2000 is a product of Speech Plus, Inc.
[4] Infovox is a product of Infovox.

a process by which a listener constructs a coherent mental representation of the propositional information expressed by a passage and relates this structure to other previously or currently available information in memory (Kintsch & van Dijk, 1978). Propositions are hypothetical, abstract units of meaning, expressing the relationship between entities or the state of some entity (Kintsch, 1974). It appears that listeners remember propositional information about a text, but not the superficial features of a text, such as the exact wording (Sachs, 1967).

Several decades of research on reading comprehension have revealed a number of factors that affect the degree of comprehension (see Kieras & Just, 1984, for reviews). These include factors operating at lexical, sentential, and discourse levels. For example, an important lexical influence on comprehension is the frequency of occurrence (in one's language) of words in a text. The higher the frequency of occurrence of words in a text, and hence the higher their familiarity, the easier one's comprehension of that text is. An important sentential factor is syntactic complexity. The more complex the syntax of a sentence, the more difficult it is to process. Still other factors influence higher levels of the comprehension process. Because it appears that readers/listeners "connect" information expressed in separate sentences, several factors appear to influence integrative proccesses. Often text leaves out details, forcing subjects to make necessary inferences to "bridge the gaps." For example, consider the following two sentences: "The burning cigarette was carelessly discarded. The fire destroyed many acres of virgin forest." In this case, one must infer that the cigarette caused the fire. It has been shown that these inferences slow the speed of comprehension (Kintsch, 1974). With proper design, one can construct messages of desired comprehension difficulty and use these to study selected aspects of the comprehension process (see Applications section below).

Most models of comprehension are based on data obtained from studies of reading, which typically try to account for only a subset of the factors known to influence comprehension (Kintsch & van Dijk, 1978; Sharkey, 1990; Thibadeau et al., 1982). Although most investigators believe that differences in comprehension between spoken and written text are minimal (Kintsch & van Dijk, 1978), the true relationship between the two is largely unknown. An important difference between the input modalities is that written text is typically static and available for re-inspection, whereas spoken language is by its very nature transitory and ephemeral. Therefore, readers have the luxury of fixating on successive words as long as they desire, and may regress back to previous text. All of the existing comprehension models address relatively restricted knowledge domains and often model data for only a single text.

Although limited in many respects, the text comprehension model of Kintsch and van Dijk (1978) is psychologically motivated and makes accurate predictions about the readability or difficulty of text (Kintsch & Vipond, 1979). This model takes as its input a list of propositions ordered as they appear in a text. The list of input propositions are presumably produced by a syntactic parser that is not specified in the model. Next, groups of propositions are connected together and to an important topical proposition by means of matches between proposition arguments. This process builds a "microstructure" with a hierarchical shape, headed by the topical proposition. The most important (uppermost) and most recent propositions are retained in STM and compared to following input propositions, and the remainder are transferred to LTM. One product of this "leading edge" strategy in matching and memory storage is that some propositions are processed more and held in STM longer than others. The model predicts that those microstructural propositions that are processed the most have the greatest chance of being recalled later.

Text often contains propositions whose arguments cannot be matched with those of propositions still in STM. The Kintsch and van Dijk model assumes that, in these instances, there is a search of LTM for propositions with matching arguments. If none are found, a "bridging inference" is executed that provides the proposition linking the intact STM microstructure and the input proposition. Both the search of LTM and the inference process are presumed to demand mental resources, as does the maintenance of the microstructure in STM. (See section 1.5.1, this chapter.)

In addition to the microstructural representation of the details of the text, there are also "macro-operators" that construct a "macrostructure," or connected representation of the global properties of the text. The macrorules operate on microstructural and macrostructural propositions to reduce the amount of information and produce the "gist" of a text. The macrostructure is related to the microstructure details and may be composed of several levels of description, headed by a macro-proposition equivalent to a passage's title. One such macro-rule, generalization, produces a macroproposition that is an accurate description of a group of related micropropositions or macropropositions. For instance, micropropositions that describe building a foundation, building walls, and raising a roof may be connected to a macroproposition representing "building a house." The same macroproposition may also be present at several levels of the macrostructure. The model predicts that the probability that a macroproposition will be remembered is related to the number of levels in which it exists.

According to the Kintsch and van Dijk model, comprehension is the process of building up a coherent, connected propositional representation of a text's meaning. An important feature of this model is that the processes, such as those that derive inferences, require attention to operate (see section below). The model is able to make accurate predictions about the recall of information from memory (Kintsch & van Dijk, 1978). In addition, the model is also accurate in predicting the readability, or difficulty of different texts (Kintsch & Vipond, 1979).

Based on previous research and theoretical work, we make a number of general assumptions about spoken language comprehension. First, comprehension is not a monolithic process, but the product of multiple, continuously-interacting processes (Liberman et al., 1967; Marslen-Wilson & Tyler, 1980). Among the major processes are peripheral and central auditory coding as well as processes related to phonetic, phonological, lexical, prosodic, semantic, syntactic, inferential, and pragmatic information (Pisoni & Luce, 1987). Second, comprehension is a nontrivial mapping of surface structure (the exact sequence of words) onto a more abstract semantic representation (the meaning of the words). Comprehension processes decode the surface structure of sentences, producing propositions representing clausal information. The propositions are connected to one another and to other propositions concerning world knowledge to represent the meaning of an utterance. Third, STM capacity is used by comprehension processes (Baddeley & Hitch, 1974; Kintsch & van Dijk, 1978). Because of the central role of STM in perception and comprehension, we review briefly several of the major findings in the literature that are relevant to the comprehension of synthetic speech. Then we return to methods of measuring comprehension.

1.5   Attention and Processing Resources

1.5.1   Limited Capacity
One of the major structural constraints on human cognitive performance is the limited attentional capacity of STM (Newell & Simon, 1972; Kahneman, 1973). STM may be conceived of as a limited reservoir of mental energy that may be allocated for various cognitive processes (Baddeley & Hitch, 1974;

Kahneman, 1973; Wickens, 1987). Cognitive processes, particularly those that require conscious effort or control, expend certain amounts of the resources (Wickens, 1987). The demands of various processes may not be apparent when they run in isolation. However, if two or more execute concurrently, and if they place demands on the same limited resources, then performance on any or all may suffer. In most natural situations, several cognitive processes operate simultaneously. For example, an individual driving an automobile can also talk and manipulate other controls at the same time, if the demands of driving and conversing are relatively low. However, if the demands of talking or manipulating controls is too great, driving or conversational performance may suffer, resulting possibly in more driving errors. Therefore, it is important to determine the resource requirements for various processes. For example, one of our research interests has been focused on whether the perception of synthetic speech demands greater resources than natural speech (Luce et al., 1983). If this is the case, there may be reason to restrict the use of TTS systems to applications where the cognitive load on the listener is relatively low.

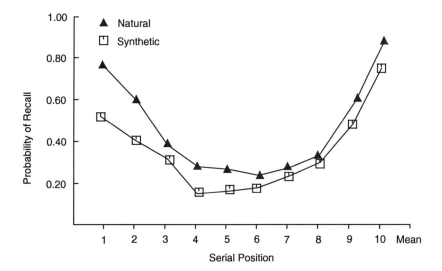

Figure 3 Probability of correct serial recall for natural and synthetic speech (Votrax) word lists. Serial position refers to the presentation order of items in the memory set. Triangles represent recall rate for natural speech and squares represent the recall rate for synthetic speech (from Luce et al., 1983).

1.5.2   Attention and Synthetic Speech

Several experiments have tested whether the perception of synthetic speech requires greater mental effort or attention than naturally produced speech. This line of research followed from earlier research using lists of spoken digits (Dallett, 1964; Rabbit, 1966). These studies demonstrated that noise-degraded digits were remembered more poorly in a recall task than undegraded digits, even though both types of stimuli were correctly identified in a labeling task with no memory constraints.

By extension, if the perception of synthetic speech requires more processing resources than natural speech, then one should be able to measure these additional demands with appropriate experimental techniques. If there are differing attentional demands for synthetic speech compared to natural speech, we would expect a differential decrease in performance as the difficulty of a perceptual task is increased or as a secondary task is added which makes use of the same resources (Baddeley & Hitch, 1974; Wickens, 1987). Luce et al. (1983) tested this hypothesis. In one of their studies, subjects recalled ten word lists produced either by MITalk or by an adult male talker. Before each list of words was presented to subjects, either zero, three, or six digits were displayed in sequence on a video monitor. Subjects were required to first recall the visually presented digits in the order they were displayed and then recall the spoken words in any order. Analysis of the digit recall data indicated that not only were there more errors overall when subjects were presented with words produced by a synthesizer, but there was a significant interaction between voice and digit preload. The decrement in performance for recall of the synthetic speech increased with increasing digit load.

In another experiment, subjects were required to recall in serial order lists of words spoken by a real talker or lists produced by a synthesizer. Results from this study are presented in Figure 3. In addition to finding that words produced by a synthesizer were recalled more poorly overall than words produced by a human talker, Luce et al. also found a significant interaction between voice and serial position. That is, the difference in serial recall between words produced by a human and a synthesizer was greatest for items from early positions in the lists. Because words from early portions of the list are assumed to be recalled from long-term memory (LTM), the results suggested that increased encoding demands for synthetic speech left fewer resources for the transfer of items into long-term memory (Murdock, 1962).

In a recent follow-up study, Lee and Nusbaum (1989) studied changes in capacity demands of synthetic speech as a function of practice. Subjects were tested using a word monitoring task before and after three days of identification training with phonetically balanced words produced by a Votrax synthesizer. During pre- and post-training tests, subjects monitored a list of words for a particular target. Subjects studied two or five visually displayed numbers before the list of words was presented, and recalled them after hearing the list. Although there was an effect of digit load on recall accuracy, there was no effect of training. Word monitoring accuracy improved after training and was higher when there was only a two-digit load, a finding that was consistent with the digit recall data. Monitoring latency decreased after training, and was shorter with only a two-digit load. There was a significant interaction between the effects of training and load on monitoring performance. The effects of training were much larger for the two-digit load condition. Based on these results and the results from a second control experiment, Lee and Nusbaum concluded that with training their subjects diverted "spare" resources (the total amount available minus that for the two-digit recall task) to acoustic-phonetic processing, which produced shorter monitoring latencies. According to Lee and Nusbaum, synthetic speech does not require more attention than higher-quality speech. However, during their initial exposure to synthetic speech, subjects erroneously devote extra attention to it anyway, an "error" that is corrected with practice.

In summary, the available evidence indicates that the perception of synthetic speech requires greater processing resources than natural speech. Because the stimuli in these experiments were simple word lists, the increased demands appear to arise during the acoustic-phonetic analysis of the input signal. In addition, more recent data indicate that given appropriate training, subjects may devote more effort to encoding processes, thereby increasing performance. The following section reviews empirical data suggesting that other comprehension processes may also make use of the same central resources of working memory.

1.5.3   Attention and Comprehension

Consistent with Kintsch and van Dijk's model (1978), several studies have demonstrated that comprehension requires attention. In one early experiment, Baddeley and Hitch (1974) presented three types of passages to subjects, one sentence at a time, and later administered a comprehension test. One half of the subjects were required to remember six different digits during each sentence. After the completion of the sentence, subjects attempted to recall the digits in ordered sequence. Baddeley and Hitch found that both comprehension and ordered digit recall were worse compared to a control condition in which subjects recalled the digits immediately after their presentation. Two other experiments replicated the major finding with different comprehension tests, memory load techniques, and text variables. Based on their results, Baddeley and Hitch concluded that comprehension requires the same resources (attention) as do other cognitive processes. Consequently, comprehension performance may suffer if there are other concurrent tasks that also compete for the same processing resources.

Other studies have examined the capacity requirements of some of the subprocesses involved in comprehension. Britton, Holdredge, Curry and Westbrook (1979) asked subjects to read passages with or without titles while they listened for randomly-occurring auditory clicks. Subjects performed more poorly on the click detection task when titles were provided, while comprehension performance also increased. The authors concluded that readers consumed STM capacity while performing the inferences made possible by the titles' context. Therefore, it is likely that some portion of the attentional demands observed by Baddeley and Hitch may have been used for deriving inferences in comprehension.

1.5.4   Summary

There are a variety of available TTS systems that vary in the sophistication of their synthesis algorithms. These computational differences determine the similarity between the output of TTS devices and natural speech. Several lines of data suggest that the perception of synthetic speech entails the use of more resources than natural speech. A distinct line of psycholinguistic inquiry has demonstrated that comprehension processes also require attentional resources. However, little research has examined whether the demands imposed by synthetic speech compete for common resources also used in comprehension. The implications of such an interaction are paramount in applications of this technology. Recognizing this, Luce et al. (1983) issued the following caveat:

> "We believe that increased processing demands for the encoding and rehearsal of synthetic speech may place important constraints on the use of various voice-response devices in high information load situations, particularly under conditions requiring differential allocation of attention among several sensory inputs."

Because comprehension performance may vary as a function of cognitive demands, it is clear that observed performance on listening tasks may not be predicted simply from estimates of segmental intelligibility. Instead, one must also consider concurrent cognitive demands of the environment as well as properties of the spoken text itself.

In the next section, we examine methods that have been developed to assess comprehension of spoken language. Then we discuss several recent studies on the comprehension of synthetic speech.

2.   Measures of Comprehension

Attempts to objectively evaluate comprehension date back at least to the 1800's and are closely related to the development of intelligence testing. Around 1900, the U.S. educational system began developing comprehension tests in order to place students in appropriate classes (Johnston, 1984). This educational tradition has yielded many "standardized" tests that are available in published form. More recently, cognitive psychologists and psycholinguists have developed measurement instruments to assess both the mechanisms and products of comprehension (Levelt, 1978; Carr, 1986). A fundamental distinction has been drawn in comprehension research between successive and simultaneous measures of comprehension. Successive measures of comprehension are those made after the presentation of the linguistic materials. Simultaneous tasks, on the other hand, measure comprehension in real-time as it takes place and usually require subjects to detect some secondary event occurring during the time that the comprehension process takes place (Levelt, 1978). Although this distinction theoretically partitions measures into dichotomous categories, in reality, experimental tasks form a continuum that varies in terms of how close in time the measures follow the presentation of stimulus materials.

2.1   Successive Measures

Historically, successive measures have been used to study comprehension and language processing much more often than simultaneous measures. Primarily memory tests, successive measures are appropriate for evaluating what information is abstracted and remembered from text. However, these techniques fail to provide information about whether the observed effects arise during the initial process of comprehension or later during memory storage and retrieval (Levelt, 1978). In addition, successive measures appear to be less sensitive than simultaneous measures, due to memory decay and reconstruction of information that was not part of the original materials.

2.1.1 Recall

In comprehension tasks that use recall measures, subjects may be asked for verbatim recall, to provide a written summary, or they may be given verbal cues to recall. The linguistic stimuli employed in recall studies have often been connected passages of meaningful text. Bartlett (1932) presented short stories to readers and asked them to reproduce them after varying time intervals. He found that subjects not only failed to recall some material from the passages, but they also committed systematic errors suggesting that memory distortions had occurred. Ambiguous portions of the stories were often deleted, new information was added that did not appear in the original passage, and more contemporary terminology was introduced in lieu of antiquated phrases.

More recently, Kintsch and others have developed techniques for objectively scoring the semantic content of texts and recall protocols (Kintsch, 1974; Kintsch & Keenan, 1973; Kintsch et al., 1975). First, passages are decomposed into their essential propositions or ideas. Later, the recalled information is decomposed into its propositional structure and compared to structures obtained from the original passages in order to derive a measure of recall of the propositional content of the passage. Kintsch's research has shown that subjects construct information in recall protocols as well as add metastatements about the text. The probability of these additions increases as a function of the length of the retention interval (Kintsch & Van Dijk, 1978; Levelt, 1978). Thus, the originally comprehended information may be distorted considerably when recall methods are used to measure comprehension.

2.1.2 Recognition

Several types of recognition tests have been devised to assess language comprehension, including word and sentence recognition, and multiple choice tasks. In general, research has demonstrated that recall is a less sensitive measure of retention than recognition (Crowder, 1976; Klatsky, 1980).

Word recognition tasks are assumed to assess memory for specific phonological or semantic entities, both of which may be evaluated by the use of rhyming or semantically similar foils (Brunner & Pisoni, 1982). False recognition of rhyming foils indexes memory for the phonological properties of similar target words. False recognition of semantic foils indexes memory for the conceptual properties of similar target words.

Sentence recognition tasks are assumed to assess memory for higher levels of representation, such as propositions derived from text. Appropriate foils may evaluate memory for different properties of sentences. For example, Sachs (1967) presented probe sentences visually after subjects had heard short passages containing embedded "critical" sentences in different locations. The probe sentences were either identical to the critical sentences, identical in meaning but expressed in a different form, or completely different in meaning. Although subjects almost always rejected probe sentences expressing different ideas than the critical ones, they often incorrectly recognized probe sentences expressing the same ideas as critical sentences in a different syntactic form. This effect was magnified with increasing delays between the critical and probe sentences. These results demonstrate that listeners abstract and remember the meaning of a sentence or passage, but rapidly forget surface structure.

One of the oldest recognition tasks used in comprehension studies is the multiple choice test (Johnston, 1984). After linguistic materials are presented, a question or statement is displayed which either may be completed (in the case of a statement) or answered (in the case of a question) by choosing one of a number of alternatives. One attraction of multiple choice testing is its ease of administration, as compared to other contemporary assessment techniques. However, due to the number of alternatives typically presented, response latencies may be so long and variable as to be unreliable.

2.1.3 Sentence Verification

The sentence verification task (SVT) has been used for a variety of purposes in psycholinguistic research. It may be regarded as a comprehension measure near the border between simultaneous and successive measures. In this task, a test sentence is presented to subjects who are required to judge whether it is "true" or "false." Since the judgments are often trivial (e.g., "A robin is a bird") and error rates are relatively low, the main dependent variable of interest is response latency. This paradigm has been used extensively to study sentence processing (Gough, 1965), semantic memory (Collins & Quillian, 1969), and the influence of intonation contour on the speed of comprehension (Larkey & Danly, 1983).

2.2 Simultaneous Measures

Simultaneous, or "on-line," measures provide an experimental methodology to study comprehension processes as they occur in real-time. In contrast to successive techniques, simultaneous measures of comprehension are assumed to be less contaminated by post-perceptual processes that operate at the time of retrieval. However, they are less appropriate for determining what information has been extracted and retained by the subject. There are two major classes of simultaneous measures that have been developed—target monitoring and reading times.

2.2.1 Monitoring Tasks

Simultaneous tasks usually require subjects to detect some secondary event occurring during the time that the primary comprehension process takes place. Under the assumption that monitoring draws from the same attentional resources as comprehension processes, changes in monitoring error rates and latencies have been used as an index of processing load during comprehension.

The phoneme monitoring task was first developed by Foss (1969; Hakes & Foss, 1970) and has been used extensively ever since to study on-line comprehension processes (Cutler, 1976; Marslen-Wilson & Tyler, 1980; Shields et al., 1974). The speed of phoneme detection is influenced significantly by the properties of the target-bearing word, such as its frequency of occurrence (Morton & Long, 1976).

Word monitoring tasks have also been used in studies of language processing (Blank, Pisoni & McClaskey, 1981; Brunner & Pisoni, 1982; Marslen-Wilson & Tyler, 1980; Morton & Long, 1976). In both procedures, subjects make a response when a designated target is detected in a sentence or passage. For example, Foss and Lynch (1970) used the phoneme monitoring task to determine whether sentence structure influenced comprehension. They presented either right-branching or self-embedded sentences[5] to subjects who were required to monitor for word-initial /b/ phones. Response latencies were longer for the self-embedded sentences, suggesting that they were more difficult to process than the right-branching sentences. Word monitoring tasks have also been modified to assess memory for phonological or semantic properties of spoken materials (Marslen-Wilson & Tyler, 1980).

---

[5] An example of a right-branching sentence is: "The child ate the rotten peanut and became ill." The self-embedded version of the same propositional statement would be: "The child, after eating the rotten peanut, became ill."

2.2.2 Reading Times

A commonly used psycholinguistic technique is the measurement of self-paced reading times (see Kieras & Just, 1984, for several reviews). These methods include the measurement of eye fixations and other techniques in which subjects are allowed to control the presentation of successive fragments of text. The dependent variable in all cases is the amount of time that subjects spend reading various portions of text, although sometimes successive tests are combined to insure that readers are actually comprehending the text. Multiple-regression analyses correlate the reading times with independent measures of lexical and textual characteristics, such as word frequency and syntactic structure. These studies have demonstrated that reading times are sensitive to a variety of textual variables that play an important role in current models of comprehension.

3. Comprehension of Synthetic Speech

Most studies examining comprehension of synthetic speech have employed successive measures. A few recent studies have also used simultaneous measures. The following section reviews studies utilizing sentence-length and passage-length materials. The next section describes a recent study using both successive and simultaneous measures.

3.1 Successive Measures

3.1.1 Sentence Verification

In recent studies, transcription responses and sentence verification judgments were obtained for the same set of sentences in order to evaluate the relationship between intelligibility and comprehension (Manous et al., 1985; Pisoni & Dedina, 1986; Pisoni et al., 1987). These studies have shown that verification response latency can be used to index speech quality, and that the relationship between segmental intelligibility and comprehension is less than perfect. For example, Manous et al. (1985) presented sentences produced by two natural talkers and five TTS systems (DECtalk-Paul, DECtalk-Betty, Infovox, Prose, and Votrax Type-n-Talk[6]). The sentences were either three or six words in length and expressed either true or false information with respect to general world knowledge.

Figure 4 shows error rates on the transcription task. Transcription accuracy was generally lowest for Votrax and Infovox synthetic speech and was

---

[6] Votrax Type-n-Talk is a product of Votrax.

lower for the six-word sentences than for the three-word sentences. In addition, an interaction was observed between voice and sentence length for the false sentences. That is, errors rates were greater for the longer sentences, but only for sentences produced by the Votrax and Infovox system. The results are consistent with the assumption that Votrax and Infovox speech, longer sentences, and "false" sentences place greater processing demands on listeners than do natural speech, short sentences, and true sentences, respectively, and that the demands manipulated by these factors tax a common resource pool. As processing demands increase, differences between natural and synthetic speech become larger.

Figures 5 and 6 display accuracy and latency data, respectively, from the sentence verification task (SVT). Analysis of variance on both sets of data revealed main effects of voice and interactions between voice and sentence length for false sentences. The subjects who listened to the Votrax sentences were less accurate and slower to respond compared to the subjects who listened to the other speech. In addition, the decreased accuracy associated with the longer sentences was especially marked for Votrax sentences. Post-hoc analysis of the latency data discriminated three groups of voices: natural speech, high-quality synthetic speech (DECtalk and Prose), and moderate-to-poor quality synthetic speech (Infovox and Votrax).

Taken together, the transcription results demonstrate that words in sentences spoken by natural talkers are recognized better than words produced by low-quality synthetic systems. The verification data also demonstrate that sentences produced by natural talkers are comprehended faster and more accurately than sentences produced by TTS systems. The interactions between voice and sentence length noted by Manous et al. provide additional support for Luce et al.'s (1983) conclusion that encoding synthetic speech incurs greater processing costs, and that these demands may interact with the demands imposed by other task variables, such as those influencing comprehension.

Manous et al. (1985) also computed correlations between transcription accuracy (error rate), verification accuracy, and verification latency. Considering only the true sentences, transcription error rate and verification accuracy were highly correlated ($r = -.86$). For false sentences, transcription error rate and verification latency were also highly correlated variables ($r = +.75$). Therefore, comprehension performance for isolated sentences appears to be predicted fairly well from segmental intelligibility measures.

Because the patterns of verification performance observed in the Manous et al. study could have been due to misidentified words, Pisoni et al. (1987) carried out another study that was designed specifically to dissociate intelligibility from comprehension performance. Natural and synthetic sentences generated by DECtalk-Paul were initially prescreened using a transcription task. A final set of sentences was selected so that all of them were transcribed nearly perfectly. These sentences contained predicates that were either predictable or not predictable in the sentence frame. Table 1 lists examples of the two different sentence types. After hearing each test sentence, subjects were required to first judge its truth value and then write a transcription in an answer booklet. Verification latency data from this study are presented in Figure 7.

There was no effect of voice, predictability, or length on the verification accuracy data, a result that was consistent with the screening treatment. However, significant effects of all three variables were observed for the verification latencies. The synthetic sentences were verified slower than the natural sentences, even though, according to the transcription scores, the component words were recognized equally well. Longer sentences were verified slower than shorter sentences, and sentences with unpredictable predicates were verified slower than those with highly predictable predicates. No interactions were observed between any of the main variables.

Table 1
Stimulus materials from Pisoni, Manous & Dedina (1987).

A. Three-word, false, high-predictability sentences

1. Men wear dresses.
2. Circles are square.
3. Sandpaper is smooth.
4. Winter is hot.
5. Screaming is soft.

B. Six-word, true, low-predictability sentences

1. Fish can swim but can't smoke.
2. Smoking is bad for your teeth.
3. Our alphabet has 26 characters.
4. A triangle has only three vertices.
5. Hawaii's a good place to sunbathe.

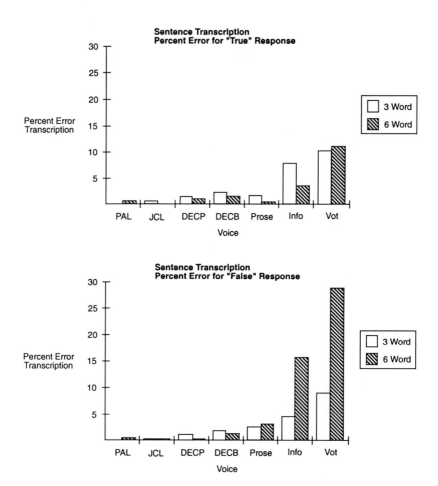

Figure 4   Percentages of errors obtained in a sentence transcription task for "True" responses (top panel) and "False" responses (bottom panel) for seven different voices. Open bars represent data for three-word sentences and striped bars represent data for six-word sentences (from Manous et al., 1985).

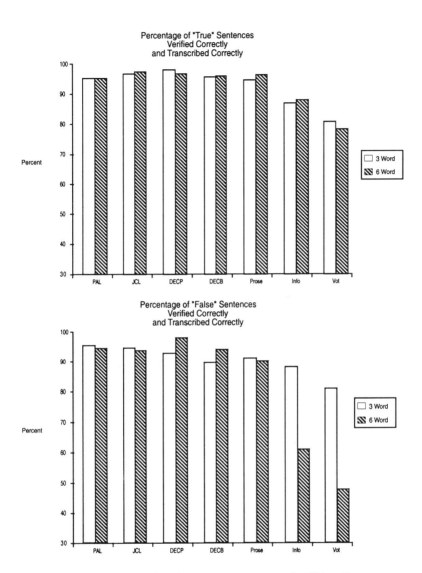

Figure 5 Sentence verification accuracy scores for "True" responses (top panel) and "False" responses (bottom panel) for seven different voices. Open bars represent data for three-word sentences and striped bars represent data for six-word sentences (from Manous et al., 1985).

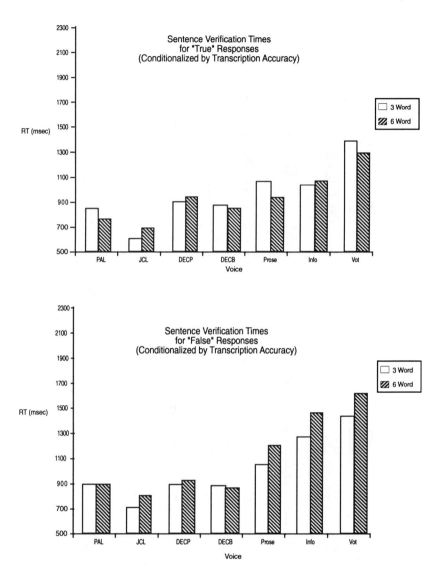

Figure 6   Sentence verification latency scores (in ms) for "True" responses (top panel) and for "False" responses (bottom panel) for seven voices. These latencies are based on only the trials in which the subject responded correctly and also transcribed the sentence correctly. Open bars represent latencies for three-word sentences and striped bars represent latencies for six-word sentences (from Manous et al., 1985).

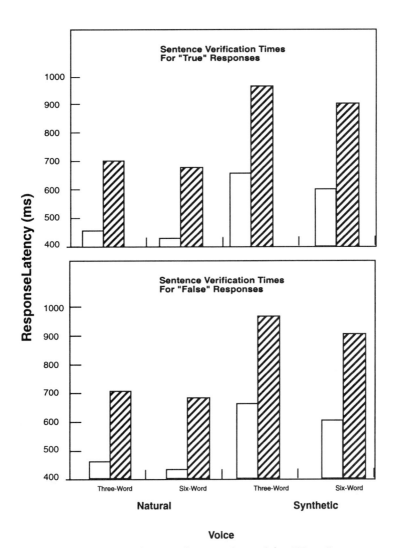

Figure 7 Sentence verification latency (in ms) for "True" responses (top panel) and "False" sentences (bottom panel) for natural and synthetic (DECtalk) speech. Open bars represent latencies for sentences in which the predicate was not predictable from the sentence context, and striped bars represent latencies for sentences in which the predicate was predicatable from the sentence context (from Pisoni et al., 1987).

The voice effect suggests that synthetic speech, even very high quality synthetic speech that can be transcribed accurately, requires more encoding time. In this situation, segmental intelligibility measures did not provide a basis for the accurate prediction of comprehension performance.

Based on the results of Manous et al. using the SVT, Schmidt-Nielson and Kallman (1987) conducted an experiment using the same methodology with digitally encoded speech stimuli. Subjects verified sentences that differed in their truth value and the degree to which their subjects and predicates were associated. Sentences were produced by a male talker and then processed digitally. The experimental sentences presented to subjects were either the original unprocessed versions or LPC-encoded copies. The LPC-encoded versions had either 0%, 2% or 5% bit errors added as encoding noise.

Analysis of accuracy and latency data revealed effects of voice, noise, relatedness, and practice. Accuracy was higher and latency was shorter for high-relatedness sentences, for sentences with less coding noise, and sentences from the second half of the testing session. Using previously obtained DRT intelligibility scores (see Voiers, 1983, for a description of the technique), Schmidt-Nielson and Kallman estimated that an increase of one percentage point in intelligibility accuracy was related to a decrease of 10-20 ms in verification latency.

The results of this study show that when listeners are presented with degraded signals, they perform much better with constraining contextual information. Pisoni et al. (1987) did not find an interaction between sentence voice and predictability. However, the difference in results may be accounted for by stimulus and subject state variables. For example, Pisoni et al. used highly-intelligible synthetic speech which was not degraded, a different form of sentence predictability, and relatively unpracticed subjects. Schmidt-Nielson and Kallman suggested that when subjects first listen to processed speech, they devote most of their available attention to acoustic-phonetic processing. After a period of familiarization, listeners reallocate resources from acoustic-phonetic processing to generate lexical and phonemic expectations to aid the listener in extracting the message.

Taken together, these recent experiments suggest that sentence verification is a sensitive measure of comprehension. All of the studies demonstrated differences between natural speech, synthetic speech and processed natural speech. Interestingly, Pisoni et al. (1987) showed that verification latency was sensitive to differences in voice quality even after the segmental intelligibility of the two sources had been equated. These findings suggest that the speed and efficiency of comprehension may vary substantially for different voice output devices, even if intelligibility is equivalent. However, the precise locus of these effects is still unknown. It is quite possible that the differences may arise simply from the increased perceptual encoding demands of the synthetic speech. If so, the increased encoding demands may limit higher levels of processing, such as those involved in parsing, semantic activation, or inference-driving. Research is currently underway on these problems and any definitive answers must await the outcome of these studies.

In summary, the interactions observed between voice and the other variables are consistent with a limited capacity resource framework. Manous et al. (1985) found an interaction between voice and length of sentences— performance was particularly poor for long sentences produced by the Votrax synthesizer. This finding suggests that processing synthetic speech and processing longer sentences both impose demands on the same limited pool of processing resources. This view is supported by results from similar studies of processed natural speech which found interactions between voice and sentence length (Pisoni & Dedina, 1986) and voice and subject-predicate relatedness (Schmidt-Nielson & Kallman, 1987).

3.1.2 Comprehension of Fluent Connected Speech

The first study to investigate the comprehension of fluent synthetic speech was carried out by Nye, Ingemann & Donald (1975). The outputs of two synthesizers, the Haskins parallel formant synthesizer and the OVE-III serial formant synthesizer were compared to natural speech. Two passages over 1500 words in length were selected from a published reading test. Each passage was followed by 14 multiple-choice questions. A separate test indicated that subjects could not answer the questions on the basis of world knowledge alone. After each passage was presented, subjects were given as much time as needed to answer as many questions as possible.

The results showed no difference in performance between conditions in terms of accuracy. However, there was a difference in terms of the amount of time needed to answer the questions after replaying portions of the passage. Subjects were nearly 25% slower answering the subset of questions following synthetic passages (*mean* = 6.27 *s*) compared to natural passages (*mean* = 4.51 *s*). However, since the natural passages were spoken at a faster rate and were therefore physically shorter than the synthetic passages, subjects may have been able to review the natural passages more quickly, thus accounting for the observed latency differences.

In another early study, McHugh (1976) used eight passages from the Diagnostic Reading Scales, a standardized comprehension test, to study the comprehension of Votrax synthetic speech. Two of the passages were presented as practice and six were presented for the experiment proper. Each of the passages was a short narrative story and each was followed by a series of cued recall questions (e.g., "How much did Bob pay for the plum?"). Seven versions of the paragraphs were presented to subjects, six produced by a Votrax synthesizer and one produced by a human talker. The Votrax versions differed in their stress patterns, which were altered either by hand or by rule. A random stress condition was also included. The stress patterns generated by rule varied in sophistication from relatively crude and mechanical rhythms to relatively natural prosody. For example, one algorithm created sentences by alternating stressed and unstressed syllables, while another made use of syntactic information. Voice (talker and stress-algorithm) was varied as a between-subjects factor.

McHugh's results revealed no differences between the different voice conditions—all were comprehended equally well in terms of scores on the recall questions. Data from the two practice passages were analyzed separately. The results showed that the natural passages were comprehended better than some Votrax versions, such as the "untreated" monotone version. However, the natural practice passages were not comprehended any better than the hand-altered Votrax passages with correct English stress patterns. The differences in performance between the practice and test data suggest that even moderate amounts of familiarity and practice are sufficient to allow listeners to quickly learn to process even poor-quality Votrax synthetic speech.

Pisoni and Hunnicutt (1980) reported the results of a study designed to assess the comprehension of MITalk (Allen et al., 1987). Different groups of subjects listened to either MITalk or natural passages, or, in a control condition, read the same passages. The materials were derived from a variety of published reading comprehension tests. Each passage was followed by a series of multiple-choice questions. Accuracy data from this study are presented in Figure 8. Overall, the reading group performed at a higher level than the MITalk or natural groups. However, when the data were divided into first and second halves of the test session, an interaction between voice and session emerged. Reading and natural speech performance were nearly the same in both halves, but performance for the MITalk group increased dramatically in the second half of testing. As in the McHugh (1976) study, there appeared to be rapid perceptual learning which compensated for early differences in performance.

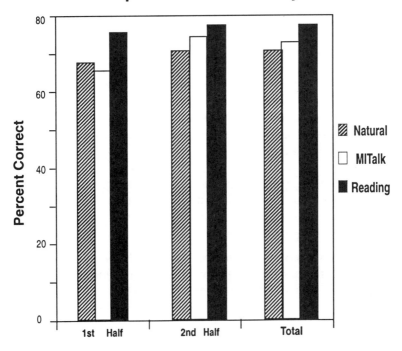

Figure 8 Comprehension accuracy for questions following passages of natural speech, synthetic (MITalk) speech, and type-written text for the first and last halves of the testing session. Striped bars represent accuracy for questions following natural speech passages, open bars represent accuracy following MITalk passages, and the filled bars represent accuracy in a reading control group (from Pisoni & Hunnicutt, 1980).

Jenkins and Franklin (1981) conducted two experiments on the comprehension of synthetic speech. In one experiment, the hand-applied stress and random stress versions of McHugh's Votrax stimuli were presented to subjects for subsequent free recall. Only three of the original passages were tested. No significant difference in performance was observed between natural speech and Votrax synthetic speech.

In a second experiment, natural and synthetic speech versions of a passage were presented twice to one group of subjects for an intelligibility test and to a second group of subjects for a comprehension test. The synthetic speech was produced using Haskins Laboratories' Speech Synthesis. Two subgroups of synthetic speech listeners were used—those with and without practice. The practiced subjects in this experiment had been tested with twenty passages a week prior to the actual testing. Trial 1 data revealed relatively small but reliable differences in performance between the natural and synthetic conditions. However, Trial 2 data revealed no difference between the natural and practiced synthetic subjects. Therefore, intelligibility differences were eliminated with even modest training. The comprehension test produced comparable results. That is, recall performance on Trial 1 and Trial 2 was better for the natural group compared to the unpracticed synthetic group, but the natural speech group was not significantly different from the practiced synthetic group. Again, initial differences in comprehension between natural and synthetic speech decreased with relatively little practice.

Luce (1981) compared recognition memory for different types of information in passages of natural speech or MITalk synthetic speech. After each passage was presented, a series of verification sentences was displayed on a video monitor in front of each subject. Different sentences probed the listener's memory for either lexical information or for different types of propositional information in the text base. Lexical items were verified faster than propositional information, but no differences were observed between natural and synthetic speech. However, verification accuracy was worse for the MITalk passages compared to the natural passages. Finally, Luce observed an unexpected interaction between voice and sentence type for the accuracy data. Accuracy was better for MITalk compared to natural speech for the "surface" sentences, which probed lexical memory, but was worse for MITalk compared to natural speech for the propositional sentences. Luce suggested that subjects listening to the MITalk passages allocated a greater proportion of their resources to acoustic-phonetic processing, which resulted in a more durable memory code for lexical information. Consequently, fewer resources were available for processing propositional information, a strategy that produced a more fragile propositional memory code.

Hersch and Tartarglia (1983) studied the comprehension of DECtalk-Paul and DECtalk-Betty at several presentation rates. The data were compared to previous data collected with natural speech by Fairbanks, Guttman & Miron (1957). Subjects were presented with short passages over a telephone. After each of the passages, a series of questions was presented that either assessed memory for explicitly stated information or required inferences based on information from the passage. The results indicated that comprehension of the synthetic passages decreased faster as a function of presentation rate than the natural speech (Fairbanks et al., 1957). Hersch and Tartarglia argued that this finding reflected the increased encoding demands for synthetic speech compared to natural speech. In addition, comprehension accuracy was higher for the male voice, with more practice, and for inferential questions. However, the authors observed that subjects knew the answers to the inferential questions without hearing the passages. While overall accuracy increased across testing blocks, the differences in performance between female and male voices decreased across testing blocks.

As part of a larger study, Schwab et al. (1985) assessed the comprehension of passages of Votrax synthetic speech as a function of training. During the same sessions, subjects were given both intelligibility and comprehension tests. Pre-training and post-training tests consisted of presentations of Votrax passages followed by verification statements assessing different levels of comprehension. On each of the training days, four passages were presented, each followed by a series of multiple-choice questions. One group of subjects was trained with Votrax stimuli, another group was trained with natural speech stimuli, and a third group, the control group, was given no training at all. All groups performed better on the comprehension test before training, and no reliable effect of training condition was observed across any of the comprehension measures. In addition, an examination of the training data revealed no difference between the Votrax and natural speech groups, nor a significant increase in performance across training sessions. No interaction was observed between voice and sentence type, as Luce had found earlier. It is possible that subjects in this study reached a training plateau by virtue of the segmental tests by the time of comprehension testing. Alternatively, as Schwab et al. suggested, these tests may have been too sensitive to subject differences, and the difficulty of the various passages may have been confounded with the day of training and/or testing. In any event, it is not clear why the earlier Luce findings were not replicated in this study.

Another investigation of comprehension of synthetic speech was conducted by Moody and Joost (1986). They compared comprehension of
passages of natural speech, DECtalk-Paul, 9600 bps digitized speech, 2400
bps digitized speech, and a reading control. Passages and multiple-choice
questions were drawn from study guides for three standardized exams: the
GED (a high school equivalence exam), the SAT (an undergraduate entrance exam) and the GRE (a graduate school entrance exam). A fourth
factor of question type was analyzed separately. Analysis of the accuracy
data indicated that voice, exam type, and length all exerted significant
effects on performance. Natural speech was comprehended better than
either DECtalk-Paul or 2400 bps digitized speech. Oddly, the SAT was the
most difficult type of passage, followed by the GRE, and finally the GED.
Finally, the moderate length passages were comprehended better than the
long and short passages, which did not differ.

Moody and Joost (1986) also classified the experimental questions by the
type of information processing required for their correct solution. Some of
this information included use of world knowledge, recognition of information explicitly stated in the passage, and the drawing of inferences from
textual information. Based on assumptions of the amount of mental effort
required to answer the questions, the questions formed a difficulty gradient from those requiring use of world knowledge to those that required
subjects to make difficult inferences.

The results showed that subjects were correct on 100% of the world
knowledge questions and only 27% of the low inference questions. Further
analyses showed that the advantage of natural speech over synthetic
speech became smaller as the difficulty of the questions increased. Comprehension performance was better for natural speech compared to synthetic
speech for questions which tested memory for explicitly stated information
but not for questions requiring inferences.

The results of this study should be viewed with some caution, however.
First, question type was poorly controlled and possibly confounded with
passages in this study. Second, text difficulty was also poorly controlled.
This was confirmed by the unexpected rank ordering of perceived difficulty and performance as a function of passage type. Finally, the specific
interaction reported between question type and voice appears anomalous.
As Pisoni et al. (1987) observed, "We do not know of any current theory of
human information processing or language processing that would predict

the results observed by Moody & Joost." In retrospect, however, it appears that the effect of voice may have been the most robust result of the study.

The comprehension studies summarized above may be classified into three broad categories. First, two studies reported reliable effects of voice on accuracy, but no training effects (Luce, 1981; Moody & Joost, 1986). Second, three studies reported performance differences between voices when synthetic speech was first encountered during the experiment, but the differences became smaller with even moderate exposure or training (Jenkins & Franklin, 1981; McHugh, 1976; Pisoni & Hunnicutt, 1980). Finally, Schwab et al. (1985) found no comprehension differences between passages of natural and Votrax speech, nor a learning effect on the comprehension of passages of Votrax speech, even after two weeks of training. Taken together, these studies suggest differences in comprehension between natural and synthetic speech, but the results appear to be extremely variable from study to study. Obviously, further research with greater experimental control is necessary to provide more reliable information about the comprehension of synthetic speech, particularly long passages of connected fluent speech.

3.2   Simultaneous Measures

In this section we summarize the results from two recent experiments that represent the first reported use of on-line methods to study differences in the comprehension of passages of natural and synthetic speech (Ralston et al., 1990). Both studies made use of the same passages produced by the same sources and made use of the same post-perceptual recognition memory task. Items on the recognition memory task were prescreened in order to eliminate questions that were so easy that subjects could correctly answer them without listening to the passages. Finally, an abbreviated form of the MRT was presented to listeners in both experiments, allowing correlational analyses between segmental intelligibility and several comprehension measures.

The first experiment combined an on-line word monitoring task with a recognition memory task to assess comprehension differences between natural and synthetic speech. Several short passages were produced either by a Votrax synthesizer or an adult male talker. All passages were adapted from published reading comprehension tests for fourth grade and college level readers. Before a passage was presented, either 0, 2 or 4 target words were displayed for 30 seconds on a video monitor. Subjects were then required to listen to a passage for comprehension and to simultaneously monitor for the word targets. Subjects pressed a response button to signal their detection of any of the target words. After each passage, subjects judged whether information in visually-presented test sentences had occurred in the previous passage. Half of the sentences assessed memory for specific words, and half probed memory for propositional information.

Monitoring accuracy data are presented in Figure 9 as a function of voice, target set size and sentence type. Monitoring accuracy was higher for targets in passages of natural speech than in passages of synthetic speech. Accuracy also decreased with increasing target set size. Thus, word monitoring performance in this task was affected by both speech quality and concurrent memory load. There was also a significant interaction between target set size and text difficulty, but post-hoc tests failed to reveal any significant pair-wise differences.

Figure 10 displays latency data for correct detections. Monitoring responses were faster for words in passages of natural speech compared to passages of synthetic speech, suggesting that speech quality affects the rate of comprehension. Latencies were also faster in the two-target condition compared to the four-target condition, suggesting that memory load also affects the speed of comprehension. Monitoring responses were faster for the fourth-grade passages than the college-level passages, confirming our assumption that this linguistic variable loads STM. Finally, there was a significant interaction between voice and text difficulty. The increase in latency from fourth-grade to college-level text was larger for the Votrax passages than the natural passages. This result suggests that perceptual encoding and comprehension processes compete for common STM resources.

Figure 11 displays accuracy data for the recognition memory test as a function of the four independent variables. Subjects performed more accurately when the sentences followed passages of natural speech compared to passages of synthetic speech. There was also an interesting interaction between voice and sentence type. While subjects listening to natural passages performed equally well on the two types of sentences, subjects listening to passages of synthetic speech were less accurate on proposition-recognition sentences. This result is similar to the earlier findings reported by Luce (1981).

Analysis of other factors indicated that accuracy was lower for the college level passages than the fourth grade passages. Finally, accuracy was lower for the four target condition than the zero or two target conditions,

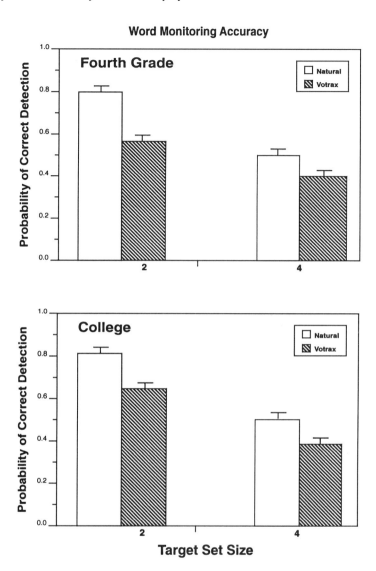

Figure 9 Word monitoring accuracy (probability of a correct detection) as a function of target set size. The upper panel shows data for fourth-grade passages and the lower panel shows data for college-level passages. Open bars represent accuracy for passages of natural speech and striped bars represent accuracy for passages of Votrax synthetic speech. Error bars represent one standard error of the sample means (from Ralston et al., 1990).

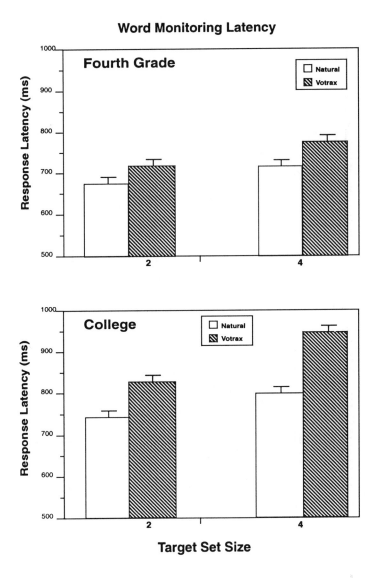

Figure 10   Word monitoring latency (in milliseconds) as a function of target set size. The upper panel shows data for fourth-grade passages and the lower panel shows data for college-level passages. Open bars represent latencies for passages of natural speech and striped bars represent latencies for passages of Votrax synthetic speech. Error bars represent one standard error of the sample means (from Ralston et al., 1990).

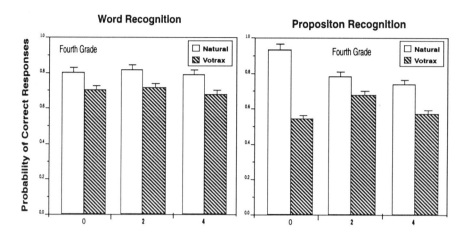

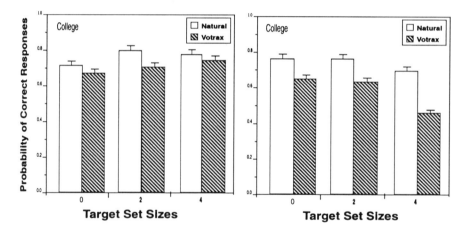

Figure 11 Recognition memory accuracy (probability correct) as a function of target-set size. The panels on the left show data for word-recognition sentences and the panels on the right show data for proposition-recognition sentences. The upper panels show data for fourth-grade passages and the lower panels show data for college-level passages. Open bars represent accuracy for sentences following passages of natural speech and striped bars represent accuracy for sentences following passages of Votrax synthetic speech. Error bars represent one standard error of the sample means (from Ralston et al., 1990).

suggesting that the monitoring task made use of the same limited capacity as comprehension processes.

In summary, the overall picture of the results suggests that the comprehension of passages of poor quality synthetic speech is slower and less accurate than the comprehension of passages of natural speech. The recognition memory data indicate that memory for linguistic information in passages of synthetic speech was also degraded in some way. The recognition memory data also reveal that propositional information derived from passages of synthetic speech was particularly poor. This result provides support for an earlier speculation of Pisoni (1982), who suggested that subjects may listen and process synthetic speech differently than natural speech. In particular, listeners may allocate more attention to processing the acoustic-phonetic structure of synthetic speech than the content or meaning of the message. With more attention devoted to acoustic-phonetic processing, fewer resources are available to allocate to comprehension and memory processes, thus producing a less complete and more fragile memory representation of the propositional information.

Finally, correlations were computed between MRT accuracy and the various comprehension measures. The magnitudes of the coefficients were generally moderate ($r = -.31$ to $r = .47$) and highly significant. Although statistical comparisons between the two studies are not possible, the values are generally smaller than those reported by Manous et al. (1985). These results suggest that the comprehension of passages of connected speech requires processing beyond lexical and sentential levels of analysis. Because these processes rely on information and knowledge not contained in the speech waveform, expectations about the overall level of comprehension performance may be predicted only moderately well from estimates of segmental intelligibility.

To obtain additional converging evidence, a second experiment was conducted with exactly the same stimuli. However, the passages were presented one sentence at a time in response to button presses by the subject. This technique is analogous to the self-paced sentence-by-sentence reading task used extensively with written texts (see Kieras & Just, 1984, for extensive reviews). This technique had first been modified and used with spoken texts in a study by Mimmack (1982). In the present study, the length of time between the presentation of a sentence and the following button press served as the dependent variable. Several studies have demonstrated that sentence reading times are sensitive to a number of linguistic variables that underlie text difficulty (see Haberlandt, 1984, for an exhaustive listing).

The sentence listening times are displayed in Figure 12 as a function of voice and text difficulty. Both the voice of the passage and the difficulty of the text had a significant effect on sentence listening times. Response times were slower for passages produced by a synthesizer than by a natural talker and were slower for the college text than for the fourth-grade text. That text difficulty had a significant effect on the sentence listening times suggests that subjects were not pressing the button indiscriminately and that the measure itself is a valid index of spoken language comprehension. Therefore, the on-line data from both experiments suggest that comprehension proceeds more slowly for passages of synthetic speech than for passages of natural speech

The results from the recognition memory task were largely the same as in the first experiment. Of greater interest, though, was the finding of an interaction between voice and sentence type, an interaction that was also found in the word monitoring experiment. In order to characterize this interaction, difference scores were computed for each subject by subtracting accuracy for the proposition-recognition sentences from the accuracy for the word-recognition sentences. Figure 13 displays the results of this analysis, as well as comparable data from the zero-target condition in the word monitoring experiment. An ANOVA on the combined data revealed that the effect of voice was highly significant. The cross-over interaction observed in these data is the same as that observed by Luce (1981)—subjects listening to natural speech were more accurate for proposition-recognition sentences and subjects listening to Votrax speech were more accurate for word-recognition sentences. The data are consistent with the hypothesis that comprehension is constrained by a limited capacity of processing resources that can be allocated to various comprehension sub-processes as well as other cognitive processes. Subjects listening to synthetic speech apparently allocate a greater proportion of the available resources to acoustic-phonetic processing, leaving relatively fewer resources for analysis of the linguistic meaning of the passage.

Correlations were again computed between MRT accuracy scores collected at the beginning of the experiment and the comprehension measures. The magnitude of the coefficients was again moderate ($r = -.40$ to $r = .63$) and highly significant. Their size again reinforces the conclusion that comprehension performance can be predicted moderately well at best on the basis of estimates of segmental intelligibility derived from isolated words. The

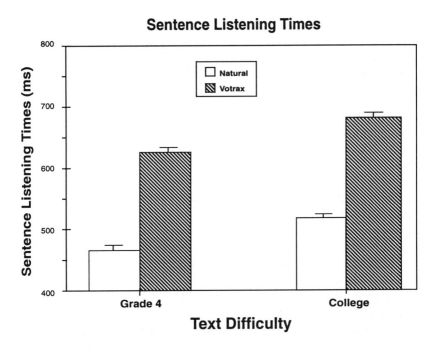

Figure 12 Sentence-by-sentence listening times as a function of voice and text difficulty. Open bars represent response latencies for passages of natural speech and striped bars represent response latencies for passages of synthetic speech. Error bars represent one standard error of the sample means (from Ralston et al., 1990).

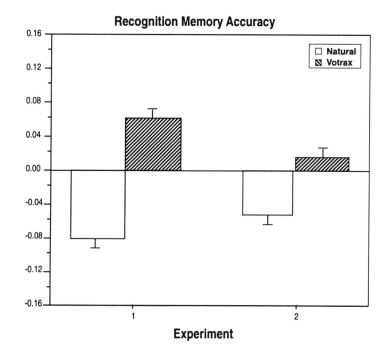

Figure 13 Accuracy difference scores (probability correct) for both the word monitoring (Experiment 1) and the sentence-by-sentence listening time (Experiment 2) experiments. Differences were computed by subtracting proposition-recognition accuracy from word-recognition accuracy. Open bars represent differences for sentences after passages of natural speech and striped bars represent differences for sentences following passages of synthetic speech. Error bars represent one standard error of the sample means (from Ralston et al., 1990).

unaccounted variance in comprehension performance presumably is due to subject-to-subject variance in the comprehension processes operating beyond the level of word recognition.

4.   Summary and Conclusions

Although our knowledge about the comprehension of synthetic speech remains incomplete, several conclusions may be drawn from the studies reviewed above. Many other questions can be identified for future research. Based on the studies considered earlier, we examine the following issues: efficiency of comprehension, attentional demands, the role of perceptual learning and applications of the research. Finally, we discuss extensions of these findings and suggest several new areas for research.

4.1   Efficiency of Comprehension

Early comprehension studies failed to uncover reliable differences in performance between natural and synthetic speech (Jenkins & Franklin, 1981; McHugh, 1976; Nye et al., 1975; Pisoni & Hunnicutt, 1980; Schwab et al., 1985). However, more recent studies examining the comprehension of isolated sentences and connected discourse have reported unambiguous differences in both accuracy and latency measures when more sensitive dependent measures are used (Luce, 1981; Moody & Joost, 1986; Manous et al., 1985; Pisoni et al., 1987). Several of these differences have been replicated and extended in the recent studies carried out in our laboratory using on-line tasks combined with a post-perceptual memory test.

The failure of earlier studies to find significant differences in comprehension between natural and synthetic speech may be due to a variety of factors including selection of stimulus materials and specific testing techniques. For example, most studies using passages of fluent connected speech relied on published multiple choice tests to assess comprehension. The accuracy of responding to these questions appears to be closely related to prior real-world knowledge. Such an effect would increase within-groups error variance and would serve to obscure any true differences in comprehension performance between conditions. This observation suggests the need for better experimental controls in comprehension research. One control procedure is to pre-screen test questions and discard those items that subjects can correctly answer without listening to the corresponding passages. Although this technique works in a "statistical" sense over a number of subjects, there are no guarantees for all individuals. Because of this problem, other techniques may be preferable. In particular, the use of passages referring to fictional events increase the probability that subjects make use of information acquired through comprehension of test passages.

4.2 Capacity Demands

The results of earlier recall experiments suggested that perceptual encoding of synthetic speech incurs a greater processing load than natural speech (Luce et al., 1983). However, it is difficult to extrapolate these results directly to a comprehension task. To the extent that connected discourse is informationally redundant or otherwise easy to process, one would expect comprehension demands to be minimized. In this case, context-guided expectations might serve to neutralize or cancel the encoding demands of synthetic speech. Therefore, we would expect that the demands of processing and comprehending synthetic speech would be more apparent as the complexity or difficulty of the text increases. Based on the available evidence, the effects of attentional load on comprehension are ambiguous, but suggest that the increased load does affect comprehension in some manner. Considering verification studies using isolated sentences, one report found an interaction between voice and load (Manous et al., 1985) while another did not (Pisoni et al., 1987). The two studies of passage comprehension involving the manipulation of cognitive load reported interactions with voice (Moody & Joost, 1986; Ralston et al., 1990). However, as noted above, there are reasons to view the Moody and Joost results cautiously. In contrast, our recent studies revealed that the increase in monitoring latencies observed with synthetic speech was greater for college-level passages, a result that is consistent with limited capacity expectations. In addition, our replication of the interaction between voice and sentence type in the recognition memory task is consistent with a limited capacity model. Future research should examine this issue in greater detail because it has important ramifications for the application of speech I/O technology in high information/workload environments (Pisoni et al., 1985).

4.3 Training Effects and Perceptual Learning

Another important issue deals with the effects of training and perceptual learning on comprehension of synthetic speech. A number of studies have examined short-term training and have found reliable effects on comprehension (Jenkins & Franklin, 1981; McHugh, 1976; Pisoni & Hunnicutt, 1980). Several researchers have concluded that practice effects in comprehension reflect the learning of new mapping rules which relate the acoustic structure of a novel synthetic voice to known phonemic categories (Lee & Nusbaum, 1989; Schwab et al., 1985). This acoustic-phonetic relearning presumably involves processing costs that impact on other cognitive activities (Luce, 1981; Pisoni, 1982). Listeners may also learn perceptual segmentation strategies through training (Greenspan et al., 1988). However, Lee and Nusbaum (1989) recently suggested that processing synthetic speech does not require more attention than processing natural speech, but that listeners presented with synthetic speech initially misallocate resources. They argue that training only helps listeners efficiently re-allocate attention.

At the present time, no attempts have been made to train subjects to asymptotic levels of performance or to determine whether differences in comprehension between natural and synthetic speech will still be present after extensive training with these systems. However, studies utilizing connected discourse have implicitly assumed that training effects have been minimized by virtue of the explicit training at the beginning of testing sessions. Clearly, this is an empirical issue. In fact, no training studies, either with isolated words, sentences, or passages, have demonstrated that subjects reach a performance plateau. It is important to determine whether the attentional load imposed by encoding processes or by comprehension processes diminishes with training or whether the load remains. Based on considerations of the results of Lee and Nusbaum (1989) and Schmidt-Nielson and Kallman (1987), subjects may re-allocate "spare" resources from acoustic-phonetic encoding to more abstract cognitive processes. If so, we would predict that comprehension performance for passages of natural and synthetic speech would converge, and that the previously observed interaction between voice and recognition sentence type would disappear.

4.4   Applications

The results discussed in the present chapter demonstrate that the comprehension of connected synthetic speech is correlated with segmental intelligibility. This conclusion argues against the use of low- to moderate-quality synthetic speech for applications requiring very high levels of comprehension. The word monitoring and sentence verification data summarized above demonstrate that comprehension of synthetic speech proceeds at a slower rate than natural speech. Therefore, particularly low-quality synthetic speech may also be inappropriate for applications requiring rapid responses. Finally, several studies have shown that comprehension of connected synthetic speech may incur greater processing costs than natural speech. Thus, poor-quality synthetic speech also may be inappropriate for applications using difficult text, such as that of a data-base retrieval system, or with other competing tasks that place significant demands on working memory, such as in a cockpit, air traffic control tower, or battlefield management system.

All of these reservations may be modified after we gain a better understanding of the effects of training and perceptual learning on comprehension. Many of the major effects associated with the comprehension of synthetic speech (lower accuracy, slower processing, and increased cognitive load) may be eliminated with appropriate practice (Lee & Nusbaum, 1989). If these effects disappear with training, the only limiting factors for applications would be practice and exposure.

Certain listener populations, such as young children, elderly adults (Humes et al., 1990) or non-native speakers (Mack, 1989), may experience difficulty comprehending synthetic speech (Greene & Pisoni, 1988). Capacity limitations and processing speed are known to be more constrained compared to college-age listeners who are typically used in these experiments (Greene & Pisoni, 1988; Salthouse, 1988). The same capacity arguments may apply to listeners or listening situations that degrade speech signals. This includes the hearing-impaired community, which is becoming increasingly dominated by older presbycutic listeners. Capacity limitations may also play an important role with signal degradations, such as noisy communication channels or reverberant environments.

4.5   Future Directions
Several problems still need to be studied. These may be grouped into the following major categories: capacity demands, training effects, memory decay and generalization.

4.5.1   Capacity Demands
As indicated above, the extent to which encoding demands compete with other comprehension processes for limited STM capacity is still a topic of great interest. While sentence verification experiments have found interactions between voice and memory load variables (such as sentence length), the evidence from studies conducted with fluent connected speech is somewhat equivocal. Therefore, further studies should be conducted with passage-length materials. These studies will help answer a number of basic questions (i.e., "Which cognitive mechanisms make use of limited attentional capacity?") as well as applications questions (ie., "Is the comprehension of synthetic speech compromised by difficult text or competing tasks?"). We

consider here possible methodological improvements for investigating the role of text difficulty and competing cognitive tasks as they relate to capacity demands in comprehension. Either of these techniques may be combined with simultaneous measures to provide a more sensitive index of comprehension processes.

Previous studies utilizing passages of varying difficulty have also used a different set of comprehension questions for each passage. One experimental strategy which circumvents this confound is to express the same propositional information in different texts varying in surface structure complexity. In this manner, the same post-passage sentences or questions could be used, yielding better control of textual difficulty.

The "digit preload" technique is a well-known method which may also be used to assess the extent to which the comprehension of synthetic speech competes with other cognitive tasks (Baddeley & Hitch, 1974; Luce et al., 1983). For example, subjects could be required to memorize a variable-sized set of digits before listening to natural or synthetic passages for comprehension. Interactions between digit set size and voice would provide strong evidence that both variables draw on a common resource pool.

Another issue related to capacity limitations deals with listener fatigue or habituation. Assuming that there are increased processing demands for synthetic speech, one might expect that listeners would become mentally fatigued, and consequently that performance would decline more rapidly as a function of time. As a test, one could examine performance over time as a function of voice (see Mack, 1989, for preliminary data on this issue).

4.5.2   Training Effects

From an applications perspective, it is important to determine the time-course of training effects and asymptotic levels of comprehension performance as well as capacity demands. For example, a system that yields initially poor comprehension performance may, with exposure and training, ultimately yield high comprehension performance. This information, as well as costs associated with training, should be weighed with other factors when selecting a particular TTS system.

4.5.3   Memory Decay

The increased processing load for synthetic speech may also lead to poorer memory for comprehended information. This possibility is suggested by earlier studies demonstrating poorer STM retention of degraded natural (Dallett, 1964; Rabbitt, 1966) and synthetic word lists (Luce et al., 1983). In addition, there may be LTM losses for comprehended information even when original comprehension levels for synthetic speech are equivalent to those obtained for natural speech. Such a result would indicate a subtle, but important effect which should be considered in application decisions. A simple way to test this would be to administer comprehension tests at variable intervals after spoken passages to assess long-term retention. To our knowledge, studies of long-term retention have not been carried out yet with passages of synthetic speech or low-bit rate coded speech.

4.5.4 Generalization
A more global issue that has received relatively little attention to date is the generality of the results obtained with synthetic speech. Are the results obtained with synthetic speech also found with other types of processed speech? At the level of segmental intelligibility, the answer is clearly "no." Nusbaum, Dedina & Pisoni (1984) demonstrated that perceptual confusions are dramatically different for DECtalk and noise-degraded natural speech CV syllables. We might expect that confusion patterns would vary with the various speech output devices, reflecting specific acoustic-phonetic synthesis rules for TTS systems, specific interactions between digital-encoding techniques, or interactions between different types of noise. However, other phenomena, such as those related to capacity demands and listener fatigue (Luce, 1981; Ralston et al., 1990; Schmidt-Nielson & Kallman, 1987) have not been investigated in studies with natural, synthetic, vocoded, and noise-degraded speech. Future research should determine whether these effects reflect general adaptive strategies of listeners to degraded or impoverished speech signals or whether they too are specific to the particular output device using synthetic speech.

4.5.5 Miscellaneous Issues
Evaluation studies of synthetic speech with special user populations have received attention recently (Greene & Pisoni, 1988; Humes et al., 1990; Mack, 1989; Ozawa & Logan, 1989). These have included studies with children, elderly listeners, and non-native English speakers. Further research is necessary to determine the extent of their deficits and how it affects on comprehension.

Likewise, demanding or stressful environments, such as noisy or reverberant sound fields, should be studied. Because these environments may be relatively common in application settings, it is important to assess their impact on performance. Noisy and reverberant environments degrade the quality of speech signals, and therefore are expected to degrade perceptual performance. Part of the expected performance decrements may be due to relatively "low-level" effects, such as degrading the physical signal or auditory masking. However, there may also be more central contributions to performance decrements, particularly attentional constraints.

Finally, emphasis should be placed on implementing voice technology using synthetic speech in real-world applications, especially when an operator is required to carry out several simultaneous cognitive tasks. Although laboratory studies have demonstrated differences in performance between natural and synthetic speech, there is a paucity of data collected in "natural" situations. Data-base query systems, computer-aided instruction, and voice mail are reasonable starting points for applied research on synthetic speech.

In summary, this chapter has reviewed research on the comprehension of synthetic speech carried out over the last 15 years. A large number of studies have demonstrated differences in segmental intelligibility between natural and synthetic speech. However, the evidence regarding comprehension has been less compelling. This is especially true with respect to comprehension of passages of fluent connected speech. Although the accumulated evidence to date indicates reliable differences in comprehension between natural speech and a wide variety of different kinds of synthetic speech, the results are quite variable across different studies, suggesting that important methodological factors need to be controlled before true differences in comprehension performance can be uncovered. In older comprehension studies that used successive measurement techniques, the results have been mixed. On the other hand, in recent comprehension studies that used on-line simultaneous measurements, the results show reliable effects that are moderately correlated with segmental intelligibility scores. When segmental intelligibility is equated between natural and synthetic speech, differences in comprehension performance have still been observed suggesting a general attenuation of the processes used to construct semantic and syntactic representations from acoustic-phonetic information contained in the speech signal. Additional research is needed to further understand the locus of these differences in comprehension performance. Because spoken language processing is extremely robust, it is often difficult to observe differences in comprehension without using fine-grained simultaneous measurement techniques.

5. References

Allen, J., Klatt, D.H. & Hunnicutt, S. (1987). *From Text to speech: The MITalk system*. Cambridge, UK: Cambridge University Press.

Allen, J. (1981). Linguistic based algorithms offer practical text-to-speech systems. *Speech Technology*, **1**, 12–16.

American National Standards Institute (1969). *Methods for the calculation of the articulation index*.

Baddeley, A.D. & Hitch, G. (1974). Working memory. In G.H. Bower (Ed.), *The psychology of learning and motivation, Vol. 8*. New York: Academic Press.

Bartlett, F.C. (1932). *Remembering*. Cambridge: Cambridge University Press.

Blank, M.A., Pisoni, D.B. & McClaskey, C.L. (1981). Effects of target monitoring on understanding fluent speech. *Perception & Psychophysics*, **29**, 383–388.

Britton, B.K., Holdredge, T., Curry, C. & Westbrook, R.D. (1979). Use of cognitive capacity in reading identical texts with different amounts of discourse level meaning. *Journal of Experimental Psychology: Human Learning and Memory*, **5**, 262–270.

Brunner, H. & Pisoni, D. B. (1982). Some effects of perceptual load on spoken text comprehension. *Journal of Verbal Learning and Verbal Behavior*, **21**, 186–195.

Carr, T.H. (1986). Perceiving visual language. In K.R. Boff, L. Kaufman & J.P. Thomas (Eds.), *Handbook of perception and human performance, Vol. II*. New York: Wiley.

Collins, A.M. & Quillian, M.R. (1969). Retrieval time from semantic memory. *Journal of Verbal Learning and Verbal Behavior*, **8**, 240–247.

Crowder, R.G. (1976). *Principles of learning and memory*. Hillsdale, NJ: Lawrence Erlbaum.

Cutler, A. (1976). Phoneme-monitoring reaction time as a function of preceding intonation contour. *Perception & Psychophysics*, **20**, 55–60.

Dallett, K.M. (1964). Intelligibility and short-term memory in the repetition of digit strings, *Journal of Speech and Hearing Research*, **7**, 362–368.

Egan, J.P. (1948). Articulation testing methods. *Laryngoscope*, **58**, 955–991.

Fairbanks, G., Guttman, N. & Miron, M.S. (1957) The effects of time compression upon the comprehension of connected speech. *Journal of Speech and Hearing Disorders*, **22**, 10–19.

Foss, D.J. (1969). Decision processes during sentence comprehension: Effects of lexical item difficulty and position upon decision times. *Journal of Verbal Learning and Verbal Behavior*, **8**, 457–462.

Foss, D.J. & Lynch, R.H. (1970). Decision processes during sentence comprehension: Effects of surface structure on decision times. *Perception & Psychophysics*, **5**, 145–148.

Gough, P.B. (1965). Grammatical transformations and speed of understanding. *Journal of Verbal Learning and Verbal Behavior*, **4**, 107–111.

Greene, B.G. & Pisoni, D.B. (1988). Perception of synthetic speech by adults and children: Research on processing voice output from text-to-speech systems. In L.E. Bernstein (Ed.), *The vocally impaired: Clinical practice and research*. Philadelphia: Grune & Stratton.

Greenspan, S.L., Nusbaum, H.C. & Pisoni, D.B. (1988). Perceptual learning of synthetic speech produced by rule. *Journal of Experimental Psychology: Human Perception and Performance*, **14**, 421–433.

Haberlandt, K. (1984). Components of sentence reading times. In D.E. Kieras & M.A. Just (Eds.), *New methods in reading comprehension research*. Hillsdale, NJ: Lawrence Erlbaum.

Haggard, M., Ambler, S. & Callow, M. (1970). Pitch as a voicing cue. *Journal of the Acoustical Society of America*, **47**, 613–617.

Hakes, D.T. & Foss, D.J. (1970). Decision processes during sentence comprehension: Effects of surface structure reconsidered. *Perception & Psychophysics*, **8**, 413–416.

Hersch, H.M. & Tartarglia, L. (1983). *Understanding synthetic speech*. User Research Group, Corporate Research & Architecture, Maynard, MA: Digital Equipment Corporation.

Hoover, J., Reichle, J., van Tasell, D., & Cole, D. (1987). The intelligibility of synthesized speech: Echo II versus Votrax, *Journal of Speech and Hearing Research*, **30**, 425–431.

House, A.S., Williams, C.E., Hecker, M.H. & Kryter, K.D. (1965). Articulation-testing methods: Consonantal differentiation with a closed-response set. *Journal of the Acoustical Society of America*, **37**, 158–166.

Humes, L.E., Nelson, K.J., & Pisoni, D.B. (1990). Recognition of synthetic speech by hearing-impaired elderly listeners. Submitted to the *Journal of Speech and Hearing Research*.

Jenkins, J.J. & Franklin, L.D. (1981). Recall of passages of synthetic speech. Paper presented at the Psychonomics Society Meeting, November, 1981.

Johnston, P.H. (1984). Assessment in reading. In Pearson, P.D. (Ed.), *Handbook of reading research*. New York: Longman.

Kahneman, D. (1973). *Attention and effort*. Englewood Cliffs: Prentice-Hall.

Kieras, D.E. & Just, M.A. (1984). *New methods in reading comprehension research*. Hillsdale, NJ: Lawrence Erlbaum.

Kintsch, W. (1974). *The representation of meaning in memory*. Hillsdale, NJ: Erlbaum.

Kintsch, W. & Keenan, J.M. (1973). Reading rate as a function of the number of propositions in the base structure of sentences. *Cognitive Psychology*, **5**, 257–274.

Kintsch, W. & van Dijk, T.A. (1978). Toward a model of text comprehension and production. *Psychological Review*, **85**, 363–394.

Kintsch, W. & Vipond (1979). Reading comprehension and readability in educational practice and psychological theory. In L.G. Nilsson (Ed.), *Perspectives on memory research*. Hillsdale, NJ: Erlbaum.

Kintsch, W., Kozminsky, E., Sterby, W. J., McKoon, G. & Keenan, J.M. (1975). Comprehension and recall of text as a function of content variables. *Journal of Verbal Learning and Verbal Behavior*, **14**, 196–214.

Klatsky, R.L. (1980). *Human memory*. San Francisco: Freeman.

Klatt, D.H. (1987). Review of text-to-speech conversion for English. *Journal of the Acoustical Society of America*, **82**, 737–793.

Klatt, D.H. (1988). Review of selected models of speech perception. In W.D. Marslen-Wilson (Ed.), *Lexical representation and process*, Cambridge: MIT Press.

Larkey, L.S. & Danly, M. (1983). Fundamental frequency and sentence comprehension. In *MIT Speech Group Working Papers, Vol. II.*

Lee, L. & Nusbaum, H.C. (1989). The effects of perceptual learning on capacity demands for recognizing synthetic speech. *Journal of the Acoustical Society of America*, **85**, YY10.

Levelt, W.J.M. (1978). A survey of studies in sentence perception. In W.J.M. Levelt & G.B. Flores d'Arcais (Eds.), *Studies in the perception of language*. New York: Wiley.

Liberman, A.M., Cooper, F.S., Shankweiler, D.P. & Studdert-Kennedy, M. (1967). Perception of the speech code. *Psychological Review, 74*, 431–461.

Logan, J.S., Greene, B.G. & Pisoni, D.B. (1989). Segmental intelligibility of synthetic speech produced by rule. *Journal of the Acoustical Society of America*, **86**, 566–581.

Luce, P.A. (1981). Comprehension of fluent synthetic speech produced by rule. *Research on speech perception progress report no. 7* (pp. 229–241). Bloomington, IN: Speech Research Laboratory, Psychology Department, Indiana University.

Luce, P.A., Feustel, T.C. & Pisoni, D.B. (1983). Capacity demands in short-term memory for synthetic and natural speech. *Human Factors, 25*, 17–32.

McHugh, A. (1976). Listener preference and comprehension tests of stress algorithms for a text-to-phonetic speech synthesis program. Naval Research Laboratory Report 8015.

Mack, M. (1989). The intelligibility of LPC-vocoded words and sentences presented to native and non-native speakers of English. *Journal of the Acoustical Society of America*, Suppl.1, **86**, NN8.

Marslen-Wilson, W. & Tyler, L.K. (1980). The temporal structure of spoken language understanding. *Cognition, 8*, 1–71.

Manous, L.M., Pisoni, D.B., Dedina, M.J. & Nusbaum, H.C. (1985). Comprehension of natural and synthetic speech using a sentence verification task. *Research on speech perception progress report no. 11*, (pp. 33–58). Bloomington, IN: Speech Research Laboratory, Psychology Department, Indiana University.

Miller, G.A., Heise G.A. & Lichten, W. (1951). The intelligibility of speech as a function of the context of the test materials. *Journal of Experimental Psychology, 41*, 329–335.

Miller, G.A. & Isard, S. (1963). Some perceptual consequences of linguistic rules. *Journal of Verbal Learning and Verbal Behavior,* **2**, 217–228.

Mimmack, P.C. (1982). Sentence-by-sentence listening times for spoken passages: Text structure and listener's goals. Unpublished M.A. Thesis, Indiana University.

Moody, T.S. & Joost, M.G. (1986). Synthesized speech, digitized speech and recorded speech: A comparison of listener comprehension rates. *Proceedings of the Voice Input/Output Society,* Alexandria, VA, 1986.

Morton, J. & Long, J. (1976). Effects of word transition probability in phoneme identification. *Journal of Verbal Learning and Verbal Behavior,* **15**, 43–51.

Murdock, B.B. Jr. (1962). The serial position effect of free recall. *Journal of Experimental Psychology,* **64**, 482–488.

Newell, A. & Simon, H.A. (1972). *Human problem solving.* Englewood Cliffs, NJ: Prentice-Hall.

Nusbaum, H.C, Dedina, M.J. & Pisoni, D.B. (1984). Perceptual confusions of consonants in natural and synthetic CV syllables. *Research on speech perception progress report no. 10* (pp. 409–422). Bloomington, IN: Speech Research Laboratory, Psychology Department, Indiana University.

Nye, P.W. & Gaitenby, J. (1973). Consonant intelligibility in synthetic speech and in a natural speech control (Modified Rhyme Test results). *Haskins Laboratory Status Report on Speech Research SR-33* (pp. 77–91). New Haven, CT: Haskins Laboratories.

Nye, P.W., Ingemann, F. & Donald, L. (1975). Synthetic speech comprehension: A comparison of listener performances with and preferences among different speech forms. *Haskins Laboratories: Status Report on Speech Perception SR-41* (pp. 117–126). New Haven, CT: Haskins Laboratories.

Ozawa, K. & Logan, J.S. (1989). Perceptual evaluation of two speech coding methods by native and non-native speakers of English. *Computer Speech and Language,* **3**, 53–59.

Pisoni, D.B. (1982). Perception of speech: The human listener as a cognitive interface. *Speech Technology,* **1**, 10–23.

Pisoni, D.B. & Dedina, M.J. (1986). Comprehension of digitally encoded natural speech using a sentence verification task (SVT): A first report. *Research on speech perception progress report no. 12* (pp. 3–18). Bloomington, IN: Speech Research Laboratory, Psychology Department, Indiana University.

Pisoni, D.B. & Hunnicutt, S. (1980). Perceptual evaluation of MITalk: The MIT unrestricted text-to-speech system. *IEEE International Conference Rec. on Acoustics, Speech, and Signal Processing,* (pp. 572–575).

Pisoni, D.B. & Luce, P.A. (1987). Acoustic-phonetic representations in word recognition. *Cognition,* **25,** 21–52.

Pisoni, D.B., Manous, L.M. & Dedina, M.J. (1987). Comprehension of natural and synthetic speech: Effects of predictability on sentence verification of sentences controlled for intelligibility. *Computer Speech and Language,* **2,** 303–320.

Pisoni, D.B., Nusbaum, H.C. & Greene, B.G. (1985). Perception of synthetic speech generated by rule. *Proceedings of the IEEE,* **11,** 1665–1676.

Pollack, I. & Decker, L.R. (1958). Confidence ratings, message reception, and the receiver operating characteristic. *Journal of the Acoustical Society of America,* **30,** 286–292.

Rabbitt, P. (1966). Recognition: Memory for words correctly heard in noise. *Psychonomic Science,* **6,** 383–384.

Ralston, J.V., Pisoni, D.B., Lively, S.E., Greene, B.G. & Mullennix, J.W. (1990). Comprehension of synthetic speech produced by rule: Word monitoring and sentence-by-sentence listening times. Submitted to *Human Factors.*

Sachs, J.S. (1967). Recognition memory for syntactic and semantic aspects of connected discourse. *Perception & Psychophysics,* **2,** 437–442.

Salthouse, T.A. (1988). The role of processing resources in cognitive aging. In M.L. Howe & C.J. Brainerd (Eds.), *Cognitive development in adulthood.* New York: Springer-Verlag.

Schmidt-Nielson, A. (this volume). Intelligibility testing for speech technology. In R. Bennett, A. Syrdal & S. Greenspan (Eds.), *Behavioral aspects of speech technology: Theory and applications.* New York: Elsevier.

Schmidt-Nielson, A. & Kallman, H.J. (1987). Evaluating the performance of the LPC 2.4 kbps processor with bit errors using a sentence verification task. NRL Report No. 9089, Washington, D.C., Naval Research Laboratory.

Schwab, E.C., Nusbaum, H.C. & Pisoni, D.B. (1985). Some effects of training on the perception of synthetic speech. *Human Factors, 27,* 395–408.

Sharkey, N.E. (1990). A connectionist model of text comprehension. In D.A. Balota, G.B. Flores d'Arcais & K. Rayner (Eds.), *Comprehension processes in reading.* Hillsdale, NJ: Lawrence Erlbaum.

Shields, J.L., McHugh, A. & Martin, J.G. (1974). Reaction time to phoneme targets as a function of rhythmic cues in continuous speech. *Journal of Experimental Psychology, 102,* 250–255.

Syrdal, A.K. (this volume). Text-to-speech systems. In R. Bennett, A. Syrdal & S. Greenspan (Eds.), *Behavioral aspects of speech technology: Theory and applications.* New York: Elsevier.

Thibadeau, R.H., Just, M.A., & Carpenter, P.A. (1982). A model of the time course of and content of reading. *Cognitive Science, 6,* 157–203.

Voiers, W. D. (1983). Evaluating processed speech using the Diagnostic Rhyme Test. *Speech Technology, 1,* 30–39.

Wickens, C.D. (1987). Information processing, decision making, and cognition. In Salvendy, G. (Ed.), *Handbook of Human Factors.* New York: Wiley Interscience.

Wingfield, A. & Klein, J.F. (1971). Syntactic structure and acoustic pattern in speech perception. *Perception & Psychophysics, 9,* 23–25.

Chapter 7

Human Factors in Lifecycle Development

John C. Thomas
Director, Artifical Intelligence
NYNEX Corporation

1. Introduction And Motivation

It needs hardly be said that voice systems, to be used and useful, need human factors input as do all computer human-interaction systems. Indeed, given the rate of change of voice technology and the fact that many voice applications provide special challenged (e.g., display-free phones, information overload in cockpits), it is especially important that voice systems be well suited to the real users using a system for real tasks in their real environment. This much admitted, the question now become exactly who should do exactly what, where, when, and at what cost to achieve what results? In this chapter, I will attempt to answer these questions in the following manner. First, I will present a normative model of the stages of lifecycle development. It is well-understood that a descriptive model of how development actually proceeds would show that people often skip many of these stages. Nevertheless, it is useful for the practitioner to understand what should happen and to understand the penalties for skipping stages.

After presenting the general model, I will delve into each stage and describe the role(s) that the human factors professional (HFP) can play, the most applicable techniques, and the kinds of knowledge that can be bought to bear. I will also comment on the likely consequences of skipping or skimping on a particular stage. I shall, of course, put special emphasis throughout on those problems having to do with Speech. Nevertheless, this chapter dos not focus on underlying technology or on the technical aspects of human factors methodology. Rather, it is primarily a chapter about *management*. It is intended as a guidebook for managing the development process of speech products. Although aimed primarily at the human factors professional, it is hoped that this chapter would also be profitably read by any development manager.

It might be useful for the reader to be aware of the author's background and biases at the outset. First, I feel that basic science, at least in psychology, progresses best when dealing with problems as close to the real world as possible. Second, I believe behavioral scientists should take a very active role throughout development and not limit themselves to being evaluators. Third, I have trouble playing the "If only the bad guys didn't" game. I've worked in both academic and industrial jobs, in leading-edge research in speech synthesis, in the development of novel voice services, and in the deployment realities of off-the-shelf technologies. I've worked in Line and Staff jobs at several levels of management. I've tried to understand both a marketing pull and technology push. So there are no "bad guys" left; I've been all of them! My third bias then, stated another way, is that the human factors professional (HFP) operates best when he or she realizes that not only are "end users" not evil or stupid when they make mistakes—neither is "management" or "Marketing" or "the academics" or "developers" or "technology gurus." The design and deployment of a voice system is a cooperative work of art amongst many types of professionals; there will always be a negotiation process involved at each of the stages I am about to describe. The best the HFP can do is to do the best they can do. They may not win every argument, but the resulting product will be much higher quality for their efforts.

2. A normative model of life cycle development.

I believe that it is useful to separate the following stages of development: (See Table 1).

A few explanatory comments are in order. First, a later stage may always cause fall-back to any earlier stage. Thus it is possible that something may happen during deployment that causes one to re-design, invent something new, or even redefine the problem. Obviously, for reasons of cost and time, one wants to fall back a few rather than many steps. It is precisely to avoid a long fall back that one uses *rapid* prototyping and evaluation.

Second, this is a normative model. I am suggesting that problem finding, formulation, and post-mortem be viewed as explicit stages; in practice, they seldom are. In fact, some developments of voice products could often be described as going through these stages: design, build, test under very idealized conditions, selectively report results, sell, deploy, go bankrupt,

Table 1

Stages of Development

- Problem Finding
- Problem Formulation
- Invention
- Design
- Prototyping
- Evaluation
- Redesign
- Testing
- Deployment
- Observation in the Field
- Post - Mortem

and re-organize the company. I am strongly suggesting that many of the technical and business failures are due to such a development process rather than the normative model suggested here.

Third, "Design" differs from "Invention" in that "Design" captures compositional notions; it attempts to solve a complex of demands and results in a specific product. "Testing" here refers to something like In-house testing or Beta testing of the real product, while "evaluation" is of a prototype. The other terms are fairly self-explanatory and should become clear in the context of the specific subsections.

3. Problem Finding

Perhaps the most important difference between the opportunities education typically provides (at lest for the first 17 years) and the opportunities life provides is in the relationship of solver to the problem finding process. In school, we are "given" problems "to solve." And if we solve them faster, we get a better grade, or get to play baseball sooner, or win the teacher's praise. We certainly are led to think we should feel bad if any of our problems are left unsolved, and it certainly never, never occurs to most students to find extra problems. Yet, in life, finding problems no-one else yet perceives is potentially the beginning of a significant breakthrough in knowledge, or enjoyment. So strong is the influence of early education though, on the way we view the desirability of problems, that most adults in business do not seek problems; indeed, they hide from them.

In traditional life cycle development, the closest thing to "problem finding" is "Marketing." Too often in practice, marketing studies are confined to penetration rates or revenue projections of existing solutions or their close relatives. What I am suggesting is a deeper look to find problems; perhaps where the end-user, consumer, or client does not yet recognize their existence.

In such an activity, the HFP should play a key role. However, while the background knowledge of human behavior and the techniques of behavioral science are useful, the role is one that traditional education does not coach or model (but, see Norman, 1988). Instead, the appropriate role here is to critique. Everything is fair game; especially the things we take as givens. An example may be instructive. Typically, we try to design computerized voice systems toward the ideal of human-human voice communication. Consider, however, some of the limitations of human-human voice communication. I speak at the same rate at which you are forced to listen. While, *if* I am a good mimic, I may connote different characters and accent, I cannot change my vocal tract arbitrarily, nor the material out of which it is made. *Nor can I move in arbitrary ways through space.* We do not typically think of these as "problems" with the human speech producing apparatus. But, they are—or can be.

Potential advantages of synthesized speech over natural human speech are that synthesized speech can be made arbitrarily fast; it can speak with a large number of identifiable voices; and it can speak from a large number of separate and identifiable locations. We could imagine developing an artificial audio "space" that represented an industrial organization. Each subunit could be clued to say its name and function; spatial location would illustrate the degree of interaction among subunits; and voice quality could cue a number of dimensions about the organization while speaking rate might illustrate the rate of activity. Such a device might or might not prove useful to someone attempting to understand a complex organization. The point here is simply that one should not assume *a priori* that a voice communication system that mimics, say a CEO, in explaining the organization sequentially in one voice in one location is necessarily best. We should actively look for problems. Behavioral scientists can help do this by focussing on mismatches—in this case the mismatch between the listener's ability to localize sound, differentiate voices, and comprehend speech at over 500 words per minute and the speaker's limitation in being in one place, speaking with one voice, and only at 100-250 words per minute.

Let us examine some techniques for discovering problems. A technique already common is to look for mismatches. One may consider mismatches not only between listener and speaker, but between vision and hearing.

Such "problems" could lead to use of the McGurk (1976) effect to increase the intelligibility of synthesized speech, to spatial auditory arrays, or to the auditory analogue of the Pulfridge pendulum or contrastively, the problem of McGurk for independent (non-yoked) audio-visual communication.

A different approach is to focus on dissatisfactions. Whenever people are dissatisfied, angry, hurt, anxious, frustrated, etc., there is a tendency to blame someone. One can also use such events as triggers to understand how the *system* contributed to the dissatisfaction. This in turn can lead to a consideration of how to fix the problem.

A variant of this proposal is to focus on special groups as a prod to invention; e.g., the telephone was invented while looking for an aid to the deaf. Focussing on the difficulties of the blind, the deaf, the very old, the very young, the non-reader, the aphasic, or the very highly verbal could lead to a number of interesting new inventions.

Another technique is to force a breakthrough. We become accustomed to working up to certain standards—it becomes acceptable practice. But suppose you require people to accomplish the same things twice as quickly? Or, with one hundredth the rework? Or with ten times the accuracy? Now, *presume* that the reason this cannot currently be done is the lack of a system. What would that system have to do or look like? Alternatively, imagine the difficulty is due to certain flaws in the existing system. What are those flaws? How can the current system be changed to bypass, eliminate, or correct for the flaws?

It is expected that in this stage of development—really pre-development— the designer will rely on general knowledge about the world as well as technical knowledge about human capabilities. In addition, problem finding is such an unusual activity, learning and using special techniques may be appropriate (e.g., see Stein 1974, 1975).

In this section, I have stressed that the human factors professional may have the background and talent to *identify* problems. Once a problem is identified, it may be fairly trivial to solve it, or, more often, it may require a lengthy traversal through all the succeeding stages of development outlined below. I believe that the human factors professional should more often be inventor as well as an evaluator of technology. Landauer (1987) made a similar point in his plenary address at CHI and gave several examples of inventions that sprang from an understanding of the problems people have in doing things.

4.   Problem Formulation

Problem solving in school not only ignores problem finding; it typically also ignores the very important step of problem formulation. Because nearly every one is trained under such a system, people typically continue to ignore this stage in the business, military, and interpersonal arenas as well. In school, the context of being in a statistics class and having just learned how to calculate z-scores and being given all (and only) the information necessary to calculate z-scores practically guarantees that the correct formulation of a problem is to find z-scores. (Under these circumstances, if students are given the following problem, most will calculate z-scores. "Harry scored 95 on a certain test and Frank a 68. If the mean of the scores for the whole class was 80 and the standard deviation 9 points, who scored higher—Harry or Frank). In business, the context is determined by corporate culture, roles, respnsibilities, budget, tradition, etc. Indeed, the constraints on what is perceived as the problem are so great, one should probably not spend a great deal of time consciously trying to reformulate every problem—only those that are central to the business or to one's own role demand careful attention to this generally overlooked stage of problem solving.

The problem formulation stage can include decisions about what constitutes the context (what will not be changed) and what constitutes the problem to be solved. In addition, one may put constraints on the solutions, the givens, and the allowable transformations. In the terms of a developer, such constraints might include the items shown in Table II.

Table II
Possible Constraints
on developing a new Voice Product

• Limited Budget	• Compatible with Our Software
• Limited Space	• Runs on Our Machine
• Limited Time	• Costs < $2000
• Runs in Real Time	• Fits in 64K Memory

The human factors professional may often serve the role of someone in a team who may formulate the problem differently. As such, he or she must realize that people may be resistant to new or alternative formulations. One approach is to lead people to consider *additional* interpretations. This will probably reap a richer yield than attempting to *supplant* the traditional interpretation. Another useful technique is to introduce explicitly a set of techniques for creativity (e.g., Stein, 1974, 1975) assuring everyone at the outset that there will later be a time for everyone to critique, organize, and select. In general, the idea is to have development team members participate in a sequence of *roles* that correspond appropriately to the various stages of the development process. Otherwise, it often happens that some people will *always* act critical throughout the development process; others will always be arguing for complete new directions even long after such new directions are feasible. Having these behaviors associated with *people* regardless of the problem solving stage, rather than roles often produces interpersonal conflicts as well as inefficiencies.

5. Invention

I am using "Invention" here to cover several separate processes. These include: focusing on a portion of the goal, generating ideas to meet that portion of the goal, evaluating the match of idea to goal, looking at the remaining mismatches, generating new ideas, and very importantly, integrating various subsolutions into an overall solution. A greater explication of these steps, and advice on how computers may support these steps may be found in Thomas (1989). Design, described in the next section, is concerned with a particular product or service. Invention then, is more generic. The main point of this section is that human factors professionals can and should take an active role in the invention process and not limit themselves to evaluating inventions (or, more often, specific designs). Landauer (1987) makes a similar case and, in fact, this group had "invented" several interaction techniques as well as designed prototypes.

There are of course, inventions that could not have been made without very specialized knowledge, e.g., of electronics, tire-making processes, or how drill bits operate. But there are other inventions that depend on knowledge of human perceptual and cognitive systems. In the case of voice technology, most inventions are limited to better methods of coding speech, translating from text to speech, or translating from speech to text. Once we consider additional problems however, and leave the notion that naturally occurring human conversation is ideal, many additional invention opportunities arise. Examples of this type of thinking can be found in Edwards (1989), and Gaver (1989). The Audio Distribution System (Gould and Boies, 1983) and the Olympic message System (Gould and Boies, 1984) are two fairly well-known examples in which human factors professionals invented and then developed specific products (as well as tested and redesigned).

Another role for human factors specialists would be to design procedures and artifacts to aid in the invention *process*. Most human factors work is concerned with products that will have hundreds, thousands, or even millions of users. There is certainly leverage to improving productivity or safety in such cases. But there would also be great leverage in improving the effective invention capability of an Edison. So far as I am aware, few human factors professional have seriously tackled the problem of creating special tools and environments for and outstanding individual inventor, scientist, or other professional by taking into account the specific aspects of that person's tasks, abilities, and context.

While we generally think of "speech technology" as recognition, synthesis, or voice messaging, other technologies are also possible. For example, a flexible synthesizer may also be used for non-speech audio data displays. One might also find application for a recognizer of other than speech sounds (e.g., congestion or crash detectors at intersections). One might develop a "mood detector" based on voice. And speaker identification/ verification is already a useful technology. Perhaps there is use for a language detector or an accent detector. The point is that the HFP should consider during invention a wide variety of options.

6.   Design

In designing a particular product or service, there may or may not be what is generally called invention involved. A useful product may simply be a fairly straightforward selection and arrangement of things that already exist. The human factors professional is critical during the design phase in several ways: Product Definition, Initial Design, and Usability Criteria.

6.1   Product Definition

First, it will be crucial to ensure that some reasonable work gets done to define users, tasks, and contexts of use. Such work may be directly under the supervision of human factors groups; more likely, Marketing will be responsible. If such is the case, the human factors professionals should help ensure that the marketing work is sound. This involves a delicate political balancing act. The Marketing organization is an important ally in that they will care more about usability and fight for it on their own more than will Development organizations. However, unguided, there are predictable and common difficulties they pose for human factors professionals. Marketing will tend to use methods like focus groups that can easily overstate how much people will actually use a product and how important certain features are. As a result, Marketing-driven requirements (≠market-driven requirements!) will tend to include too many features and will tend to include more users and more contexts than the product will be used in. In addition, there will tend to be too much emphasis placed on people's interpretations and explanations for their behavior (ct. Nisbett and Wilson, 1977). Another difficulty is that Marketing organizations. who tend to be allied with and come from sales, will tend to conflate requirements with the features of competitor's products. "Product XYZ is said to be easy-to-use and they have Windows, Icons and Mice, so if we add Windows, Icons, and Mice to our product it will also be easy-to-use." Finally, in the process of trying to resolve differences in approach between human factors professionals and the Marketing organization, the Marketing people typically do a vastly better job of "selling" their viewpoint. They understand their audience, their presentations are polished, and when they get challenged directly, they back off and dance back later. In contrast, too often, the human factors professional gives the same type of presentation that they would to a colleague; they do not put sufficient time into organizing and practicing the presentation; and when challenged directly, they alienate the decision maker, or their needed allies in Marketing, or both!

The major pieces of advice for dealing with this situation are fairly obvious but include the following. 1) Become friends and allies with Marketing and get involved early in advising on their efforts. Do not attempt to take over their job; show respect for their methods, but understand and be frank about the limitations of such methods (as well as your own!). "Focus groups are a great way of getting user input early on—what we've also found is that the total set of features people claim they'll pay for and use tends to be a bit larger than what happens in the field." 2) Work on a long long-term plan to understand more about marketing and sales and help them understand why usability cannot be guaranteed by including a set of features. 3) Work together on a plan to visit, collect field data, and observe actual users in actual use situations (See section 12.0. 4) Work together on sales materials. Usability can help sell products. Sales people can help train users— especially in why and when to use system. 5) If and when you do have to compete, keep it friendly, but win. Remember that your presentation needs to show work and be geared toward the audience and purpose. Do not lose your executive audience by presenting information at a level of detail appropriate to the Human Factors Society Annual meeting (even there, attendees enjoy legible slides). In other words, use the basic principles of human factors engineering.

6.2 Initial Design
A second major involvement of human factors professionals during design is in the initial design itself. While interactive prototyping and testing (Thomas, 1983; Gould and Lewis, 1983) will be critical, the human factors

professional has four approaches to impacting initial design and ideally all should be used. First, he or she should make sure that some basic principles of human capabilities are a part of the education of people likely to be involved in design. Second, there should be come design *guidelines* to serve as defaults when there is not specific reason to do otherwise. For example, audio instructions should be of the form, "From Interstate 684 North, turn right onto Interstate 84 East From Interstate 84 East take exit 2..." Such guidelines are most effective when incorporated into a tool to help designer and implementers. They help prevent mindless inconsistencies and focus design discussions on new issues. (See Table III for example guidelines). Guidelines should not, however, be used as rules of the universe; the field is too new and the particular circumstances of users, tasks and context can easily overpower the utility of overall consistency (Grudin, 1989). As should also be obvious, these guidelines often represent trading relations, common words are easier to access in long-term memory but tend to occur as multiple parts of speech and be more acoustically confusing because they are short.

TABLE III

- Provide high level maps of system—visually if the system is complex

- Use medium length words

- Use distinctive stimuli to differentiate warnings, prompts, feed-backs

- Use frequently used words

- Avoid negations

- Avoid long string of nouns (also known as the "Long Noun String Confu sion Avoidance Principle")

- Avoid words with multiple parts of speech ("Run Time Buffer"?)

- Verb-Object statements are easier that conditional ("Enter First names" better than "if first name, then enter")

- Use consistent command patterns ("Forward/backward," not as "next, back")

- Avoid ambiguous words ("Last" = "Final" or "Previous")

- Avoid "Telegraphese" (Memory cheap keep short unneeded)

Design problem solving involves attempting to satisfy tradeoffs among a large number of interacting variables. Design is never easy but an important principle for maximizing the ultimate chances of success is what I term the "Principle of Coverance." Basically, this means that it is critical to cover *all* aspects of design as early as possible in the design process. From a usability standpoint, it is obviously vital to get information about actual use into the design process. This is why it is critical to have HFPs involved in design, to do rapid prototyping and evaluation, etc. What may be less obvious to the HFP is that it is also critical for usability to get every other important function involved in design. Thus the HFP should attempt to get manufacturing, sales, and suppliers involved in design as early as possible. If such people are *not* involved early, their constraints will be applied late in development and adding constraints late will require changes in other aspects of the design. These changes will fall disproportionally on those aspects of the design that *can* change with the least short term organizational impact. The aspects of design that *can* change with new requirements are typically the user interface and documentation!

Any last-minute variation in the interface based on the needs of manufacturing, sales, or suppliers will tend to destroy any elegance, consistency, or over-arching metaphor that has been designed into the interface.

Let us examine a specific example. You are part of a design team and construct a phone-based service that includes a fair number of audio prompts and menus. The user may use simple voice commands (for rotary dial users) or touch tone input. You build, test, and refine a prototype. Everything looks fine. Because your company does not manufacture, you must buy the hardware platform from an outside vendor. Late in development you discover that the chosen vendor's hardware *cannot handle voice input during voice output*. This means even experienced users of rotary phones will have to listen through each audio menu in its entirety before responding. Now, you have to scramble. Do you make shorter prompts thus penalizing ease-of-learning? Do you provide two different interfaces— one for rotary customers; one for touch-tone customers? Do you try to change vendors? The point is that the hardware vendors got involved *too late*. If legal constraints prevented their early involvement, someone on the design team should have taken the *role* of vendor advocate with knowledge of what is possible.

The design of every new product or service has implications for sales, service, maintenance, your suppliers, other products, and so on. Anyone whose function will be impacted by the product should be brought into the design process as early as possible. This will increase the conflict during design and probably increase the time to design but will decrease the times in subsequent development stages and improve the quality of the design.

The third role for the human factors professional during initial design is to ensure that it is flexible enough to accommodate any changes occasioned by feedback form usability testing. For example, if every separate user error is separately flagged, and later tests show that all these various error messages are confusing and that a single error message is preferable, it is fairly trivial to collapse the error messages that are presented to a single message. If however, all errors are structurally routed to one place where a single error message is presented the the user and later testing shows that users need to have five different error messages, this will be a much harder change to implement. More generally, you should push for an architecture that separates user interface decisions from the underlying code, though cogent arguments have been made on both sides of the User Interface Management System issue (Olsen, 1987). Other architectural suggestions are made in TABLE IV.

TABLE IV
Architectural Guidelines

- Consider "Wizard-of-Oz" prototyping (see below) for capabilities that are difficult to implement and the team disagrees on the value of.

- Use high level prototyping languages initially.

- Never let a bad feature slip by now to be fixed later. Insist on quality throughout.

- Consider writing user manuals first—to drive architecture.

- Circulate to all development team members a description of the product from the end-user's perspective.

- Define the end-user(s), task(s), context(s).

- Provide a "Home Base."

- Provide "Undo" Capability

- Use table-driven interface.

- Put all messages in one place in the code.

- Use variable length fields for messages, prompts, etc.

6.3 Usability Criteria

The third major task of the HFP during design is to engineer a consensus on usability criteria. As pointed out by Butler (1985), the development process is always under the pressure of limited resources—limitations in time, expense dollars, capital dollars, and people. Under these circumstances, if management is to make informed judgements about tradeoffs in resource allocation between usability and other considerations, acceptable, *quantified* usability criteria are a necessity.

It is clear from this description that the design phase is certainly filled with work for the human factors professional. Those tasks need not all be done by one person; indeed probably cannot be.

7. Prototype

Fred Brooks, in *The Mythical Man-Month* (Brooks, 1982) states "You will build a prototype. The only question is whether you'll sell it as a product." There are many reasons for building a prototype; testing usability is a key one, but not the only one. Others are to understand how various components interact, to visualize additional users and markets, and to test how the system will interact with other systems (electrical, social, physical, etc.).

From a usability standpoint, prototyping is a necessity. Though intuition, guidelines, and modelling can greatly reduce the space of design alternatives, only testing real users really using the system can reveal whether the usability criteria are being met; if not, where the major difficulties are; and in what directions solutions lie. There are a large number of pototyping tools available. Certainly, rapid prototyping and evaluation is more feasible now than previously. There may still be cases, however, where "Wizard-of-Oz" prototyping will be required. This term, coined by Kelley (1984), refers to using a human being to simulate some of the functionality of the system. Such a technique can be useful because the person can be quickly "programmed" to behave in a number of different ways and to exhibit functionality that would be difficult or impossible for the machine (e.g., continuous, very large vocabulary, speaker—independent speech recognition). The technique can also be useful as a way of anchoring the value of an extreme case. For instance, one could compare performance among a cheap text-to-speech synthesis system, an expensive text-to-speech system, and normal human voice. Looking at the difference on performance and preference between normal human voice and synthesizers can reveal what the value would be of a perfectly natural synthesizer. The human voice could also be processed in various ways to simulate some current synthesizer limitations.

Prototyping can exist at various levels of versimultitude. For instance, many of the features of Query By Example were tested with pencil and paper (Thomas and Gould, 1974). The Audio Distribution System (ADS) vocabulary and mnemonics were sometimes tested with pencil and paper; and indeed, even probable social impact was studied indirectly by pencil and paper (Thomas, 1983). ADS Interactions were further studied with a CRT based simulator. (Richards, Boies, and Gould, 1986). Others (Savage, 1984) have studied menu structures with pencil and paper prior to implementation. Obviously, the investigator who uses such indirect means needs to use judgement about which test results are applicable to the real interface. If "send" is a more intuitive command than "transmit" on a visual display, the same is likely to be true for the Audio Distribution system once it is implemented with audio menus. On the other hand, one can *see* 20 menu items on a screen; it would be foolhardy to conclude from good results on such a system that one could have these 20 items in an audio menu. Similarly, and equally clearly, visual presentation will not tell you about auditory confusions (though these should be predictable on the basis of analysis). Even a working prototype with real audio may not reveal timing problems. A real system, under heavy load conditions, may take too long to respond and confuse the user in ways not observed with a laboratory prototype. If the means, variances and contingencies of system response times can be modelled in a prototype, more realistic results will be observed.

8. Evaluation

After building a prototype, (or a set of prototypes) one then wants to observe people who are representative of real users, performing tasks representative of their real tasks. Often, this is done in a laboratory setting (Hirsch, 1981). In addition to performance data and subjective questionnaires, one can employ think-aloud methods or other variations to gain more insight into user difficulties. An alternative is to work with users in their real environment. This avoids many the problems of extending laboratory results to the real world (Thomas and Kellogg, 1989; Spitz, 1991).

To take an obvious example, a phone-based service may enable users to perform very well in a quiet laboratory setting; the synthetic speech may be as intelligible as human speech. But, if users in the real world will be using the systems under noisy conditions with a high short term memory load from additional unrelated tasks, the synthetic speech may be very disruptive relative to human speech (Silverman,). If the synthetic speech is listened to on many occasions throughout an eight-hour day, there may also be fatigue factors that would be unobserved in an hour long laboratory experiment. Furthermore, if the users of the system are socially isolated apart from phone contact, and the point of the speech synthesis system is to remove the "nonproductive" social chit-chat that accompanies human-human conversations, productivity gains in the real world may be more than offset by the cost of decreased social cohesion. It might also be the case that part of the social "chit-chat" actually carries vital though hard-to-formalize information about the emotional states of the interacting parts of an organization. The point is not that laboratory evaluations are useless; only that one needs to understand the real contexts of use and interpret laboratory evaluations in that light. A combination of methods probably makes the most sense; particularly if one keeps track of the relationship between what happens in the laboratory and what happens in the real world (Thomas and Kellogg, 1989).

9. Redesign

The concept of rapid prototyping, evaluating, and redesign is widely accepted among HFPs. While there are numerous techniques for evaluation, judging *how* to redesign on the basis of evaluation results is largely a creative act. Obviously, if there is a particular term, command, icon, or menu structure that is confusing, one wants to consider changing that item. There are several complications, however. First, the *cause* of confusion need not be local to the behavioral evidence of confusion (cf. Lewis, 1989). Second, even if one is confident what is causing a problem (e.g., a particular icon is confusing) and even if one has a decent guess about *why* it's confusing (e.g., it destroys an overall metaphor), the solution is not necessarily obvious (a new icon may be *more* confusing). Third, even if one makes a change to solve a local problem, it is far from clear what the net effect will be of an *ensemble* of changes.

For example, suppose an audio interface uses several different synthetic voices for different portions of the interface. Testing may reveal that one of the voices is distinctly more intelligible than any of the others. An obvious ploy is to use the highly intelligible voice everywhere. Unfortunately, this may cause a new problem; people may now be confused about "where they are" in the interface. Overall performance may actually drop. Hence, several iterations may be necessary. Preparing developers for this and getting their concurrence *early* in development is crucial.

10. Testing

The term "Testing" here refers to final Quality Control testing against the agreed-upon usability criteria. This is different form the interactive evaluation testing that is part of the design-prototype-evaluate cycle discussed in section 7. While evaluations can, and probably should be done by someone on the design team, the acceptance testing should be done by someone *not* on the design team. While there are a variety of methods for doing interactive evaluations (laboratory tests, simulations, expert intuitions, story board, etc.) the portion of acceptance testing that is concerned with usability should be empirically testing under conditions approximating as closely as possible real world conditions.

There are often a sequence of acceptance tests; e.g., lab test, alpha test, beta test. Usability should be measured in *all* these phases. In addition, the HFP should make sure that real users with no hints from the development staff are able to do whatever installation, configuration, diagnosis, and maintenance tasks it is assumed they will do with the real product. In other words, do not limit acceptance testing to end use but include all ancillary tasks as well. The HFP should also seek to ensure that tests include a number of major anticipated environments. All the documentation for a particular speech synthesis device a few years ago implicitly presumed that the device would be connected to that manufacturer's terminal though it operated via a standard interface and many of the devices actually sold are connected to other terminals. This made it very confusing for a large number of application developers though the synthesis itself was high-quality.

11. Deployment

It should be obvious from earlier parts of this chapter that HFP should be involved form the *beginning* of the development process. Nevertheless, there are significant contributions that can be made even during deployment. The manner in which the product is advertised, sold, and supported can do a lot to help or harm usability as well as the perception of usability. One particularly important consideration is that a product sold for purposes, or to users, or in contexts that it was not designed or tested for, has no guarantees of usability. A second consideration is that, at small cost, sales and support activity can be used to gather information about how the product is used, who the real users are, and what their problems are. Depending on the nature of the system, it may well be worthwhile for HFPs to be involved in some early deployments. Not only may ideas be generated for additional systems, but simple work aids may be designed that will greatly enhance performance.

12. Observation in the Field

Perhaps of all the steps for the HFP, observation in the field is the most important. There is simply no way, absent such observation, to design intelligent laboratory experiments, gain intuitions relevant to design considerations, see new problems to be solved, understand the goals and contexts of users and to understand and improve the relationship between laboratory experiments and what happens in the real world.

Perhaps a few examples will help motivate this emphasis. Field observations by the IBM Hursley human factors group reveals that users of a color display occasionally complained that the display was too dim and had no idea that it was possible (and very easy) to turn up the display by a knob right on the front of the display. The point is that the HFP would typically test the usability of products given that they were properly adjusted; they would not purposely misadjust the machine and then see whether users would spontaneously correct it.

Similarly, in the laboratory, you typically test a product or service in the manner it is *designed for*; not in the manners it is actually used in. Thus, it is easy to see why a usability test would not reveal the "dangers" of having the top of the printer spring up for service, spilling hot coffee in the process. The printer top is not designed to hold coffee. It just turns out that people do that in the real world.

In evaluating and testing for the Audio Distribution System, mnemonics were found which enabled people easily to associate the function of a command with its name. What real world observation revealed, however, is that this is but part of the problem. Perhaps more significant, a necessity for a new tool introduced via old hardware (the desk phone) for dicretionary use, is to induce people to even think about using the tool in the course of their on-going behavioral patterns.

To measure how effectively someone in the laboratory remembers that one uses *S to send a message tells us nothing about whether a user in the real world will think to use ADS instead of writing a memo.

13. Post-Mortem

Everyday observation suggests that typically, after reaching a goal (e.g., developing a product, solving a problem) people celebrate, rest, and begin toward a new goal. A very atypical behavior recommended by Polya (1956) is to take a retrospective objective look at the process used to reach the goal and determine what was done correctly, what was done incorrectly, and other ways one might have succeeded. In particular, the HFP should pay particular attention to : 1) how conclusions reached by empirical study might have been arrived at more quickly, 2) which guidelines were useful, useless, or counterproductive and what new guidelines might be added, 3) what bottlenecks existed and how they might have been avoided or overcome, 4) what important differences in behavior occurred in the lab versus the real context of use and how these might be anticipated next time. As in the case of redesign, one cannot write a prescription for finding ways to improve how things are done. But it is useful to take this perspective: "How could we have been more productive; more accurate; more insightful." In other words, *presume* there is a better way and set out to find it.

There are two somewhat similar processes often engaged in at the end of a project. One is publicity; a success provides an opportunity to advertise success and part of that story is why one was successful. A second is credit (or blame) assignment by management. When a project terminates, it is time to reward and punish. These two processes have their uses and are probably inevitable but neither should be confused with the open, honest post-mortem look I am suggesting. If you contaminate the post-mortem with trying to look good, you'll gain little as a problem solving HFP. Similarly, when you *do* take an honest look, *think* about how and what to reveal for the purpose of publicity and credit assignment. In the ideal case where you work in an ideal organization for an ideal manager, you would tell all; the Corporation and the world would gain from your experience. But make sure before taking that leap that the ideal conditions or something close to it actually exists.

14. Special Problems With Voice

Much of what has been said up to this point is generally applicable with respect to the issue of incorporating good human factors into the design and deployment of any product. In this section, however, I will focus on issues more specifically related to speech.

14.1 Testing for Technologies that Do Not Exist.

Speech recognition, speech synthesis, and even particular varieties of speech encoding and decoding are technologies that are continually evolving. For this reason, and in contrast with more established technologies, the human factors professional may be asked to evaluate interfaces based on performance standards that do not exist at the point in the development cycle where user interface testing should ideally begin. Human beings are capable of dealing quite well with natural language. One strategy for dealing with this dilemma then, is to have a person simulate a proposed system. For example, Thomas (1976) tested the feasibility and helped develop system requirements for a natural language interface prior to the capability of such a system by having a person simulate this interface using a set of restricted rules. Gould, Conti and Hovanyecz (1983), used a similar methodology to find out which of several possible directions to push the IBM Speech Recognition effort. In this case, as well as in others, it was necessary to artificially introduce errors in the human transcription process, in order to simulate possible performance levels of speech recognition system to be developed. While it will seldom be possible to simulate precisely all the error patterns and timing interactions that a real system will eventually exhibit by using a human being, one may nevertheless get a much better feel for user's reactions to a system than if such methodologies where not used at all.

Another difficulty stemming from the fact that voice technologies are rather new and in many cases even novel for users and laboratory subjects is that familiarity with these new technologies can be a rather large effect. For example, listeners who have not had previous experience with a speech synthesizer many adapt rather significantly even during the course of a single experiment. This makes comparisons of the intelligibility or natural-ness of speech synthesis devices using a Within-Subjects design difficult. However, it is also true that there are large individual difference in the ability to understand synthesized speech. This makes Between-Subjects designs difficult. Worse, it makes extrpolation to the real world difficult since it is seldom possible to obtain a truly random and representative sample.

A third challenge is that voice is often simply more difficult to deal with technically. One can easily prepare, edit, store and randomly display visual stimuli. In contrast, all these operations tend to be lengthy and require special (often expensive) equipment, in the case of speech. Depending on the nature of studies one needs to do, it may make sense to work with another lab or to do a number of preliminary studies with easy-to-make materials. In addition to the special problems of *how* to use speech tech-nologies, there is the more fundamental question for the HFP of *whether* to use them. Some specific applications for the technologies are shown in Table V below. A more fundamental analysis is to consider the character-istics of speech technologies and the user's tasks and look for a match. Advantages of Speech Synthesis, for instance, are shown in Table VI while Table VII shows some relative advantages of synthesis and recorded voice.

TABLE V
"Applications of Speech Technology"

- Generalized Content "Eavesdropping"-seeing organizational, societal trends
- Talking piece-parts that self-instruct
- Voice verification of credit cards
- Automatic routing of vocal communications
- Fire alarms
- ATM by phone
- Auditory data playout
- Teaching foreign language
- Auditory fb for motor learning
- House reminders
- Repair request dialogue
- Talking yellow pages
- Driving instructions
- Personalized audiotapes
- Automated Psychotherapist
- IRS dialogue
- Airline dialogue
- Improved coding
- Wake me up calls
- Reminders
- Key entry
- Audiotext interaction

TABLE VI

Synthesis Advantages
  - Ubiquity of telephone
  - Convenient, cheaper output
  - Eyes free/hands free
  - Omnidirectional signal
  - Multichannel stimulus
  - Alternate channel for
    -non-readers
    -young
    -blind
    -overload

TABLE VII

Recorded Speech vs Synthesis

  - Totally recorded messages are
    -natural
    -intelligible
    -hard to edit
    -very hard to update
  - Recombinant recorded messages are
    -almost natural
    -intelligible
    -limited in scope
  - Synthesis (Text-to-Speech) is
    -flexible (prototype messages)
    -easy to edit
    -cheap to update
    -fairly intelligible
    -not natural
    -requires more attention

Similarly, recognition tends to be a useful technology when the vocabulary is limited or speaker training is feasible, when eyes and hands are otherwise busy, when errors are not disastrous, when high throughput is useful, and when the environment is quiet. Obviously, there are a number of tradeoffs and other issues including the cost of the recognition device, error recovery procedures, and training the recognizer. To make intelligent judgements about such issues and tradeoffs the HFP must get fairly heavily involved in understanding the technology and even specific devices. For example, how quickly can new "active" vocabulary items be down-loaded in response to user input? What is the machine's speed of recognition? Are confidences for other choices available from the recognizer for combination with other information for the application? Does the recognizer adapt?

It should be clear that the roles of the HFP suggested in this chapter are many and varied—none are trivial. HFPs should be involved throughout the development process and will have to emphasize quite different skills at various times. The HFP will have to be creative and critical; be able to run controlled laboratory experiments and make insightful observations in the field; be able to help manage the entire development process to ensure a quality process. To make intelligent decisions about speech systems, the HFP will have to understand not only the application(s) and human perceptual, motor, and cognitive abilities but also be conversant with the technologies and be able to give excellent presentations! This will prove to be challenging and fun.

References

Brooks, F. *The Mythical Man-Month*. Reading, M.A.: Addison-Wesley, 1982.

Butler, K.A. Connecting Theory and Practice: a case study of achieving usability goals. *Proceeding of the 1985 SIGCHI Conference*, 1985, San Francisco, CA. 85–88.

Buxton, W., Bly, S. A., Frysinger, S.P., Lunnery, D., Manxur, S.L. Mezrich, J.L., & Morrison, R.C. (1985). Communicating with sound. *Proceedings of the '85 ComputerHuman Interaction Conference*. San Francisco, ACM

Carroll, J.M. and Rosson, M.B. "Usability Specifications as a Tool in Interactive Development," in *Advances in Human—Computer Interaction*, H. R., Hartson, ed., Ablex Publishing, Norwood, N.J., 1985.

Card, S.K., Moran, T.P., and A. Newell. *The Psychology of Human—Compute Interaction*, Hillsdale, N.J.: Erlbaum, 1983.

Edwards, Alistair S.N., Soundtrack: An Auditory Interface for Blind Users. *Human Computer Interaction*, 1989, 4(1), 45–66.

Gaver, W.W. The SonicFinder: An Interface That Uses Auditory Icons. *Human—Computer Interaction*. 1989, 4(1), 67–94.

Gould, T.D., Conti, J., & Havanyecz, T. (1983). Composing letters with a simulated listening typewriter, *CACM*, 1983, 26(4), 295–308.

Gould, J.D. and Lewis, C.H. Designing For Usability—Key principles and what designers think. IBM—Research Report, RC-10317, 1983.

Gould, J.D. & Boies, S.J. Human Factors of the 1984 Olympic Message System. *Proceedings of the Human Factors Society—28th Annual Meeting*, 547-551, 1984.

Gould, J.D. and Boies, S.H. Human Factors challenges in Creating a Principal—Support Office System: The Speech Filing—System Approach, *ACM Trans. Office—Information Systems*, Oct. 1983. pp. 273–298.

Grudin, J. The case against user—interface consistency. *MCC Tech Report No. ACA-HI-002-89*, 1989.

Halstead-Nussloch, R. The design of phone-based interfaces for consumers. *Proceedings of the ACM SIGCHI Meeting*, 34–352, 1989.

Hirsch, R. S. Procedures of the human factors Center at San Jose. *IBM Systems Journal*, 1981, 20, 123–171.

Kelley, J.F. And interactive design methodology for user-friendly natural-language officeinformation applications. *ACM Transaction of Office Information System*, 2, 26–41.

Landauer, T.K. Psychology as a mother of invention. *Proceedings of the ACM SIGCHI Meeting*, 333-335. 1987.

Lewis, C.H. Generalization, consistency, and control. Presented at the ACM SIGCHI Meeting, Austin, Texas, May 1-5, 1989.

McGurk, H. & MacDonald, J. Hearing lips and seeing voices, *Nature*, 1976, 264, 746-748.

Manheimer, J. M., Burnett, R.C. and Willers, J.A. A case sturdy of user interface man-agement system development and application. *Proceedings of the ACM SIGCHI Meeting*, 127-132, 1989.

Nisbett, R.E. and Wilson, T.D. Telling more than we can know: Verbal reports on mental processes. *Psych. Review*, 1977, 84, 231–259.

Norman, D.A. *Psychology of Everyday Things*. New York: Basic Books, 1988.

Olson, D.R. Panel: Whither (Or whether) UIMS Proceedings of the ACM SIGCHI meeting on Human Factors in Computing Systems, 1987, 311–315.

Polson, P.G., & Keiras, D.E. A quantitative model of the learning and perform-ance of text editing knowledge. In L. Borman & B. Curtis (Eds.), *Proceedings of the 1985 ACM Human Factors in Computing Systems*. New York, NY: ACM, 1985.

Poyla, G. *How To Solve It*, Princeton: Princeton University Press, 1956.

Richards, J.T., Boies, S.J. And Gould, J.D. Rapid Prototyping And System Development. *Proceedings of the ACM SIGCHI Meeting*, 1986, 216-220.

Rosson, M.B. (1985). Using synthetic speech for remote access to information. *Behavioral Research Methods, Instruments, and Computers, 17*, 250-252, 1985.

Sanders, M.S. and McCormick, E.J. *Human Factors In Engineering And Design*, New York: McGraw—Hill, 1987.

Savage, R., Habinek, J.K., and Barnhart,T.W. The design, simulation, and evaluation of a menu-driven user interface. In J. Thomas, and M. Schneider, (Eds.) *Human Factors in Computing Systems*, Norwood, N.J.; Ablex, 1985.

Sorkin, R.D. and Kistler, D.S. and Elvers, G.C., An Exploratory Study of the Movement-Correlated Cues in an Auditory Head-Up Display, *Human Factors*, 1989, *31*(2), pp. 161-166.

Stein, M.I. *Stimulating Creativity*. New York: Academic Press. 1974.

Stein, M. (1975). *Stimulating Creativity, Volume 2: Group procedures*. New York: Academic Press.

Stewart, C.J., & Cash, W.B. (1974). *Interviewing: Principles and Practices*. Dubuque, IA: William C. Brown.

Tappert, C. Cursive script recognition by elastic matching. *IBM Journal of Research and Development, 26*, November, 1982.

Thomas, J.C. and Gould,J.D. A psychological study of Query By Example, *AFIPS Conference Proceedings*, 1975, *44*, 439-445.

Thomas, J.C. An analysis of behavior in the hobbits-orcs problem. *Cognitive Psychology, 6*, 257-269, 1974.

Thomas, J.C. A method of studying natural language dialogue. *IBM Research Report*, *RC-5882*, 1976.

Thomas, J.C. Cognitive psychology for the viewpoint of wilderness survival. Paper presented at the American Psychological Association, San Francisco. (Available as IBM T.J. Watson Research Report RC-6647), Yorktown Heights, NY: IBM, 1977.

Thomas, J.C. Psychological issues in the design of data base query languages. In M.E. Simes & M.J. Coombs (Eds.), *Designing for human-computer communication*. London: Academic Press, 1983.

Thomas, J.C. Studies in Office Systems: The Effect of Communications Medium on person perception. *Office Systems Research Journal*, 1983, 1(2), 75–88.

Thomas, J.C. Goodness (human factors) does not equal degree (quantification). *Contemporary Psychology*, *29*(2), 119–120, 1984.

Thomas, J.C. Organizing for human factors. In Y. Vassilou (Ed.), *Human factors and interactive computer systems*. Norwood, NJ: Ablex Publishing Corp., 1985.

Thomas, J.C. Problem Solving by Human—Machine Interaction. In *Human and Machine Problem Solving*, K.J. Gilhooly (ed.). London: Plenum, 1989.

Thomas, J.C., & Carroll, J.M. Human factors in communication, *IBM Systems Journal*, *20*(2), 237-263.

Thomas, J.C., Kellogg, W.A., *Minimizing Ecological Gaps in Interface Design*. IEEE Software, 78-86, January, 1989.

Thomas, J.C., Klavans, J., Nartey, J., Pickover, C., Reich, D., & Rosson, M.C. WALRUS: A development system for speech synthesis (MIB T.J. Watson Research Report RC-10626), Yorktown Heights, NY: IBM, 1984.

Thomas, J.C., Lyon, D., & Miller, L.A. Aids for problem solving. (IBM) T.J. Watson Research Report RC-6468), Yorktown Heights, NY: IBM, 1977.

Thomas, J.C., Rosson, M.B., & Shodorow, M. Human Factors and synthetic speech. In B. Shackel (Ed.) *INTERACT '84*. Amsterdam: Elsevier, 1985.

Thomas, J., Klavans, J., Nartey, J., Pickover C., Reich d., & Rosson, M.B. (1984). WALRUS: A development system for speech synthesis. *IBM Research Repot*, *RC-10626*.

Thomas, J.C. The computer as an active communications medium. *Proceedings of the 18th Annual Meeting of the Association for Computational Linguistics.* (pp. 83-86). ACL, 1980.

Wickens, C.D., Sandry, D., & Vidulich, M. Compatibility and resourcecompetition between modalities of input, central processing, and output: Testing amodel of complex task performance. Human Factors, 25, 227-248, 1983.

Williges, B.H., & Williges, R.C. Dialogue design considerations for interactive computer systems. In F.A. Muckler (Ed.), *Human factors review.* Santa Monica, CA: The Human Factors Society, 1984.

Williges, B.H., Schurick, J.M., Spine, T.M., & Hakkimen, M.T. Speech in human—computer interaction. In R.C. Williges & R.W. Ehrich (Eds.), *Human—computer dialogue design.* Amsterdam: Elsevier, 1985.

Winograd, T., & Flores, R. Understanding computers and cognition. Norwood, NJ: Ablex Publishing Corp, 1986.

Witten, K.H. *Principles of computer speech.* Academic Press: London, 1982.

Wright, P., & Reid, R. Written information: Some alternatives to prose for expressing the outcomes of complex contingencies. *Journal of Applied Psychology, 57,* 160-166, 1973.

Yetton, P.W., & Vroom, V.H. *Leadership and decision making.* Pittsburgh, PA: University of Pittsburgh Press, 1973.

Zimmer, A.C. (1984). A model for the interpretation of verbal prediction. International Journal of Man—Machine Studies, 20, 121–134.

Chapter 8

Technical Issues Underlying the Development and Use of a Speech Research Laboratory

H. S. Gopal
University of California, Santa Barbara

1. Introduction

Speech research is a multidisciplinary field. Speech scientists, linguists, engineers, mathematicians, psychologists, neuroscientists, hearing scientists and other professionals study various aspects of speech process for different purposes. One purpose of this research is theoretical - to understand the basic processes involved in speech communication. For example, speech scientists, psychologists and linguists develop theories which attempt to relate articulatory, acoustic and auditory attributes of the various speech sounds with their psychological and linguistic function. Psychologists study speech with an attempt to understand the processes involved in the perception or production of speech. Neuroscientists and hearing scientists are interested in the representation, coding and analysis of speech by the human auditory system. Another purpose of speech research is practical: engineers are interested in modelling the process of speech communication in order to utilize this knowledge for various applications. These applications include the efficient coding and transmission of speech, systems that recognize speech or generate synthetic speech, and prosthetic devices that aid speech- or hearing-impaired individuals. Speech-language pathologists and otolaryngologists are interested in understanding speech production so that this knowledge can be applied in the diagnosis and remediation of speech impairment. Thus, speech research has attracted the interest of several different professions.

Advances in our understanding of the fundamental processes of speech communication and application of speech research have been heavily dependant upon the instruments that are used to study speech. These instruments capture, analyze and quantify various aspects of the speech signal. Oscillographs, tape recorders, the sound spectrograph, the "Pattern Playback" device, and recently, digital analysis of speech have formed the backbone of instrumentation used for speech analysis and have provided us with much of our existing knowledge about speech. The objective quantification of speech and the study of the acoustic correlates of speech with their linguistic function could not be accomplished without the tools used to measure and analyze speech. A basic understanding of the instruments used in the acoustic analysis of speech is fundamental to speech research.

The purpose of this chapter is to provide an exposition of the basic concepts involved in the instrumentation used for the acoustic analysis of speech. The instrumentation used for the study of speech production (such as kinematics, physiology, etc.) is entirely omitted here, even though there is some overlap in the instrumentation used between these fields. Given the impact of digital technology on speech research, the emphasis is on the instrumentation used in the computer analysis of speech. This new generation of tools - inexpensive but powerful high-performance computer workstations, analog-to-digital (A to D) and digital to analog (D to A) converters, digital-signal-processing (DSP) chips - are having a major impact on speech research and the methods used in speech research. It is recognized at the outset that no one software/hardware system will meet the needs of all speech researchers. This chapter emphasizes only key issues which are of general relevance to the computer-aided analysis of speech (both hardware and software considerations) and in the associated instrumentation, such that it may be useful to a wider audience. In this sense, the scope of the present chapter is quite limited. It is directed at a non-technical or non-engineering audience, although the basic principles are relevant to several groups of researchers, including engineers.

This chapter is organized as follows: Section 2.0 outlines the basic requirements of a speech research lab. Section 2.1 discusses the issues involved in capturing the speech signal using microphones and recording it onto a medium. Section 2.2 deals with the basics of data acquisition by computer and the digital representation of speech. This section presents the concepts of analog-to-digital conversion, sampling, etc. Section 2.3 describes low-pass filtering and considerations in choosing a filter. Section 2.4 deals with considerations in choosing a relatively inexpensive computer for speech research. Section 2.5 discusses some of the speech analysis software that is currently available and the desirable features of such software. Section 2.6 describes outputting the digital signal and considerations such as digital-to-analog conversion, low-pass filtering, and the transducers used to listen to the speech sound. Section 3 is a brief discussion of the types of applications wherein such instrumentation may be employed successfully. Finally section 4 describes a functional speech research lab that is in use for various types of speech research.

2. Requirements

The requirements of a basic speech research system for acoustic analysis of speech is illustrated by a block diagram in Figure 1.

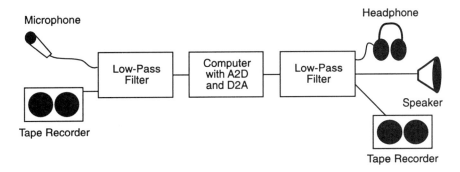

Figure 1: Block diagram of a basic speech research lab

Considerations involved in the choice and usage of each of these major components is described below.

2.1 Input Source

In the analysis of speech, a faithful recording of the speech signal is critical. This involves transducing the acoustic speech signal into an electrical form and recording it onto a medium for later retrieval. The speech signal is either recorded onto a tape recorder or directly input to a computer. The choice of a transducer is vital to a faithful recording of speech. A simple definition of a transducer is a device which converts one form of energy to another. A microphone which converts sound energy into electrical energy is a transducer. A speaker is another example of a transducer. Following a general discussion of transducers, specific aspects of microphones will be discussed.

There are several general considerations in evaluating a transducer. First, amplitude linearity is an important factor. This means that the output of the transducer must be proportional to the amplitude of the input signal.

Changes in the amplitude of the actual speech signal ought to be mirrored proportionally by the transducer in order to render a faithful representation of the signal. Otherwise amplitude distortion results. Linearity deviations of less than 1% across the range of input values are desirable. Secondly, the frequency response of the transducer is a critical factor. The frequency response must be equal to or greater than the input signal . This means that the transducer must be capable of responding to all the frequencies present in the input signal in the same way. A flat or linear response in the frequency range of the signal of interest is very desirable. Most transducers for music have a broader range frequency response than those used for speech. Thirdly, sensitivity of the transducer is another important factor. The transducer must be capable of responding to very small and very large changes in the input signal. The dynamic range of the transducer must be at least equal to the dynamic range of the input signal. These are some of the important factors that ought to be considered in the choice of a transducer.

Microphones convert pressure variations of sounds or pressure differences to electrical energy. Pressure microphones respond to pressure variations in the sound field in front of a built-in diaphragm, whereas pressure gradient microphones respond to the pressure differences across the built-in diaphragm. Pressure microphones are omni-directional in that they respond to sound coming from any direction. Pressure gradient microphones are directional in that they typically respond best to sound coming from directly in front of them. They are useful in reducing the amplitude of unwanted background signals from other directions. Directional microphones are also sensitive to the angle of incidence of the sound with reference to the diaphragm. Some respond best to sounds directly in front of them while others respond best to some other angle. These are usually specified in the technical manual of the microphones. The distance from the sound source (speaker's mouth) to the microphone should be kept constant during recording. A fixed distance of about 6 to 8 inches is a good placement. Variation in this distance causes unwanted fluctuations in the amplitude of the signal. Therefore, it is preferable to have a boom-mounted microphone which can be attached to the talker's head, thereby maintaining a constant distance between the microphone and the source.

There are several types of microphones, including crystal microphones, dynamic microphones, condenser microphones, and electret microphones. The two types preferable for speech research are the electret and condenser microphones. The condenser microphone provides more precise measurements than any of the other microphones but is quite expensive. Table 1 provides a listing of some of these microphones. They usually have a very flat frequency response ranging from 20 Hz to 20,000 Hz or even higher depending on their diaphragm diameter size. Because they dissipate their output energy rapidly (due to high output impedance) and generate a low output voltage, they invariably require a pre-amplifier which is either attached to the microphone or is attached separately. The preamplifier amplifies only the voltage and not the current output from the microphone, in addition to providing impedance matching. Usually the output signal quality stays high for about 10 feet or so from the microphone/preamplifier set-up. Condenser microphones are recommended for high-quality signal capture and analyses (such as calibration, etc.). The electret microphone is quite similar to the condenser microphone, provides comparable quality of

Table 1: Some Options for Microphones and Their Suppliers

Manufacturer	Model	Type	Price*	Comments
AKG Acoustics 77 Selleck Street Stamford, CT 06902 203-348-2121	C414 B-ULS	Pressure-Gradient	n/a	Excellent
	C568	Condenser	n/a	Excellent
Ariel 433 River Road Highland Park, NJ 08904 201-249-2900	DM-N Digital	Microphone	n/a	Excellent
Audio Technician 1221 Commerce Drive Stow, OH 44224 216-686-2000	ATM-33R ATM-31	Condenser Condenser	$250 $250	Very Good Very Good
Electro-Voice 600 Cecil Street Buchanan, MI 49107 616-615-6815	RE11	Cardioid	$222	Good
Radio Shack (any local dealer)	33-1073	Cardioid	$59	Average
Sennheiser 6 Vista Drive Old Lyme, CT 06371 203-434-9190	several		$400	Excellent
Shure 222 Harrey Ave. Evanston, IL 60202 708-866-2000	SM81 545 series 546 series	Condenser Cardioid Cardioid	$500 $150 $150	Excellent Good Good

* All prices are approximate.

performance and costs considerably less. Electret microphones are ideal for quick, preliminary data capture and piloting purposes, although they also may be used for research purposes.

Given a high-quality microphone, the speech signal should be recorded in a sound-treated booth or in a very quiet room. Other instruments in the room (especially computer monitors) can be very noisy and cause a degradation in the signal of interest. It is best to keep all CRTs as far away from the microphone as possible. Particularly painful is the low-frequency 60 Hz hum that is usually due to lack of proper grounding of the instruments. Care must be taken to ground the instruments to avoid this unwanted signal to be superimposed on the speech signal. This signal is either recorded onto a medium (e.g., tape) or directly fed into the computer (after Analog-to-Digital conversion). Input of the speech signal into the computer should be flexible. That is, there should be provision for either direct input or line input (via tape recorder). For the purposes of this chapter, it is assumed that the speech signal will be first recorded onto a tape-recorder and then fed into the computer.

Obtaining a high-quality recording of the original signal is critical for later acoustic analyses. With the current advances in technology, the difference between high fidelity cassette and reel-to-reel tape recorders is getting smaller. Reel-to-reel tape recorders still offer a wider frequency response when recording at higher speeds (7.5 ips). For very low frequency recordings (such as those of chest movements during speech or even d.c. signals), an FM (frequency modulated) tape-recorder is desirable. These tape-recorders are rather expensive, but they capture the low-frequency signals much better than non-FM tape-recorders.

There are several considerations in selecting and using a tape-recorder. The number of channels available for recording will depend on the number of signals to be recorded simultaneously. Usually, these vary from one to four. It is preferable to have at least a two-channel recording capability. The number of tracks will also determine the quality of the signal. A full track reel-to-reel will provide a one channel high quality recording of the signal. A half-track recorder provides up to 2 channels, and a quarter track up to 4 channels. The greater the number of tracks, the poorer is the quality of the signal recorded. Recording speed is another factor. While this is not an option on cassette recorders whose speed is set at 3 3/4 ips (inches-per-second), reel-to-reel recorders offer speeds of 1 7/8, 3 3/4, 7 1/2 ips and in some cases 15 ips. The faster the speed of the recorder, the wider the frequency response. Usually a half-track 2 channel, reel-to-reel tape recorder is preferred for high quality recording. With the availability of Digital-Audio-Tape recorders (DATs), none of the above considerations become that important. In DATs which provide for 2-channel recording, the signal of interest is usually digitized using a 16 bit Analog-to-Digital converter, with a fairly high sampling frequency (44.1 kHz). DATs offer recording quality that is far superior to either the reel-to-reel or cassette recorders. At the time of this writing, only professional quality DATs are available in the USA. These are rather expensive, although their prices are dropping considerably. Recently, less expensive models have been introduced. These DATs, in addition to being used to record the speech signal, could also be used as tape back-up systems for the computer once the drivers become commercially available. Table 2 provides a list of some of the tape recorders and DATs that are available and their features.

Some useful hints for proper recording are as follows. Make sure that the microphone is a fixed distance from the source, about 6-8 inches. During recording, set the volume control (or record level) such that the needles on the VU meter or the lights on record level are in the mid-range and do not ever fall in the red or overload region. All recording must be done in a very quiet room or in a sound-treated room. If using a reel-to-reel recorder, the faster tape speed is recommended (7.5 ips). The signal from the microphone being fed into the tape-recorder must be of sufficient strength. That is, if one is using a condenser microphone, then a good-quality pre-amplifier (or a mixer) must be used. These pre-amplifiers (or mixers) usually have independent gain controllers for each channel of input. The output of pre-amplifiers is fed into the line input of the tape-recorder. If a mixer is used, then one can combine more than one input source signals. Each of these inputs is fed into a separate input channel of the mixer which amplifies each of the signals in addition to providing an impedance match. The mixer then provides one common output signal of sufficient signal intensity which can be either recorded onto a tape-recorder or fed into the computer.

Once the signal is recorded onto a tape-recorder or a DAT, the signal can be analyzed later on the computer. The first step involves getting this analog signal from the tape-recorder onto the computer in a digital form. The signal must be low-pass filtered and then digitized and stored on the computer. Before describing the characteristics of these processes, a brief review of the basic principles involved in data acquisition is provided.

2.2 Basic Principles of Data Acquisition
Analog signals are representations of the physical word, and are usually represented as continuous signals. A digital representation of the analog

Table 2: Some Options for Tape Recorders and Their Suppliers

Manufacturer	Model	Type	Price	Comments
Otari 3798 Vintage Park Dr. Foster City, CA 94404 415-341-5900	MX-55-N B5050 Mark III	1/4" 2 track, 2 channel 1/2" 4 channels	$4000 $4000	Excellent
Marantz 20325 Nordhoff St. P.O. Box 2577 Chaptsworth, CA 91313	PMD-430 PMD-420	DAT DAT	$400 $350	
Nakamichi 19701 South Vermont Ave Torrance, CA 90502 213-538-8150	CR-7A CR-3	Cassette Cassette	$1600 $800	
Panasonic One Panasonic Way Secaucus, NJ 07094	SV-3500 SV-250	DAT DAT	$2300 $2300	Excellent Excellent
Racal Recorders Inc. 18 Technology Dr., St. 100 Irvice, CA 92718 714-727-3444	several	Reel-to reel	$3000	Very Good
Revox 1425 Elm Hill Pike Nashville, TN 37210	MK-II	Reel-to reel	$3500	Excellent
Sony 1600 Queen Anne Rd. Teaneck, NJ 07666 800-328-SONY	PCM-2500 PCM-108M -CD -D3 (walkman)	DAT DAT DAT	$2800 $3000 $850	Excellent Excellent Excellent/ portable
Sharp (local dealer)	SX-D100(BK)	DAT	$2700	Excellent
Tascam Photo & Sound Co. 9956 Baldwin Place El Monte, CA 91731 818-575-1924	32 112	2-track 2 channel Cassette	$2000 $679	Good Good
TEAC Co. 7733 Telegraph Rd. Montebello, CA 90540 213-726-0303	22-2	 DAT	$1200 $2400	 Excellent
Yamaha Photo & Sound Co 9956 Baldwin Pl. El Monte, CA 91731 818-575-1924	KX1000 112	Cassette Deck Cassette	$749 $679	Very Good Good

signal consists of representing the signal in terms of a sequence of discrete numbers. That is, each number defines or specifies the signal at a single instant in time, and the signal between two consecutive instants in time is unspecified or not represented. A digital signal represents the signal in discrete rather than continuous terms. The individual numbers are referred to as "samples" of the input signal. Thus, the analog signal is digitized into a series of numbers using a binary system to represent those numbers. In a computer, the analog signal is stored as digital values or numbers. The process of converting analog signals into discrete or digital signals is called Analog-to-Digital (A/D) conversion, and the device used is called an A/D converter. The A/D converter usually is offered as an add-on board to most computers, although in some instances, the A/D chip is built into the computer system. A/D conversion represents the changing amplitude (or voltage) of the signal in terms of a number. There are several important considerations in the choice and usage of an A/D converter for speech research.

2.2.1 Resolution
Resolution is specified as the number of bits on the A/D converter, for example, a 12-bit or a 16-bit A/D converter . This resolution of the A/D converter is a function of 2 raised the power of the number of bits of the A/D converter. Thus, a 1-bit converter provides only two steps of resolution ($2^1 = 2$); a 2-bit converter provides 4 levels of resolution ($2^2 = 4$), and so on. For speech signals, a 12-bit converter is acceptable, providing a resolution of 1 in 4096 parts, and for psychoacoustic research, a 16-bit converter is preferred. If the input signal has a range of 20 volts (+/- 10 volts) and a 12-bit A/D converter is used, the resolution is 20 volts/4096 = 4.88 mV (milliVolts). That is, the input level signal is coded or represented in steps of 4.88 mV, which is the smallest difference in level that can be encoded by this 12-bit A/D converter. Most A/D converters operate on a straight linear binary coding of the input signal, rather than Pulse Code Modulation (PCM) or mu-law coding, because it preserves signal integrity. This is particularly critical for acoustic-phonetics, speech perception, and psychoacoustic research, and not as critical for engineering applications. However, an 8-bit PCM converter provides the equivalent dynamic range of a 12- or 13-bit linear A/D converter, and is adequate for a number of applications. In PCM, larger amplitude values are represented in equal logarithmic steps rather than in equal absolute steps.

2.2.2   Sampling Rate

Sampling rate refers to the rate at which the A/D converter samples a signal for digitization. The choice of an appropriate sampling frequency is dependent on the frequency range of the signal used. In order to faithfully represent any frequency component in the input signal, there are mathematical rules that govern the number of samples required for this purpose. This is referred to as the Nyquist theorem on sampling frequency. In an ideal situation, the sampling theorem tells us that the sampling rate must be at least twice the highest frequency contained in the input signal. Usually, the input signal is low-pass filtered such that no frequencies higher than the highest frequency of interest are contained in the signal input to the A/D converter. However, due to the limitations of A/D converters and low pass filters, a higher sampling frequency is used. For example, if the highest frequency of interest is 6 kHz, then the A/D converter must sample this signal at 13.2 kHz (6 kHz * 2.2 = 13.2 kHz). For purposes of speech research, sampling frequencies of 16 kHz or 20 kHz are preferred. For most engineering applications, an 8 kHz sampling frequency is typically used. Because certain consonants (such as [s]) have energy in the high frequencies around 6 to 8 kHz, a higher sampling frequency of about 16 kHz is desirable for most purposes of research, while the lower sampling frequency of 8 kHz is adequate for most vowel sounds. Most modern A/D converters provide sampling frequencies up to 150 kHz. Analyses of infant speech, fricatives, and female speech require sampling frequencies greater than 10 kHz. If a sampling frequency lower than two times the highest frequency of interest is used, parts of the original signal are represented as being lower in frequency than they really are resulting in distortion of the real signal. The introduction of low frequencies that do not actually exist in the original speech signal is referred to as ALIASING, and the distortion as alias frequencies. This is an auditory analogue to the visual aliasing effect you have undoubtedly noticed in films, where fast turning wheels can appear to be turning slowly in the reverse direction of their acutal movement.

Thus it is important to use a high enough sampling frequency. The range of sampling frequencies provided must be programmable. That us, it should be possible to choose any given sampling frequency through software depending upon the situational need. Since low-pass filtering of the signal before passing it to an A/D converter is a critical step, low-pass filtering is discussed later in this section.

2.2.3 Triggering Options

Most A/D boards provide for either internal or external triggering. Triggering is the process which signals the A/D board to commence conversion or digitizing. If there is a provision for external triggering, then A/D conversion can be started when the external trigger (like pushing the return key on the computer keyboard) is applied. If there is no external triggering, then the card must be informed through software as to when to begin the conversion - usually based on detecting some specified point on the voltage rise of the incoming signal.

2.2.4 Number of Channels

Most A/D converters provide more than one channel for converting signals. That is, more than one signal can be digitized at the same time. These channels are provided as either Single-Ended (SE) or Differential-Input (DI). Typically, A/D cards provide 16 SE or 8 DI channels. In single-ended input, there is one common signal ground, and the signal is the difference between the input signal and the common ground. In differential input mode, two channels are used to convert a single signal input. The difference between the two channels is used to represent the signal to be digitized. When more than one channel is being converted, the A/D rapidly steps through each of the channels successively. The converted signals are stored as one continuous stream of multiplexed signals. The software keeps track of the input channel number and the signal value of the channel. Input signals are then retrieved by way of demultiplexing, whereby each channel and its corresponding digital signal is stored separately. The advantage of multiplexing is that when there is a need to digitize more than one channel, as in research on speech physiology, where the speech signal is sampled simultaneously with various physiological measures, a single card can handle several simultaneous conversions.

2.2.5 Input Voltage Range

Most A/D converters accept an input signal within a certain voltage range. Values exceeding this range can destroy the A/D card or components in this card. These are specified as +/- 5 Volts (a 10 volt range) or +/- 10 Volts (a 20 volt range). For most speech research purposes, these two input ranges are typical.

2.2.6 Direct-Memory-Access (DMA)

When data is being acquired at fast rates (greater than 10 kHz), it becomes essential to use the DMA mode of conversion wherein the converter directly deposits the samples into some memory location in RAM (Random-Access-Memory), entirely bypassing the CPU (Central Processing

Unit) of the computer. If a non-DMA mode is used, each sample converted by the A/D has to be moved from the registers in the converter by the CPU to a memory location in the RAM before the A/D can begin its next conversion. For higher sampling rates, this becomes too demanding on the CPU and there is a possibility of losing some of the original input signal. In order to prevent this, the DMA-mode of transfer of the A/D converter releases the CPU to do other chores and directly writes to RAM. A number of manufacturers also provide software (called drivers) that automatically transfer the data from the A/D to the hard-disk. This is eventually limited by the speed capabilities of the hard-disk, the disk controller and the disk driver. For most speech research purposes, direct-to-disk A/D conversion is available for sampling frequencies up to 100 kHz, and in some cases for even higher sampling frequencies. There is a major consequence of this process. If the direct-to-disk option exists, then data can be acquired or digitized for an unlimited time interval, constrained only by the memory available on the hard-disk. If this option does not exist, then the duration of the input signal that can be digitized is limited by the available RAM on the computer. For example, if only 1 MByte of RAM is available for data capture and storage, then using a sampling rate of 10 kHz, 50 seconds of continuous speech can be digitized. (Each sample takes up 2 Bytes on a 16-bit computer. Thus 10,000 samples per second take up 20,000 Bytes for 1 second of speech. Given 1,000,000 Bytes in a MByte, this amounts to 50 seconds worth of speech.) On the other hand, if one has 40 Mbytes of hard-disk space available, then 40 times more continuous speech can be digitized.

The above are some of the important considerations to be taken into account in the choice of an A/D converter card. Table 3 provides a listing of some of the commercially available A/D converters and their features.

2.3   Filters and Low-Pass Filtering

In order to prevent aliasing during the process of converting an analog signal into digital form on a computer, the analog input signal is first low-pass filtered before it is sent to the A/D converter. This is usually done by a separate filter device outside of the computer and the A/D card, although recent A/D cards have an option for a filter card "daughter board" to be attached to them to alleviate the need for a separate external filter. The input signal from the tape recorder is fed into the Low-Pass filter. The input signal must be low-pass filtered and this low-pass cut-off frequency (f_l) must be set at the highest frequency of interest (or f_l = sampling frequency/2.2). This ensures that no frequencies above the highest frequency of interest are

Tabel 3:   Sample options for A/D and D/A Converters

Manufacturer	Model	A/D (bits)	SF	D/A (bits)	SF	Computer	Price*
ADAC	5025MF	12	100k	12	100k	PC	$1150
70 Tower Office Park	5045	16	16k	12	16k	PC	$2400
Woburn, MA 01801							
508-935-6669							
Analog Devices	RTI-81	12	27k	12	27k	PC	n/a
One Technology Way	RTI-815	12	58k	12	58k	PC	n/a
P.O. Box 9106							
Norwood, MA 02062							
617-246-0300							
Ariel	DSP-16+	16	50k	16	50k	PC	n/a
433 River Road	DSP-32C	16	100	16	100k	PC	n/a
Highland Park, NJ 08904	DSP-56						
201-249-2900							
Biopac Systems	MO100	16	50k	12	50k	Mac	$3000
5960 Mandarin Dr., St. D5							
Goleta, CA 9317							
805-967-6615							
Burr-Brown	PCI-200041C	12	89k	12	32k	PC	$1500
Box 11400	PCI-701C	12	70k	12	70k	Mac	$1000
Tuscon, AZ 85734							
602-746-1111							
Data Translations	DT2801-A	12	27.5 k	12	29.5	PC	$1000
100 Locke Dr.	DT2821-F	112	150 k	12	130k	PC	$1600
Marlboro, MA 01752	DT2821-G	12	250k	12	130k	PC	$2200
508-481-3700	DT2823	16	100k	16	100k	PC	$2600
	DT2211	12	20k	12	50k	PC	$1000
	DT2221-F	12	40k	12	130k	PC	$2300
	DT2827	16	100k	12	130k	PC	$3200
	DT2211	12	20k	12	20k	Mac	$1000
	DT222X	16	750k	12	130k	Mac	$3000
GW Instruments	MacAdios-II	12	80k	12	80k	Mac	$1500
35 Medford St.	MacAdios/16	16	55k			Mac	$2000
Somerville, MA 02143							
617-625-4096							
GreenSpring	1260	12	65k	12	65k	Mac	$1495
1204 O'Brien Dr.			on-board DSP processor				
Menlo Park, CA 94025							
415-327-4096							
MetraByte/	DAS-20	12	100k	12	100k	PC	$1500
Keithley/ASYST/DAC	DAS-16F	12	100k	12	100k	PC	$1115
440 Myles Standish Blvd.	DAS-HRES	16	20k	16	20k	PC	$2000
Taunton, MA 02780	DAS-50	12	1MHz			PC	$2200
508-880-3000	MBC-625	12	140k	12	140k	Mac	$1500
National Instruments Lab	NB	12	62k	12	62k	Mac	$1500
6504 Bridge Point	MB-A2100	16	48k	16	48k	Mac	$695
Austin, TX 78730							
512-794-0110							
RC Electronics		12	1MHz	16	250k	PC	$2500
5386-D Hollister Ave.							
Santa Barbara, CA 93111							
805-964-6708							
Spectral Innovations	DSPSE/30	16	128k	16	128k	Mac	$2500
292 Gibraltar Dr. St. A4							
Sunnyvalt, CA 94086							
408-727-1314							
Strawberry Tree	ACM2-12	12	10k	12	12k	Mac	$800
160 S. Wolfe Rd.							
Sunnyvale, CA 94086							
408-736-3083							

* All prices are approximate.

input to the A/D converter. In this way, aliasing is minimized. Certain specifications of a low-pass filter must be taken into consideration:

2.3.1   Programmable Cut-Off Frequency

Programmable filters are preferable to and much more expensive than fixed-frequency cut off filters. The cut-off value depends on the highest frequency of interest in the input signal. The following three cut-off frequencies are the most often used in speech research: 4.8 kHz, 7.5 kHz and 9.6 kHz (used in conjunction with sampling frequencies of 10 kHz, 16 kHz and 20 kHz, respectively.)

2.3.2   Roll-Off Frequencies

Since all devices are real-world devices, there is "leakage" of frequencies beyond the cut-off frequencies. That is, unwanted frequencies do pass through the filter. The amplitude of these "unwanted" frequencies is indicated by the roll-off, which indicates how much attenuation (or decrease in amplitude) occurs in the frequencies beyond the cut-off frequencies. A very steep roll-off (about 96 dB/octave) indicates that frequencies beyond the cut-off value are present only at minimal amplitudes. For purposes of speech, a minimum of 48 dB/octave is typically used, although 96 dB/octave is preferable. One may simply cascade two 48 dB/octave filters to obtain 96 dB/octave roll-off. Again, the steeper the roll-off frequencies, the more expensive the filters tend to be. For psychoacoustic experiments with speech stimuli, a 96dB/octave roll-off is desirable.

2.3.3   Input Voltage Range

As with A/D converters, filters also have an input voltage range, and values exceeding this range can either destroy the filter or distort the output signal. It is important to make sure the input voltage range of the filter matches that of the A/D card. For most speech research purposes, either a +/- 5 or +/- 10 Volt range is typically used.

2.3.4   Active or Passive Filters

Active filters contain an amplifier along with the filter, and thus provide selective amplification of the desired signal. They have a wide dynamic range, good linearity, and perform better that passive filters. All active filters require a power source. Most active filters provide a much higher role-off rate (around 96 dB/octave) than passive filters. Passive filters on the other hand do not require an external power source. They usually work by cutting out the amplitude of the unwanted frequencies. However, passive filters are not as selective as active filters. That is, in the process of filtering, some of the input signal is attenuated. Either type of filter is acceptable for speech research. Gain control options on the filters (on both the input and output side) are useful to provide an added level of amplification. It is preferable to use the gain control during the input stage of the filter rather than during the output stage of the filter in order to prevent distortion of the signal. If the signal is amplified after filtering, one would also be amplifying the noise in the electrical circuitry and may end-up introducing unwanted frequencies. Again, these are only some of the important considerations in the choice of a low-pass filter. Table 4 provides a listing of some of the commercially available low-pass filters and their features.

2.4 Computer Systems

The choice of a computer system is the most difficult decision in designing a speech laboratory. There are several options that could be pursued depending in part on budget. The discussion here is confined to microcomputers because they are very common, very inexpensive and fairly adequate for purposes of speech research. One must bear in mind that given the falling prices on some high-performance workstations such as Sun Sparc-Stations, VAX work stations and others, they may increasingly be the computers of choice. The two main groups of microcomputers considered are the IBM-PC or compatible group and the Apple Macintosh group. In the PC group, an AT (or clone) using the Intel 80286 as the CPU ought to be considered as a minimum, but again Intel 80386-based PC's are a better option. The 286-based PC's are 16-bit computers whereas the 386-based PCs are 32-bit computers. These 32-bit PC's are much faster and provide much higher performance for a minimal difference in price. Either of these two scenarios ought to be considered with a numeric co-processor or Floating-Point-Processor (FPU), the 80287 chip or the 80387 chip. The 32-bit PC's have enough power to run most speech analyses programs fast enough for a number of applications. However, none of these can cope with the demands of multi-user or multi-tasking environments, and are strictly single-user options. The PCs are run under Disk-Operating-System (DOS) and thus are constrained by the 640 KByte memory barrier. Even though memory expansion facilities are available, the problem of the 640 KByte memory limitation with DOS continues to pose hardships to speech researchers.

The Apple Macintosh group of computers are much easier to use and preferable in a number of ways. They have a better graphic interface and provide good grey scale displays of the speech signal. The Mac II is a 32-bit system (using the Motorola 68020 chip for its CPU) and ought to be

Table 4: Sample Options for Low-Pass Filters

Manufaturer	Model	Type	Price*	Comments
Analog Devices One Technology Way P.O.Box 9106 Norwood, MA 02062 617-246-0030	several	n/a	$700	n/a
Ariel 433 River Road Highland Park, NJ 08904 201-249-2900	several	n/a	$500	Very Good
B&K 185 Forest St. Marlborough, MA 01752 508-481-7000	several	n/a	$1300	Very Good
Frequency Devices 25 Locust Street Haverhill, MA 01830 508-374-0761	LP-BU8 9002 848DOW 900	8-pole 48dB/Octave Dual Channel 48 to 80dB/Octave 80dB/Octave 48dB/Octave	$1000 $2495 $300 $750	Very Good Excellent Good Good
Ithaco, Inc. 735 W. Clinton St. P.O. Box 6437 Ithaca, MY 14851 800-847-2080	several	48dB.Octave	$1900	Very Good
Kron-Hite Avon Industrial Park Avon, MA 02322 508-580-1660	3905 3916	57dB/Octave 115dB/Octave	$1900 $2800	Very Good Very Good
Precision Filters, Inc. 240 Cherry St. Ithaca, MY 14850 607-277-3550	Several	200dB/Ocatve	n/a	Excellent
Rockland 10 Volvo Dr. Rockleigh, NJ 07647	2382 2582 2762	Dual Channel 48 dB/Ocatave Dual Channel 48dB/Octave Dual Channel 94 dB/Ocatve	$3000 $3250 $3500	Very Good Excellent
Stanford Research Systems 1290 Dreamwood Ave. Sunnyvale, CA 94089 408-744-9040	SR640	Dual Channel 115dB/Octave	$3000	Excellent
TTE (local dealer)	J97E	Low-Pass	$300	Excellent

* All prices are approximate.

considered as a minimum system. There are advanced models in the Macintosh group such as the Mac IICx, CXi and Fx which are all more powerful that the Mac II. Most of the advanced models come with an FPU, and if one is using a Mac II it is highly recommended to use it with an FPU. A Mac II system is quite adequate for most speech analyses.

There are general factors, regardless of the system one prefers, that ought to be considered. The list of factors is a long one, and only the most important ones are considered here. First, the amount of RAM to be used is an important factor. One should consider buying as much RAM as one can afford, with a minimum of 4 to 8 MBytes. Given the low-cost of RAM, this is not an expensive option. Second, an FPU is a must and care should be taken that it matches the speed of the computers CPU. Thirdly, the type of display or monitor is also important. An Enhanced-Graphics Monitor (EGA) or a Virtual Graphics Monitor (VGA) should be considered a minimum. Along with the monitor, the appropriate video-board or adapter card ought to be purchased. These video-boards have built-in Video-RAMs. Typically the low-cost boards have 128 KBytes of Video-RAM, and the cost goes up for higher RAM. For spectrographic displays, a greyscale or color monitor with a resolution of 8-bits per pixel is very useful. This provides 256 shades of grey, which is essential for a usable spectrographic display.

Fourth, a large hard-disk is a must. A minimum of 80 Mbytes ought to be provided, although a 300 MByte or 600 MByte disk should be considered as the prices of hard disks have plummeted. Digitized speech uses up a lot of disk space, and it is very easy to run out of space even with a 600 MByte hard disk. When using a hard disk, the average access time of the disk (along with its controller card) must be considered. Current hard disks provide an average access time of about 16 to 18 ms, which is adequate for speech purposes. A problem exists in using these large disks with DOS, as DOS 3.3 requires that the disks be partitioned into 32-MBytes units. This problem is easily alleviated by purchasing separate inexpensive software to manage large disks which are not partitioned into small units but still communicate with DOS. Fifth, backing up these disks is a very important consideration. Backing up such large disks (or even a 32-MByte disk) on floppies is a nightmare and shouldn't even be considered. There are several solutions, such as streaming tape back-up units, DATs (4mm and 8mm), VCR back-up units, and erasable optical disks. There are many inexpensive streaming tape back-up units that are available which are easy to use and back-up disks as large as 150 MBytes onto one tape. Additionally, DATs are becoming increasingly available as options for tape back-up. A single DAT can back-up 1.2 GBytes of data. Tape back-up is a very critical factor to consider since hard disks crash frequently. Sixth, using a mouse for manipulation of speech data is recommended as a very convenient tool. While these are very inexpensive options, several factors need to be considered in the purchase of a mouse, such as a bus mouse or a serial mouse, the number of buttons on the mouse, mechanical vs. optical mouse, and whether or not the speech analysis software package makes use of the mouse.

Given the advances in technology and the decline in the cost of computers, one should seriously consider high-performance, relatively inexpensive workstations such as the Sun SparcStation, and VAX workstations, over the PC's. These workstations are comparable in cost to a fully-loaded 386-clone but provide a level of performance that is 5 to 10 times higher than those of the PCs. The standard configuration of a workstation has about 8 MBytes of RAM, with a sophisticated graphics processor, a processor speed of about 12 MIPS (Millions of Instructions per Second), a 17- or 19-inch color monitor, a mouse, and extensive hardware and software as part of the standard equipment. The trade-off is that these workstations are demanding in their upkeep and have proprietary bus standards that exclude third-party providers for A/D converters and other hardware. Most of these tend to be UNIX-based systems and are thus less user-friendly than the Mac Operating System. Given the commercial availability of the latest and most powerful speech signal processing software on these workstations (such as Waves+ and SPIRE), these workstations are probably the most desirable computer choice and are an indication of the future direction in speech research.

Regardless of the type of computer chosen, there are enough options in the market today to satisfy a wide range of speech researchers with very different needs. The response time, ease of use of the system and efficient management of computer resources are dictated and restricted by the system used.

2.5   Speech Software

The most critical part of the instrumentation for speech research is the actual speech software itself. There are several different speech analysis software packages with vastly varying capabilities and flexibility. Some of these packages are highly system specific while others have packages for various systems. Rather than discuss each of these packages here, only design features of generic speech analysis software will be discussed. These features are considered highly useful and desirable across many different speech research settings. Where appropriate, mention will be made of those packages that provide some of these options. Table 5 is a fairly comprehensive list of the currently available speech software for some of the different systems. Packages such as ILS, CSpeech, MicroSpeech Lab, Vishranth Speech System, Realtime Speech Lab, and Hyperception for the PCs; the MacSpeech Lab and Mac Recorder for the Macintosh computers; ILS, Waves+ and SPIRE for the Sun and Dec Workstations are some of the packages currently available. Each of these packages has its own merits and limitations, and users should choose the one that best fits their needs.

Some desirable features of speech analysis packages are listed below:

2.5.1   Ease of Recording:
It should be easy to digitize the analog speech signal either into a file on the hard disk or to the RAM of the computer to be divided up and stored in different files later. This step involves setting up the A/D converter with the desirable sampling frequency and the low-pass filter with an appropriate cut-off frequency and specifying the number of channels of data being acquired, the duration or length of the speech signal that is being acquired, and the name of the file where it is to be stored. Options should be available for specifying these settings either interactively (preferably using a menu) or by setting these up in a batch file without having to go through the menu every time for storing the signal in different files. Additionally, it should be possible to create several different consecutive files at a time (using numbers for filenames) and to specify the size of each of these files rather than being limited to creating only one file at a time.

2.5.2   Options in Displaying the Digitized Speech Signal:
It should be possible to have an instantaneous display of the waveform (the time series signal) while or immediately after recording. This permits easy and instantaneous re-recording of the signal if it is warranted. Other options should include the capability of displaying the signal from a file; displaying portions of the signal or the complete signal; controllable display size or scalable, single/dual/multiple waveform display options; cursor control - separate left and right cursors; time-instant and time-interval measurements with cursors; provision for labeling portions of the waveform (phonetic labeling for example) and for storing the portion as a segment into another file with time measures; easy playback of segments between cursors, cut and paste, save and/or zero segments, insert segments rescale or pre-emphasize portions of the waveforms between cursors, etc. All of these features are useful in both acoustic phonetics and speech perception research.

Table 5: Sample Speech Analysis Software

Manufacturer	Model	Type	Price*	Comments
Ariel Corporation 433 River Road Highland Park, NJ 0894 201-249-2900	Speech Station	PC	n/a	analysis and syntheisis
Farallon Computing 2000 Powell St, Suite 600 Emeryville, CA 94608 415-596-9000 (any Mac dealer)	MacRecorder	Mac	$189	analysis
GW Instruments 35 Medford St.' Somerville, MA 02143 617-625-4096	MacSpeech Lab-II	Mac II	$4500	analysis
Hyperception 9550 Skillman LB 1255, Suite 316 Dallas, TX 75243 214-343-8525	Hypersignal Plus	PC	$1000	analysis
Kay Elemetrics 12 Maple Ave. P.O. Box 2025 Pine Brooks, NJ 07058 800-289-5297	Computerized/ Speech Lab	PC	$5950	analysis
Laboratory Micorsystems 450 Cloud Dr. #11 Baton Rouge, LA 70806 504-926-8671	APRLS (Acoustic- Phonetic Research Laboratory System	PC	$2500	analysis and synthesis
Paul Malenkovic Drpt. of EECS University of Wisconsin Madison, WI	C-Speech	PC	n/a	analysis
Robert Morris Systems Engineering MacKenzie Bld. Rm. 377 Carleton University Ottawa, Ontario, K1S 5B6, Canada	Realtime Speech Lab	PC	n/a	analysis
Signal Technology Inc. 120 Cremona Dr. P.O. Box 1950 Geleta, CA 93116 800-235-5787	ILS-PC	PC	$1000	analysis and synthesis
Software Research Co. 3939 Quadra St. Victoria, B.C. Canada V8X 1J5 604-727-3744	MicroSpeech Lab	PC	$2000	analysis
Spectrum Signal Processing Inc. 460 Totten Pond Rd. Waltham, MA 02154 800-323-1842	Speech Workstation (with DSP board)	PC	$4715 $5996	analysis
UCLA - Phonetics Lab Drpt. of Linguistics UCLA 405 Hilgard AVe. Los Angeles, CA 90024-1543	speech software	Mac	$95	analysis and synthesis
Voice & Speech Systems Bangalore, India 560-003	Vishranth	PC	$1600	analysis/ syntheses
Washington Research Laboratory 600 Pennsylvania Ave. S.E. Suite 202 Washington, DC 20003 202-547-1420	ESPS Waves+	SparcStation SparcStation	$6000 $2500	Excellent Excellent

* All prices are approximate.

2.5.3   Types of analyses of the speech signal

This is probably one of the most critical features of any software package. For most speech research purposes, multiple windows with each window showing the results of a separate selectable analysis is a very useful feature. For instance, one could have a spectral slice (DFT of a section of the signal) and a wide or narrow band FFT in another window for the same interval of data, a window with the signal magnified or expanded in the time domain, and another window with a wide band or narrow band spectrogram display. Each of these analysis windows ought to have scalable size, and it should also be possible to specify the analysis parameters for each of the analyses separately with the help of pop-down menus. Equally critical would be the availability of time-aligned cursors such that by moving a cursor in one of the windows, there is appropriate movement of the cursor in each of the different windows.

Specifically for speech, analyses should include information about both the vocal tract function and laryngeal function separately. The following analyses and options are useful and yield information about the vocal tract: *LPC analysis of speech* yielding a section- or continuous-display of LPC formants as a function of time; *Spectrographic analysis* including wide- and narrow-band displays with the option of overlaying format tracks on the spectrograms; *format tracking* with and without bandwidths; and *3-dimensional displays* of amplitude-spectrum or LPC-spectrum as a function of time are all required features. For each of these analyses it should be possible to specify the number of points (or window duration) over which the analysis operates, zoom function, cursors, selection of number of coefficients, frequency bandwidth or resolution of the spectrographic analysis, etc. Provision should exist for saving the output of each of these analyses in a separate file. The following analyses and options are useful and yield information about laryngeal functioning. Fundamental frequency extraction as a function of time (with intensity values optional); scalable displays of this analysis; availability of a cursor aligned with the fundamental frequency display, waveform and spectrogram; inverse filtering resulting in the residual signal which reflects the acoustic structure of the glottal signal, etc. Fundamental frequency analysis has been one of the most challenging of speech analyses for most existing software packages and is fraught with many errors and imprecision particularly for high-frequency pitch analyses (female and children speech). Thus these analyses are somewhat suspect in most packages.

2.5.4   Digital Filtering

Digital filtering through software is a required feature of most signal processing packages. Options should exist to design the required filter with user-selectable specifications. It should be possible to input a sampled data file to such a software filter and output the result of this process in another file.

2.5.5   File Manipulation

File manipulation, file editing, file import and export, header management, and program control are critical issues. One of the tasks in speech research is to take the obtained analysis data and subject it to certain statistical analyses using a different software package. It is not always easy to import/export the speech files (data or analysis files) to ASCII formats or to manipulate their headers to adapt it for other needs. Although some vendors do provide rudimentary file manipulation routines, obtaining clear documentation on these issues is extremely important. For the analysis of multiple speech files for extraction of formant frequencies or fundamental frequency, batch processing is a boon, but not all packages offer this option. It is extremely painful to analyze thousands of speech files (which is typically the case in phonetic and speech research) one at a time in an interactive environment when all that one needs is a similar analysis on a group of speech files. Thus the option of batch processing or interactive processing is a very useful feature.

A major limitation of most commercially available packages for the microcomputer world is that the options are limited, fixed, and thus inflexible. It is very hard to customize the analysis parameters or display options as is warranted by researchers' needs. The situation may be acceptable for a number of applications but soon one runs into severe limitations with such software. Some vendors do provide the source code but at an exhoribitantly high price. For most research purposes, the lack of custom tailoring or flexibility in the software is a major hindrance and can severely limit the type of research being pursued. Additionally, technical support offered for a number of the packages is severely limited. A willingness to help, but with severe limitations in understanding researchers' needs seems to be more often the rule. Access to a users' group or pursuing these issues before purchasing decisions are made may help to some extent. Obtaining a publishable quality plot of the spectrograph displays is unsatisfactory with a vast majority of these programs. Although this is more a problem of availability of a printer adequate to faithfully represent the shades of grey as discernable contrasts on the plot, it continues to be a source of concern.

Even laser quality printers seem inadequate in capturing grey-scale resolution. There is much to be desired with this particular need of most researchers.

2.6 Speech Output and Signal Generation (Speech Synthesis)

The computer is an ideal device for generating signals (and speech) for a number of reasons. It provides a high degree of precision, flexibility and stability. Stimuli of a high degree of complexity can be produced easily. One can control and manipulate individual parameters. This usually consists of the user specifying the relevant parameters as a function of time. The software converts these parameters and generates a digital waveform, wherein the signal is specified in terms of discrete values or numbers representing voltage as a function of equally spaced time intervals. This sequence of numbers is output to a D/A converter which takes the discrete values and generates a continuous or analog output that is low-pass filtered (and smoothed) and results in the actual analog signal.

Considerations discussed for the A/D converter are equally applicable to the D/A converters. Issues such as resolution (number of bits), sampling frequency, number of channels and triggering options also apply to D/A converters, but there are some additional considerations that have to be taken into account for D/A converters. Some D/A boards have an on-board deglitcher. These are very useful when listening to the signal from the computer output. When listening to any audio signal, if the onset amplitude is quite high or the maximum value of the signal is reached very quickly, it introduces unwanted "clicks" at the beginning of the signal. One way to eliminate these clicks is by use of an on-board deglitcher. In the absence of a deglitcher, the output signal must be ramped through software. That is, the amplitude during the first few milliseconds of the onset of the signal must be allowed to grow gradually. Additional when a D/A converts a number to a voltage, this change does not always occur instantaneously and does not always remain stable at that voltage until the next conversion of a sample occurs. This transition from one voltage to the next is accompanied by unwanted transient voltages which can have a high magnitude. These are also referred to as "glitches" and contribute to distortion noise in the output signal which can be crucial for perception experiments (psychoacoustic and speech perception experiments). These glitches are related in a non-linear fashion to the step-size of the converter.

For such problems too, an on-board deglitcher is a very useful solution. It is extremely important to use a D/A converter that uses a straight linear conversion (as opposed to PCM) for speech perception and psychoacoustic experiments. Converting data using a linear signal in logarithmic steps defeats the purpose of sound amplitude or intensity discrimination tests. For such purposes, a 16-bit D/A converter is much preferred over a 12-bit converter. Such fine-scale discriminatory tasks are seldom used in speech perception experiments and thus a 12-bit D/A converter usually suffices.

The output from the D/A converter is low-pass filtered and smoothed and results in the output analog waveform in an electrical form. The factors to be considered using this low-pass filtering are the same as those discussed in section 2.3. Now all that needs to be done to listen to the signal is to pass it through a transducer to convert the electrical energy back into sound energy. This is accomplished by passing the output signal from the filter into an amplifier and then either into a loudspeaker or a headset. Alternatively, the signal from the filter may be recorded on a tape recorder (or a DAT). The factors involved in the selection of a transducer at the output end are essentially the same as those discussed for the input end. Essentially, the frequency response of the transducer, desired power output and impedance matching with the amplifier are factors to bear in mind. Table 6 provides some examples of loudspeakers and headphones.

Table 6: Sample Options for Head Phones

Manufacturer	Model	Type	Price*	Comments
Koss (local dealer)	several		$150	OK
Radio Shack (local dealer)	Nova-45		$40	OK
Sennheisser 6 Vista Drive Old Lyme, CT 06371 203-434-9190	HD430 HD540		$200 $400	Excellent Excellent
Telex Photo & Sound Co. 9956 Baldwin Place El Monte, CA 91731 818-575-1924	500 PH-6	130 ohms	$57 $125	OK Good

* All prices are approximate.

3.   Areas of Speech Research and Its Applications

There are several areas and applications of speech. In speech science and acoustic phonetics, the basic goal is to relate the acoustic attributes of speech sounds with their linguistic units (or other relevant dimensions). Here various aspects of the speech signal are employed to study such relationships. Formant frequencies, formant transitions, spectra of vowels and consonants, and various temporal measures are some essential acoustic attributes of sound. Engineering applications typically consist of speech coding, text-to-speech synthesis (TTS), automatic speech recognition (ASR), and Voice I/O systems. In speech coding, the goal is to come up with efficient ways of encoding the speech signal—either in the time domain and/or the spectral domain - such that a minimal number of bits are used for storage and transmission. In TTS, the goal is to generate intelligible, natural sounding speech output from text input for purposes of communication. Thus the computer-generated speech should contain detailed acoustic properties that are important in distinguishing speech sounds. In speech recognition, the goal is to analyze the speech signal to determine the message. For psychologists, the goal is to investigate how humans produce and perceive speech. Thus experimentation with synthetic and natural speech is an important capability. Hearing scientists and neurophysiologists are concerned with characterizing how speech is represented in the human auditory nervous system. Here, digital generation of acoustic stimuli (both speech and non-speech) and experiments that determine minimal detectable differences between various types of acoustic signals (including speech stimuli), analysis of responses, phase locking, etc. are important. For speech-language pathologists and otolaryngologists, the goal in acoustic analysis of speech is to assist them in diagnosing and aiding impaired populations. Analyses of infant cries and early vocalizations may help in the diagnosis of laryngeal/vocal tract impairment, deafness at birth, and so on. In therapy, one could use acoustic analyses of speech for an objective determination of the acquisition of sounds and in suggesting articulatory maneuvers that match a desirable given acoustic pattern which is usually associated with such movements. Diagnosis of voice disorders and their treatment is another good example of applications of this research. These are some of the applications of speech research for which laboratory instrumentation has become indispensable.

4.   A Description of a Functional Speech Lab

In putting together most of the information above, I though it best to use the example of my laboratory, at the University of California in Santa Barbara, in demonstrating the choice and configuration of most of the equipment above. A schematic representation of the lab is shown in Figure 2. This lab is configured with three different types of computer systems - a 386 PC-based system, a Macintosh II based system, and a Sun SparcStation based computer system.

All speech data is acquired in a sound-treated room (IAC double-walled) using a Shure condenser microphone (M267). This microphone is attached to a Shure mixer which has 4 inputs (M467) and one output. The output of the mixer is fed either into a Panasonic Digital-Audio-Tape (Model SV3500) or an Ampex reel-to-reel tape recorder. The speech signal (either from the mixer or the tape-recorder) is then fed into a programmable low-pass filter (Standard Research Systems Model SR650). This is an active filter with two input and two output channels and separate gain controls at the input and output ends, and has a roll-off of 115 dB/Octave. The low-pass filtered signal (usually filtered at 9.6 kHz) is fed into a screw-terminal panel which is connected to an A/D card housed in a computer.

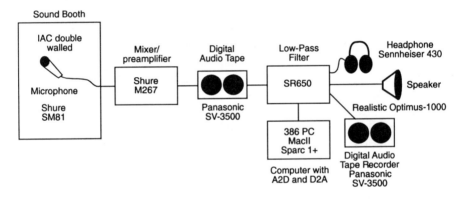

Figure 2: Block diagram of the speech science lab at UCSB

Each of the computers (with the exception of the Sun SparcStations) have a 12-bit A/D card which contains 2 12-bit D/A converters and 8 digital I/O outputs. These boards also contain an on-board deglitcher in the D/A conversion state. On the PC, the DT2821-F16-SE model (from Data Translations, Inc.) A/D card is used. This card has a maximum programmable sampling frequency of 150 kHz with DMA. On the Macintosh, the MacAdios A/D card is used (from GW Instruments, Inc.). This card is capable of a maximum sampling frequency of 80 kHz. The recorded speech signal is usually sampled at 20 kHz on both these computers.

The PC-computer system consists of a 386 clone with an FPU (or the math co-processor) running under DOS 3.3. It has a RAM of 4 MBytes, a 702 MByte SCSI Hard-Disk with a 150 MByte streaming tape drive. It also consists of 2 floppy drives, 1.2 MByte high-density drive and a 360 KByte drive. It has a VGA monitor with a video-card which has 256 KBytes of Video-RAM, and an enhanced keyboard. Several different speech analysis packages are used in this lab. On the PCs, ILS and VSS are typically used. The Macintosh system consists of a Mac II (68020 CPU with an FPU), 4 MBytes RAM, a 40 MByte Hard disk, an 8-bit/pixel video card with color graphics monitor and the MacOS. On this system, the MacSpeech Lab and the MacRecorder are used for speech signal analysis. The Sun SparcStations are equipped with a 104 MByte SCSI hard disk, 8 MBytes of RAM, an 8-bit/pixel color graphics monitor with a graphics accelerator card from Sun Microsystems, and the SunOS as the operating system. On this system the ESPS signal processing package (Entropics, Inc.) and Waves+ (Entropics) speech analysis package are used.

On the output end, speech data from the computer is output through the same card(s) which have both A/D and D/A, passed through the same low-pass filter and then fed into an amplifier (Realistic STA-2380). From the amplifier, speech is heard via headphones (Sennheisser 430) or via two loudspeakers (Realistic Optimus-1000)

Various types of speech research are being pursued in this lab. Primarily, all of the research involves the acoustic analysis of speech and digital generation of speech and other acoustic stimuli. Experiments dealing with analysis of infant cries (normal, deaf and hearing-impaired infants), formant frequency analysis of different sounds across several speakers and languages, acoustic analysis of the speech of neurogically impaired populations, psychoacoustic experiments using speech and speech-like stimuli, speech perception experiments, analysis of voice (and its disorders), study of glottal source function of adults and children, are examples of some of the ongoing research in this lab.

5. References

Cooper, F.S. (1983). Some reflections on Speech Research. In *The Production of Speech*. Ed: Peter F. MacNeilage. New York: Springer-Verlag.

Curtis, J.F. (1987). *An Introduction to Microcomputers in Speech, Language, and Hearing*. Boston: Little, Brown, Co.

Curtis, J.F. and Schultz, M.C. (1986). *Basic Laboratory Instrumentation for Speech and Hearing*. Boston: Little, Brown, Co.

Davis, R.O. (1986). Digital Signal Processing in studies of Animal Communication including Human Speech. *Computer Methods and Programs in Biomedicine*, **23**, 171–196

Decker, N.T. (1990). Instrumentation: An introduction for students in the speech and hearing sciences. New York: Longman (Addison-Wesley).

Everest, A.F.

O'Shaughnessy, D. (1987). *Speech Communication: Human and Machine*. New York: Addison-Wesley, New York.

Talkin, D. (1989). Looking at Speech. *Speech Technology*, pp. 74–77, April/ May.

Users Manual for ILS-PC V6.0, volumes 1 and 2 (1986). Signal Technology Inc. Goleta, California.

Users Manual, Entropics (1989).

Chapter 9

Speech Recognition[1]

Diane Kewley-Port
Indiana University

1. Introduction

If computers could recognize and understand speech, there would be a revolution in the way in which humans use computers. Computers, or devices controlled by computers, could be used in very different environments than are now possible, and by ordinary people who find computers and advanced technology incomprehensible or threatening. Unfortunately, present speech recognition technology is far from the ideal goal of understanding speech by all persons in all settings.

Speech input systems can be divided into two types: speech *recognizers* and speech *understanding* systems. The task of a speech recognizer is simply to identify the words spoken without interpreting their meaning in a sentence. Recognition output would be very useful if speech recognizers could identify words in fluent speech for any talker. Some of the more advanced (and costly) recognizers on the market today approach this goal. However, for most commercial speech recognition systems, the goal of speech recognition has been subdivided into smaller goals which the present technology is capable of handling in a cost-effective way.

Very few speech understanding systems are currently being marketed. In addition to associating the acoustic input with a particular vocabulary item, speech understanding systems need syntax (parsers) and semantics (dictionaries) to assign meaning to speech input. The focus of the present

[1] This manuscript was prepared with the help of support from grants from the National Science Foundation, ECE 84-19339, and the Air Force Office of Scientific Research.

chapter is to discuss the problems related to speech recognition, not speech understanding. However, since speech understanding is the primary problem being addressed in current research, a few comments about the state of this effort will be made. Laboratory systems are investigating vocabularies from 1,000 words (Lee, 1990) to 60,000 words (Deng et al., 1989), with corresponding accuracies between 95% and 75%. Commercial systems include one with a 40,000 word dictionary (DS200, $33,900; Meisel et al., 1989) and systems targeted for more specific tasks, such as radiology reports (VoiceRad, $30,000; Joseph, 1989) or a voice-driven typewriter (DragonDictate, $9,000; Baker, 1989).

Speed, cost, and accuracy are all issues that are not satisfactorily resolved for either laboratory or commercial speech understanding systems. The intent of this chapter is to provide background information on why the speech recognition task alone is so difficult, and then to describe the algorithms that have been proposed to simplify the problem.

1.1 Special Considerations of Natural Speech for Speech Recognizers

The problems a machine has in understanding language are somewhat similar to those of adults learning a foreign language. Remarks such as "the words all run together," "my vocabulary is just too small," and "I can't understand all these different dialects" apply equally well to machines and foreign language learners. Some of these problems have been studied by phoneticians and speech scientists interested in speech acoustics. Since engineers building speech recognizers have had to find solutions to these problems—solutions that usually mean limiting the generality of the speech recognized we need to consider some of these problems in detail.

One of the biggest puzzles in speech science is how the human listener easily identifies words within a normally-spoken sentence when there are no obvious features marking word boundaries in the speech signal. Linguists generally agree that the smallest segment of sound that can differentiate words is the phoneme. Phonemes are classified as consonants or vowels. Acoustically, the phonemes in words run together, reflecting the continuous movement of the gestures in speech. This phenomenon is referred to as coarticulation. While computer algorithms can locate many phoneme boundaries quite accurately (Mermelstein, 1975; Haltsonen, 1981; Blomberg and Elenius, 1985), in general it is much more difficult to reliably locate word boundaries, except where there are long syntactic pauses. The fact that speech cannot be easily segmented into words is probably the most important problem to be solved in speech recognition.

Other major problems facing speech recognition relate to the tremendous *variability* observed in normal speech. That is, normal listeners are able to correctly perceive speech even though many types of variability exist, for example speakers talking at different rates or speech that is distorted by a variety of environmental factors. Some significant categories of variability to be discussed here include speaker differences, dialect variation, speaking rate differences, and token-to-token variation. Speaker variability refers primarily to the fact that differences in the size of the vocal tract between speakers, from large males to small children, directly affect the frequencies observed in the speech signal (Wakita, 1977). Most noticeable are the differences in pitch of the voice between men, women and children. In addition, the frequencies important for specifying male vowels are much lower than those of females which are in turn lower than those of children (Peterson and Barney, 1951). The overall effect of these frequency differences is very large. Many speech scientists have tried to develop algorithms for mapping these frequency differences into one "normalized" phonetic space, but they have not been able to match human performance (Neary, 1989). As we shall see, the solution to the speaker variability problem is one of the major differences between speech recognizers.

Speaker differences such as dialect, speaking rate, and voice characteristics (pitch, hoarseness etc.) are often thought of as properties that identify the speaker is and these properties are important in speaker verification. Speaker differences are generally considered to be problems for speech recognizers, and require solutions that enable a recognizer to "learn" to handle a particular voice (i.e. ignore speaker differences).

Token-to-token variability refers to the normal variation observed when one speaker repeats a word many times. Small but significant differences in the temporal structure and energy levels within a word occur for each repetition. Various schemes for normalizing these time and energy differences have been proposed. Since speech recognition cannot be successful without accounting for token-to-token variability, all speech recognizers incorporate algorithms to handle this problem.

2. Subdividing the Speech Recognition Problem

Given the many difficulties facing engineers trying to build accurate and fast speech recognizers, it is not surprising that the first successful algorithms could recognize only a few words (the ten digits), spoken clearly, in isolation by one speaker (Denes et al., 1960; White and Neely, 1976). As systems improved, names were given to specific recognition problems to differentiate between systems. Currently, a speech recognizer can be defined by identifying the particular problems it has solved. For example, the first recognizers were "small, fixed vocabulary," "speaker dependent," "isolated word" recognizers. Below we consider the particular subdivisions of speech recognition problems used in research and development. Unfortunately, marketing fact sheets often obscure exactly what speech recognition problems a particular device is designed to solve.

Continuous, connected and isolated (or discrete) are terms that refer to how the problem of word boundaries has been handled. *Isolated word recognition* requires about a half-second (500ms) or greater pause be inserted between spoken words. *Connected word recognition* only requires a very short pause be inserted between rather carefully spoken words. *Continuous speech recognizers* require no pauses between words, and accept fluent speech pronunciation.

Restrictions on the *size and nature of the vocabulary* of words differentiates speech recognition devices. Vocabulary size is usually divided into small (100 to 200 words), large (about 1000 words) and very large (5000 words or greater) vocabularies. While the size of the vocabulary poses obvious restrictions on speech recognition, the nature of the vocabulary should also be considered. One primary consideration of vocabulary size is the extent to which users may specify their own vocabularies. For example, two quite different sizes of fixed vocabularies are required for recognition of digits or alarm messages, versus the operation of voice-driven typewriters. Fixed vocabularies are usually found for devices tailored to a specific task that need to be extremely reliable across talkers. Large fixed vocabulary systems (1,000 to 5,000 words) have been designed, but their structure usually makes it difficult for users to add their own words (Lee, 1990).

When users choose their own vocabularies, they may choose simple word lists, or organize the lists according to some *rules or syntax*. For example, vocabularies may contain over 200 words, but may be subdivided into separate lists or nodes in which words on one node may follow only those on another node. In this case, the user designs the syntax and structures the vocabulary in a way that is useful and consistent for a particular task. This syntax may not conform closely to accepted rules of English grammar of the type incorporated into speech understanding systems (Wilpon, Rabiner and Martin, 1984). The user's syntax has the effect of reducing the total number of words that must be considered by the recognizer at any one time, thereby improving the speed and accuracy of the recognizer. This concept will be more fully discussed later.

Another major subdivision of recognizers specifies whether they can identify speech from many talkers (*speaker independent*), or only one speaker at a time and are *(speaker dependent.)* Clearly, users of speech recognizers would prefer speaker independent systems, but these algorithms are far more difficult to construct at acceptable levels of accuracy (Rabner and Wilpon, 1987). Recognizers that claim speaker independence are usually not, in fact, totally independent of such things as a talker's dialect and individual voice characteristics. Typically speaker independent systems still require a short training period, called enrollment, to adjust to each talker.

Speaker dependent recognizers generally use stored *templates* (i.e. examples of the speakers utterances) created specifically for each talker. A problem associated with such systems is how the templates are created, and how long it takes to make them for vocabularies of 100 words or more (Rabiner and Wilpon, 1980). Although speaker dependent systems are not generally as desirable as speaker-independent systems, they have proven to be quite useful in many applications.

3. Overview of Recognition Algorithms

This section will introduce some of the basic concepts involved in speech recognition algorithms. This overview is divided into four sections: Endpoint detection, speech coding, recognition algorithms, and second level algorithms.

3.1 Endpoint Detection

Speech recognizers must determine the beginning and end of a speech event in the acoustic input (Lamel et al., 1981; de Souza, 1983). Even in the simplest case of isolated word recognition, algorithms must distinguish environmental noises, coughs, lip-smacks etc. from words. In addition, speech signal levels can change substantially with the distance between the microphone and the lips. Even more troublesome are the high levels of background noise commonly found in offices or factories. One step toward solving the endpoint problem is to provide users with a close-talking microphone that attenuates environmental noise, and then mount it on a head-set to maintain a fixed distance between the mouth and microphone. Frequently, the effect of noise is further reduced by sampling background noise and subtracting it from the input. Endpoint-detection algorithms are used to isolate speech and exclude non-speech sounds, which are too short or too soft. Although these techniques correctly exclude most non-speech sounds, they can also incorrectly reject some speech sounds such as low-level fricative *f* and *h*. While other techniques, such as backsearching algorithms, may improve the detection of low-level fricatives, users are usually encouraged to avoid these phonemes in their recognition vocabularies.

One different approach to the endpoint detection is called word-spotting. Word-spotting algorithms have been developed for systems using stored templates for recognition (Christiansen and Rushforth, 1977; Higgins and Wohlford, 1985). Recognition is then performed by a pattern matching process in which the input is continuously compared to the stored templates. As the input slides by the templates, a word is spotted when a matching score exceeds some criteria. This approach not only bypasses the endpoint problem but, in fact, works on continuous speech as long as the number of templates to be recognized in the continuous input is fairly small. In some systems templates can be formed from short phrases or sentences, as well as words; this can extend the applicability of word-spotting systems.

3.2 Speech Coding
The amount of information in the input speech signal is usually coded and significantly reduced to gain efficiency in recognition. The form of this speech coding is dependent on the *linguistic units* of speech chosen as the basis for subsequent recognition algorithms. In isolated word recognition, the unit chosen is typically the whole word. In continuous word recognition, the initial coding unit is typically smaller than the word, for example diphones (two-phoneme pairs) (Rosenberg et al., 1983), phonemes or acoustic features. These units serve as the basis for recognizing larger linguistic units (e.g. syllables) until, ultimately, words are identified.

A common recognition method is to store a coded representation of speech units as templates for comparison with incoming speech. Templates include diphones, demi-syllables, syllables, words or even phrases and sentences. Speech is pre-processed to generate a normalized form and then processed further for recoding and comparison to specific templates.

Preprocessing slices the speech waveform into segments 5 to 40 msec long. In one class of methods, each time slice is coded as a set of energy values in certain frequency regions; for example, as formant values or as the output values of a filter bank (Dautrich et al., 1983). Filter banks that model the spectral properties of the human ear (auditory front-ends) have been investigated in recent years. In several cases, improvement in recognition accuracy was obtained using the auditory front-ends, even when the remainder of the algorithm was held constant (Cohen, 1989; Hermansky, 1990).

In another class of methods, the time slices are analyzed by statistically based models of speech such as linear prediction analysis. The output-vector values, or linear prediction coefficients (LPC), from these algorithms can serve as codes for speech templates. Almost two decades of research has been spent on implementing and improving LPC speech recognizers (for a review see O'Shaughnessy, 1987, Chapters 8 and 10). While some of the earliest commercial recognizers (the IBM system found in the Speech-Viewer speech training aid and The Speech Board by Texas Instruments) were based on LPC algorithms, they are implemented currently in some of the most sophisticated systems (SPHINX; Lee, 1990).

Recognition methods that use phonetic coding use different kinds of algorithms from those discussed above. Basically these methods follow a series of steps analogous to traditional linguistic analysis (Cole et al., 1986; Zue, 1985). First, a number of acoustic parameters that can serve to distinguish between *phonemes* are measured. These are then combined using a set of rules that determine a set of possible phonemic segments associated with the speech signal. Any portion of the speech waveform can be associated with several possible phoneme candidates which are rank ordered in probability. Another set of rules are subsequently applied in conjunction with a dictionary (lexicon) to identify the words consistent with high probability phoneme choices. Many phonetically-based systems are in fact speech understanding systems, and therefore another level of rules corresponding to syntactic analysis is invoked to make a final deter-mination of the sentence or phrase spoken.

Thus there is a clear distinction between phonetically based systems and other recognizers. Phonetic recognizers depend on a large set of complicated linguistic rules to analyze and manipulate incoming acoustic information. For this reason they require a massive amount of computational power. In addition, phonetically-based systems have *fixed* vocabularies which are integral to the rules of the system and in particular the structure of its lexicon. Therefore, to make phonetic recognizers marketable, the vocabu-laries need to be quite large (Meisel, 1989)

3.3 Recognition Algorithms
Once the speech has been coded, the task of the recognizer is to determine whether the incoming speech signal contains one of the words in its vocabulary. This task has two components, one that reduces variability in the temporal structure of the same word in different utterances, and another that contains the decision rules to identify the word.

Algorithms that remove variability in temporal structure can be divided into (1) those in which coding units are allowed to overlap and unit timing is treated as asynchronous, and (2) those in which coding units are distinct segments and time-slices and unit timing is treated synchronously. On the whole, *phonetically-based* algorithms treat time asynchronously, with rules resolving temporal order of the segments found at higher levels of the analyses.

The majority of speech recognizers today, however, rely on *synchronous*, template methods. In these methods the algorithms generally warp time in such a way that the beginnings and ends are aligned, and the time-slices in between are aligned in a non-linear way. Simple algorithms involve time-normalization for those portions of the input speech signal that are relatively constant. Following the time-alignment, a *goodness-of-fit* metric is used by a pattern recognition algorithm to determine which template most closely corresponds to the incoming, coded signal. These metrics are typically mathematically based, e.g. Euclidian distances. More recently perceptually based metrics have been developed (Hermansky, 1990).

More complex algorithms incorporate the time-alignment and pattern-recognition algorithm. For example, there is a class of *dynamic time-warping* algorithms that calculate measures of the difference between each time-slice of the spoken utterance and the word template to produce a metric representing the path through the alignment space with the smallest total difference (Sakoe and Chiba, 1987). While these methods can work well with isolated words, they have the disadvantage of tending to ignore temporal information from speech which can specify some phonemic differences ("bit" versus "bid") or prosodic information such as stress assignment (e.g. "the *record* is black" versus "they *record* music"). Furthermore, they are not terribly effective with vocabularies that are distinguished by consonants with rapid spectral transitions, such as the alphabet (Furui, 1986).

Another class of algorithms is based on interconnections of nodes through a network. The most common and well developed of these algorithms are called Hidden Markov Models (HMM) (Rabiner et al., 1983; Picone, 1990). In these algorithms, a set of nodes is chosen that is appropriate for a particular vocabulary. Five nodes, for example, could represent a vocabulary with words containing five or fewer phonemes. The nodes are ordered and connected from left to right, with recursive loops allowed. Recognition is based on a transition matrix of changing from one node to another and on a second matrix representing the probability that a particular set of co-eds (e.g. LPC) will be observed at each node. These matrices are generated iteratively from speech input during a training period. HMM recognizers are particularly well-suited for speaker-independent recognition because the speech used during training can be from multiple talkers.

Speech recognizers based on HMM algorithms are currently the type being most actively pursued commercially and in the laboratory. These include commercial large-vocabulary, speaker-independent, connected-word systems (*DragonDictate*, Baker, 1989; Tangora, Jelinek, 1985) and labora-tory-based large-vocabulary, speaker-independent, continuous speech systems (Schwartz et al., 1985; *Sphinx*, Lee, 1990).

The newest algorithms applied to speech recognition are also based on networks, but the nodes are more interconnected than for HMM. These algorithms are variously called (artificial) neural networks, parallel distrib-uted processes or connectionist models (Lippmann, 1987; Lippmann, 1989).

In neural networks, nodes exist in several layers. Input nodes receive information, usually as coded speech. The network is updated synchro-nously at time intervals (for speech, every 5-20 ms), receiving new inputs and propagating information through the rest of the network. The output nodes represent output status, or response, which signals that a particular event has been recognized. Between the input and output nodes are one or more *hidden layers* of nodes. Connections between nodes may go forward towards output nodes, sideways within hidden layers, or backwards, and can be recursive or have delays built in. The networks are roughly analo-gous to biological neurons such that information is passed as the result of the weighted sums of firings of input connections to a node, causing that node to fire if a threshold is exceeded.

Neural networks are being applied to a variety of speech tasks. They have been particularly successful with accurate recognition of some of the most difficult phoneme identifications, such as stop consonant pairs (Elman and Zipser, 1988; Waibel, 1989a), nasals and sonorants (Watrous, 1990), and fricatives (Waibel, 1989b). Much of the success of the neural network approach appears to derive from recursive or time delay networks, which are well suited to ignoring the temporal variability that is undesirable in speech (Waibel, 1989b), while capturing the temporal features that mark prosodic distinctions within words or groups of words (Port, 1990). It is widely expected that significant progress in phonemic speech recognition will be made through neural network algorithms (Lippmann, 1989).

3.4 Second Level Algorithms

The recognition methods discussed so far (excluding phonetic methods) work well for small vocabularies and isolated words. As vocabularies exceed 100 words, performance will improve by adding another level of structure to the recognition system. This may be done in many ways. In some systems, a second level is built into the first-level algorithms. For example, input signals may be sorted into sets of acoustic pattern possibilities according to gross acoustic features (e.g. words beginning with fricatives versus stops). After this gross partitioning, the recognition algorithms perform a detailed analysis to determine which words the input matches within each partition (Zue, 1985).

Alternatively, syntactical or grammatical restrictions on word order might be built into word recognition. In this approach, recognition of a word is aided by knowing that it is preceded or followed by other words. Such analysis can be useful for smaller vocabulary systems in which fixed types of natural sentences (e.g. questions only) are to be recognized. A similar approach is to allow the user to specify a (perhaps artificial) syntactic structure for a particular vocabulary. For example: "INSERT ... PART A ... PART B" instead of "Take Part A and insert it into Part B". In this case the second level of processing is left to the user who may develop a specified syntax for faster recognition.

In connected- or continuous-speech recognition, second level algorithms are essential for processing input at all levels of analysis (Lee, 1990). In continuous-speech systems there are usually many linguistic levels developed as separate program modules, and the more complex systems are more properly called speech understanding systems. These levels interact both from the bottom up, and from the top down. For example, suppose the specific speech recognition problem is an airline reservation system (Levinson and Shipley, 1980). In such cases, knowledge about other words in the sentence (e.g. "a frequent...") may be used at a semantic or pragmatic level to help make decisions at lower levels (e.g. next word probably begins with "f", i.e. flier). Future success of speech understanding systems will depend on the successful integration of information between these processing levels.

4. Defining Your Speech Recognition Needs

How can a potential user evaluate the performance of a product before purchasing it? Most systems advertise 98 to 99 percent accuracy, without much explanation on how this performance was determined. Performance standards for the industry have been needed for a long time, and are now being actively developed by the National Bureau of Standards using their data base. However, since standards are not presently available, the sections below are designed to assist readers in interpreting the marketing literature, and in evaluating and possibly modifying their applications for a particular recognizer. Appendix B lists some of the recognizers currently being marketed.

4.1 Application Environment

Choosing a speech recognizer requires a careful analysis of the application environment. One approach would be to identify the recognition problems that *must* be solved in this application, following the subdivisions described in Section 2. Can this application use isolated words as input, or must it use continuous speech? Or could users adapt to connected word recognition with the requirement that little pauses be inserted between words? Very few continuous speech recognizers are on the market, and they are expensive ($4,000 to $50,000). Continuous speech recognition would probably be chosen, therefore, only when no other type of recognizer provides an acceptable solution.

Another consideration is the relative value of mediocre performance that can be provided by a low cost ($600) recognizer. Whereas such performance might rule out a speech recognizer in some cases, in other applications, such as with the physically handicapped, reduced performance would be outweighed by the gain in communication at an affordable price.

4.2 Vocabulary

Many applications can use a fixed vocabulary recognizer. The advantage of such systems is that they can be honed for high accuracy with a particular vocabulary. Such systems include those that recognize only ten digits, specialized vocabularies (for example, radiology), as well as some with rather large vocabularies for dictation. The choice of the vocabulary affects both the accuracy of word recognition and the recognition response time. That is, the smaller the vocabulary, the better the recognition performance (and the lower the cost). Some applications require that a vocabulary of a particular size and type be used, e.g. in an electronic mail system, a text editor, or a spreadsheet interface. In these cases, the maximum allowable vocabulary storage available in the recognizer must fit the application. Users should consider, however, that systems often allow several different vocabularies to be stored. When it is easy to switch between vocabularies, the absolute size of the vocabulary is not as important.

If vocabulary items can be selected by the user, best performance is achieved for acoustically distinct words. One classic example of the limitation of speech recognition is the inability to identify the letters of the alphabet. This is because many of them are acoustically very similar, such as the "e-set" consisting of {b, c, d, e, g, p, t, v, and z}. In fact, the e-set and the set of 39 alphadigits have become almost standard vocabularies for testing recognition performance. Since recognizers are generally inaccurate when acoustically similar words make up the vocabulary, potential users must determine whether this constraint is acceptable for the application.

4.3 Speaker Dependence and Training Methods

Most speech recognizers on the market are *speaker dependent* and must be trained to recognize individual users' voices. There are only a few speaker independent systems available, and even they usually need some training (enrollment) to adapt to a new speaker. If a particular application requires speaker independence, for example a voice warning system, then the limitations of the available systems must be carefully considered.

Training methods for speaker-dependent methods should be considered before selecting a recognizer. When the user selects the vocabulary, templates associated with each word must be trained. This process usually requires at least three repetitions of each word. Once a person has made the templates for a vocabulary, they are stored in a file or on a separate mini-cartridge which can be retrieved by the user. Of course, separate template files must be made for each user. For vocabularies greater than 100 words, this can be a fairly tedious process. Once it is done, however, updating procedures are usually provided to easily make small changes in the vocabulary, or to handle problems with poor templates.

For fixed vocabularies, and especially large vocabularies, the training methods consist of obtaining a sample of each person's speech. This could take the form of reading a specific subset of the vocabulary, or perhaps reading some material for some length of time until the system reaches a reasonable criteria of recognition performance. These systems are delivered with "appropriate" templates already stored for each word. There might be just one of these prototype templates for each word, or there might be several representative templates for each. The task of the training process is to adapt the recognizer to each voice. Some of these systems continue to adapt to the talker while in use. In many of these systems, the training process needs to be repeated each time the talker changes, as there is no procedure for storing many individual training histories.

5. Future Speech Recognition Systems

Given the limitations of the speech recognition algorithms today, there is plenty of room for improvement. The largest research efforts are devoted to large and very large vocabulary systems (Baker, 1989; Deng et al., 1989; Lee, 1990). There are many researchers who believe that present speech recognition technology, which is based on statistical methods, cannot be simply improved on to achieve the goal of reliable, large vocabulary, continuous speech recognition. This goal can only be achieved, it is thought, by using phonetically based recognizers, or perhaps using neural networks, with the addition of a top-down, speech understanding system incorporating linguistic and pragmatic knowledge. The government is funding the development of such systems at MIT and Carnegie-Mellon University, among others. Unfortunately, progress toward completing these systems is slow, and cost-effective commercial products cannot be expected in the near future.

6. References

Baker, J. (1989). DragonDictate—30K: Natural Language Speech Recognition with 30,000 words. *Proceedings of Eurospeech 89*, European Conference on Speech Communication and Technology, Paris.

Christiansen, R. & Rushforth, C. (1977). "Detecting and locating key words in continuous speech using linear predictive coding," *EEE Trans.ASSP*, 25, 361–367.

Cohen, J.R. (1989). "Application of an auditory model to speech recognition," *Journal of the Acoustical Society of America* 85, 2623–2629.

Cole, R., Stern, R. & Lasry, M. (1986). "Performing fine phonetic distinctions: templates vs. features," *Invariance & Variability in Speech Processes*, (J. Perkell & D. Klatt, eds.) Erlbaum: Hillsdale, NJ, 325–341.

Dautrich, B., Rabiner, L. & Martin, T. (1983). "On the effects of varying filter bank parameters on isolated word recognition," *IEEE Trans.ASSP*, 31, 793–807.

Denes, P. & Matthews, M.W. (1960). "Spoken digital recognition using time-frequency pattern matching," *Journal of the Acoustical Society of America*, 32, 1450–1455.

Deng, L., Lennig, M. & Mermelstein, P. (1989). "Use of vowel duration information in a large vocabulary word recognizer," *Journal of the Acoustical Society of America*, 86, 540–548.

Elman, J.L. & Zipser, D. (1988). "Learning the hidden structure of speech," *Journal of the Acoustical Society of America*, 83, 1615–1626.

Furui, S. (1986). "Speaker-independent isolated word recognition using dynamic features of speech spectrum," *IEEE Trans.ASSP*, ASSP-34(1), 52–59.

Ghitza, O. (1987). "Auditory nerve representation criteria for speech analysis/synthesis," *IEEE Trans.ASSP*, 35, 736–740.

Haltsonen, S. (1981). "Improvement and comparison of three phonemic segmentation methods of speech," *Proc. IEEE Int. Conf. ASSP*, 1160–1163.

Hermansky, H. (1990). "Perceptual linear predictive (PLP) analysis of speech, " *Journal of the Acoustical Society of America*, 87, 1738–1752.

Higgins, A. & Wohlford, R. (1985). "Keyword recognition using template concatenation," *Proc. IEEE Int. Conf. ASSP*, 1233–1236.

Jelinek, F. (1985). "The development of an experimental discrete dictation recognizer," *Proc. IEEE*, 73, 1616–1620.

Joseph, R. (1989). "Large vocabulary voice-to-text systems for medical reporting," *Speech Technology*, 4 (4), 49–51.

Lamel, L., Rabiner, L., Rosenberg, A. & Wilpon, J. (1981). "An improved endpoint detector for isolated word recognition," *IEEE Trans. ASSP*, 29, 777–785.

Lee, K., Hon, H. & Reddy, R. (1990). "An overview of the SPHINX speech recognition system," *IEEE Trans. ASSP*, 38(1), 35–45.

Levinson, S.E. & Shipley, K.L. (1980). "A conventional-mode airline information and reservation system using speech input and output," *The Bell System Technical Journal*, 59(1), 1980.

Lippmann, R.P. (1987). "An introduction to computing with neural nets, " *IEEE ASSP Mag.*, 4–22.

Lippmann, R.P. (1989). "Review of neural networks for speech recognition," *Neural Computation*, 1, 1–38.

Meisel, W.S., Fortunato, M.P. & Michalek, W.D. (1989). "A phonetically-based speech recognition system," *Speech Technology*, 4(4), 44–48.

Mermelstein, P. (1975). "Automatic segmentation of speech into syllable units," *Journal of the Acoustical Society of America*, 58, 880–883.

Neary, T. (1989). "Static, dynamic, and relational properties in vowel perception," Journal of the Acoustical Society of America, 85, 2088–2113.

O'Shaughnessy, D. (1987). *Speech Communication: Human and Machine,* Reading, MA: Addison-Wesley Publishing Company.

Peterson, G.E. & Barney, H.L. (1952). "Control methods used in a study of the vowels," *Journal of the Acoustical Society of America,* 24, 182.

Picone, J. (1990). "Continuous speech recognition using hidden Markov Models," *IEEE Trans. ASSP,* ASSP-7, 26–41.

Port, Robert (1990). Representation and recognition of temporal patterns. *Connection Science* (2) 1–2, 151–176.

Rabiner, L. & Wilpon, J. (1980). "A simplified, robust training procedure for speaker trained, isolated word recognition systems," *Journal of the Acoustical Society of America,* 68, 1271–1276.

Rabiner, L., Levinson, S. & Sondhi, M. (1983). "On the application of vector quantization and hidden Markov models to speaker-independent isolated word recognition," *Bell Sys. Tech. Journal,* 62, 1075–1105.

Rabiner, L.R. & Wilpon, J.G. (1987). "Some performance benchmarks for isolated word speech recognition systems," *Computer Speech and Language,* 2, 343–357.

Sakoe, H. & Chiba, S. (1978). "Dynamic programming algorithm optimization for spoken word recognition," *IEEE Transactions on Acoustics, Speech, and Signal Processing,* ASSP–26, 43–49.

Schwartz, R., Chow, Y., Kimball, O., Roucos, S., Krasner, M. & Makhoul, J. (1985). "Context-dependent modeling for acoustic-phonetic recognition of continuous speech," presented at the IEEE Int. Conf. Acoust., Speech, Signal Processing, April 1985.

de Souza, P. (1983). "A statistical approach to the design of an adaptive self-normalizing silence detector," *IEEE Tans. ASSP,* 31, 678–684.

Waibel, A., Hanazawa, T., Hinton, G., Shikano, K. & Lang, K. (1989a). "Phoneme recognition using time-delay neural networks," *IEEE Trans. ASSP,* ASSP–37, 328–339.

Waibel, A., Sawai, H. & Shikano, L. (1989b). "Modularity and scaling in large phonemic neural networks," *IEEE Trans. ASSP,* ASSP-37, 1888–1897.

Wakita, H. (1977). "Normalization of vowels by vocal-tract length and its application to vowel identification," *IEEE Trans. ASSP*, 25, 183–192.

White, G.M. & Neely, R.B. (1976). "Speech recognition experiments with linear prediction, bandpass filtering, and dynamic programming," *IEEE Trans. ASSP*, 24, 183–187.

Wilpon, J., Rabiner, L. & Martin, T. (1984). "An improved word-detection algorithm for telephone-quality speech incorporating both syntactic and semantic constraints, " *AT&T Bell Labs Tech. Journal*, 54, 297–315.

Zue, V. (1985). "The use of speech knowledge in automatic speech recognition," *Proc. IEEE*, 73, 1602–1615.

7.1 Annotated References

For a review of a the ARPA speech understanding project which highlights many of the difficulties of constructing this type of system see: Klatt, D.K. (1977). "Review of the ARPA understanding project," *Journal of the Acoustical Society of America 62*, 1345–1366.

This collection includes some of the most important early technical papers on speech recognition: Dixon, N.R. & Martin, T. B. (1978). *Automatic Speech and Speaker Recognition*, IEEE press, Selected Reprint Series.

This book broadly covers issues on speech recognition: Lea, W.A. (1980). *Trends in Speech Recognition*, Prentice Hall, Englewood Cliffs, NJ.

For a more technical review of the following types of recognizers, see: Rabiner, L.R. & Levinson, S.E. (1981). "Isolated and connected word recognition-theory and selected applications," *IEEE Trans, on Communications 29*, 621–659.

For a current technical tutorial on speech recognition, especially research on continuous speech recognition see: Vaissiere, J. (1985). "Speech Recognition: A Tutorial," in *Computer Speech Processing*, F. Fallside and W. Woods (eds.), Prentice Hall International, Englewood Cliffs, NJ.

This magazine is devoted to speech applications, especially reviews of current products: *Speech Technology*, published by Media Dimensions, Inc., 42 East 23rd Street, New York, NY, 10010.

Chapter 10

Psychological and Human Factors Issues in the Design of Speech Recognition Systems

Demetrios Karis and Kathryn M. Dobroth
GTE Laboratories Incorporated

1. Introduction

During the past decade, automatic speech recognition (ASR) technology has improved at a dramatic rate. However, spoken interaction with machines that use ASR continues to be quite different from natural conversations that occur effortlessly between humans. To carry on a conversation with a human, a machine will obviously need to do much more than recognize individual words; it will need to produce speech, to understand what is being said to it, and to have extensive knowledge of conversational dynamics and discourse structure. Integrating these capabilities into a single system will require developments in the fields of artificial intelligence, natural language processing, computer science, digital speech processing, and the behavioral sciences.

In this chapter, we will argue that it is important to understand human conversational behavior even when designing simple systems that employ ASR. We provide examples from efforts to automate services with speech recognition, and analyze in detail the problems encountered in attempts to introduce automation over the public switched telephone network (PSTN). Although the PSTN imposes its own set of severe constraints on speech recognition systems, we focus primarily on the psychological and human factors issues that should generalize to all ASR applications. When effective speech-based interfaces are developed, individuals will be able to interact with computers via a telephone to perform a wide variety of tasks, including querying databases, performing financial transactions, and receiving assistance from expert systems about tasks that involve repair or diagnosis (of anything from cars to computers to humans).

We begin by reviewing current telephone-based applications: the problems encountered, and the lessons learned. Our review is limited, to some extent, by the lack of complete documentation on most field trials. We also provide descriptive data from over 500 recorded telephone service transactions. These data describe some of the acoustic characteristics of users' environments, as well as several aspects of human conversational behavior. In discussing field trials, we propose a broad perspective for system evaluation and demonstrate how focusing on recognition performance alone can lead to misleading estimates of system performance. Throughout the paper we assume that a decision has already been made to use ASR as a central part of an automated system, and we do not compare the relative merits of speech recognition to other techniques, such as tone dialing from push-button phones.

Human conversation is a collaborative process with great flexibility. In our longest section, on user-interface design, we argue that if automated systems are to succeed they must incorporate some of the flexibility of human conversations, especially with respect to error recovery. User-interface principles or guidelines may be useful at times to a system designer, but the only way to ensure the quality and efficiency of a user interface is through an iterative design process. We are currently engaged in a project to introduce automation using ASR, and we discuss the five-stage approach that we have adopted, which is based in part on published accounts of previous field trials, as well as current techniques for user-interface design. We end by describing more advanced capabilities that will be required for both near- and far-future applications, identifying areas where research is needed, and discussing the difficult problems that must be overcome. To give a general idea of the vocabulary requirements of future systems, we present data on the number of words telephone customers use when calling a customer service center to install or disconnect service.

2.   Current Applications

The reason for introducing automation is primarily to save costs. Telephone operator services, for example, are often targeted because of the large potential savings for telephone companies; one estimate of the cost savings from automating all collect calls within the local access and transport area (LATA) exceeds 200 million dollars nationwide each year (Lennig, 1989). To be successful, new applications should also, of course, benefit customers. Most new services would eliminate waiting for an operator or service representative, and would provide 24-hour access. As the success of automatic teller machines attests, these two attributes alone can lead to favorable customer evaluations. In addition, given estimates of the work force available for operator-level jobs, it may be hard to maintain current staff levels without automation.

There has already been a wide variety of application trials involving automation using ASR over the PSTN. The largest trials, primarily by AT&T, Bell Communications Research (Bellcore), and the regional Bell operating companies (RBOC's), involve automating operator services. These include automating the verification of collect and third number billed calls (Bellcore: Adams and Lewin, 1989; Bell-Northern Research: Lennig, 1989; International Telecharge, Inc.: Tagg, 1988), intercept operator number identification (where an operator asks, "What number did you dial?")(NYNEX: Levas, 1988; Rubin-Spitz and Yashchin, 1989; Yashchin *et al.*, 1989), directory assistance call completion (Basson *et al.*, 1989), and identifying the type of 0+ call intended (Mikkilineni and Perdue, 1989). Other trials have included speech-recognition-based directory assistance for 976 services (Lennig and Mermelstein, 1988), voice dialing by speaking digits (Gagnoulet, 1989), data entry by merchants for American Express credit authorization (Bounds and Prusak, 1989), a stock quotation system (AT&T: Mikkilineni and Perdue, 1989), collecting seven-digit telephone numbers for recognition experiments (Wilpon, 1985), and voice dialing by speaking a name (Chang *et al.*, 1989; see also Immendorfer, 1985; Rabiner *et al.*, 1980). An automated alternate billing service offered by Northern Telecom is now in operation in several regions of the country, including most of the Midwest in the Ameritech RBOC's region (Bossemeyer *et al.*, 1990; Murphy *et al.*, 1991). In this service, the billed party is asked whether he or she will accept the charges by responding "yes" or "no." Operator number identification, incorporating continuous digit recognition, is also currently in operation (Schrage *et al.*, 1990).

In many field trials, services are often simulated by using a human instead of an ASR device. Callers think they are interacting with a completely automated system because they hear only recorded prompts, but their verbal responses are recognized by a human listener, not a machine. The human listener types commands into the system based on the caller's responses, and these commands lead to the playing of new recorded prompts. Such simulations are used to record the caller's responses in order to evaluate the automatic speech recognizer off-line, or to evaluate the effectiveness of automation using ASR. (This procedure is discussed in more detail in Section 7.)

From the available data on field trials and laboratory simulations, which are often found only in conference proceedings, it is clear that successful applications using currently available technology must involve highly constrained interactions between a caller and the automated system. Vocabulary size must be quite small and is generally limited to a subset of "zero," "oh," 1-9, "yes," "no," and a small set of other words. All current applications are intended for speaker-independent recognition except one, voice dialing, in which a residential user must train the recognizer before use. The recognizer can be located either in the central office or on the customer's premises. In addition, most systems require users to speak isolated words or digits (where isolation is usually defined as including pauses of at least 200 ms between words). Interacting with the system must be very simple, and users should be able to recover from errors and be able to reach a human operator if desired.

3.   The Physical and Acoustical Environment

3.1   The Public Switched Telephone Network (PSTN)

The nature of the PSTN and the user population combine to create enormous problems for introducing automation using ASR. Although we focus in this paper on the human user of these systems and the nature of verbal communication, it is worth briefly listing the problems introduced by telephone transmission. First, of course, the reduced bandwidth of 300 - 3400 Hz cuts out much of the high frequency components of some speech sounds. This problem may eventually disappear with the introduction of Integrated Services Digital Network (ISDN) if the increased bandwidth is used to extend the range to 7000 Hz. Since complete ISDN coverage to residential customers will take decades to implement, the near-term implications of ISDN will affect only business customers. There is also a great deal of variability in frequency characteristics and gain of transmission lines. In one field trial, for example, signal-to-noise ratios varied from 10 to 60 dB (Wilpon and Rabiner, 1983). There may be echo and crosstalk, as well as a variety of noises that can be superimposed over speech, including loud static, pops and clicks, tones, and humming (Wilpon, 1985). Other sources of variability that affect the speech signal include telephone microphones (e.g., standard carbon vs. dynamic), how loud an individual speaks, and the distance between a speaker's mouth and the handset (Kahn and Gnanadesikan, 1986).

3.2   The Acoustic Environment and Human Conversational Behavior

Our focus in this paper is the end user, typically a residential telephone customer, and the problems encountered in trying to design an automated system that can be effectively used by untrained users who reflect the diversity of the general population. Three issues must be confronted: the nature of spoken language itself, the nature of the interaction between a human and a machine, and the physical environment of the user. We have been able to collect data relevant to the first and third issues by recording, transcribing, and cataloging 518 conversations (40 hours) between customers and service representatives in a GTE residential Customer Service Order Center in California. The conversations involved a number of topics, including requests for installing new service, changes in service, disconnecting service, and information. The conditions under which the recordings were made, and the dimensions on which calls were cataloged, are described in detail in Dobroth, Zeigler, and Karis (1989). In addition, several subsets of the conversations were analyzed using a software-based language analysis tool called Systematic Analysis of Language Transcripts (SALT, Miller and Chapman, 1982). SALT provided us with word lists, distribution of speech between the customer and the representative, and frequencies of speech events that were indicated in the transcripts by specialized punctuation. Our findings included the following.

- Over one-third of all calls (40.2%) contain noticeable background auditory impairment *unrelated* to telephone line quality, including talking (19.1% of all conversations), television or music (13.3%), traffic (7.1%), and other sounds (9.1%).

- Simultaneous speech is a common occurrence in human conversation: 14.4% of customer utterances and 12.1% of representative utterances from a subset of 50 conversations contained some simultaneous speech.

- Customers produce a significant amount of extraneous vocal output: 22.9% of customer utterances contained stuttering or nonword vocalizations (such as "umm"), 8.4% of customer utterances were false starts (in which they began speaking, stopped without finishing their thought, and then continued), and 2.7% of customers conversed with third parties during the interaction.

- Customers frequently use backchannels: 24% of customer speaking turns are backchannels, which are crudely defined as speaking turns that consist of one word and do not follow a question (e.g., "uhhuh").

When confronted with an automated system rather than a person, there is evidence that people will change their patterns of speaking, such as by using fewer "out-of-vocabulary" words (Mikkilineni and Perdue, 1989; Rubin-Spitz and Yashchin, 1989; see Hauptmann and Rudnicky, 1988, for an empirical investigation). However, many aspects of human spoken communication are so overlearned and automatic that they are difficult to modify, especially on the first encounter with an automated system. For example, it is so natural to speak continuously, with no pauses between words, that many people have difficulty in modifying this behavior when instructed to do so. (This problem will be discussed in detail in Section 5.)

4.   Accuracy/System Evaluation

Recognizers are usually evaluated in terms of the percentage of utterances that are accurately recognized. It is appropriate to focus on this measure of recognizer accuracy in research devoted to improving recognition algorithms, but it can be misleading to assume recognition performance is closely related to the performance of the entire system. High recognition accuracy is necessary, but not sufficient. In fact, other factors are often more important than recognizer accuracy in contributing to overall system performance. In this section, we discuss some of these factors and describe different measures of recognition performance, string accuracy, the differences between performance in the lab and in the field, and the need for multiple criteria for evaluating overall system performance.

4.1   Measures of Recognition Performance

Most published studies focus only on the percentage of correct recognition, and present little or no other data, which can make it difficult to accurately evaluate or compare recognizers. The percentage of correct recognitions can be manipulated by varying the criterion for accepting an utterance, in accord with signal detection theory. By setting a high criterion, accuracy will increase when the recognizer makes a choice, but the number of rejections, or deletion errors, where the recognizer detects an input but is unable to make a choice, will also increase. For example, when the recognizer was forced to make a decision, Wilpon (1985) found a 14% error rate (0% no decision), which decreased to 10% errors with 9% no decisions, and 1% errors with 60% no decisions. There is also a trade-off between rates for false acceptance and false rejection (see Lennig, 1990, for trade-off curves) and most system designers usually consider reducing the false acceptance rate as critical. If a person says "no" and the recognizer output is "yes," there is a false acceptance; if the recognizer rejects the input there is a false rejection.

In addition to reporting correct recognition and rejection rates, it is important to report substitution and insertion errors (Pallett, 1985). Insertion errors occur when the recognizer reports a word in the absence of any verbal input, whereas substitution involves replacing the word actually spoken with another word.

4.2 Accuracy of Strings Versus Isolated Digits or Words

If the success of a single transaction involves entering a string of digits or words, then it is string accuracy that is important, not the accuracy of an isolated utterance. Assuming independence, the accuracy of recognizing a string of N isolated utterances is the average accuracy for an isolated utterance raised to the Nth power. Thus, for a recognizer that is 95% accurate on isolated digits, performance on a 10-digit string will fall to $(.95)^{10}$, or 60%, while 99% accuracy for isolated digits falls to a level of 90% for string accuracy. Improvements in three areas will increase string performance: the recognizer itself, the use of higher level knowledge such as syntax, and effective error recovery strategies.

4.3 Recognizer Performance in Lab Versus Field

Given the problems recognizers face from the telephone network and the general public, it is not surprising that there are dramatic differences in performance between laboratory and field settings. For example, with voice dialing, errors increased from 8% to 25% from lab to field settings (Gagnoulet, 1989). When comparing recognition performance for isolated digits recorded over the PSTN to digits in the Texas Instruments database, which was recorded in a lab by 105 speakers (Yashchin *et al.*, 1989), digit accuracy decreased from approximately 90% for the lab recordings to 70% for the recordings made over the PSTN. Thus, performance data from both lab and field should be collected. In the lab, experiments can be conducted to isolate the effects of particular variables on recognizer performance, whereas only through field studies can an accurate assessment of recognizer performance be made. Some of the problems involved in transmission can be simulated, but there are no simulations that also include the ranges of background noise found in customers' homes, along with speaker variability and failure to interact with the system as intended. Since template sets created under laboratory conditions perform poorly in the field (Wilpon, 1985), template sets should be constructed from speech recorded over the PSTN under actual operating conditions. It may not be necessary, however, to recreate templates for different regions of the country (Wilpon, 1985; see also Barry *et al.*, 1989).

In most cases, little data are published from actual field trials, and care must be taken in evaluating published error rates. For example, Lynch (1989) reports an error rate of less than 1% from a database recorded over the PSTN (using an algorithm developed by Rabiner *et al.*, 1988). The database contained 1200 connected digit strings from each of 50 naive subjects. This level of performance is deceptively high, however, because 21% of the strings contained "gross mispronunciations" that were removed prior to analysis.

4.4 The Need for Multiple Criteria

Multiple criteria are necessary when evaluating the results of an automated application. Performance in completing the transaction successfully is generally of greatest importance from a human factors perspective, but other perspectives are also important. For example, customers' attitudes toward the system and their level of satisfaction should be assessed. One possible effect of customer attitudes on system performance is that some customers may abandon the call and hang up when they find themselves interacting with an automated system instead of with a human operator. Customers may even be dissatisfied with systems that are convenient and easy to use if these systems fail to meet all the customers' goals. For example, if it is important for someone to receive an apology from a service representative for a company mistake, then interacting with a machine will probably be unsatisfactory. There are also a variety of other factors, often application specific, that may be important in evaluating an automated system. In automating operator number identification, for example, the call duration (holding time) is important because it can affect trunk occupancy rates and switch capacity (Levas, 1988); replacing operators with an automated system will save money but, if holding times increase, lower labor costs may be offset by the need for higher capital expenditures.

When all of the factors that we have discussed are viewed together, it is clear that the success of the automated system as a whole is quite different from the accuracy rate of the recognizer alone. In one recent study, where recognition performance is reported as 98% correct, system performance is at less than 60% (Wilpon *et al.*, 1988). Also consider the AT&T field trial designed to collect seven isolated digits in order to test recognizer performance under real world conditions (Wilpon, 1985). When confronted with an automated system, 20% of the callers immediately hung up, on 31% of the calls an operator had to intervene, on 7% a human observer listening to the speech to check recognizer performance was unable to understand what was said, and on 4% of the calls the caller spoke more than seven digits. This removed 62% of the calls. Of the remaining 38% of the calls, 65% contained only isolated digits as required by the recognizer. Only these calls, 25% of the total, contained acceptable input, and once string recognition performance was considered, the percentage of all calls that could be accurately handled fell to 11%. Another constrained application is intercept operator number identification, where the caller needs only to respond with the digits of the called number. In the NYNEX field trial, since only 39% of callers responded with a telephone number, Levas (1988) estimated a speech automation rate of 0 to 20% after recognition performance is also considered. In trials to automate 0+ dialing, customers are prompted with the message, "At the tone, please say collect, calling card, third-number, person, or operator." Only between 60 and 70% responded with a correct word as an isolated utterance (Mikkilineni and Perdue, 1989; Wilpon *et al.*, 1988).

5. Typical Problems Encountered in Current Systems

Field studies have revealed a number of serious problems that are not directly related to recognizer performance. In particular, there are two common problems that can have serious consequences. The first is the tendency to speak in a continuous manner, which is so strong that it is difficult to override. For example, in one large study, where 1,364 customers were requested to speak the digits of the telephone number they were dialing with pauses between each digit, only 37% left appropriate pauses between digits (Yashchin *et al.*, 1989). Although most studies reviewed here used recognizers that require isolated input, there are now speaker independent continuous digit recognizers on the market that appear promising (e.g., Voice Processing Corporation; see Vitale, 1989).

The second serious problem is that users often respond with words and utterances not included in the vocabulary. Out-of-vocabulary responses can be a major problem even with a yes/no vocabulary, and there are also problems with pronunciation. When explicitly instructed to respond with "yes" or "no," users will frequently say "yeah," "sure," and "okay." Even "yes" often becomes "yes'm" or "yay-es" (Adams and Levin, 1989). "Yes" can be distorted in so many ways that "okay" is sometimes suggested as an alternate (Adams and Srenger, 1988; Adams and Lewin, 1989). This solution does not always work, however, because "yes" and "okay" are not completely interchangeable. In most situations involving verification (e.g., "Do you still live at 1234 Main Street?"), "okay" is not an acceptable affirmative response. In AT&T trials to automate identifying 0+ calls ("At the tone, please say collect, calling card, third number, person, or operator"), 19% of callers responded with an invalid word in one study (Mikkilineni and Perdue, 1989) while in another (reported in Bennett *et al.*, 1989, p. 29), 37% of callers "added extraneous utterances (e.g., *please* or *uhh*) or paraphrased the keywords (e.g., saying *reverse the charges* instead of *collect*) or said nothing." Even with reprompting, 40% still did not respond with an isolated item. In another application involving a financial information service (Mikkilineni and Perdue, 1989), users were given written instructions and lists of stocks, each associated with a number. When callers were asked for a stock number, 14% responded with an out-of-vocabulary word and 8% gave no response. Recent advances in recognizing key words in multiword phrases (wordspotting) may aid in solving this problem (Wilpon *et al.*, 1990).

There are also problems associated with an individual's reaction to automated systems. Customers may hang up ("abandon" the call) when they realize they have contacted a machine. As discussed above, this occurred on 20% of the calls in Wilpon (1985) and in up to 63% of calls in the NYNEX study on operator number identification (Levas, 1988). In the NYNEX study, 22% of the customers hung up when they reached a human operator who asked for the number they were dialing. This jumped to 40% when callers were asked for the number by an automated system, and 63% when the system asked them to "dial one" (in order to determine if the call was from a phone with tone dialing capability). Another problem is that callers may not realize at first that they are interacting with a machine, and engage in a conversational style that is beyond the capabilities of the system (e.g., by interrupting or restating questions, Adams and Lewin, 1989). Using a synthetic speech greeting is one way to specify immediately that a machine will be involved in the interaction but there is little research to back up the usefulness of this technique.

Timing of conversational turns is another prevalent problem because people are not used to speaking at only designated times and have a tendency to speak before system prompts. Studies of speaker turn-taking have found that the interval between two speakers is often less than 50 ms (Walker, 1982). Listeners use a variety of cues to decide when a speaker will reach a turn-transition point where it is appropriate to take the floor. In many situations, listeners do not wait and either interrupt the speaker or talk simultaneously. As mentioned previously, in a subset of our conversation database, simultaneous speech occurs on 12.1% of the service representatives' utterances. Most current systems are unable to process speech input as they play speech prompts, and interruptions or simultaneous speech usually cause problems.

Problems often arise in recognizing the variety of ways in which people speak number strings. Telephone numbers, for example, are usually spoken as single digits ("four-four-three-five-eight-six-six") while, in other cases, especially for dollar amounts, words and numbers are mixed ("four million, four hundred and thirty-five thousand, eight hundred and sixty-six dollars"). In one application for credit-card authorization (Bounds and Prusak, 1989), the system designers tried to get merchants to speak dollar amounts as digits by varying the prompts. After several attempts, they gave up and argued that the answer lay in adapting the system to recognize numbers the way people naturally speak them, with an extended vocabulary and natural language processing, rather than trying to change users' responses.

6. User-Interface Design

People will always make errors — in speaking, in recognition, in understanding, and in action — regardless of whether they are interacting with another human or with an automated system. Errors can be reduced by good design, but never eliminated. The goal should be to create a system that allows a user to recover easily after taking some action that the system considers inappropriate. We take the position that if people have difficulty completing a transaction with an automated system, then the system is at fault, not the user, and therefore "training" or "educating" the user is not the solution. We believe that the solution is to incorporate good error recovery techniques in the final product, as well as following an iterative design process that involves testing the system during development to eliminate most system errors before final deployment. Since inexpensive, low-fidelity prototypes can be very effective in many situations (Fay *et al.*, 1990; Virzi, 1989), and because a fairly large percentage of user-interface problems can be identified by running a small number of subjects (Nielsen and Molich, 1990; Virzi, 1990), an iterative design process need be neither extremely expensive nor time consuming.

In developing a user interface, emphasis should be on principles of design and usability rather than adherence to any particular set of specific user-interface guidelines. Principles of design include focusing early on the users of the system and the tasks they will perform, collecting performance data using simulations and prototypes when possible, and iterating the process of collecting data, identifying problems, and modifying the system (Gould and Lewis, 1985; see Williges, Williges, and Elkerton, 1987, for a description of six "fundamental" principles of human-computer dialogue design). During the design process, a basic set of usability principles should be kept in mind, such as that provided by Nielsen and Molich (1990), and reprinted here:

- Use simple and natural dialogue.

- Speak the user's language.

- Minimize user memory load.

- Be consistent.

- Provide feedback.

- Provide clearly marked exits.

- Provide shortcuts.

- Provide good error messages.

- Prevent errors.

Evaluation need not be expensive nor time consuming to uncover a number of potential problems. Asking subjects to identify problems in a user interface design after giving them only a written description may uncover many of the major problems, and can be useful even with a small number of untrained users as subjects (Nielsen and Molich, 1990).

6.1   Dialogue Control

Conversation involves constant collaboration between participants, not an alternation between two states, one in which information is transmitted, the other in which it is received. Designing human-computer interaction based on this type of model may be adequate for command-based keyboard applications but will lead to serious problems in speech-based applications. Researchers now postulate that conversation proceeds along two separate, but simultaneous, levels (Schoeber and Clark, 1989; Waterworth, 1982). On one level, conversational participants accomplish tasks by asking questions, providing information, and indicating their intentions. Cox (1982) calls these "goal oriented acts." On the other level, people take extra conversational steps whose sole purpose is to control the flow of the interaction and to ensure that previous utterances have been understood. Examples include utterances such as "What?," "Slow down, please," "Did you get that?," "Okay, go on," or "I'm not sure I understood the first part of your explanation." These extra steps are called "dialogue control acts" (Cox, 1982; Waterworth, 1982). Their primary purpose is to prevent errors and allow for easy correction when errors do occur. Speakers can explicitly assert their level of recognition or understanding, or imply it indirectly.

Clark and Schaefer (1987, pp. 22-23) present an example centered around the utterance, "I just saw Julia." A listener could assert directly, "I didn't hear the last word," or provide the same information by asking, "You just saw what?," which also serves as proof that the listener correctly recognized the first three words. Asking, "And how is she?" implies the previous statement was both recognized and understood, while allowing the speaker to continue without saying anything is an implicit acceptance. Using dialogue control acts, a speaker can check whether the listener has understood while a listener can ask for information to be repeated, elicit additional information, control the rate of information delivery, or stop the flow of information when what has already been presented is sufficient.

A common approach to investigating the effects of dialogue control is to compare task performance in interactive conditions, where subjects can speak to each other freely, with performance in non-interactive conditions (Krauss and Weinheimer, 1966; Oviatt and Cohen, 1989; Schoeber and Clark, 1989). The presence of dialogue control acts seem to have three major effects on conversational behavior. First, speakers use fewer words. Second, participants can prevent communication errors by acknowledging and verifying previous utterances. Third, detection and recovery from errors is facilitated when the error recovery process is integrated into communication. Our perspective is that the more we can incorporate natural dialogue control techniques into an automated system, the easier the system will be to use and the easier it will be to recover from errors.

In typical interactions with automated systems there is an opening greeting, service identification, and instructions from the system, followed by a request from the user (Cox, 1982). How the interaction then proceeds, including the acceptable input vocabulary and output messages to the user, is defined by the dialogue structure. Dialogue control also includes how feedback is presented and how errors are handled. Dialogue control in current automated systems is severely impoverished compared to that exercised effortlessly by humans in normal conversations. This lack of capability leads, we believe, to much of the dissatisfaction customers often express after interacting with automated systems or when asked their opinion of future systems. Error recovery and feedback are part of dialogue control but are treated separately below, because with the limited intelligence presently available in automated systems these capabilities will probably be implemented independently. (See Young and Proctor, 1989, and Waterworth and Talbot, 1987, for research systems that provide considerable flexibility in dialogue structure for interactions with databases via telephone.)

6.1.1   Feedback and Timing

It is important that systems provide feedback to users, especially when the system is designed to be used by novices, so that users know their utterances have been recognized correctly. Feedback can be provided by repeating the input in a confirmatory phrase or as tones to indicate that the system has accepted the input as valid. Feedback provided concurrently (e.g., after each digit as opposed to after a string of digits) can be used to regulate the timing of the interaction, and also to catch errors at an early stage (Jones, Hapeshi, and Frankish, 1989). However, tones used to control the pace of the interaction are often judged to be unacceptable when they are presented immediately after individual responses (see Mulla and Vaughan, 1985). It is natural to group digits when speaking, and systems can be designed to provide feedback whenever a speaker pauses. In one such system (Tagg, 1988), if the speaker paused after saying "Five, one, two," for example, the system would respond "Five, one, two. Say 'yes' if correct, 'no' if wrong." This has the advantage of adapting to the speaker's style, but is slow. The system could be streamlined by omitting the "yes" response as a requirement; if the string was correct, the speaker could just continue the input, or give an appropriate command word. Otherwise, the speaker would respond "no." This technique can be used with either isolated or continuous speech recognizers. For the voice-dialing trial in France (Gagnoulet, 1989; Poulain and Tirbois, 1988), it was decided that speaking isolated digits was too slow to satisfy users. Since complete continuous recognition was not technically possible, callers were instructed to enter two digits at a time, such as "thirty-eight," or "fifty-two." This was reported to work well because speaking telephone numbers as a sequence of two-digit numbers is common in France. This requires, however, a vocabulary of about 30 words. In reciting credit card numbers in the United States, customers usually segment the digits into groups of three or four, and leave pauses between groups (Holmgren, 1983). This is probably influenced, to some extent, by the way digits are grouped on the card.

In general, the more words verified by a single feedback message the better, provided error rates are low (i.e., constant correction is not needed) and users feel confident with the system. Although the techniques described above may be required to ensure adequate levels of accuracy with current technology, they are unsatisfactory because they depart so radically from normal conversational behavior. It is unnatural, and inefficient, to explicitly verify every utterance. Eventually, explicit feedback will be required only when the user requests it. For a large part of a conversation, the continued coherence of the dialogue will provide implicit feedback that previous utterances have been processed correctly, as in human conversations. When the ASR system is uncertain about what the user said, it will ask for confirmation.

6.1.2. Error Recovery

Effective and efficient error handling has been a major problem for most automated systems. Human error recovery involves complex interactive processes acting continuously as part of dialogue control, but there are a variety of simple techniques that can be used in automated systems. For example, several error recovery or repair subdialogues can be designed, based on where in the dialogue the error occurs. These can revert to a smaller vocabulary to achieve higher recognition accuracy and can be combined with additional information or instructions (Cox, 1982). A recognizers' internal estimate of accuracy should interact with a dialogue control subsystem if possible. For example, when a recognizer makes a decision with a high level of confidence, no confirmation would be given and the dialogue could proceed. When a decision is made with less confidence, the system could respond with "Did you say —," rather than the typical request to repeat the word (Leiser and Brooks, 1988). If the first choice is rejected, the system can be designed to receive another input immediately after the "no" instead of including an additional prompt. For example, the system would be prepared to recognize "Thursday" in the following interaction. System: "Did you say 'Tuesday'?" User: "No, Thursday."

After the user identifies a mistake by the recognizer and speaks the word again, recognition systems can be designed to choose the next most likely word rather than making the same error twice. Consider the following scenario in the French system for voice dialing (Poulain and Tirbois, 1988): a user says "eighty" but "eighty-one" is recognized and displayed on an LCD as feedback for the subject. The user says "correction" and then "eighty." If "eighty-one" is again the best match, the recognizer should instead choose an alternative based on word scores and/or a confusion matrix, rather than making the same mistake a second time.

The careful analysis of human error recovery will provide ideas that may be implemented using current technologies. For example, when Clark and Schaefer (1987) analyzed 602 British Telecom directory assistance calls, they found that phone numbers were presented either all at once by the operator (e.g., "Cambridge one two three four five") or in installments ("one two [yes] three four five [yes]...," where "yes" is spoken by the customer). When numbers were presented all at once (83% of all cases), customers always responded vocally, either to acknowledge that they had correctly understood the number (83% of the time) or to initiate error recovery (17%). The majority of the responses involved the customer repeating all or some of the numbers back to the representative, indicating acknowledgment with final falling intonation and potential error with final rising intonation. This behavior was consistent across acknowledgments and error recovery initiations. The rest of the time, customers used phrases that were independent of the content of the transaction, such as "Right" or "Thank you" for acknowledgment, or "What did you say?" to initiate error recovery.

We see two implications in these data for error recovery techniques by spoken language systems. First, the majority of acknowledgments and requests for clarification depend on interpretation of intonation; the actual words in the request are often completely dependent on the content of what has been communicated (i.e., the listener repeats some of the speaker's words). Spoken language systems must be able to interpret the ways that people use intonation as well as to produce utterances whose intonation accurately reflects intent. Second, listeners appear to prefer to use recovery techniques that require the least amount of effort. In 57% of the error recovery initiations in the Clark and Schaefer (1987) study, customers indicated partial hearing by repeating a subset of the numbers with final rising intonation (e.g., "four five?"). The interpretation is that these customers do not necessarily want to start over at the beginning of the previous utterance, they just want the end repeated or verified. During partial recognition failures, the system could repeat what was recognized and then request, by adjusting prosody (pitch, loudness, duration), that the customer only repeat the section of the utterance that the system has failed to recognize.

6.1.3 Exiting the System
It should be possible to exit the system from any point and reach a human operator. This is especially important in services for the general public, and where callers do not know before calling that they will be interacting with an automated system. Although recognizers continue to improve dramatically, for the present some speakers will need to be transferred to an operator because the recognizer has trouble recognizing their speech. Simpson, McCauley, Roland, Ruth, and Williges (1987) estimate that 25% of the general population exhibits low consistency in pronunciation, and it may be many years until recognizers can deal with this variability.

6.2 Convergence

Convergence is the process by which conversational participants adopt aspects of one another's speech during the course of a conversation. Convergence has been documented in experimentally elicited conversations between humans in terms of lexical choice (Schoeber and Clark, 1989) and descriptions of game coordinates (Garrod and Anderson, 1987). Convergence in lexical choice (Holmgren, 1983), syntactic structure (Leiser, 1989), and intonation (Leiser *et al.*, 1987) has been found in interactions between humans and computers. By exploiting convergence of lexical choice, it is sometimes possible to modify a user's vocabulary by carefully choosing the system's responses. Holmgren (1983), for example, found that when 0 was spoken as "zero" in feedback messages, the percentage of subjects saying "zero" as input increased from 30% to 70% over twelve trials. Zoltan-Ford (1984) found experimental evidence that subjects interacting with an inventory control program modeled the style of their inputs on the program's outputs. Subject messages contained 60% more words when subjects heard "conversational" output phrases from the program versus terse messages. Subject input was also shaped by the program's error messages. For half of the subjects, input was acceptable only if it matched the vocabulary and message length used by the program. When input did not match, error messages were provided that contained the appropriate input format. Subjects in this condition generated over twice as many messages that conformed to the program's messages. These studies support the position that convergence in human-computer interaction can be useful for constraining the speech of the user without imposing unnatural, explicit constraints.

6.3 Combining Input: Voice and Tone Dialing

Although many applications can be automated using tone dialing input from push-button phones (DTMF), a frequent objection is that there is still a large percentage of rotary, or pulse dial, phones in operation. This is considered to be an additional reason for the use of speech recognition, especially in applications that could involve any telephone customer, such as accepting collect calls. For more specialized applications in industry, a high percentage of users will have tone dialing capability and, by combining voice and tone input, it may be possible to develop a more streamlined and efficient interface, given current ASR capabilities. Numbers can be entered quickly via push-buttons, while commands can be entered by voice, and information that may be beyond a recognizer's capability, such as street addresses, can be recorded for later transcription. In this way, a hybrid system can be created that can handle more complex problems than would be possible with voice input alone.

6.4   Prompt Messages

The general usability principles presented previously can be applied to prompt messages. Prompt messages should consist of simple and natural dialogue, should be expressed in language familiar to the user, should minimize the user's memory load, and should not use different words to mean the same thing. Several studies have demonstrated the importance of prompt wording for the success of the interaction (Gellman and Whitten, 1988; Yashchin *et al.*, 1989), and others have reported problems arising from ambiguous prompts. For example, in a phone-in competition designed to collect a large sample of speech from a diverse population (Millar *et al.*, 1988), callers recorded a slogan about telephone banking. When asked, "Would you like to record your slogan again?," the designers expected either "yes" or "no." To their surprise, some people started to speak their slogans immediately. The recommendation that "Instructions should be <u>very</u> clear, easy to follow, and short" (Adams and Lewin, 1989) is widely accepted, but what is not universally accepted is that the evaluation of clarity must involve users' perceptions and performance, not just the designer's opinion.

In designing prompt messages for an automated voice operated intercept service, the NYNEX field trial (Levas, 1988; Yashchin *et al.*, 1989) varied several prompt parameters, including speed (fast, slow), verbosity (wordy, concise), and prosodic modeling (whether or not the prompt contained pauses between words). Customers preferred the wordy prompts, prompt speed did not affect the accuracy with which the response was recognized, and normal prosody (no pauses) was preferred. The optimal dialogue was fast and wordy. Unfortunately, it may not be possible to generalize across applications. Preference and performance may be influenced by the nature of the application and the experience of the user. A short, constrained dialogue may require prompts that differ from those needed for a long, more flexible dialogue, and interfaces designed for frequent users will have to have additional features, such as the ability to choose a more streamlined set of prompts.

7.   Developing Automation with ASR: A Five-Stage Approach

From a user-interface perspective, we propose five stages for developing a new automated system that incorporates ASR. There are many variations to this approach, and whether ours is preferable to others must await further study. While reading the stages below, consider the automation of a service currently performed by an operator or service representative.

7.1 Stage 1

The first stage involves understanding the architecture of the service contact as it presently occurs between humans—the nature of the dialogue, the information exchanged, the vocabulary used, the time required, the frequency of confusions and misunderstandings, and so on. This stage includes a systematic acquisition and analysis of conversation data recorded at the application site, as well as studying procedure manuals and interviewing customer representatives and their supervisors. The aim is not necessarily to model the human-computer interaction after the human-human interaction, but to collect basic information about the nature of the task itself and the type of difficulties that presently occur. Some difficulties discovered in the human-human interaction will disappear with a constrained human-computer dialogue, while others, such as those related to misunderstanding the meaning of information provided, are independent of the interface and will present a problem to any type of automated system.

We used both the actual recordings of the conversations as well as transcripts to gather information in this stage. Our first step was simply to listen to the recorded conversations and catalog them. This did not require much time, and allowed us to calculate summary statistics for variables such as the average duration of the transactions, the percentage of volume accounted for by various call types, the number of callers with accents, and the number of calls made from severe acoustic environments. In the second step, we had the calls transcribed and then analyzed them with transcript analysis software. The second step was admittedly much more time consuming than the first step, but yielded valuable information about the size and characteristics of customer vocabulary. Having the transcripts available also greatly facilitates the systematic study of the architecture of service transactions. In the final step, the transcripts were used to help locate particular samples of speech in the recordings (e.g., all digit strings). These samples can now be acoustically analyzed to study variables such as customer input levels, and can also be used for template construction or to calculate rough estimates of recognizer performance.

7.2 Stage 2

Based on the information collected in stage 1, a preliminary dialogue for the user interface can be designed in stage 2, and a prototype of the system developed and tested in the lab using a "Wizard-of-Oz" technique. In this technique, a test subject hears recorded prompts and speaks to the system, thinking that it contains an ASR device; in reality, there is a human hidden from the user replacing machine recognition. The human observer, who is trained to simulate the capabilities of the proposed recognizer, acts as an intermediary between the subject and the system, inputting control commands, based on the subject's responses, or error messages reflecting recognition problems. For example, if the recognizer accepts only isolated words and the user speaks continuously, the human intermediary would reject the input. To investigate users' responses to recognizer problems, appropriate input can also be occasionally rejected. In this and succeeding stages, detailed subject performance data are collected and analyzed.

7.3   Stage 3
Based on the performance data collected during initial testing in stage 2, the user interface can be refined and then tested with actual customers at the application site using the Wizard-of-Oz technique described above. There are four reasons not to use the actual recognizer during this stage. First, the interface is not yet complete, particularly with respect to error recovery. Second, the human intermediary can change roles, if necessary, and talk directly with customers who are unable to complete their transactions. This capability may aid in gaining management approval for this stage of the field trial. Third, the recognizer has not yet been tested off-line with speech collected at the application site. Fourth, the human intermediary can simulate different levels of recognition errors for later evaluation. During this stage, user-interface modifications can be made and evaluated rapidly and iteratively. Note that from a customer's perspective, this system is indistinguishable from one that is completely automated, except when problems occur and the human intermediary intervenes.

7.4   Stage 4
Recognizer performance is evaluated in the lab using speech recorded at the application site during stage 3. This stage can start before stage 3 ends. The results of these tests are needed to determine the type and extent of error recovery procedures needed, and for estimating system performance.

7.5   Stage 5
A decision can be made on whether the system should be implemented based on system performance with near perfect recognition accuracy (from the human intermediary, stage 3 above), system performance with different levels of recognition errors (induced by the human intermediary, also from stage 3), and recognizer performance in the lab using realistic input obtained in the field (from stage 4). If implementation proceeds, the complete system, including the recognizer, is installed at the field site. Initially, human operators can monitor the system performance and intervene if required. Performance assessment should continue as before, with

information on every transaction collected. During initial evaluations, observers can listen to the entire transaction and rate recognizer performance and system performance on several measures, as well as rating customer attitude. If feasible, call-back interviews with callers should be arranged.

If possible, the laboratory prototype is updated using information gathered at the application site in stage 3, and new ideas are then tested first in the lab. It is possible to collect far more information from a lab prototype than from a field trial. Think aloud protocols can be collected in which subjects describe their thought processes as they interact with the system. Subjects can also be interviewed afterwards, and the effect of repeated exposure to the system can be examined by including multiple trials.

8.   Future Systems and Their Requirements

The ultimate goal of automatic speech recognition is often described as allowing natural, effortless communication between humans and machines. This requires human-level abilities in a wide variety of domains, not just speech recognition. Communication, in one view, "is not accomplished by the exchange of symbolic expressions. Communication is, rather, the successful interpretation by an addressee of a speaker's intent in performing a linguistic act" (Green, 1989, p. 1). Consider, for example, the utterance "Can you reach the hammer?" In most situations, this is interpreted as a request that you pass the hammer, not a question as to whether or not it is within your reach. Understanding the intent of a speaker is only one of several exceedingly difficult problems that future systems must overcome. In the next section we outline several others.

8.1   Conversational Computer Systems

There are four basic components to a conversational computer system, all highly interconnected: 1. speech recognition, 2. language comprehension (semantic interpretation), 3. understanding conversational dynamics and discourse structure, and 4. speech production (synthesis). Sophisticated systems cannot be developed around recognizers that rely only on the acoustical properties of speech. Syntax is already being used extensively in many research settings, including Carnegie Mellon (Rudnicky and Stern, 1989), Bolt, Beranek, and Newman (Makhoul, 1989), Stanford Research Institute, AT&T, Texas Instruments, and IBM, as well as in some commercial products. Eventually, however, recognizers must be combined with a system that has general world knowledge in order to consider the context of the utterance at levels much higher than syntactic, including the nature of the topic, the knowledge and background of the speaker, and perhaps even the time, location, and social situation.

People do not focus on identifying individual words or sentences, they focus on trying to understand the meaning of an utterance and the *intent* of the speaker. Many utterances do not, by themselves, contain enough information for accurate recognition, even by humans. Consider a classic example in the speech recognition field, the utterance "jeet." If you say "jeet," a listener will be unable to recognize this utterance as a standard word, and will not know what you mean. However, if you normally eat at noon, and if at noon a colleague steps into your office, carrying a small paper bag, and says, "Jeet yet?," you will probably know, first, that this is a contraction of "Did you eat yet?," and second, that the intent of this speech act is to invite you to lunch. Going from "Jeet yet?" to "If you have not yet eaten lunch, would you like to have lunch with me?" requires a lot of intelligence, which we tend to take for granted.

Language comprehension, the second component in a conversational computer system, involves a large collection of skills, abilities, and knowledge, and the complexities of creating a machine that understands language are similar to creating human-level machine intelligence. Natural language processing, another term for this area, is a major topic within artificial intelligence and computational linguistics, but natural language interfaces are still very limited and work well only in constrained domains (see Allen, 1987, for a review, and the journals *Computational Linguistics* and *Artificial Intelligence* for current research).

The third component required for automated conversational systems, knowledge of conversational dynamics, has received the least attention. "Effortless" spoken communication with machines will mean that the machine must have extensive knowledge of conversational dynamics and structure, including knowledge on turn-taking, backchannels ('uh-huh," "I see"), error recovery, simultaneous speaking, and interruptions. For example, the system should be able to determine when a speaker has finished a speaking turn or come to a "turn transition point" (using, perhaps, some combination of pitch, amplitude, and duration, as well as syntax), and should also be able to signal turn-transition cues in its responses to the user.

Our knowledge of the fourth component, speech synthesis, is improving rapidly, but extensive work is still required to produce human-sounding speech. Controlling the intonation, amplitude, and timing of synthetic speech will require complex models of speech production, as well as theories that relate speech production to language comprehension and conversational dynamics.

As conversational interfaces are incorporated into automated systems, new problems may arise. For example, when a system exhibits language capabilities by recognizing and producing speech, users may attribute more intelligence to the system than it really possesses and assume, incorrectly, that it also possesses other sophisticated cognitive abilities. Users may then talk in a more natural manner, expecting human-level abilities in error correction, problem solving, and natural language understanding. The dialogue will then "derail" when the system is unable to process the user's language.

8.2 Vocabulary Requirements

What are the vocabulary requirements for automated conversational systems? Our approach is to assume that vocabulary size should not surpass that of human-human conversations in the same domain. By characterizing vocabulary in the customer service contacts we recorded, we can obtain a fairly accurate estimate of the upper bounds of the vocabulary requirements for automated systems. We analyzed vocabulary in a subset of 52 conversations between telephone customers and service representatives in which customers disconnected service (N=28) or ordered new service (N=24). Two measures of vocabulary are commonly used: *types* (the number of different words) and *tokens* (the total number of words). The number of types used by a single customer ranged from 60 (tokens = 97) for a disconnect lasting 2:24 (2 minutes and 24 seconds) to 348 (tokens = 1531) for an installation order lasting 17:44. The mean number of types and tokens for disconnects and installations, per conversation, are presented in Table 1. Although considerable effort has been devoted to developing large vocabulary speech recognizers (some with up to 30,000 words), we found that less than 1,200 different words were used in the 24 installations we studied. Similar vocabulary requirements were reported in another domain, air-travel planning, where 1,076 different words were used in 48 conversations between travel agents and their customers (Kowtko and Price, 1989).

There are several questions we can address with our vocabulary data. For example, how large should a recognizer's vocabulary be to recognize some chosen percentage of the customer's words? This number can be estimated for disconnects by examining Figure 1, where number of different words is plotted against the cumulative percentage of total words used by customers. With a vocabulary made up of the 100 most frequently used words, slightly over 70% of all words are recognized, while with a 200-word vocabulary, 80% are recognized. Recognizing 90% requires about 350 words and, at this point, it becomes increasingly difficult to recognize a greater percentage of words, because new words added to the vocabulary are used infrequently in the conversations.

Table 1:   Mean Number of Types and Tokens per Conversation for Disconnects and Installations

	Disconnects	**Installations**
	N = 28	N = 24
Types		
M(SD)	105 (33)	188 (70)
Tokens		
M(SD)	214 (105)	534 (325)
Total types	763	1164
(all conversations)	(76 proper nouns)	(117 proper nouns)

Note. Total types refers to the number of different words used in all disconnects or all installations.

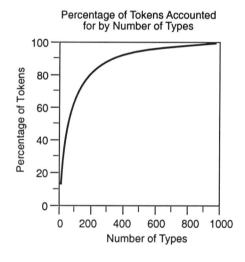

Figure 1   Types (different words), ranked by frequency, are represented along the X-axis, while the cumulative percentage of tokens (total words) used by customers is on the Y-axis. The curve represents the percentage of total words used by customers accounted for as a function of vocabulary size. For example, the 50 most frequently used words account for 56.8% of all words used. These data come from 28 calls in which telephone customers talk with service representatives to disconnect phone service.

9. Conclusions

During 1990, simple operator services were automated using a combination of automatic speech recognition and touch tone input. During the next decade, the automation of services using speech recognition will increase dramatically, and attempts will be made to automate fairly complex transactions. Advances in speech recognition technology are obviously needed, along with advances in artificial intelligence and natural language processing, but of equal importance is the overall design of these systems with respect to their capabilities for interacting with users. Future systems must take into account human conversational behavior, which we have described, as well as principles of user-interface design. An iterative design process will also be essential, and we have outlined a five-stage approach that should eliminate serious problems before a system is implemented. It is hard to predict exactly when fully conversational computer systems will be developed — in part because it is difficult even to specify what capabilities such systems will have. It is clear, however, that our ability to talk with computers to obtain services or information will improve significantly in the immediate future. The effectiveness of these systems, and their acceptance by the public, will depend in large part on the extent to which they have been designed to accommodate some of the flexibility inherent in human communication, rather than trying to force users to follow a script in which they are rigidly constrained in what they can say, and when they can say it.

10. Acknowledgments

We would like to thank David Fay, Sol Lerner, Bob Virzi, Lydia Volaitis, and Bonnie Zeigler for their comments on an early draft of this paper. Lydia Volaitis, in particular, helped us during the course of several hours of discussion on language processes and automation using speech recognition.

11. References

Adams, L. T., and Lewin, L. M. (1989). The human interaction component of incorporating speech recognition technology into the telephone network. *Conference Record of the International Conference on Communications*, 1, 1.1.1–1.1.6.

Adams, L. T., and Srenger, E. (1988). Considerations for speech recognition systems in automated telephone services. *Proceedings of the Annual Meeting of the American Voice I/O Society*.

Allen, J. (1987). *Natural Language Understanding*. Menlo Park, CA: The Benjamin/Cummings Publishing Company, Inc.

Barry, W. J., Hoequist, C. E., and Nolan, F. J. (1989). An approach to the problem of regional accent in automatic speech recognition. *Computer Speech and Language*, **3**, 355–366.

Basson, S., Christie, O., Levas, S., and Spitz, J. (1989). Evaluating speech recognition potential in automating directory assistance call completion. *Proceedings of the Annual Meeting of the American Voice I/O Society*, 271–276.

Bennett, R. W., Greenspan, S. L., Syrdal, A. K., Tschirgi, J. E., and Wisowaty, J. J. (1989). Speaking to, from, and through computers: Speech technologies and user-interface design. *AT&T Technical Journal*, Sept/Oct, 17–30.

Bossemeyer, R. W., Schwab, E. C., and Larson, B.A. (1990). Automated alternate billing services at Ameritech. *Journal of the American Voice I/O Society*, **7**, 47–53.

Bounds, A., and Prusak, M. (1989). Implementing speech recognition in an operational environment. *Proceedings of the Annual Meeting of the American Voice I/O Society*, 3–7.

Chang, H., Smith, A., and Vygotsky, G. (1989). An automated performance evaluation system for speech recognizers used in the telephone network. *Conference Record of the International Conference on Communications*, **1**, 1.2.1–1.2.5.

Clark, H. H., and Schaefer, E. F. (1987). Collaborating on contributions to conversations. *Language and Cognitive Processes*, **2**, 19–41.

Cox, A. C. (1982). Human factors investigations into interactions with machines by voice. *International Conference on Man/Machine Systems*, 254–257.

Dobroth, K. M., Zeigler, B. L., and Karis, D. (1989). Future directions for audio interface research: Characteristics of human-human order-entry conversations. *Proceedings of the Annual Meeting of the American Voice I/O Society*, 277–282.

Fay, D. Hurwitz, J., and Teare, S. (1990). The use of low-fidelity prototypes in user interface design. *Proceedings of the 13th International Symposium on Human Factors in Telecommunications*, 23–31.

Gagnoulet, C. (1989). Voice replaces dial in new public phones. *International Voice Systems Review*, **1**, 1.

Garrod, S. and Anderson, A. (1987). Saying what you mean in dialogue: A study in conceptual and semantic coordination. *Cognition, 27,* 181–218.

Gellman, L. H., and Whitten, W. B. (1988). Simulating an automatic operator service to optimize customer success. *Proceedings of the 12th International Symposium on Human Factors in Telecommunications.*

Gould, J. D., and Lewis, C. (1985). Designing for usability: Key principles and what designers think. *Communications of the ACM, 28,* 300–311.

Green, G. M. (1989). *Pragmatics and Natural Language Understanding.* Hillsdale, N.J.: Lawrence Erlbaum Associates.

Hauptmann, A. G., and Rudnicky, A. I. (1988). Talking to computers: An empirical investigation. *International Journal of Man-Machine Studies, 28,* 583–604.

Holmgren, J. E. (1983). Toward Bell system applications of automatic speech recognition. *The Bell System Technical Journal, 62,* 1865–1880.

Immendorfer, M. (1985). Voice Dialer. *Electrical Communication, 59*(3).

Jones, D., Hapeshi, K., and Frankish, C. (1989). Design guidelines for speech recognition interfaces. *Applied Ergonomics, 20,* 47–52.

Kahn, D., and Gnanadesikan, A. (1986). Experiments in speech recognition over the telephone network. *Proceedings of the International Conference on Acoustics, Speech, and Signal Processing,* 729–732.

Kowtko, J. C., and Price, P. J. (1989). Data collection and analysis in the air travel planning domain. *DARPA Speech and Natural Language Workshop.* Los Altos, CA: Morgan Kaufmann Publishers, 119–125.

Krauss, R. M., and Weinheimer, S. (1966). Concurrent feedback, confirmation, and the encoding of referents in verbal communication. *Journal of Personality and Social Psychology, 4,* 343–346.

Leiser, R. G. (1989). Exploiting convergence to improve natural language understanding. *Interacting with Computers, 1*(3).

Leiser, R. G., and Brooks, P. (1988). Natural language voice control of telecommunications services: Desirability and feasibility. *Proceedings of the 12th International Symposium on Human Factors in Telecommunications.*

Leiser, R. G., de Alberdi, M. J. I., and Carr, D. J. (1987). Generic issues in dialogue design for speech input/output. In F. Laver and M. A. Jack (Eds.), *Proceedings of the European Conference on Speech Technology,* Volume 2. Edinburgh: CEP.

Lennig, M. (1989). Using speech recognition in the telephone network to automate collect and third-number-billed calls. *Proceedings of Speech Technology '89*,124–125.

Lennig, M. (1990). Putting speech recognition to work in the telephone network. *IEEE Computer*, **23**, 35–41.

Lennig, M., and Mermelstein, P. (1988). First public trial of a speech-recognition-based 976 directory. *Proceedings of Speech Technology '88*, 291–292.

Levas, S. (1988). Automation potential of operator number identification (ONI) intercept services. *Speech Technology*, Mar./Apr., 26–29.

Lynch, J. F. (1989). A speaker independent connected digit recognizer for use over telephone lines. *Proceedings of Speech Technology '89*, 137–145.

Makhoul, J. (1989). Toward spoken language systems. *Speech Technology*, Apr./May, 34–36.

Mikkilineni, R. P., and Perdue, R. J. (1989). Experiences with implementing automatic speech recognition in the public telephone network. *Proceedings of the American Voice I/O Society*, 27–32.

Millar, P. C., Cameron, I. R., Greaves, A. J., and McPeake, C. M. (1988). Phone-in competitions: A development and evaluation tool for voice-interactive systems. *British Telecommunication Technology Journal*, **6**(2), 98–104.

Miller, J., and Chapman, R. (1982). Systematic analysis of language transcripts (SALT). Unpublished manuscript, University of Wisconsin.

Mulla, H., and Vaughan, J. F. (1985). Application of speech recognition and synthesis to PABX services. *Electrical Communication*, **59**(3).

Murphy, M., Bielby, G. , Roe, B., Read, K. O'Gorman, A., and Lennig, M. (1991). Automation of alternate billed calls using speech recognition. *IEEE Communications Magazine*, **29**(1), 25–29.

Nielsen, J., and Molich, R. (1990). Heuristic evaluation of user interfaces. *Proceedings of the ACM CHI'90 Conference on Human Factors and Computing Systems*, 1–5.

Oviatt, S. L., and Cohen, P. R. (1989). The effects of interaction on spoken discourse. *Proceedings of the 27th Annual Meeting of the Association for Computational Linguistics*, 126–134.

Pallett, D. (1985). Performance assessment of automatic speech recognizers. *Journal of Research of the National Bureau of Standards*, **90**(5), 371–387.

Poulain, G., and Tirbois, J. (1988). A voice actued (sic) callbox: Design and evaluation. *Proceedings of the 12th International Symposium on Human Factors in Telecommunications*.

Rabiner, L. R., Wilpon, J. G., and Rosenberg, A. E. (1980). A voice-controlled, repertory-dialer system. *The Bell System Technical Journal*, **59**, 1153–1163.

Rabiner, L. R. , Wilpon, J. G., and Soong, F. K. (1988). High performance connected digit recognition using hidden Markov Models. *Proceedings of the International Conference of Acoustics, Speech, and Signal Processing*, 119–122.

Rubin-Spitz, J., and Yashchin, D. (1989). Effects of dialogue design on customer responses in automated operator services. *Proceedings of Speech Technology '89*, 126–129.

Rudnicky, A. I., and Stern, R. M. (1989). Spoken language research at Carnegie Mellon. *Speech Technology*, Apr./May, 38–43.

Schoeber, M. F., and Clark, H. H. (1989). Understanding by addressees and overhearers. *Cognitive Psychology*, **21**, 211–232.

Schrage, J., Yashchin, D., and Ortel, W. (1990). VOIS — voice operated intercept services: Service description and preliminary experience. *Proceedings of the Annual Meeting of the American Voice I/O Society*, 179–184.

Simpson, C. A., McCauley, M. E., Roland, E. F., Ruth, J. C., and Williges, B. H. (1987). Speech Controls and Displays. In G. Salvendy (Ed.), *Handbook of Human Factors* (pp. 1490–1525). NY: John Wiley and Sons.

Tagg, E. (1988). Automating operator-assisted calls using voice recognition. *Speech Technology*, Mar./Apr., 22–25.

Virzi, R. A. (1989). What can you learn from a low-fidelity prototype? *Proceedings of the Human Factors Society 33rd Annual Meeting*, 224–228.

Virzi, R. A. (1990). Streamlining the design process: Running fewer subjects. *Proceedings of the Human Factors Society 34th Annual Meeting*, 291–294.

Vitale, T. (1989). Application-driven technology: Automated customer name and address. *Proceedings of the Annual Meeting of the American Voice I/O Society*, 33–40.

Walker, M. B. (1982). Smooth transitions in conversational turn-taking: Implications for theory. *The Journal of Psychology*, **110**, 31–37.

Waterworth, J. J. (1982). Man-machine speech "dialogue acts." *Applied Ergonomics*, **13**, 203–207.

Waterworth, J. J., and Talbot, M. (1987). *Speech and Language-based Interactions with Machines: Towards the Conversational Computer.* NY: John Wiley and Sons.

Williges, R. C., Williges, B. H., and Elkerton, J. (1987). Software Interface Design. In G. Salvendy (Ed.), *Handbook of Human Factors* (pp. 1416–1449). NY: John Wiley and Sons.

Wilpon, J. G. (1985). A study on the ability to automatically recognize telephone-quality speech from large customer populations. *AT&T Technical Journal*, **64**, 423–451.

Wilpon, J. G., DeMarco, D. M., and Mikkilineni, R. P. (1988). Isolated word recognition over the DDD telephone network—results of two extensive field studies. *Proceedings of the International Conference on Acoustics, Speech, and Signal Processing*, 55–58.

Wilpon, J. G., Mikkilineni, P., Roe, D. B., and Gokcen, S. (1990). Speech recognition: From research to the real world. *Proceedings of the Annual Meeting of the American Voice I/O Society*, 103–108.

Wilpon, J. G., and Rabiner, L. R. (1983). On the recognition of isolated digits from a large telephone customer population. *The Bell System Technical Journal*, **62**, 1977–2000.

Yashchin, D., Basson, S., Lauritzen, N., Levas, S., Loring, A., and Rubin-Spitz, J. (1989). Performance of speech recognition devices: Evaluating speech produced over the telephone network. *Proceedings of the International Conference on Acoustics, Speech, and Signal Processing*, 552–555.

Young, S. J., and Proctor, C. E. (1989). The design and implementation of dialogue control in voice operated database inquiry systems. *Computer Speech and Language*, **3**, 329–353.

Zoltan-Ford, E. (1984). Reducing variability in natural-language interactions with computers. *Proceedings of the Human Factors Society 28th Annual Meeting*, 768–772.

Chapter 11

Voiced Mail: Speech Synthesis of Electronic Mail

Chris Schmandt
Massachusetts Institute of Technology

In recent years we have seen an increasing number of telephone-based interactive speech systems. These systems use touch tones for user input and recorded speech segments for output. They are becoming pervasive; in a recent week I encountered them when I called my bank, my mortgage company, one of my airline frequent flier numbers, and a toll-free number giving the bus schedule to Boston's airport. Few of these systems employ text-to-speech synthesis; this is due largely to the poorer intelligibility of synthesized speech as compared to recorded speech. But recorded speech cannot be used in every application for which speech output is desired. This chapter considers some issues in the design of phone-based interfaces using text-to-speech synthesis for access to human-authored data. The particular application to be described in detail is a voice interface for reading electronic mail.

1. Applications of Synthetic Speech

Despite improvements in speech synthesis, synthetic speech is still of much lower quality than most recorded natural speech. This diminished quality may be measured as decreased intelligibility of individual words, poorer performance by subjects in listening comprehension tests, subjective evaluations of voice preference, or the cognitive load placed on the listener trying to understand synthetic speech (See Schmidt-Nielsen and Ralston, et al., chapters, this volume.) This suggests that whenever possible, recorded speech should be used instead of synthetic speech. Recorded speech is used in a wide range of telephone-based applications with a limited message set. One such example is the telephone number playback for directory assistance. After an initial dialog with a human operator, a recording plays the requested number. Examples are also seen in more fully automated systems, the so-called "audio-text" services, in which a caller uses touch tones to select information for playback (weather forecasts, highway conditions, movie theater show times, etc.). If recorded speech is both of better quality and suitable for such a wide range of applications, what role is left for synthetic speech?

Text-to-speech can be useful in three specific applications. The first is when the system has limited range of possible output phrases, but a large number of data items which can fit into the output, such as street names, surnames from a telephone book, or user IDs on a computer system. In this case, it may be impractical to record and store the large number of words. Additionally, if the underlying database changes, it may be difficult to add new recorded words, as these should ideally be in the same voice as the rest of the utterances and the person who spoke the original recordings may not be available.

The second application is one in which the system has a relatively small vocabulary size but may deliver a large number of possible responses, such as reporting the status and contents of various orders to a salesman while traveling. The problem with recorded speech in this situation is one of prosody; simply concatenating a series of words, spoken in isolation, results in very choppy prosody as compared to whole spoken sentences. In such cases, the attitude of the service users may be the leading factor in choosing choppy digitized speech versus smoother but possibly less intelligible synthetic speech.

The third and final application of synthetic speech is speaking human-authored text. Here there is no question of using recorded speech, as the message set is highly variable and not predictable. Example applications include proofreading, describing entries in a calendar, or reading electronic mail over the telephone, the application to be described in this chapter.

2.   Limitations of Synthetic Speech Output

For the majority of these services, the only reason for speech output is to provide *remote access*, i.e, interaction over a telephone. Unless the user is visually impaired, any of the three types of output described above will be more effectively read than heard. Speech, especially synthesized speech, is a difficult output medium to employ successfully. Why?

Speech is *transitory*. Once spoken, it is gone. Text can be printed and carried about, e.g. phone lists and driving directions. Also, speech is *serial*, implicitly including a time dimension as it is fundamentally a time-varying signal. Text, either printed or on a display, can be perused in whatever random order the user desires. If a list of options or a whole sentence contains something the user does not understand, it is easy to re-read a portion of the screen. In a voice interface, with no means to guess at what point the listener became confused, it is necessary to repeat the entire passage. Finally, speech is *slow*, much slower than any competent reader. Most commercial synthesizers operate in the 150 to 200 word per minute range; people can read several times faster than this. Even the nearly obsolete 300 baud modem can transmit text almost twice as fast.

Two other factors are more unique to synthetic speech. The first of these is intelligibility. Because of limitations in both the text-to-phoneme rules, as well as phoneme realization in the common parametric synthesizers, they achieve limited intelligibility (Pisoni, *et al.*, November 1985; Pisoni, 1983, also see the Ralston, *et al.* chapter, this volume). Of course, intelligibility is a function of many variables, including user experience, the size of the vocabulary, and predictability of the text. Proper nouns, such as names, are even less likely to be pronounced correctly (Murray, 1985), but of course may represent a large fraction of the utterances in some applications. And, if the synthesis system is reading human-authored text, typographic errors and misspellings are always possible; with electronic mail they are common.

Another significant characteristic of synthetic speech is an increase in *cognitive load* when listening to it (Luce *et al.*, 1983). Perhaps because the cues to differentiate phonemes are not as rich as in natural speech, more processing of the incoming speech is required, taxing short-term memory. Short-term memory is a limited resource, so this listening task conflicts with other tasks, such as remembering which choice to make in a menu or what step of a task is being performed. This may result in increased difficulty performing complex tasks with synthetic speech.

Any good user interface to a synthetic speech system must compensate for these limitations if the resulting application is to gain widespread acceptance. Of course, acceptance will depend on other factors as well, such as how necessary is the service provided by the application, or what special advantage can be gained from remote telephone access to the service.

In this chapter we will consider a specific service, remote access to electronic mail, from the point of view of the limitations mentioned above. It is vital to acknowledge the problems with synthetic speech output, and factor this into each stage of the design process. With some luck, this knowledge may result in a useful system. Of course, feedback from users and iterative design to overcome unforeseen problems is always helpful.

3.   Voiced Mail Operation

Any speech application must successfully solve a real need. The system described here was built in 1983, when modems were usually 300 baud and home computers almost non-existent. Even in a research lab at a leading university, relatively few system users had terminals at home; certainly students did not. At the Architecture Machine Group (now the Media Laboratory) at M.I.T, where this system was built, heavy use was made of electronic mail for all aspects of laboratory administration, making mail access particularly useful. In this decade of laptop computers and portable modems, full voice access to electronic messages may be less useful than it was five years ago.

Voiced Mail was a system that used touch tones as input and synthetic speech as output to provide remote telephone access to electronic mail. It was a subscriber system, with one phone number being used for access by a group of users. Voiced Mail worked in parallel with an existing mail system, operating on the same text database as the users normal terminal-based mail reading program. A limited repertoire of reply messages could be generated automatically.

To use Voiced Mail, one would call a telephone number and be greeted by a *login* prompt. The caller would enter his or her user ID using touch tones, with one key press per letter. After entering a password, the user would be greeted, told how many new messages awaited reading, and the system would start reading the messages. While reading a message, various telephone keys could be used to jump ahead to the next message or group of messages (see below), repeat part of a message, get more information about the message (*envelope* style information such as date and time transmitted and received), or generate a reply.

In its later stages, this project also used digital speech recording to allow voice responses to be created in reply to text mail. The associated recorded voice file would be linked to a text message stored in the recipients incoming mailbox. If that user accessed messages by voice, she would hear the recorded reply. With text access, she was simply informed that a voice message had been recorded and instructions were given for retrieving the recording (the recipient was not limited to the set of Voiced Mail subscribers, but could be anyone capable of sending a subscriber a text message). Most of the functionality of Voiced Mail was subsumed by *Phone Slave*, a conversational answering machine also employing both voice and text messages (Schmandt, 1984 and Schmandt, 1985).

A typical session might run something like:

```
Welcome to Voiced Mail. Please log in.
```

> user presses 4-3-3-5 (sequence for "geek," the user's login).

```
Hello Chris Schmandt. You have twelve new messages. <pause>
Four from Walter Bender. <pause>   Message one. This is a
very long message; it's about window system subroutines...
```

> user presses 1 (next message).

```
Message two. It's about the new conference room.   <pause>
Can we get together tomorrow afternoon to decide about
chairs?
```

> user presses 7 (affirmative reply).

```
Message sent. Message three. It's about Monday's demo...
```

> user presses 4 (next sender).

```
Two messages from Barry Arons. <pause> Message one.
It's about the pizza recipe...
```

The remainder of this chapter will deal with some of the design decisions made with Voiced Mail in the attempt to overcome some of the limitations of synthetic speech.

3.1   Text Filtering

Since speech is slow, it is worthwhile to consider every opportunity for trimming text from the message to be synthesized. With electronic mail, a good example is the message headers. Figure 1 shows the complete body of text associated with an internet mail message. Note in particular that less than half the text is the message body itself. Many of the header fields are of interest only to a system administrator maintaining the mailer program. Even the ones that are of interest to the recipient, such as the sender and date/time received, are in a format inappropriate for a synthesizer.

3.1.1 The "From": field usually contains the sender's real name, in some form, as well as the sender's return email address. A return address may be unpronounceable, because computer names may be cryptic acronyms. Even where they can be spoken, they will not come out "right." In internet host names, for example, the "." character is pronounced "dot"; but a synthesizer will likely call it "period," further reducing intelligibility.

3.1.2 The "Date": field is given in a format including time in hours, minutes, seconds, tenths of seconds, etc. While it is easy to skip most of this information when reading, it is painfully slow to listen to it. Voiced Mail reduced dates to short, relative forms, such as "This morning at 10:15," or "Yesterday afternoon at 1:15." In fact, these dates were not presented unless requested with the "More Info" key. Only rarely does the date of a message matter to the recipient.

```
>From dcj@Sun.COM Tue Aug 22 15:53:21 1989
Received: by media-lab (5.57/4.8)
id AA11928; Tue, 22 Aug 89 15:53:15 EDT
Received: from snail.Sun.COM (snail.Corp.Sun.COM) by
Sun.COM (4.1/SMI-4.1)
id AA24516; Tue, 22 Aug 89 12:53:51 PDT
Received: from jacksun.sun.com by snail.Sun.COM (4.1/
SMI-4.1)
id AB18658; Tue, 22 Aug 89 12:51:56 PDT
Message-Id: <8908221953.AA06751@jacksun.sun.com> To:
Chris Schmandt <geek@media-lab.media.mit.edu> Subject:
possible bug in fax.c
In-Reply-To: Your message of Tue, 15 Aug 89
            12:43:41  -0400.
            <8908151643.AA27528@media-lab>
Date: Tue, 22 Aug 89 12:53:13 PDT
From: dcj@Sun.COM Status: RO

Fax couldn't find my ~/.fax_sig file, and dumped
core on my 386i. This is a nice addition to rolo!
Don
```

Figure 1: An electronic mail message, including the full header.

Voiced Mail removed all header information. Instead, some of the information was presented in the message preamble, e.g. "Message 5: from Don Jackson. It's about a possible bug in fax.c."; but, most of it was not available.

3.2 Message Ordering

Most text and voice mail systems present messages in the order they were received; some systems allow the sender to mark a message as "urgent." Text mail reading programs usually include some summary display, perhaps with one line per message, showing date, time, and part of the subject line (as in Figure 2). With Voiced Mail we chose to not implement a summary mode, as it still would take an excessive amount of time to hear. Instead, messages were grouped according to the sender, and, for each sender, presented in the order in which they were received (a user defined configuration list could easily have identified the most important correspondents for earliest presentation, but we did not implement this). Senders with the most unread messages were presented first. Touch tone commands allowed the caller to move forward and backward either by message or by sender.

```
 224   hulteen@apple.com Fri May 11 13:47 16/482 "Re: visits'
 225   cahn Sat May 12 03:54 28/845 "references"
 226   ackerman@ATHENA.MIT.EDU Sat May 12 13:30 38/1330 "sv"
 227   sheldon Sun May 13 05:53 20/821 "caldummy on 386"
U230   geek Sun May 13 22:43 14/339 "tix"
 231   howcome Mon May 14 10:27 19/418 "Re: X11r4"
 233   leyna Mon May 14 11:30 22/739 "Ira Marks/Strategic Alternati"
N234   jrd Mon May 14 12:15 12/327 "Bennett email"
N235   leyna Mon May 14 12:17 16/439 "support staff lunch"
N236   barons Mon May 14 12:54 16/578 "book comments"
```

Figure 2: Email message summarization, from a text-based mail program.

The logic to this message ordering was to minimize the cognitive load on the caller. Multiple messages from the same sender are likely to be related, so it can aid comprehension to present them together. Since the reply mechanism was awkward, it was useful to hear the complete set of messages before replying; otherwise the time spent replying to the first message is wasted if a subsequent message renders the reply unnecessary. This was also true for reading text messages back in the days of slow modems.

In fact, there are some cases where it might be more useful to group messages according to subject. For example, there may be a mail thread about a meeting agenda with messages from each participant. Or, the listener may have been copied on messages between two other users that are really a dialog between them. Voiced Mail did not support sorting by subject, however.

3.3   Intelligibility Issues

As already noted, speech synthesis is not noted for correct pronunciation of surnames. Synthesizers are also likely to mispronounce acronyms as well as local jargon. A common approach in synthesizer text processing rules is to spell a word that is not obviously pronounceable, which works in many circumstances (MBTA, CTA, VMS). But this fails in others, such as MIT, which should be pronounced "m-i-t," not like "mitt." But this is not always enough. On the operating system (Magic 6) under which Voiced Mail ran, mailboxes were called "mbx's" because of their file name extension. This word was pronounced by system users as "mubix"; a message about "your m-b-x" would be cryptic at best. And then there are some words spoken with a hybrid of words and letters, such as the common Unix mail defaults file, ".mailrc", which is pronounced "dot mail r-c."

The only way to cope with these problems was with a local exception lexicon. This involved building up a file of substitutions; words would be replaced by a phonetic spelling to give correct pronunciation. Although some synthesizers now offer an on-device exception lexicon, this tends to be implemented in a rather weak manner in which the phonetic spelling is substituted only if the word matches the lexicon entry exactly. Thus, if "mbx" is in the lexicon the substitution occurs; but, if "mbxs" is sent to the synthesizer, no substitution is done. So, it may be more useful to implement the exception lexicon as a filter in the computer anyway. Of course, the optimal place for such a dictionary would be in the synthesizer's internal morpheme dictionary, which would be consulted after the affixes had been removed from the incoming text.

Any system that talks needs to support some form of repetition, which is not trivial if the user can interrupt at any point in what might be a lengthy text passage. Synthesizers support text input buffering because speech is so slow. Simply because a word has been sent to the device does not mean it has been spoken yet. Most synthesizers support some form of synchonrization marker, which the host can insert in its output periodically, and which will be acknowledged when that point in the text passage is spoken.

Voiced Mail inserted "sync" markers between every independent clause. This was part of its tokenization of the input mail passage, involving checking each word in the lexicon and noting punctuation indicating clause boundaries. When the user hit the "repeat" key, the program tried to figure out which clause was currently being spoken and would play it again. Of course, there can be a bit of skew between speech output and user response because the user may listen to the entire sentence before deciding it was unintelligible, and then may take reaction time to press the key. The synthesizer and computer input/output system may introduce further delays. If "repeat" is detected too close to a clause boundary, both the preceding and following clauses are re-played.

Voiced Mail would initially play text relatively fast (180 or 200 words per minute) to minimize listening time. The first repetition of a clause would cause it to be re-synthesized at 120 words per minute. If another repetition was requested during this time, the sentence was spelled letter by letter. This speed variation was an attempt to trade time for intelligibility.

In fact, spell mode is not very useful. It is absurdly slow and quite hard to follow. Recently we developed a better scheme. Only one level of repetition is supported, at the slow rate. During this playback, certain words are spelled; the words chosen for spelling are those not found in the dictionary of the local spelling checker program. This enables precise designation of those words most likely to need spelling, i.e., proper nouns and typographic or spelling errors by the original human author. For example, on first playback the sentence might be, "This is a tset message from jrd." Repetition would play, "This is a t-s-e-t message from j-r-d," at a slower rate.

3.4 Advantages of Multiple Media

Recognizing that an immediate reply is one of the most valued features of electronic mail, Voiced Mail initially supported generation of a text reply in one of three forms. These forms were:

```
In response to your message about <insert subject here>
my answer is yes.

In response to your message about <insert subject here>
my answer is no.

In response to your message about <insert subject here>,
please call me at <a number then entered by the caller>.
```

However, this reply mechanism, which used up three valuable keys on the telephone, was almost never used. Why? Correspondents rarely give such unequivocal answers, and, if traveling, are rarely at a telephone long enough to receive a return call.

Late in the project, just before its transition to Phone Slave, we added the facility to record a voice reply to a message. The sender then received a text message both indicating that a voice reply had been sent, and giving instructions as to how to access the system. Included in the message was a unique, one time only password, which would allow the caller to leave a follow-on (voice) reply. In other words, anyone who could send me email, could hear my voice reply. This was all possible because the mail software could easily determine a valid return address for a text message, and all of the voice storage was local on our computer system.

Of course, the recipient of such a reply could be a subscriber to Voiced Mail. Our subscribers were much more likely to read mail as text, in their offices; there was no reason to choose the synthetic voice presentation when a terminal was available. But, if they did encounter a recorded reply during a voice session, the program detected that this was a form message it had sent itself and would instead say something like, "Message 4 is a voice message from Walter...", and play it.

Once recording a reply became an option, the reply mechanism was invoked more often, although shortly thereafter the system was discontinued.

This is an example of a common problem. The telephone keypad can be fine for interacting with a menu or selecting one of a predetermined number of items, but it is notoriously poor for data entry. The solution of allowing the underlying computer database to support multiple media, i.e., both text and recorded voice, is attractive, at least from the point of view of the user. We are currently employing this strategy in several other applications, such as the voice interface to a personal appointment calendar.

3.5   Flow of Presentation in a System Without Menus
One of the more pernicious problems with voice interfaces is how long it takes to get anything done. The problem can be compounded by having to listen to a host of prompts or choose the next action at many points in a menu hierarchy. There has been much debate as to the number of items that can be presented at one time in a menu. The numbers usually cited are three or four (for example, see Gould, 1987), although, as pointed out by Englebeck and Roberts (1989), there is no hard and fast rule, as it depends on user

experience and familiarity. This makes menu design a difficult compromise between novice users and experienced users, particularly since novices require considerable familiarity with an application before they become adept at interrupting. Voiced Mail was an attempt at an opposite extreme from menu based systems, and used no menus. Instead, we took a flow oriented approach and optimized the interface to perform, by default, the most common path of user interaction.

With electronic mail, the user's task is primarily to read messages. Replying is a strong secondary function, even less important for Voiced Mail, simply because it supported only a minimal set of replies, at least initially. So, once logged in, Voiced Mail reported how many messages had arrived, and started presenting them. Commands (such as "next" and "previous") were always available to interrupt this default behavior.

The system would tell what it was about to do, pause briefly to allow the user to digest this information and possibly skip to the next operation, and then continue. Wherever it seemed useful, the system would present auxiliary information that might influence the user's choice, e.g., "Message 5. This is a very long message about window system subroutines." An early version of Voiced Mail went too far in minimizing the amount of text being spoken. If a message was very short (determined by number of characters), the subject line would not be spoken at all. The logic here was that the subject was useful mainly as a filter, i.e., to determine whether to listen to the attached message at this time. But this approach fails badly on a message such as the one in Figure 3!

```
Message 141:
>From derek Thu Mar 15 18:05:25 1990
To: geek Subject: Metal-Oxide Varistor
Date: Thu, 15 Mar 90 18:05:21 EST

It's here... The one for the telephone system...
I'll leave it in the sound room on the middle
shelf...
```

Figure 3: For some messages, the subject field is essential.

If the user made no response after logging in, the system would play all the user's messages, indicate that it was available for other operations, such as sending a message, and then time out and exit. If the user did interrupt with some other task, most likely replying to a piece of mail, Voiced Mail would keep track of its state when interrupted (e.g., playing message 7), and, when the interruption was completed, return to this point and resume playing messages.

3.6 Simple Command Set

One consequence of avoiding menu-based interaction is that it is easier for an interface to be modeless. In a modeless interface all commands are always active, the interface has a single state, and each user input always causes the same response. With a heavily moded voice system, particularly one based on hierarchical menus, the user may have difficulty remembering where he or she is amongst these menus, or even what operation is in progress. Of course, without menus, the user must remember the commands. In practice this was not overly bothersome. A list of commands was always available with a "help" key, and since users were all familiar with electronic mail, they knew what functionality to expect.

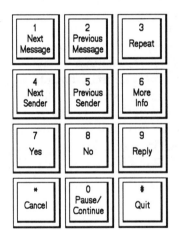

Figure 4: The Voiced Mail command set on the telephone keypad.

But, as mentioned above, there is some need to minimize the number of options at each step in menu presentation. This directly conflicts with the application developer's desire to include maximum functionality in the system. With Voiced Mail we chose to err on the side of ease of use over functionality, and, in doing so, limited the number of available commands so that each touch tone key had a single, consistent meaning throughout a session. These commands were always active; the system was always interruptible and would perform some consistent action in response to user input.

Figure 4 shows the Voiced Mail command set, and how it was mapped onto the keypad. Note the geographic correspondence between the "next" and "previous" choices for choosing a sender or a message.

4.   Voiced Mail Today

In many ways, Voiced Mail is dated, mostly by the rise in laptop use, combined with decreased cost and size, plus increased speed, of modems. There are few situations in which one would prefer synthetic speech access over text access, although sometimes we do dream about hearing our mail while stuck in traffic or taking a shower.

There actually may be places for lower quality interfaces. While traveling I have become accustomed to reading mail with a laptop. This tends to be the kind of activity performed at the end of the day from a hotel room, while synthesized mail would provide access from any telephone. Once logged in, it is tempting to "catch up," but when one receives 50 to 100 messages a day, this ends up consuming a lot of time.

Certainly one of the advantages cited by voice mail users is that they can drop in on their mailbox whenever it is convenient during the day. Perhaps an interface which is less conducive to browsing, combined with a good message filter, such as the Information Lens (Malone, 1987), might be helpful. One clear observation about Information Lens is that users are capable of formulating rules, and may have different mail filtering rules for different circumstances, e.g. normal daily use as opposed to having just returned to the office from a week's vacation (Mackay, 1988).

Although Voiced Mail did gain acceptance, its user community was relatively small and certainly far from computer naive. No strong claims are being made here about the viability of this particular user interface: Our users were computer programmers who show a remarkable tolerance for less than optimal user interfaces! On the other hand, it does reveal some of the trade-offs to be made in the design space for synthetic speech and telephone based systems. Such systems are developing an almost generic interface, modeled as the user listening to a menu and selecting an option. Other presentation styles may offer improved interfaces at least with more advanced applications.

5.   References

Englebeck, G., & Roberts, T. L. (1989). The effect of several voice-menu characteristics on menu-selection performance. Technical report, *US West Advanced Technologies*.

Gould, J. D., Boies, S. J., Levy, S., Richards, J. T., & Schoonard, J. (1987). The 1984 Olympic message system: A test of behavioral principals of system design. *Communications of the ACM, 30(9)*, 758–769.

Luce, P. A., Feustel, T. C., & Pisoni, D. B. (1983). Capacity demands in short-term memory for synthetic and natural speech. *Human Factors, 25(1)*, 17–32.

Mackay, W. E. (1988). How information lens users use rules. *Human Factors in Computer Systems—CHI'88 Conference Proceedings*, 211–216.

Malone, T. W., Grant, K. R., Turbak, F. A., Brobst, S. A., & Cohen, M. D. (1987). Intelligent information-sharing systems. *Communications of the ACM, 30(5)*, 390–402.

Pisoni, D. (1983). Perception of speech: The human listener as a cognitive interface. *Speech Technology, 1*, 10–23.

Pisoni, D. B., Nusbaum, H. C., & Greene, B. G. (1985). Perception of synthetic speech generated by rule. *Proceedings of the IEEE, 73(11)*, 1665–1676.

Schmandt, C., & Arons, B. (1984). A conversational telephone messaging system. *IEEE Trans on Consumer Electr., CE-30(3)*, xxi–xxiv.

Schmandt, C., & Arons, B. (1985). Phone slave: A graphical telecommunications interface. *Proc. of the Soc. for Information Display, 26(1)*, 79–82.

Spiegel, M. F. (1985). Pronouncing surnames automatically. *Proceedings of 1985 Conference, American Voice I/O Society*.

Chapter 12

The Design of Spoken Language Interfaces*

Alexander I. Rudnicky
Carnegie Mellon University

This chapter describes how a speech application using a speaker-independent continuous speech recognition system is designed and implemented. A voice spreadsheet application is described and evaluation techniques are discussed.

1. Introduction

The ability to use speech enhances the quality of communication between humans, as reflected in shorter problem-solving times and in general user satisfaction (Chapanis, 1981, pp.65–114). Unfortunately, these benefits have not yet been realized for human-computer communication because of the inherent limitations of early speech recognition technology. Recent advances in speech recognition technology (Lee, 1989) have made it possible to build "spoken language" systems that permit natural interaction with computers. Spoken language systems combine a number of desirable properties. Recognition of *continuous speech* allows users to use a natural speech style. *Speaker independence* allows casual users to easily use the system and eliminates training as well as its associated problems (such as drift). *Large vocabularies* make it possible to create habitable languages for complex applications. Finally, a *natural language* processing capability allows the user to express him or herself using familiar locutions.

---

*The research described in this chapter was sponsored by the Defense Advanced Research Projects Agency (DOD) ARPA Order No. 5167, monitored by SPAWAR under contract N00039-85-C-0163. The views and conclusions contained in this document are those of the author and should not be interpreted as Agency or the US Government.

The availability of such features as speaker-independence and continuous speech removes a number of restrictions that have limited the usefulness of speech interfaces (but for the same reasons have simplified the development of such interfaces). Speaker-independence makes a system accessible to casual users who do not need to commit to an enrollment procedure, as do users of speaker-dependent systems. Similarly, the ability to process continuous speech removes a major restriction on the user (separating words by silences) and allows fairly natural communication of complex information.

Removing these restrictions complicates the interface design process. To preserve the naturalness of communication, the designer must make an effort to define an expressive system language that allows natural modes of expression. The system design must also minimize a system's attentional requirements, so the user can concentrate on the task rather than on the operation of the speech system. This latter goal requires the system to handle a variety of phenomena related to spontaneous speech, such as pauses in the middle of an utterance and the intrusion of both environmental and talker-generated non-speech sounds.

We would like to understand the design of spoken language systems for complex problem-solving environments in which the user can take advantage of speech to control a variety of applications. To develop an understanding of such environments, we built a voice-operated spreadsheet program and studied users interacting with it. In this chapter we describe the techniques used for developing and evaluating this system. We present a rather detailed description of each step in the process, since any implementation of a spoken language system meant for working environments requires an approach similar to the one described.

Since we were interested in examining a voice interface to basic spreadsheet functions, we chose to work with *sc*, a UNIX[1]-based spreadsheet similar in functionality to VISICALC[2], an early spreadsheet program. To have speaker-independent and continuous speech recognition, we adapted the SPHINX recognition system for use with the spreadsheet.

2.   Task Analysis

The suitability of speech for a particular application should be established. Although speech is clearly a desirable input medium, it does not follow that

---

[1] Unix is a trademark of AT&T
[2] VISICALC is a trademark of VISICORP.

it should be used in all cases. Moreover, potential interactions between different input modalities must be considered during the design process. A drawing program is a good example of a system where the decisions on how to use speech are clear-cut. Components of a drawing program that produce graphics are clearly unsuited for voice control and are more efficiently done through direct manipulation as afforded by a mouse or similar device. On the other hand, discrete inputs such as selecting modes seem to be well suited for voice. Combining voice and manual input may produce benefits that are difficult to realize using a single modality. For example, conventional mode selection strategies require the user to either release the mouse in order to key in mode changes, or move the pointer to a menu panel. The availability of a parallel voice channel eliminates the resulting disruption.

In the case of the spreadsheet, we felt that all its functionality, command function invocation and numeric data entry could be controlled by speech. The one exception is the input of arbitrary text information since current recognition technology does not allow the incorporation of novel items into the recognition lexicon.

In our experiments with the system we simulated the ability to define arbitrary words by including a vocabulary keyed to the tasks we gave our subjects (personal finances). When the area of application is well-defined, a suitable vocabulary can be built into the system, and would give the user the flexibility to use intuitively preferable modes of expression, i.e., keyed to the conceptual categories being worked with (such as meaningful cell labels) rather than the abstractions provided by the base system (row and column coordinates).

3. Language Design

Once the functionality suitable for speech control has been identified, the language to be understood by the system can be developed. A spoken language is unique and differs significantly from other varieties of language. Consider the difference between expressing something verbally and writing it out. Written language allows one to choose expressions carefully and to revise the presentation until it is satisfactory. In spoken language, particularly if production is spontaneous, presentation will be very different. It will use different argument structures, grammatical constructs and word choices. The design of a recognition language must capture the properties of spoken language.

A spoken language interface also needs to do more than provide a direct translation of commands designed for another modality. For example, keyboard command languages are often designed to minimize the number of keystrokes required. Such a goal may not be relevant for a speech command language, where the effort of producing an entry is less. Speech would also differ from menu-driven interfaces, where limited real-estate (and other considerations) might force the design of complex menu trees, necessitating a succession of interactions to produce a result that could otherwise have been achieved by a single voice command. Spoken language allows (and encourages) the user to express requests more abstractly, in terms of desired effects rather than component actions. Language design needs to reflect this.

The proper choice of language for an interface is not obvious from a simple survey of an application's functionality. We have found that the most useful approach is to record the language of users while they perform tasks using the system and to use this as a basis for developing a spoken language suitable for the application. It is necessary to observe a variety of users, since individuals may display idiosyncratic behavior that is not representative of a user population.

3.1 The "Wizard" paradigm

The design of a spoken language system is a chicken-and-egg problem. It is not possible to understand how best to design such a language without knowing how people wish to interact with a particular application. On the other hand, it is not possible to observe interactions unless the system is available.

Our solution to this program is to build a simulation of the target and to observe users interacting with it. The speech data collected from such a study can then be analyzed and a speech language developed. The function of the speech recognizer and parser is carrier out by human operator, hidden from the user, who is unaware of the operator's intervention. This form of simulation has recently come to be called the "Wizard" paradigm.[3]

---

[3] The term comes from a character in L. Frank Baum's Book for children, *The Wizard of Oz* book. The wizard being someone who manipulated a large statue from behind a curtain, leaving observers with the impression that they were speaking to the statue itself. The "Wizard of Oz" Story was also the source for the no longer favored term "pnambic experiment" (for "Pay No Attention to the Man Behind the Curtain"), another allusion to the Wizard of Oz.)

We have used different forms of the Wizard paradigm, from fairly elaborate simulations that presented the user with a complete illusion of a functioning system (see e.g., Hauptmann and Rudnicky, 1988) to informal situations designed to elicit speech more characteristic of human-human exchanges (see Rudnicky *et al.*, 1989).

To develop a spoken language for the spreadsheet program, we used a series of simulations in which participants performed several well-specified tasks. To see whether the complexity of the task had any influence on language, we used both a financial data entry task and a planning task. In the former, people were asked to enter information characteristic of an individual's monthly finances into a pre-programmed spreadsheet. In the planning task, people were given a filled financial spreadsheet and were asked to modify it to satisfy certain constraints (e.g., decreasing expenses by a total amount). Interestingly, subjects in both experiments produced similar protocols, invoking the same facilities in both cases. The only difference was a small increase in "speculative" constructions for the planning task (*"What if rent were changed to $500?"*). Significantly, subjects used language appropriate to the known functionality of the system and did not, by virtue of using speech, expect expert-system-like properties of the spreadsheet.

Table 1: An excerpt from a protocol transcription

under cable, enter fifteen dollars even [*]

oka:y, go to the next screen [*]

oka:y unde:r . movies . . in the entertainment, section, subsection .

enter twenty-eight fifty [*]

oka:y . . u:h in the . FOOD subsection under HOSting [*]

enter . on the line above that, enter a hundred seventy-five dollars [*]

okay, go down to the oh wait

on the CLOthing . entry [*]

ente:r . sum of . eighty-five, eighty-nine, twenty-four [*]

[click] okay

and, under gasoline, enter twenty-two fifty [*]

okay . uh . next screen [*]

Notes: The transcription, in addition to recording the speech produced, attempts to indicate additional phenomena of interest, primarily prosody and extraneous events. The [*] mark indicates the point in time at which the "system" is responding. A comma (,) indicates a boundary mark, either a short pause or an inflection. Capitalization (e.g. CLOthing) indicates emphatic stress. Items in square brackets (e.g., [rustle] describe extraneous audible events.

3.2 Protocol Transcription

All speech produced during these sessions was recorded on tape and later transcribed. Table 1 shows an excerpt from a transcription. The system of annotation chosen provides detailed information about the contents of subjects' utterances. In addition to information about the lexical and syntactic choices made, the transcript allows for analyses of pause location, emphasis, and interjection. Information about these phenomena is desirable since all have consequences for the operation of a speech recognition system.

Transcription, in the course of spoken language system development, actually has two uses. The first is for the initial language analysis being described in this section. The second is for evaluation purposes, where the goal is to match the output of a recognition system to what was actually spoken. The requirements for this second transcription style are more rigid and some additional distinctions need to be made, such as between words that are in the recognition lexicon and those that are not. The following guidelines were used for the evaluation portion of this study:

1. An *event* is audible acoustic energy delimited by silences or by other labeled events. When two events overlap, preference is given to the lexically meaningful element (e.g., word over noise), or to the element attributable to the nominal session talker. Otherwise, the most salient event (as judged by the transcriber) is given preference. No attempt is made to further code overlapping events.

2. *Transcribe all words.* If a particular word is not recognizable, a guess is made, based on the transcriber's best understanding of the context of occurrence, both sentential and task, in which the word occurs. If a word or phrase cannot be identified then the "++MUMBLE+" marker is used. If a word is mispronounced but is nevertheless recognized correctly, it is transcribed as if it were spoken correctly. If it is misrecognized, it is transcribed as heard.

3. *Label all other audible events.* At the least level of detail, these can be identified by a cover symbol ("++Noise+"). We have found, however, that it is useful to label separately those events that occur frequently enough to be of interest in themselves, such as breath noises or telephone rings.

4. *If the system recognizes an interrupted word correctly, then the word is transcribed as if it were spoken in its entirety.* This convention is

arbitrary and obviously hides information about interrupted words that are nevertheless correctly recognized.

5. *Utterances that produce no recognizer output are eliminated from the transcript.* In our system, this consisted of zero-length "utterances" that result from malfunctions in endpoint detection. A record of these utterances should be kept, so that relevant statistics can be calculated.

6. By convention, *any utterances at the beginning of the session that reflect the user's unawareness that the system just went live are eliminated.* This speech consists of interactions with the experimenter and typically reflect the user's unawareness that the period of instruction has ended. Since the user is not "using" the system, this convention is justified. A record of such deletions is kept, however.

7. *Extraneous noises are always transcribed if they affect the recognition.* Otherwise, noises are transcribed only if, in the opinion of the transcriber, they are sufficiently prominent ("loud enough"). Certain noises, in particular inhalations and exhalations at the start and end of an utterance, are not typically transcribed.

The above guidelines could be equally applicable to transcriptions produced at the exploratory stage. These guidelines and related issues are discussed in greater detail in Rudnicky and Sakamoto (1989).

Table 2: Utterance categories in the spreadsheet task.

DATA ENTRY:	Numeric
	Absolute Locate and Enter
	Relative Locate and Enter
	Symbolic Locate and Enter
	Symbolic Locate and Enter (no keyword)
	Absolute Locate and Enter (reverse order)
	Relative Locate and Enter (reverse order)
	Symbolic Locate and Enter (reverse order)
MOVEMENT:	Absolute screen movement
	Relative screen movement
	Explicit screen movement
	Screen positioning
	Absolute movement
	Symbolic movement
	Compound position

CORRECTION:	Simple deletion
	Keyword at head
	Mid-utterance correction
	Keyword at end
	Replacement
	Implicit correction
	Prosody
MISCELLANEOUS	
COMMANDS:	Screen refresh
	Addition of row/column
	Labeling new row
	String formatting

3.3 Language Analysis and Design

On first examining the transcripts we found such a wide variety of locutions that little consistency seemed to be present. A detailed analysis however, revealed that the language was quite consistent and could be classified into a compact set of categories. These are shown in Table 2. Examples of utterances for one of the categories, DATA ENTRY, are shown in Table 3. A more detailed discussion of these categories can be found in Rudnicky (1989).

These regularities made it possible for us to define a manageable language for the spreadsheet task. Spoken language design should not mean that every locution encountered in the simulation should be made part of the language. Rather, the goal should be to ensure that all major categories are represented. As long as the user has available the proper *modes* of expression, and as long these modes are derived from the actual productions of users, users should be able to remain within the minor syntactic and lexical bounds imposed by the designer.

Table 3:   Examples of entries in the DATA ENTRY category.

DATA ENTRY

Numeric
> sixty-five hundred dollars

Absolute Locate and Enter
> uh go down to line six and enter four thousand five hundred

Relative Locate and Enter
> on the next line enter seventy-five ninety-four

Symbolic Locate and Enter
> go to the cell for my salary and enter the amount six thousand five hundred
> under credit card enter the amount zero

Symbolic Locate and Enter (no keyword)
> food two seventeen and eighty-five cents plus two hundred forty-six dollars

Absolute Locate and Enter (reverse order)
> enter six thousand five hundred in column b row 6

Relative Locate and Enter (reverse order)
> enter seven hundred and forty-eight fifty-seven there

Symbolic Locate and Enter (reverse order)
> fifteen dollars under bank charges

Once this analysis is complete, lexicon and grammar can be defined. The lexicon specifies all words that the recognition system must be able to recognize. The choice of a lexicon is important, since it defines the composition of the training materials for the recognizer. Since training represents a major time and resource investment, it is important that it be done correctly. Grammar is somewhat more flexible, since it represents arrangement of lexical units and can be modified at any time during development.

A task language has three components: control, task-specific, and generic. This is a useful distinction to maintain, particularly if multiple tasks are being implemented. The control component provides access to general system functions, such as rejecting a misrecognition, putting the recognizer into standby mode, or quitting the system. The generic component represents language that would be of use in a variety of applications. The language of numbers is a good example of this. Finally, task-specific language designates the non-transportable component of a language, incorporating task-specific lexical items and grammatical forms.

We have developed utilities that allow us to specify language in a fairly convenient fashion. For example, grammar is expressed in the form of a Backus-Naur Form (BNF), while lexical entries are specified in terms of phonetic pronunciations. Table 4 shows a fragment of the BNF grammar for the spreadsheet. Table 5 shows some lexical items and their corresponding ARPABET specifications.

Table 4:   Excerpt from the spreadsheet BNF grammar.

<number_type> ::=   <numberstr_act> |

                       <numberstr_act> <decimal_act> <digitstr_act> |

                       <begin_digitstr_act> <decimal_act> <digitstr_act> |

                       <decimal_act> <digitstr_acts> |

                       <begin_digitstr_act> |

                       <o> <decimal_act> <digitstr_act>

To produce a knowledge base for the recognizer requires creating suitable phonetic models. Since we are working with a speaker-independent system, this requires the collection of a sufficient amount of recorded speech. We accomplish this by using the BNF grammar to generate a corpus of training utterances that can then be used as scripts for recording. Since we have control over the generation process, we can assure (by differentially weighing production rules) that sufficient instances of each word occur in the corpus. To achieve speaker-independence, we have many different individuals read sets of utterances (say, as many as might fit into a 15 minute session). The recognition system is then trained using this material. For spreadsheet training, we combined several databases, including ones containing calculator, spreadsheet, and financial management sentences (the domain used for the evaluation tasks). A total of 4012 utterances was available for training.

Table 5:   Some phonetic specifications for (using ARPABET symbols) lexical items.

BEGIN	B IX G IH N
BONDS	B AA N D Z
BOTTOM	B AA DX AX M
BREAK	B R EY KD
BY	B AY
C	S IY
CABLE	K EY B AX L

3.4 Parser Design

The parser in our original system uses a simple context-free grammar, built using the UNIX *lex* and *yacc* packages. The parsing strategy incorporated into VSC uses a two-stage parsing process to interpret a single string produced by the recognition system and to generate suitable spreadsheet commands. Figure 1 shows this process.

The first stage produces an initial analysis of the input string, to determine whether it is syntactically correct and to perform certain forms of pre-processing, such as the conversion of spoken numbers into their digit equivalent (e.g., TWELVE HUNDRED AND THIRTY FOUR into 1234). The second stage completes the parse and performs the mapping into spreadsheet system commands.

Our current parser designs are based on case-frame representations, coupled with a finite-state phrase-based recognition grammar. Case-frame parsers offer comparable execution speeds, but with more powerful language processing, better suited for spoken language.

4. The Recognition System

The voice spreadsheet uses Hidden Markov Model (HMM) recognition technology, described more fully in Lee (1989). (Also see O'Shaughnessy, Chapter 2.) The units of recognition are word, built from triphone models which are phones taken together with their immediate context (preceding and following phones). The use of triphone models allows the representation to incorporate information about coarticulatory effects and thereby increases recognition accuracy. The language designer specifies the words in the lexicon in terms of pronunciation, as shown in Table 5. Note that the pronunciation used is the most common form of the word rather than the (citation) form found in a dictionary. Determining the most common form of a word demands some investigation, often made easier by the availability of the wizard experiment recordings. However, the effort is well worth it. Experience with several recognition systems that use phonetic representations (Cohen, 1989; Lee, 1989) has shown that using the most common pronunciation increases recognition accuracy.

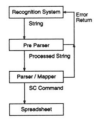

Figure 1: The parsing process in the voice spreadsheet system.

Phonetic pronunciations can be automatically transformed into triphone forms (as in Table 6), the units actually used for training the recognition system. For a task such as VSC, the initial lexicon is defined in terms of 48 phonetic labels. The actual number of triphone models trained is 971. Techniques are also available for clustering similar models, to reduce the total number of models needed. Since this clustering does not increase accuracy (Lee, 1989), we did not perform it for the current system.

Table 6:   Triphone expansion of monophone lexical items.

BEGIN	B(SIL,IX) IX(B,G) G(IX,IH) IH(G,N) N(IH,SIL)
BONDS	B(SIL,AA) AA(B,N) N(AA,D) D(N,Z) Z(D,SIL)
BOTTOM	B(SIL,AA) AA(B,DX) DX(AA,AX) AX(DX,M) M(AX,SIL)
BREAK	B(SIL,R) R(B,EY) EY(R,KD) KD(EY,SIL)
BY	B(SIL,AY) AY(B,SIL)
C	S(SIL,IY) IY(S,SIL)
CABLE	K(SIL,EY) EY(K,B) B(EY,AX) AX(B,L) L(AX,SIL)

The recognizer uses grammatical constraints to reduce search and to increase recognition accuracy in the process. These constraints are expressed in the form of a word-pair grammar, derived from the BNF grammar. A word-pair grammar provides minimal constraint, since it only specifies which words may follow the current word, and does not incorporate more global constraints, such as would be provided by a finite-state grammar. For the VSC task, the perplexity[4] of the tasks carried out by the user is approximately 52. A finite state grammar would provide lower perplexity and would make the recognition problem more tractable. Other things being equal, it is desirable to construct languages that have low perplexity, since this insures higher recognition accuracy. An alternate method for increasing recognition accuracy would be to configure a speaker-dependent system. Our experience indicates that for a SPHINX-like system, speaker-dependent training reduces the utterance error rate by half for the spreadsheet task. This level of performance, however, requires about 1500 training utterances per talker.

5. Interface Design

To properly design a speech interface we need to consider to a number of factors, including attention management, error correction, and interaction control.

Spoken communication does not have a direct physical focus in the way that keyboard entry does. In keyboard interaction, there is little ambiguity about the user's intent to communicate—the keyboard is mechanically activated by direct contact. There is no such explicit link in the case of speech. When a user speaks, the utterance may be directed at the currently active application, but it could also have been directed to another human in the environment, or perhaps have been the result of thinking aloud. The problem is that the system does not have the concept of *attention*; it does not know when it should be paying attention to a potential input. There are a number of solutions to this problem.

The simplest is a "push to talk" system, where the user depresses a button during the duration of the utterance or presses a key just prior to speaking. Having these solutions requires the user to perform an incompatible or even disruptive act in order to signal an input to the system. We have experimented with the use of "attention" words that allow the user to activate the recognizer via a single keyword, such as LISTEN. If the recognizer is in the standby mode, it will not actively process speech until it encounters the attention word. If we also provide a keyword for switching off attention, e.g., STANDBY, then the user has been given explicit control over the system's "attention" in a manner that is consonant with the modality. (We also have found it useful to have the system enter the standby mode if the quality of recognition falls below some level, on the assumption that the user has redirected his or her attention to another listener in the environment).

A second aspect of attention control has to do with the tendency of intended utterances to map imperfectly onto *acoustic utterances*. An acoustic utterance is defined in terms of physical attributes and consists of a continuous region of acoustic energy delimited by silence. Actual complete utterances (a *logical utterance*), as a human might understand them, may consist of one or more acoustic utterances, particularly if the user pauses in the middle of an utterance to decide what to say next. A related phenomenon occurs when

---

[4] Perplexity is defined as the geometric mean of the branching factors in an utterance. Perplexity is used as an estimator of the difficulty of recognition for a particular language. The perplexity of arbitrary English text is estimated to be about 200; the perplexity of a tightly-constrained task language can be as low as 5, a value characteristic of many commercial recognition systems. While perplexity gives an indication of how difficult the recognition process might be for a particular language, it is only one determinant of difficulty. The confusability of items in the vocabulary, as well as its size will also affect recognition difficulty.

the user runs together several logical utterances into a single acoustic utterance. If this is allowed, then the system gives up a valuable input constraint, somewhat like the one exploited by discrete-word recognition systems. A proper solution to the potential lack of a one-to-one correspondence between acoustic and logical utterances is beyond the scope of a simple interface design and requires the use of a sophisticated parsing algorithm.

A third component of speech interface design is some provision for error recovery. Speech recognition systems will, for the foreseeable future, produce errors. Even if perfect recognition is achieved, the user will occasionally utter unintended commands and will need to restore the system to a previous state. As a result, it is important to provide, as part of the interface design, mechanisms for error recovery. Such mechanisms can be studied systematically. In one experiment, we compared time-to-completion for a voice spreadsheet task using two different forms of confirmation. In one mode, recognized inputs were acted upon immediately and the user had to recover from errors by re-entry of commands. In a second mode, users had the opportunity to edit an ASCII version of the utterance, presented in an editor buffer, before it was acted upon.

Table 7 shows the times to completion for these two confirmation modes as well as reference time-to-completion for keyboard entry, taken from Rudnicky (1989). There is a completion time advantage for the explicit (keyboard only) confirmation mode. This mode, however, is more awkward to use, since the flow of the interaction is interrupted by the requirement for a keyboard confirmation. Because of this, and because of the desire to implement a "pure" speech system, we chose the implicit (voice only) confirmation model and did not provide an explicit mechanism for error recovery. It is our belief that error recovery should be done entirely within the speech modality. If this is not feasible, it should be a multi-modal system that can function with minimal interruption in the flow of interaction, since such interruptions involve shifts of attention and increase the effort required to interact by speech.

Table 7:   Comparison of confirmation styles.

Input Modality	Task Completion Time (min)
keyboard only	12:39
voice and keyboard	15:16
voice only	19:21

5.1 Interaction Structure

Figure 2 shows a detailed flow diagram of the VSC interaction, showing recognition, parsing, and execution components.

The system can be in one of two major input modes: Listening and Execution. The system does all signal acquisition and recognition in the Listening mode and locks out speech input during the Execution phase. The structure of the Listening mode is shown in Figure 3. Immediately upon entry into the input loop, the system displays the "Wait..." token in the information buffer (line 2 of the spreadsheet display) and initializes the signal processing module. This step takes an average of about 200 ms, though conditions will occasionally force a longer delay. Once the system is actually listening, a "LISTEN" token appears in the display buffer. The system waits until the onset of speech energy is detected and immediately begins the recognition search. The transition to this state is indicated by the appearance of the "Recognizing..." token. Termination of the recognition process is signalled by the appearance of the recognized string on the screen. Since recognition is not real-time, this change in state may occur some (noticeable) interval after the user has finished talking. This protocol provides the user at all times with a clear indication of recognizer state, which is desirable, as the temporal uncertainties associated with speech processing exceed certain limits. In a pilot study, Rudnicky and Quirin (1990), found that users seem to cope well with delays of up to 150-300 msec. With longer delays (exceeding 600-800 msec) users found it easier to pace their interactions by means of the external indicators.

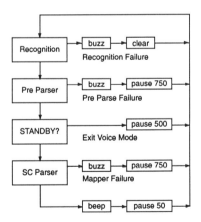

Figure 2: Interaction flow in VSC

An utterance that successfully passes through the recognition and parsing stages will result in a spreadsheet action, indicated to the user by a harmonic beep (F_0 250 Hz) of 100 ms duration. The various failure modes will generate a 100 ms buzz (F_0 100 Hz). These two signals are distinctive and give the user initial information about the success or failure of the current input. A short pause follows parser failures, so that the user has the opportunity to glance at the display buffer (and note the nature of the failure).

Given the operating characteristics of our system, we found that the inclusion of such detailed information about system state was useful to the user. A system functioning without delays and capable of high-accuracy recognition might not need to rely on many state indicators. Once systems with such characteristics are available, a systematic investigation can be undertaken.

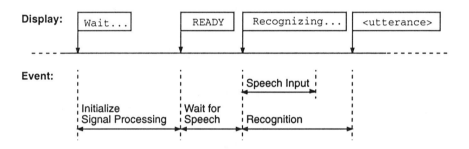

Figure 3:   Detail of the Listening Mode

6.   System Evaluation

To be informative, the evaluation of a spoken language system needs to take into account a number of dimensions, some relevant to comparisons with other input modalities, others useful for understanding the performance of the speech system itself. The potential advantage of speech input is that it can improve the performance of some complex tasks. Is the user capable of performing the task more rapidly when input is by voice? Are there fewer errors in the completed work? Does using speech interface entail less effort for the user?

Understanding the performance of a spoken language system requires the examination of a number of traditional measures, in addition to some new ones, insofar as they impact system performance. While word accuracy has been considered as a base measure of system performance, in a task situation utterance accuracy becomes more important,[5] since it has a direct impact on task throughput—each erroneous utterance requires either re-entry of the information or correction followed by re-entry. The usability of a system is also affected by the degree to which the system language is appropriate for the task and the degree to which it manages to encompass the language that the user chooses to bring to the task.

6.1 Task Completion Time

The effectiveness of a spoken language system as an interface can be evaluated by comparing the time it takes a user to carry out a set of standard tasks by voice with the time it takes to complete the same task using some other input modality, keyboard in our case. Figure 4, taken from Rudnicky, *et al.*, (1990), shows total task times for spreadsheet tasks performed by voice and by keyboard. As can be seen, these tasks take longer to carry out by voice. These data, however, confound a number of variables, in particular the performance of the speech system itself, with the effectiveness of spoken input.

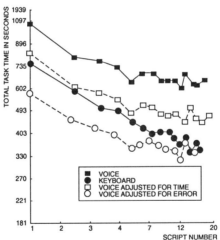

Figure 4: Task completion time.

---

[5] Word accuracy (w) is related to utterance accuracy (u) by $u = w^n$ where n is the average utterance length, in words. Systems for which interactions are limited to single words or short utterances are reasonably characterized by word accuracy. Systems that are characterized by long input sentences will exhibit much poorer utterance accuracy. The presence of extraneous sounds, as observed for the spreadsheet system, can significantly degrade system response, in comparison to evaluations performed on "clean" speech.

Two aspects of recognition system performance were poorer than desired: system recognition time, and recognition error. Due to the nature of our hardware implementation, average system response was on the order of 1.9 times real-time, the excess over real-time being attributed to speed limitations in the search component of the system (additional delays were introduced by the requirement that the end of utterance be delimited by approximately a 200 ms silence, and by a potential pipeline delay in the signal processing component of over 400 ms; intermittent delays were also introduced by network communication software). While engineering solutions exist for many of these delays, they could not be avoided in our experimental system. Figure 5 shows the distribution of delays for a typical session. Most delays fall into the range of 400-600 ms, though some delays are quite long. Some understanding of such delay distributions can be of use in evaluating the usefulness of a speech system, particularly for applications that require a fairly tight interaction loop, as is the case for a spreadsheet. Users of systems that are characterized by a less coupled interaction style (database retrieval may be an instance) may tolerate significant delays in response (see Gallaway, 1981).

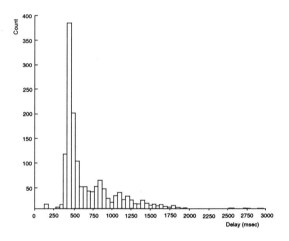

Notes: A total of 1330 delay intervals are shown here, pooling a dozen sessions from several talkers. The bin size is 50 msec. Less than 1% of the delays exceed 3 sec. These are not shown in this histogram.

Figure 5:   Distribution of system response delays.

The system under evaluation also exhibited a less than desirable error-rate, on the order of 25%, meaning that one out of every four utterances spoken by the user was misrecognized and required reentry or correction. This level of performance is not acceptable for a production system. We believe that for a task such as the spreadsheet, utterance accuracy rates of at least 90% are essential for usability and rates better than 95% are highly desirable.

We can estimate the impact of real-time performance and high-accuracy recognition by subtracting the time lost to non-real-time response and error recovery from the voice task time-to-completion. If we do so, we find that the voice-operated spreadsheet can be faster than keyboard input, indicating that on the simple criterion of time-to-completion, a voice-operated spreadsheet would represent a real improvement over keyboard input. The dotted lines in Figure 4 show the recalculated values. In the present case, we estimate that a system capable of operating in real-time and providing at least 85% utterance accuracy would produce equivalent times-to-completion for voice and keyboard. Deciding that this is actually the case, of course, would require building such a system. We are doing so.

The potential advantage of voice input is supported by an analysis of action times calculated separately for movement and entry instructions. In both cases, commands are entered more rapidly by voice. The median action time (including preparation and entry times) for numeric and formula entry is, for voice, 1906 msec, and for keyboard, 3301 msec. The total time for movements (including all delays) is 200.4 sec for voice and 202.6 sec for keyboard. The reason that total task completion times are excessive is the consequence of recognition errors and the resulting loss of time needed for reentry and correction.

In addition to examining the consequences for task performance, we also need to evaluate how well the recognition system performs with respect to several performance metrics.

6.2 Speech recognizer performance
To analyze recognizer performance we captured and stored each utterance spoken, as well as the corresponding recognition string produced by the system. All utterances were listened to and an exact lexical transcription produced. The transcription conventions are described more fully in Rudnicky and Sakamoto (1989), but suffice it to note than in addition to task-relevant speech, we coded a variety of spontaneous speech phenomena, including speech and non-speech interjections, as well as interrupted words and similar phenomena.

The analyses reported here are based on a total of 12,507 recorded and transcribed utterances, comprising 43,901 tokens. We can use these data to

answer a variety of questions about speech produced in a complex problem-solving environment. Recognition performance data are presented in
Figure 6. The values plotted represent the error rate averaged across all
eight subjects.

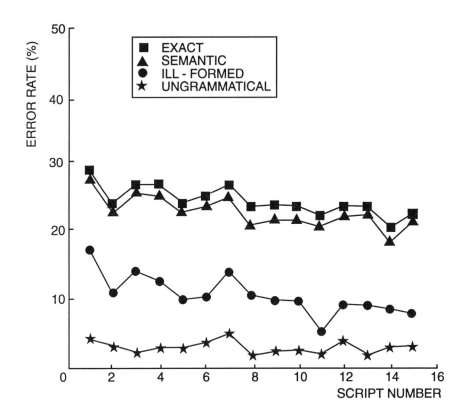

Figure 6:   Mean utterance accuracy across tasks.

The top line in Figure 6, taken from Rudnicky *et al.*, April (1990), shows exact
utterance accuracy, calculated over all utterances in the corpus, including
system firings for extraneous noise and abandoned (i.e., user interrupted)
utterances. It does not include begin-end detector failures (which produce a
zero-length utterance), of which there were on the average 10% per session.

Exact accuracy corresponds to utterance accuracy as conventionally reported for speech recognition systems using the NBS scoring algorithm (Pallet, 1989). The general trend of improvement in performance over time appears to be fairly gradual. The improvement indicates that users are sufficiently aware of what might improve system performance such that they could modify their behavior accordingly. However, the amount of control they have over it appears to be very limited.

The next line down shows *semantic* accuracy, calculated by determining, for each utterance, no matter what its content, whether the correct action was taken by the system. For example, the user might say "LET'S GO DOWN FIVE," which lies outside the system language. Nevertheless, because of grammatical constraints, the system might force this utterance into "DOWN FIVE," which happens to be grammatically acceptable and which also happens to carry out the desired action. From the task point of view, this recognition is correct; from the recognition point of view it is, of course, wrong. Semantic accuracy, relative to exact accuracy, represents the added performance that can be realized by the parsing and understanding components of a spoken language system. In the present case, the added performance results from the "silent" influence of the word-pair grammar that is part of the recognizer. Thus, grammatical constraints are enforced not through, say, explicit identification and reanalysis of out-of-language utterances, but implicitly, through the word-pair grammar. The spread between semantic and exact accuracy defines the contribution of higher-level processes and can be used to track the performance of "higher-level" components of a spoken language system.

The line at the bottom of the graph shows *grammaticality* error. Grammaticality is determined by first eliminating all non-speech events from the *transcribed* corpus then passing these filtered utterances through the parsing component of the spreadsheet system. Grammaticality provides a dynamic measure of the *coverage* provided by the system task language (on the assumption that the user's task language evolves with experience) and is one indicator of whether the language is sufficient for carrying out the task in question.

The grammaticality function can be used to track a number of system attributes. For example, its value over the period that covers the user's initial experience with a system indicate the degree to which the implemented language covers utterances produced by the inexperienced user and provides one measure of how successfully the system designers have anticipated the spoken language that users intuitively select for the task.

Examined over time, the grammaticality function indicates the speed with which users modify their spoken language for the task to reflect the constraints imposed by the implementation and how well they manage to stay within it. Measurement of grammaticality after some time away from the system indicates how well the task language can be retained and is an indication of its appropriateness for the task. We believe that grammaticality is an important component of a composite metric for the *language habitability* of a spoken-language system and can provide a meaningful basis for comparing different spoken-language system interfaces to a particular application.[6]

Examining the curves for the present system we find, unsurprisingly, that VSC is rather primitive in its ability to compensate for poor recognition performance, as evidenced by how close the semantic accuracy curve is to the exact accuracy curve. On the other hand, it appears to cover user language quite well, with only an average grammaticality error of only 2.9%.[7] In all likelihood, this indicates that users found it quite easy to stay within the confines of the task, which in turn may not be surprising given its simplicity.

When a spoken language system is exposed to speech generated in a natural setting a variety of acoustic events appear that contribute to performance degradation. Spontaneous speech events can be placed into one of three categories: *lexical, extra-lexical,* and *non-lexical,* depending on whether the item is part of the system lexicon, a recognizable word that is not part of the lexicon, or some other event, such as breath noise. These categories, as well as the procedure for their transcription, are described in greater detail in Rudnicky and Sakamoto (1989). Table 8 lists the most common non-lexical events encountered in our corpus. The number of events is given, as well as their incidence in terms of words in the corpus. Given the nature of the task, it is not surprising to find, for example, that a large number of paper rustles intrudes into the speech stream. Non-lexical events were transcribed in 893 of the 12,507 utterances used for this analysis (7.14% of all utterances).

The *ill-formed* curve in Figure 6 shows the proportion of transcribed utterances that contain extraneous material (such as the items in Table 8). This function was generated by calculating grammaticality with both non-lexical and extra-lexical tokens included in the transcription. As is apparent, the

---

[6] *System habitability*, on the other hand, has to be based on a combination of language habitability, robustness with respect to spontaneous speech phenomena, and system responsiveness.

[7] Bear in mind that this percentage includes *intentional agrammaticality* with respect to the task, such as expressions of annoyance or interaction with other humans.

incidence of extraneous events steadily decreases over sessions. Users apparently realize the harmful effects of such events and work to eliminate them (although the user does not have complete control over such events, otherwise the decrease would have been much steeper).

Table 8: Incidence of (some) non-lexical spontaneous speech tokens.

585	++RUSTLE+	4	++PHONE-RING+
206	++BREATH+	4	++NOISE+
43	++MUMBLE+	4	++DOOR-SLAM+
18	++SNIFF+	4	++CLEARING-THROAT+
13	++BACKGROUND NOISE+	4	++BACKGROUND-VOICES+
11	++MOUTH-NOISES+	2	++SNEEZE+
10	++COUGH+	1	++SIGH+
6	++YAWN+	1	++PING+
5	++GIGGLE+	1	++BACKGROUND-LAUGH+

While existing statistical modeling techniques can be used to deal with the most common events (such as paper rustles) in a satisfactory manner (as shown by Ward, 1989), more general techniques will need to be developed to account for low-frequency or otherwise unexpected events. A spoken language system should be capable of accurately identifying novel events and disposing of them in appropriate ways.

7. Summary

In this chapter we have described in detail the design and evaluation of a spoken language system whose operating characteristics approach the minimal requirements for a natural and easy to use system, incorporating speaker independence and continuous speech capabilities.

The design process is time-consuming and requires careful attention to the development of a spoken language and the training of the speech recognition component. The design of the speech interface must take into account characteristics of the speech device, such as delay and recognition error, that may make it difficult for a user to work with.

An informative evaluation of a spoken language system must provide information about the system's performance as an interface in comparison with other modalities, as well as a detailed characterization of its characteristics as a recognition system.

8. Acknowledgments

The work described in this chapter has benefited from the contributions of many people. I would particularly like to mention Bob Brennan, who implemented an initial version of the voice spreadsheet; Joe Polifroni, who performed the Wizard experiments and carried out the language analyses; and Michelle Sakamoto, who conducted the evaluation experiments.

9. References

Chapanis, A. (1981). Interactive Human Communication: Some lessons learned from laboratory experiments. In B. Shackel (Ed.), *Man-Computer Interaction: Human Factor Aspects of Computers and People* (pp. 65–114). Rockville, MD: Sijthoff and Noordhoff.

Cohen, M. H. (1989). Phonological structures for speech recognition. *Unpublished doctoral dissertation, University of California, Berkeley.*

Gallaway, G. R. (1981). Response times to user activities in interactive man/machine computer systems. *Proceedings of the Human Factors Society—25th annual meeting*, 754–758.

Hauptmann, A. G., & Rudnicky, A. I. (1988). Talking to computers: An empirical investigation. *International Journal of Man-Machine Studies, 28*, 583–604.

Lee, K. (1989). *Automatic Speech Recognition: The Development of the SPHINX system.* Boston: Kluwer Academic Publishers.

Pallet, D. (1989). Benchmark tests for DARPA Resource Management database performance evaluations. *Proceedings of the ICASSP, IEEE*, 536–539.

Rudnicky, A. I., Sakamoto, M. H., & Polifroni, J. H. (1990). Spoken language interaction in a goal-directed task. *Proceedings of the ICASSP, 4*, 45–48.

Rudnicky, A. (1989). The design of voice-driven interfaces. *Proceedings of the February DARPA Speech and Natural Language Workshop*, 120–124.

Rudnicky, A., Polifroni, J., Thayer, E., & Brennan, R. (1989). Interactive problem solving with speech. *Journal of the Acoustical Society of America, 84*, S213(Abstract).

Rudnicky, A., & Sakamoto, M. (1989). Transcription conventions for spoken language research. *Carnegie Mellon University School of Computer Science, CMU-CS-89-194.*

Rudnicky, A. I., & Quirin, J. L. (1990). *Subjective reaction to system response delay: A pilot study*. Unpublished Manuscript.

Ward, W. (1989). Modelling non-verbal sounds for speech recognition. *Proceedings of the October DARPA Workshop on Speech and Natural Language*, 47–50.

Chapter 13

Synthetic Spoken Driving Instructions by Telephone and while Driving: Implications for Interfaces

James Raymond Davis[1]
Massachusetts Institute of Technology

This chapter describes two programs—*Direction Assistance* and the *Back Seat Driver*—that use synthetic speech to provide driving instruction. Direction Assistance, the older of the two, uses the telephone, and provides directions for the entire route at the beginning of the trip. The Back Seat Driver is installed in an automobile, and gives instructions while enroute. The differences in the way these programs are used require differences in the strategies and tactics adopted in the user interface. This chapter describes these programs and the issues they address in the use of synthetic speech for interfaces. These issues should be meaningful to those building speech interfaces for other applications.

1. Direction Assistance

Direction Assistance gives spoken driving instructions over a telephone. The user enters destination and origin addresses using touch tone input, and the program finds a route, and then describes it with synthetic speech. Direction Assistance was inspired by a program written by Jane Elliot and Mike Lesk that could generate simple text instructions and draw maps. The structure of the route finder and map database of Direction Assistance is substantially similar to theirs. The Direction Assistance program differs from Elliot and Lesk's in its interface and by the higher quality of the text it produces.

Direction Assistance has four parts. The *Location Finder* queries the user to obtain the starting point and destination of the route. A location can be specified as a street address or as a telephone number. The *Route Finder* finds a simple, short route between the two points. The *Describer* generates

[1]The work reported in this chapter was completed while the author was at M.I.T., Cambridge. Curremtly, J.R. Davis works at the Design Research Institute, Cornell University, Ithaca, NY.

high quality English text describing the route. The *Narrator* recites the route to the user. A digital street map, which covers a 41 square mile area of Boston centered on the Charles River, records the name, position, and quality of each street, whether it is one-way, whether it has lanes reserved for left or right turns, and the position of features such as stop-lights, stop-signs, notable signs, and gas stations. Direction Assistance is a tool for research on two related areas. The first is the use of the telephone for accessing services from a computer. To this end, Direction Assistance is an application with an intrinsic motivation for its users. People do call it and do rely on its output. Direction Assistance helps test the limits of the kinds of interface we can construct using only synthetic speech output and touch-tone input. Second, Direction Assistance lets us investigate the generation of fluent, spoken instructions. We now consider the implications for interface design.

People use Direction Assistance by calling it on the telephone. Its input comes only from push-buttons on the telephone, and its only output is synthetic speech. The two modules that interact with the user, the Location Finder and the Narrator, have quite different behavior, because the Location Finder is input oriented, while the Narrator is output oriented. The Location Finder needs to obtain two locations, and it does this by asking questions and soliciting input. The user can specify location by giving either a street name and address number, or by giving a telephone number (the program's data base includes an inverted phone book). It needs to get several different types of input—answers to yes or no questions, telephone numbers, address numbers and street names. It has little to say, other than to guide the user through the input process. The Narrator, on the other hand, has a lot to say, and needs no input from the user. Its main concern is *flow control*, making sure that it is going as fast as the user can write, but no faster. Both of these modules also have the secondary goals of keeping the user oriented within the interaction and recovering from errors.

1.1 The initial message

Direction Assistance is designed to be used by people with no experience with computers or synthetic speech. Almost every American is at least familiar (through fiction) with the concept that computers might talk, but they are not experienced with interfaces built with present-day technology. There are lots of ways to go wrong. The interface tries to forestall some of them with its initial message:

> Hi. This is Direction Assistance. I can speak to you, but I can not hear your voice. When I ask you a question, answer me with the keys on

your telephone. If you get confused any time while you're using me, hit the key with the star or asterisk.

The initial message conveys several important ideas. First, it tells the user how to communicate. People expect to use the telephone to have conversations with people, not machines. They are only beginning to be competent with answering machines (which speak, then listen), and hardly anyone knows how to interact with a program that speaks often, but listens only for button pushes. This message says that one is to "speak" only in response to a question, and then only by pressing buttons, not by actually speaking.

The second idea is that there is always help available, and always in the same way, by hitting the "star" key. This is a surprisingly difficult concept to convey. Few users ever use the help key, even those who daily use computer systems. There are several possible explanations. First, this initial message is unexpected, and may have caught people by surprise. Second, the message has no direct relevance to the task at hand. People call Direction Assistance to get directions for driving, not instructions for using a program. Finally, people may not have understood what "star" meant. In general, it is difficult to find a universal names for the "star" key. Some people prefer "asterisk." The "number sign" key is even worse, being called "pound sign," "sharp sign," "hash" or even "tic tac toe" by different people.

1.2 Six Different Protocols for Data Entry

In order to find a route, Direction Assistance needs the user's origin and destination. To obtain these locations, it asks the user a series of questions. These questions take the form of small dialogs or protocols, each specialized for one kind of data entry. This section considers these six protocols, most of which are relevant to other applications.

The user specifies a location with a *street address number* and a *street name*, e.g. "111" and "Ivy." The user may also specify a location with a *telephone number*, which is then converted to an address using a telephone directory database which has been inverted on the phone number. This feature is not available on all implementations of Direction Assistance, as it depends on the availability of this database and upon issues of privacy. (You may not want people to be able to locate your dwelling from your phone number.) These three protocols are logically necessary for obtaining a location. The remaining three protocols are overhead—they help the user use the program, but do not contribute any direct value. In some cases (described below) the street number and name may not determine a unique location, so the user will be asked to make a *selection* from a small list of candidates.

There are actually two forms of selection, as described below. Finally, it is sometimes necessary to ask yes or no *questions*. We consider each of these in turn, starting with questions.

The interface poses a yes or no question by stating a possibility and requesting the user to hit any key if it is true, for example "If you want to enter a different address, please hit any key now." If the user takes no action within a specified time the answer is no. The wording of the message always includes the consequence of the "no" if it is not obvious. This protocol is easier to use than one that requires an explicit action for "yes" or "no" (e.g. "Press 1 if yes, 2 if no"), but can be slower, since the user has no way to directly enter a "no" answer, but must instead wait the full duration allowed for the answer. This duration must be long enough for the user to make a decision and hit the key. The present duration is three seconds, a value chosen by informal observation only.

Selection means choosing one of a small list of items. There are two types of selection. In a *sequential* selection the system slowly reads a list of choices, pausing briefly after each, until the user designates one by striking a key. This is effectively a yes or no question ("Do you want this one?") for each element of the list. In an *enumerated* selection the system reads the entire list, assigning each item a number, then asks the user to hit the key for the number of the desired item. (If Direction Assistance used the "explicit action" form of yes or no question mentioned above, it would be an example of an enumerated selection.)

Each type of selection has its advantages and disadvantages. Sequential selection is simple to use but can be very slow, since the user may have to listen to several undesired choices before hearing the one wanted. The user may also not know which choice is the best without hearing them all. For this reason, if the user makes no selection, the selection routine offers to repeat the list. Enumerated selection is harder to use than sequential selection because the user must remember and enter a number. The compensation for this complexity is that it can be faster than sequential selection. There are two reasons for this. First, the list is read faster, since the system need not pause to await a user action while reading. More importantly, if the user already knows the order of the options she or he can enter the number immediately, without waiting for the list to be read. This makes enumerated selection most appropriate when the same list of choices will be presented more than once in an interaction, or when the user is familiar with the choices.

The user enters a street address number by entering the digits, then hitting the number sign key (#). A delimiter is required because the number of digits in a street address number is unpredictable. The delimiter is the number sign key because the only other non-digit key is *, which is reserved for help. Telephone numbers require no delimiter since the number of digits in a phone number is deterministic, at least for calls within North America. (The current program accepts exactly seven digits, since one area code covers all of Boston. This would not work in New York City. The program would require a more complex algorithm, but the number of digits would remain deterministic.) If the user enters at least one digit, then pauses for more than 10 seconds, the program reminds the user to hit the number sign key when finished entering.

The user selects street names by spelling them with the letters on the keypad. Spelling words with the telephone keypad is difficult for three reasons. First, people are not familiar with the layout of the letters - they have to "hunt and peck" for letters. Second, the letters Q and Z, and the space character are missing. Finally, each of the keys has three different letters, and there is no obvious way for the user to designate which of the three is intended. Other systems have resolved this problem by using more than one button push per character, either with a shift sequence (e.g. using keys *, 0, and # to select one of the letters), by a two key sequence where the first key specifies a group of three letters and the second selects one of them (e.g. 2 1 is "A", 2 2 is "B", 2 3 is "C"), or by hitting a key N times to select the N'th letter upon it.

Direction Assistance places the letter Q on the 7 key (with PRS) and Z on the 9 key (with WXY). This means that if the user guesses that Q belongs with its neighbors, P and R, the guess will be correct. In addition, Q and Z are also on the 1 key, as this is another possible guess. It is harder to find a reasonable place for the space character (which is needed for names like "MOUNT AUBURN"). It is on the 1 key, but I don't expect users to guess this. They just have to hit the help key to find out. Users can also enter such names without the space.

Ambiguous spelling is not a serious problem for Direction Assistance. To understand why, think of the spelling scheme as actually assigning new spellings to words, thus for instance "FISH" is "spelled" "3474." Ambiguous spelling will only be a problem for those streets which have the same spelling in this reduced alphabet. Even though Direction Assistance can't tell at first whether the 3 stands for D, E, or F, when it has all four letters there is no ambiguity. To say this more formally, the spelling scheme forms a set of equivalences classes for the set of street names, and most of these classes have only a single element because of the redundancy in the way the English language uses letters in words.

Like numbers, names are delimited by the number sign. The user need only enter enough letters to be unique. This is possible because Direction Assistance stores the set of street names in a "letter tree," which is a tree where each (non-terminal) node has nine leaves, one for each digit of the telephone keypad. Terminal nodes store the word (or words) "spelled" with the corresponding digit sequence that leads from the root to the node. To determine that a word is unique at a given (non-terminal) node the program need only check that there is only one non-empty branch at that node, and at all child nodes. If the word is not unique, the program requires the user to continue spelling.

If the terminal node is ambiguous (that is, there is more than one word with the numeric "spelling") then the system asks the user to make a sequential selection among them. There are fewer ambiguous words than one might imagine at first. As a test, I encoded all the top level words in Webster's Seventh Dictionary into this spelling. After removing hyphenated, contracted, and compound words I had 48102 words. Of these, only 2158 (4.5%) were ambiguous. More than half of these had only one ambiguous alternative. The largest set had nine members: paw, pax, pay, raw, rax, ray, saw, sax, and say. Witten (1982) found 8% collisions in a 24,500 word dictionary using a similar encoding. For Boston street names, which average 7 characters, there are just 37 ambiguous sets out of 2433 names (1.5%), and the largest collision sets have three members.

1.3   Correcting errors

These protocols are designed to be as easy to use as possible when things go right, but the price of this simplicity is complexity when things go wrong. There is usually a way for the user to correct a mistake, but that way is seldom obvious. Error correction depends on which party notices the error first—the system or the user. Direction Assistance does a reasonable job of diagnosing those mistakes it catches, but leaves it to the user to fix them. The most common mistake is users forgetting to enter the closing delimiter after a number or name. If the user does nothing for ten seconds, the system reminds him or her of the need for a delimiter. The system can also tell when a user enters the number and name with no delimiter after the number, because no address number in Boston can exceed four digits. After the fourth digit, the system interrupts the user, explains the error, and asks the user to start over.

The system can also catch some spelling mistakes. If the user strikes a key sequence that cannot possibly lead to a valid word, the system immediately interrupts the user. (It can detect this case using the same mechanism used for "completion" described above.) The message given is that the name being entered is either outside the area mapped, or was misspelled, and invites the user to try again. The system cannot detect spelling errors that are nevertheless valid street names. Likewise, if the user hits the zero key ("Oper"), the system says that that key is not used for spelling, and invites him or her to hit the star key for help.

Error correction is harder when it is the user who first notices the problem. While spelling, if the user hits the zero key twice, spelling is aborted. The user is not expected to guess this, so the help message for spelling mentions it. If the user begins to enter a number, and notices a mistake in the entry, there is no "rubout" key, nor is there an "abort," because there is no key to spare. If the user simply waits and does nothing, however, the system will eventually remind him or her to hit the delimiter. If the user continues to wait, the system will timeout for a second time and ask with a yes or no question whether he or she wants to enter a different address. The user can then start over. If a mistake is made, but not noticed until after entering the delimiter (when the system speaks the number as a confirmation), there is nothing that can be done immediately, because the system is now listening for a street name. However, if the user aborts from spelling a street name, Direction Assistance asks for a new address as well.

A final possible error is that the user may enter one street name, only to have Direction Assistance find some other street than the one intended. For example, the user might spell "Alban" (a street in Dorchester, just below the southern border of the program's street map) which the system interprets as "Albany." There is nothing the user can do to correct this error. The only course of action is to hang up.

This section has described a set of protocols for querying the user for yes or no questions, selections, numbers of fixed and variable length, and names chosen from a dictionary. Most of these protocols could be useful to other applications that use synthetic speech and a telephone. The next section gives more detail about how Direction Assistance uses these protocols.

1.4 How Direction Assistance Determines Locations

After the user has specified a street number and a street name, Direction Assistance determines a location by consulting the street map database, which records the beginning and ending address numbers on every block of every street. It finds intermediate locations by interpolating along the street. It will sometimes happen that an unambiguous name has more than one referent. For example, the address "10 Beacon" could be Beacon Street or Beacon Place or Beacon Terrace. (Had the address been 100 Beacon, then Beacon Place and Terrace would have been eliminated, as these streets are quite short.) Moreover it could be the Beacon Street in Boston, Somerville or Chelsea. If the address number cannot be found on any of the street names, then Direction Assistance informs the user, and offers to accept a different number. The most common cause for this error is an error in the addresses stored in the street map.

Resolving an ambiguous reference requires the user to make a selection from the set of possible referents. Before asking anything, Direction Assistance attempts to partition the set in two different ways, by street "type" (e.g. "Street" or "Lane") and by city. If either one is a complete partition then it asks the user to make a (sequential) selection from that category. For example, given "11 Davenport" it might say "11 Davenport Street could be in Boston or Cambridge." If neither means of classification is a partition, then it asks first for the street type, and then the city. In both cases, the alternatives are presented in order of decreasing *a-priori* likelihood, that is, "Streets" come first, and "Cities" are presented in decreasing order of size. Sometimes a city is not a sufficiently fine criterion to determine a location. For instance, there are two distinct places "140 Elm Street" in Cambridge. In this case, the program uses the names of neighborhoods, as determined by the ZIP code of the two segments. It is a regrettable fact that the names of neighborhoods, as determined from ZIP code, does not always correspond with one's intuitions for the boundaries of neighborhoods, but this seems to be the best that can be done. As a final detail, when the Location Finder finds an ambiguous reference, it says "Hmmm" to provide an immediate echo to the user, just in case the process of testing for partitions takes a noticeable amount of time.

Most versions of Direction Assistance accept only addresses, but one version accepts phone numbers as well. In this case, before the user can enter a location he or she must first decide which form of address is preferred by answering an enumerated selection: "Enter 1 before a phone number, 2 before an address." This is the only place Direction Assistance uses an enumerated selection, since this is the only question Direction Assistance asks that is the same every time one uses it.

After the program has locations for the origin and destination, no further user input is required. The program finds a route, and then forms and recites text describing the route. If the user strikes any keys during this time, the system tells the user that it is ignoring this input. After reading the text, the system offers to repeat it. There is no way for the user to pause the narration or repeat parts of it. An earlier version of this program attempted to provide such features, but I removed it, because I could not design an interface that was easy enough to use to require no explanation, and I did not want to take up the user's time with a lengthy explanation before reading the directions. A preliminary experiment on the use of voice to control reading is described in Schmandt (1988). This appears more promising than using touch tones.

1.5 The Telephone is a Mixed Blessing for Direction Assistance

The great advantage of the telephone is its ubiquity. Synthetic speech makes each telephone a potential computer terminal, albeit a weak one. But the telephone has some problems of its own.

The first is that it is impossible to present a continuous *context* to the user when requesting data input. By context, I mean some continually available output that tells the user what kind and quantity of input is expected and how much progress the user has made in providing it. This kind of information is easily provided by a graphic interface such as a form filling environment or a menu. The interface always prompts for input, but the user may not understand the prompt because of noise, inarticulate speech, or inattention. Even if the prompt is correctly heard, it must also be remembered, for it is not present during the time the user is entering the data. In a graphics environment the prompt remains visible. (We might look forward to the day when telephones also have graphics, or at least alphabetic output. The AT&T 7506 ISDN telephone "terminal" on my desk has a two line, 25 character wide display on it. Unfortunately there is no way for Direction Assistance to display a message on this screen, or even determine that it is there.) The problem, then, is that the user may not know what to enter or how to delimit it. Neither of these are explicitly indicated, other than in the prompt. One possible solution is to employ acoustic icons, as discussed in Gaver (19??). The system might play a faint dial tone to indicate that a phone number was expected, and ambient street noise to indicate that an address was expected. If a closing delimiter is expected, and none arrives after a fixed delay, a timeout occurs, and the interface reminds the user that a delimiter is required. This has often been helpful.

A second problem is that programs cannot detect whether the caller is still on the line or has hung up the phone. A user might hang-up through frustration, or to recover from an error, or by accident. The only sign of a hang-up is that no input is received. As a result, the interface is more complicated than I like. Every routine that expects input must have a timeout, such that if no input occurs, the user is deemed to have hung up. This time-out adds a further complication, since the system should not hang up if the user is merely slow, so in every case where a timeout occurs, the system first asks the user to respond by striking any key. This is described by Hayes (19??) as a channel checking dialogue. This dialogue can be a problem, too, since it introduces a timing condition in input: when the dialogue occurs the user may be uncertain whether a keystroke is taken as answer to the channel checking dialogue or as ordinary input.

1.6 The Describer Produces a Text Description of the Route

Direction Assistance produces high quality text descriptions. As such, it can be considered to be a text producing system, like those of Appelt (19??), Danlos (19??), Hovy (19??), McDonald McKeown (1985), Paris (1988), Simmons and Slocum (1972) and Young and Fallside (1979). Like all these systems, it has the problems of using limited means to impart potentially unlimited information, and of conveying information in a form with no direct mapping into natural language.

In this case, the input to the Describer is a route, which is simply a sequence of street segments, each a straight line. In general, at the end of each street segment there will be more than one next possible segment, only one of which lies along the route. The simplest way to describe the route would be a sequence of alternating rotations and straight line motion. But the driver could never follow a route expressed at such a low level of geometric detail. Even if possible (if the driver were a robot), it would be useless, for the map is an abstraction, and the world is more complicated than the map. If the driver drove literally according to the map, he or she would soon have an accident. Therefore the program must produce a text for the driver to interpret, a text which may be thought of as a program in a very high level language. This requires that the program have some sense of the "programming language" for driving, for how people think about the actions of driving, for these are the terms it must use in describing the route.

An examination of people's descriptions of routes shows them broken into a series of "choice points" where the driver is to take an action other than that which he or she would ordinarily do. Route descriptions typically assume that drivers will "go straight" unless told to do otherwise. There are various kinds of choice points, and each is described in its own way. All "turns" are not alike: some will be called "turns," but others will be called "forks" or "exits." The choice of terms depends upon the topology and geometry of the intersection, the kind of streets involved, and also varies with local dialect. The task for the Describer, then, is to recognize those points along the route that are choice points, and to generate text that tells the driver what to do at those choice points. The Describer has a taxonomy of driving actions, each represented by a small "expert" called an *act*. For each choice point, the Describer determines which act best describes it. Then it asks the expert to decide whether the act taken there is obvious, that is, whether the driver can be expected to take it without being told to do so. If not, the act generates some text to describe the action.

In addition to telling the driver what to do, the act expert must also tell her when to do it. It might seem that distance traveled (as measured by the odometer) would be sufficient, but it is not, for odometers are inaccurate, and drivers do not attend to them. Nor is it enough to give the name of the next street, for some streets have no names, moreover the street signs may be missing, misaligned, or hard to see. Instead, the Describer attempts to generate a *cue* that tells the driver when to act. A cue helps the driver follow the tour. There are four kinds of cues. *Action* cues tell when to do an act. *Confirmatory* cues describe things that will be seen while following the route. *Warning* cues caution the driver about possible mistakes. A warning successfully heeded also serves as a confirmatory cue. *Failure* cues describe the consequences of missing an act, e.g. "If you see this, you have gone too far."

1.7 The Narrator Reads the Route Description

After the Describer has produced a text, the Narrator reads it. In the earliest versions of Direction Assistance, the Narrator simply sent the text to a text-to-speech system. This had the unfortunate result that the text (which was quite lengthy) was difficult to understand. One reason for this is that the text-to-speech system was unable to produce correct prosody (intentional variations of pitch and timing) for the text, because prosody depends in part on discourse-level phenomena such as topic structure and information status (Hirschberg, 19??). Such discourse information cannot be correctly computed from the text alone by present day text-to-speech systems. They are designed to make only the most neutral choices in prosody, since it is less harmful to be boring than to be misleading. This is ironic, for all of the information required for expressive prosody is present in the representations used by the Describer, only to be lost when text is generated.

The solution, as described in Davis (19??) is to make both attentional and intentional information about the route description available for the assignment of intonational features. The implementation of this intonation assignment component provides a first approximation of how recent models of discourse structure can be used to control intonational variation in ways that build upon recent research in intonational meaning. Additionally, it suggests ways in which these discourse models must be enhanced in order to permit the assignment of appropriate intonational features.

2.   The Back Seat Driver

The Back Seat Driver is the successor to Direction Assistance—it is what Direction Assistance would be if it could ride in the car with you. The Back Seat Driver knows where the car is (it uses a dead-reckoning navigation system), so it need not ask for your starting location, and it gives you instructions as you need them, instead of all at once.

Compared with Direction Assistance, the Back Seat Driver is even easier to use, because it frees the driver from having to keep track of progress along the route. The driver using a route described by Direction Assistance must decide when to take the next action, but the Back Seat Driver tells the driver when to act. In addition, the Back Seat Driver can recover from errors. Direction Assistance accepts user input only in response to prompts, but the Back Seat Driver is a conversational system, in that either party can give input at any time. To be sure, the conversation takes an odd form, in that the two parties contribute in different modalities. The Back Seat Driver contributes only by speaking, the driver by driving and/or pushing buttons. (The use of buttons is regrettable, but at the time this work was done, there was no speech recognition system suitable for real-time use in a car.)

Compared to other in-car navigation systems (which display maps, perhaps showing the position of the car or destination), Back Seat Driver provides a new and better class of service, because it provides both less and more information that a map. A computer-controlled map provides more information than the driver needs. Driving down a street, the driver does not need to know the names of the parallel streets, or even that they are there. The driver does not even need to know where he or she is. What must be known, and what the Back Seat Driver provides, is what to do. Route guidance should be procedural, not declarative, as in maps. Even those systems that find routes and display them on maps still suffer by comparison, for they continue to provide too much information, and the route guidance is still in declarative form. The driver must look at the map and interpret the route displayed there to decide what to do.

The strongest reason for using speech in the Back Seat Driver is that it makes it easy to provide procedural route guidance to the driver. A few other navigation systems provide procedural guidance in the form of arrows or icons, but doing so requires inventing a whole new graphic language. Why do so, when speech is already available? Using natural language allows the program to describe the route with great flexibility, including the ability to use a wide variety of landmarks (e.g. traffic lights, stop signs, gas stations). The following text provides an example of this power:

> Get in the left lane because you're going to take a left at the next set of lights. It's a complicated intersection because there are two streets on the left. You want the sharper of the two. It's also the better of them. After the turn, get into the right lane.

A second strong reason for using speech is that it leaves the driver's eyes free for watching traffic instead of a display. The implications for traffic safety should be obvious.

2.1 The Back Seat Driver Maintains the Driver's Sense of Co-presence

A key issue for the Back Seat Driver is to maintain the driver's sense of the program's co-presence with the driver. For the driver to have confidence in the Back Seat Driver, he or she must feel that the program is seeing the world as it changes.

One reason this is an issue is that the Back Seat Driver is not constantly providing evidence of its presence. A driver relying on a real human navigator can be assured of the navigators presence and attentiveness with little effort. Likewise, a driver using a mapping system can see the map moving using only peripheral vision. But the Back Seat Driver is not constantly talking—that would be most annoying—and so long stretches of time can go by with no evidence that the program is still running. When the program is silent, the driver may begin to wonder whether it has crashed. This was also an issue for Direction Assistance, since the route finding algorithm sometimes takes tens of seconds to find a route. In that case, it was changed to say "Still working" every ten seconds, but this would not be desirable in the car.

Failing the means to provide continual evidence of existence, the program attempts to compensate when it does speak by forming utterances which clearly show that the program is "aware" of the car's position and speed and the driver's actions.

One way this is done is by proper use of *deictic* pronouns. Deictics are words that "point" at something. The four deictic pronouns in English are "this" and "these," and "that"and "those." The difference between the first and second pairs is that the first are *proximal*, that is they refer to something close. The Back Seat Driver uses the correct deictic when referring to landmarks. If the landmark is close, it uses use the proximal form (e.g.

"these lights"); when distant, it uses a brief noun phrase (e.g. "the next set of lights"). This is important. When a driver is stopped 30 meters back from a stop light, it may be literally true to say "turn left at the next set of lights," but it will confuse the driver.

A second means of conveying co-presence is to acknowledge the driver's actions. After the driver carries out an instruction the system briefly acknowledges the act if there is time, unless the act was so simple (e.g. continuing straight) as to need no acknowledgment. This makes using the Back Seat Driver more like a conversation, one where the driver contributes by driving and the program by speaking. The driver comes to know that the program will speak when he or she does anything notable, and this makes the program's silences more tolerable while the driver is simply going straight. The acknowledgment is typically a short phrase like "Okay," but if the driver turns onto a new street that has a name, and the name has not already been mentioned, the program tells the driver the name of the street as an acknowledgement, e.g. "Now you're on Ames Street." This serves as both a confirmation and at the same time, perhaps helps the driver to learn more about the city. Those drivers who dislike acknowledgments may disable them.

Another way to acknowledge the driver's actions is to use *cue words* in the instructions. It will often be the case that the route calls for the driver to do the same thing twice (e.g. make two left turns). The speech synthesizer we use has very consistent pronunciation, and drivers sometimes get the impression that the system is repeating itself because it is in error (like a record skipping). The acknowledgments help to dispel this, but we also cause the text to include cue words such as "another." These indicate that the system is aware of its earlier speech and the driver's previous actions.

Yet another means of conveying co-presence is to make occasional remarks about the road and the route. These remarks indicate that the program is correctly oriented. As an example, when the road makes a sweeping bend to one side, the program speaks of this as if it were an instruction ("Follow the road as it bends to the right") even though the driver has no choice in what to do. The program also warns the driver about potentially hazardous situations, such as the road changing from one-way to two-way, or a decrease in the number of lanes. As with acknowledgments, these warnings can be disabled if the driver dislikes them.

The program also conveys co-presence by making "idle" remarks when the driver is on the route and the program has been silent for five minutes, and would otherwise be silent. Even though these comments (e.g. about the weather) have nothing to do with the route, they still convey information, according to the conversational theory of H. P. Grice, which holds that cooperative speakers organize their talking by means of a set of maxims (Grice, 1975). One maxim is that of *quantity*, which says: "Make your contribution as informative as is required." Normally speakers follow these maxims, but can also convey information by appearing to violate a maxim. When the program makes an uninformed remark, the driver can reason as follows: "The program, like all cooperative agencies, obeys the maxim of quantity. Therefore, if it had something important to say, it would say it. The program said nothing of great significance, therefore there is nothing urgently requiring my attention. So everything is well." At present, our "Gricean" utterances are trivial observations about the weather, but we are re-designing them to convey useful information about the city.

A final example of co-presence is the program's ability to recover when the driver does not follow the Back Seat Driver's instructions. This can happen for many reasons: the driver can make a mistake, the program (or database) can be in error, or there can be some external factor (such as an accident) that prevents the driver from doing as the program requests. When this happens, the Back Seat Driver finds a new route from the current location to the destination, while the driver is still moving. It also describes the mistake, saying something like "Oops, I meant for you to go straight." This kind of text makes clear to the driver that the system itself notices the miscommunication, without assigning any blame on the driver, and it does so in a way that allows the driver to come to better understand the system's style of giving instructions. This also shows the superior power of natural language. No iconic language is likely to be able to talk about the past or describe hypothetical actions that did not take place. The Back Seat Driver can do it with ease.

If, despite this, the driver should become anxious about the program's continued operation, he or she need merely push one of several buttons. One button, the so-called "What next?" button, gives the next significant instruction, even if the action is still quite distant. Another button, the "What now?" button, gives an instruction for the the very next intersection, even if the program considers it obvious. It would be better to use speech input for these functions, and this is a topic of ongoing research.

3. Conclusions

This chapter has described two programs that give high quality spoken driving instructions, each in its own way. Direction Assistance prompts the user for an origin and destination address using a variety of protocols for the various types of data required, finds a route, then forms a route description by classifying actions according to a taxonomy of driving terms. The Back Seat Driver builds upon this by following the driver's progress along the route, speaking when instructions are needed. Careful attention to linguistic detail is necessary to maintain the driver's sense of the program's co-presence while driving.

4. Acknowledgments

The work described here was supported by several institutions at various times, among them the Thinking Machines Corporation, the DARPA Space and Naval Warfare Systems Command, the Nippon Telegraph and Telephone Public Corporation, Symbolics, the Digital Equipment Corporation, and the Nippon Electric Company Home Electronics Division.

5. References

Grice, H. P. (1975). Logic and Conversation. In P. Cole & J. L. Morgan (Eds.), *Syntax and Semantics 3: Speech Acts* (pp. 41–58). New York: Academic Press.

Hovy, E. H. (1988). Two types of planning in language generation. *Proceddings of the 26th Conference of the Association of Computational Linguistics*, 179–186.

McKeown, K. R. (1985). Discourse strategies for generating natural-language text. *Artificial Intelligence*, 27(1), 1-41.

Paris, L. (1988). Tailoring object descriptions to a user's level of expertise. *Computational Linguistics*, 14(3), 64–74.

Schmandt, C. (1988). Employing voice back channels to facilitate audio cocument retrieval. *ACM Conference on Office Information Systems*, 213–218.

Simmons, R., & Slocum, J. (1972). Generating English discourse from semantic nets. *Communications of the ACM*, 15(10), 891–905.

Witten, I. H. (1982). *Principles of Computer Speech*. Academic Press.

Young, S. J., & Fallside, F. (1979D). Speech synthesis from concept: A method for speech output from information systems. *Journal of the Acoustic Society of America*, 66(3), 685-695.

Chapter 14

Human Factors Contributions to the Development of a Speech Recognition Cellular Telephone

Eileen C. Schwab, C.A. Ball
and Barry L. Lively[1]

In the mid 1980's the cellular telephone market began to experience explosive growth. As the market expanded, so did concerns about the risks of dialing and driving. It was believed that using Automatic Speech Recognition (ASR), whereby the caller would say a name and the appropriate number would be dialed, could significantly reduce the risks associated with cellular telephones. A speech-recognition cellular telephone, code-named "Liberty," was developed at AT&T, and contained up to twenty-one speaker-dependent vocabulary items.[2] In addition to ASR, Liberty had digitized speech to aid the user while training and using the telephone. Spoken digit feedback was also given when the user manually dialed the telephone. Other unique features of Liberty were a speakerphone designed especially for use on the highway, and a port allowing a laptop computer to communicate with other computers from the car. The product was baselined in September 1985 and announced for sale seven months later. It was reliable and easy to use, but was withdrawn from sale when AT&T chose to leave the cellular telephone market.

---

[1] The work reported in this chapter was completed while all authors were at AT&T Bell Laboratories in Indianapolis. Currently, E. Schwab works at Ameritech Services in Chicago, C. Ball works at College of St. Elizabeth in New Jersey, and B. Lively is still at AT&T in Indianapolis.
[2] Digit-dialing by voice was a possible addition to the feature set that was investigated. Our users wanted to be able to pick up the handset, say any number, and have it dialed. Digit-dialing was tested several times, with average correct recognition per digit around 92%. This meant the probability of correctly recognizing a seven-digit number would be about 56%, while a long-distance number would be correct 40% of the time. Based on this information, the decision was made to exclude digit-dialing from the initial offering of the product.

Despite its limited market appearance, the product was a human factors success for several reasons. First, product management and the development team recognized that the user interface would be critical to the success of the product. They agreed that it would be better to execute a modest feature set well, rather than a larger feature set. Second, comprehensive testing and evaluation programs were conducted to assess the technology and to address specific aspects of the human interface. Third, the human factors specialist was a member of the development team from the outset. User interface issues were thus aired among all affected parties on the team when those issues arose. Thus, no issues were dropped because of a separation between human factors and the development team.

This article concentrates on the methodologies employed in our testing program, and what was done as a result of the testing. A number of methodologies were employed to evaluate the technology and interface. Both laboratory and field studies were conducted, the latter under both controlled and naturalistic conditions. Some of the studies were designed to determine how well the ASR technology worked, and the optimum setting of various parameters. Other studies focused on optimizing the digitized speech feedback. Still other studies were conducted on the user aids for the telephone, i.e., the owner's manual and a quick reference guide. Finally, we studied the transmission quality of both the handset and the speakerphone. This paper discusses only those studies related to the speech technology. The development interval for this product was short and while some of the laboratory work to be discussed was done before product baselining, there was not time to do all the studies that we would have liked to have done. The studies we did were often small and are thus more indicative than definitive. Our intention here is to give the reader a sense of the questions we asked and how we addressed them in the context of an aggressive schedule and a very supportive design team.

The initial rendition of Liberty was an emulator of the product's capabilities; it had little resemblance to the final product. The emulator was designed for two functions: demonstrating the feasibility of a speech recognition dialer, and testing alternate features and operations. The results could then be used to create the final product. The emulator was an IBM-PC-compatible portable computer, containing a speech recognition board and text-to-speech synthesis. Its size allowed it to be installed in a car for on-the-road testing. The emulator features were: 21 speaker-dependent vocabulary items (twenty names, and a word to indicate 'redial the last number dialed'), speech prompts to guide the user and provide feedback on button presses, and beeps to indicate when a user should start and finish speaking. With these features the user could: store a name and number, change a number but retain the previously trained name (called "store-by-voice"), delete a name and number, and review a number by saying a name (called "recall-by-voice").

For safety reasons, users were encouraged to train the recognizer while the car was parked. To create an acoustic environment as similar as possible to driving on a highway, users were also asked to idle the engine and turn the climate control fan on high with the windows rolled up. Drivers don't often pay attention to it, but the inside of a car is noisy on the highway, often reaching 70 or 75 dBA. So, one of the first questions to be addressed was how accurately the recognizer would perform under conditions of highway noise. Ideally, to answer this question, we should have conducted a field study, but we were not yet ready to run subjects in a moving car. A number of laboratory studies were conducted under noise conditions which simulated a car's environment at various speeds. For this testing, we used "pink" noise colored to preserve the characteristics of a typical car with a phone on the highway. We were also careful to place the speakers so that the subject could move around a bit and still be in the "pocket" of noise at the intended level. In these studies, subjects were given a vocabulary to train and test. On each trial, the name to be said appeared on a small video screen.

The goal of the first study was to estimate the range of performance for the speech recognizer. AT&T employees trained two different vocabulary sets. One list contained dissimilar names (e.g., Scott, Eileen and Roberta), and the other contained phonetically similar names (e.g., Adam, Mom and Dad). Performance was perfect on the dissimilar names when the training and testing conditions matched, i.e., the noise simulated a parked car with an idling engine. When the simulated noise represented a car driving at 30 or 60 mph, mean correct recognitions dropped to 99.8% and 98.9% respectively. With the list of similar names, performance was much lower (82%, 83%, and 79.2% at 0, 30, and 60 mph).

Confusability was obviously going to be a concern, so we pushed the issue to the limit by testing a highly confusable (albeit unlikely) vocabulary. For this test, the vocabulary contained five names (Gary, Jerry, Terry, Barry, and Harry). The mean correct recognition rate was 36.1%. When easily pronounceable surnames were added (e.g., Gary Herman, Jerry Roberts), performance rose to 89.5% correct recognitions. Clearly, we had our first recommendation to our users: "First and last names together work better than first or last names alone." We also had a recommendation for the designers: "Help us avoid this problem in the first place by developing an algorithm that will test each new model as it is being trained against existing models for likelihood of confusion." This was done, and its appearance to the user is shown in Table 1. Testing showed that this procedure significantly reduced the frequency of recognition confusions. Another training algorithm, intended to deal with the effects of extraneous sounds during training, was also suggested and implemented. Its operation is illustrated in Table 1.

Another question concerned the stability of recognition over time. The formal testing we did here had subjects train and test a vocabulary of ten names and then test the vocabulary again, two weeks later. After training, correct recognition was at 99.6%; two weeks later it was 99.1%. Later, less formal testing greatly extended the range of model "age" and showed very little drop off with time.

At this point, the emulator was ready to be used in a car. The experimental arrangement called for a driver, an experimenter in the back seat with the computer/recognizer, and the subject in the front passenger seat holding the telephone handset while viewing a small monitor that displayed (one at a time) the names to be spoken. The session began with the car stopped in a parking lot while the subject trained the recognizer with the same ten names used in the earlier study. The driver then moved onto the road. Correct recognition on the highway averaged 98.9% under a wide range of conditions that included size of car (Dodge Aries, Chevrolet Caprice, Pontiac Firebird, Buick Riviera, or Lincoln Town Car), driving conditions (60 mph on a divided highway or stop and go traffic on a busy street), and noise levels inside the car (fan on high or low). Of course, performance varied slightly from one condition to another, but not by very much. These results suggested potentially robust recognition performance on the road.

While our testing had been focused on the speech technology, a number of human interface concerns began to surface and were addressed. It became clear that the quality of the text-to-speech feedback was unacceptable, so we decided to use digitized speech. We had the hardware and software needed to record, edit, and prepare EPROMs (erasable programmable read-only memory) needed for prompts and feedback. An employee who had done professional recording provided the voice. In selecting the form of digitized speech, the design team and project management reasoned that although some money could be saved by selecting a low bit-rate unit, the better decision would be to go with the higher quality sound of 32 kbit ADPCM. We believed that the apparent quality of the device could be strongly determined not only by recognition performance but also by the

Table 1: Representative User/System Interactions

TRAINING THE SYSTEM

Activity	User Action	System Response
Normal Training		
	Dial a number	
	Press STORE	
	Press* (see note below)	"Please say the name for this number."
	"Jim Flanagan"	"Again."
	"Jim Flanagan"	"Thank you . Stored in location 81."
Training a Name Similar to One Already in Memory		
	Dial a number	
	Press STORE	
	Press *	"Please say the name for this number"
	"Jim Bannigan"	"Again"
	"Jim Bannigan"	"Warning. Stored in location 82. That name is very similar to the name in location 81. Please change the name in location 81 or 82.
Reducing the Effect of Noise During Training		
	Dial Number	
	Press STORE	
	Press*	"Please say the name for this number"
	"Joan Smith"	"Again"
	"(Cough!) Joan Smith"	"Please repeat that"
	"Joan Smith"	"Thank you. Stored in location 83."

USING THE SYSTEM

Activity	User Action	System Response
Normal Use		
	handset	"Name please."
	"Jim Flanagan"	"Dialing 5551234."
Saying a Name Not in Memory		
	Lift handset	"Name please"
	"Carl Jones"	"Please repeat that."

sound quality of the prompts and speech feedback. We didn't have time to test this belief directly, although intelligibility testing, discussed later in this chapter, indirectly supports this assumption.

Our subjects' experiences in the laboratory and on the road revealed some incorrect assumptions about when and how to give feedback. For example, initially it seemed straightforward that when the handset is in its cradle, speech feedback for button presses (dialing a number, pressing a function button, etc.) ought to be given over a loudspeaker and when the phone is out of the cradle, it should be given over the receiver in the handset. This didn't match up with the user's need. Contrary to the instruction booklet, state laws, and perhaps good sense, users commonly dial the phone as they are driving. When they dial, they often lift the handset out of the cradle and hold it up near the steering wheel where they can see both it and the road. Speech feedback reporting the numbers as they are pressed would not help these drivers if it is given over the receiver but it does help substantially if it is given over a speaker. More will be said about the contribution of speech feedback to ease of manual dialing later in this chapter. Another naive assumption concerned the usefulness of beeps to signal the state of the recognizer. The user making a call would lift the handset and hear "Name please" followed by a beep to indicate the ready state of the recognizer. After saying a name, another beep signaled reception of the utterance, followed by "Dialing (the number)." The beeps were redundant and the subjects were irritated by them, so the beeps were eliminated. Users found some of the speech prompts to be too verbose. For example, when training a name, users had to speak the name twice. After saying the name the first time, the user would hear "Again. Please say the name that goes with this number." On the recommendation of the users, the prompt was shortened to "Again."

We continued to evaluate the technology on the road. A test list was constructed that consisted of the word "redial" and 20 names selected at random from the Indianapolis phone directory subject to the constraint that the names be easily pronounceable. Average recognition rate was 97% on the highway. The range of performance was such that some users were at ceiling, but some were at 90-93% correct. Many of the recognition errors that occurred when these people spoke arose because of differences between the way the name was spoken in training vs. use. People tended to be stilted and precise in training and relaxed and variable during testing. This resulted in some names on the list becoming more similar to one another and hence more confusable. (Maybe other names became more dissimilar.

We didn't look at that possibility.) In other cases, subjects would lengthen the pause between the first and second names, and a failure of recognition would result. This lack of consistency between the utterance in training and in later use is a common concern in the design of recognizers and supporting algorithms.

Since we were confident the technology was fairly robust across voices and vehicles, we wanted to examine the effect of user-generated name lists. We continued to test under a variety of driving conditions, and in a variety of vehicles. However, instead of being given a list of names, subjects were asked to generate their own list of names that they would train if they owned an ASR telephone. Performance for individual users ranged from 89-100% correct recognitions, with an average of 96% correct.

An interesting problem with the user-generated lists was that occasionally the user would say a name that had not been trained. For example, a person may have trained "Work" and then said "Office" while trying to dial that number. The appropriate response would be to ask the user to "Please repeat that." since the recognizer should not be able to match the word "Office" to any of the trained names. However, we learned that our erroneous "recognition" of these out-of-vocabulary items was fairly high, around 20%. If out-of-vocabulary names occur frequently, this error rate would be unacceptable. We could reduce the frequency of this type of error by manipulating the appropriate parameter, but reducing the likelihood of this kind of error would also reduce the tolerance of the system to normal variations in speech. In the laboratory, we determined the tradeoff function, but the issue of where to set the parameter was ultimately determined by field testing with experienced users.

We monitored for out-of-vocabulary items. All of these items can be called intrusions, such as substituting "Office" for "Work," or saying a name for a number that isn't in the vocabulary. However, there was a special category of intrusions that we treated separately. These were called variations and were very similar to a trained name, e.g., saying "Howard Office" when "Howard Work" is what was trained. We considered it an appropriate response if the intended number was dialed or if the recognizer asked the user to repeat what was said, and it was an error if some other number was dialed.

To estimate the magnitude of the out-of-vocabulary problem we conducted a paper and pencil study. Users were asked to list up to 20 names that they would use with a voice dialer. Then, a day or more later, we asked them to recall the names on the list. List length varied from 11 to 20 names. Of the names recalled, 3% were intrusions and 4% were variations. We then conducted a laboratory study with the recognizer, using the variations and intrusions obtained from the subjects. Each out-of-vocabulary name was tested ten times. For the variations, the recognizer responded appropriately 97% of the time. For intrusions, results depended upon the particular name. The intrusions were handled appropriately anywhere from 9 to 95% of the time, with a mean of 46% appropriate responses.

Since speech was the main communication channel in Liberty, we needed to insure that people could understand the speech prompts easily and correctly. One factor that affected comprehension was the digitization rate. The speech prompts had been digitized at 8 kHz, but there was insufficient memory to store all the prompts at that rate. A 4 kHz rate was considered, but we needed to know what effect this would have on the intelligibility and quality of the prompts. The same set of utterances was digitized at both rates, and then studies were conducted in which a number of users transcribed a random presentation of prompts while on the road. This gave a "worst-case picture" of comprehension, since users did not have a context for understanding the speech. The prompts were played over both the handset and the speaker, and each user heard only one digitized rate. The participants wrote down what they heard, and at the end of the session they answered a questionnaire concerning the quality of the speech. The results indicated a significant difference in intelligibility and acceptability of the speech rates; it was clear that the higher rate was needed. In order to encode the speech at 8 kHz, we rewrote the prompts to shorten them, and stored them without any waste. Fortunately, all the prompts fit into memory. Subsequently, the same type of intelligibility testing was performed on any changes to the prompts.

We then began a series of field trials. In the first part of these studies, the software continued to change while testing was going on. The test units were upgraded at various points in the study. Users brought into testing towards the end of the field trials had stable units with no software changes. For present purposes all field trials were combined since the important differences in speech recognition performance occurred across field trials: differences between AT&T employees and outside users. The outside users all had businesses that benefited from the use of a cellular telephone. Most had cellular service prior to being enrolled in our trials. Each participant had a Liberty installed in his/her car for two months, and was asked to use the phone on a regular basis. A number of user interface issues were to be addressed in these trials, e.g., ease of training the recognizer, usefulness of the prompts, and accuracy of recognition. A variety of methodologies was used to obtain this information, including tape recordings, interviews, and questionnaires.

For an objective record of what the participants said and how Liberty responded, a tape recorder was attached to the telephone. Whenever a button on the phone was pressed, or whenever the handset was picked up, recording would begin. Recording ceased when the handset was replaced in the cradle, when the END button was pressed, or ten seconds after the SEND signal was transmitted. Since it took more than 10 seconds for the cellular network to set up a call and contact the called party, there was no danger of recording private conversations. These tapes were changed weekly.

Interviews were conducted in the users' cars one week after important software changes. Brief scenarios were conducted to focus attention on various operations. Also, questionnaires were administered at the beginning, middle, and end of the trial. They addressed issues of overall satisfaction, perceived accuracy, reaction to prompts, feedback, and other characteristics of the human interface.

Early in the trials, we noticed a significant difference in behavior between the AT&T employees and the outside participants. The employees were stress-testing Liberty and the outside participants were using it in a more normal fashion, i.e., they were not trying to trick or break it. The employee data were therefore treated separately. The major conclusions we report are from our outside users and they are as follows:

1.   All of these users asked to keep the recognizer at the end of the trial. All were very happy with it despite the fact that recognition performance, averaging 87% over all subjects, was lower than we had seen in more controlled settings. One user averaged 62% performance and reported that "Except for one time, it worked fine." The prepotent factor here was probably the fact that the unit seldom (1% or less for most users) misdialed a number. The parameter setting used strongly biased the system to ask the user for another utterance ("Please repeat that.") unless the utterance matched one model well and the others poorly. A second factor that made a difference was the voice used for prompts and feedback. It was described as clear, nonthreatening, and mellow.

2. The system was described as easy to use. Placing a call by name dialing was rated as easy as reading the green and white destination and distance signs used on interstate highways. If the user manually dialed a number, providing spoken digit feedback made the task easier than finding and tuning a radio station not programmed on a button. Dialing without speech feedback was more difficult than finding and tuning a radio station not programmed on a button.

3. Some features were changed or dropped as a result of testing. One of the changes concerned the "Name please" repetition loop. Originally, Liberty would repeat the "Name please" prompt every five seconds until an audio event occurred. The trial indicated that this increased the error rate; users frequently took the handset out of the cradle with no intention of immediately placing a call. If background noise persisted, Liberty eventually would detect a match and place a call. Because of this, Liberty was modified so that it only repeated the "Name please" prompt twice. After two repetitions, ASR was deactivated.

Another change affected the feature set. The trial indicated that two features, "recall-by-voice" and "store-by-voice," were rarely, if ever, used. Also, "store-by-voice" was easily confused with the training procedures. Both features were dropped. In addition, we learned that the gain levels needed to be monitored and perhaps modified. Several of the field trial participants frequently heard the "Please speak louder" prompt; one person heard it on 14% of her call attempts. The field trial results also indicated that we should disable the digitized speech feedback when the phone was locked (i.e., outgoing calls could not be placed).

Liberty was developed on a very aggressive schedule and we did not get the opportunity to do the in-depth studies we would have liked to have done. Yet, it was a human factors success because everyone connected with the design recognized the importance of an easy-to-use interface. To the extent possible, Liberty was designed and built around the needs of the user. The enthusiastic response from our users confirmed the merits of this approach.

Chapter 15

Voice Quality Assessment of Digital Network Technologies

Duane O. Bowker
AT&T Bell Laboratories

1. Introduction

The engineering of global digital telecommunications networks requires thorough performance evaluation to ensure that customers' ever-increasing expectations for quality are met or exceeded. When the network applications are voice-related, as in traditional voice telephony, a thorough service performance evaluation will include formal customer opinion studies of voice quality. AT&T has a long-standing commitment to provide its customers with excellent service quality and, as part of that commitment, AT&T Bell Laboratories has been conducting formal customer-oriented voice quality evaluations on an ongoing basis for many years (Hanson, 1983).

Over the last two decades, AT&T has undertaken a massive redesign of its core telecommunications network, moving from a primarily analog network to one that is essentially all digital. This chapter discusses voice quality assessment experiments related to two classes of current digital network technologies: Echo Cancellation Systems (Section 2) and Digital Circuit Multiplication Systems (Section 3). Echo Cancellation Systems are widely used in telecommunications networks to improve the voice performance associated with long-haul facilities. Digital Circuit Multiplication Systems are used primarily in private and international network applications to increase the voice capacity of digital transmission facilities.

2. Voice Quality Assessments of Echo Cancellation Devices

Echo arises in telephony when some portion of the talker's own voice is reflected back to the talker through the telecommunications network (Gayler, 1989; AT&T, BL, 1982). These reflections generally originate from impedance mismatches either in the loop plant or at 2/4-wire hybrids, but can also originate from significant acoustic coupling between the far-end party's receiver and transmitter. If the magnitude of the reflection and the delay encountered in the echo path are each sufficiently large, the talker may experience a degraded telephone connection. To counter echo impairments of electrical origin, AT&T deploys adaptive echo cancellers throughout its long-distance network. These cancellers effectively perform a digital subtraction of the reflected signal from the true signal.

To assess the voice quality of networks with and without echo cancellation devices, pairs of trained subjects recruited from outside of AT&T engaged in a series of proof-reading exercises over telephone connections simulated in the laboratory. The proof-reading task was structured so that each subject in the conversation would have a turn to speak and was also designed to encourage double-talking (both subjects speaking simultaneously), since double-talking situations may cause particular problems for adaptive echo cancellers. Each proof-reading task took subjects from two to three minutes to complete. After each exercise, subjects rated the voice quality of the connection as either *excellent, good, fair, poor,* or *unsatisfactory*.

The network used in the study was four-wire end-to-end, i.e., there were no 2/4-wire hybrids anywhere in the connection, including the telephones themselves. Electrical echo paths for both subjects were simulated using audio splitters and mixers, allowing complete experimental control over the Echo Path Delay (EPD) and Echo Path Loss (EPL) in both directions of the connection. The simulated connections that subjects rated were varied from trial to trial according to: (1) EPD; (2) EPL; (3) activation/deactivation of echo cancellers in the connection; and (4) single or multiple cancellers in the connection. Results presented below are from an experiment that included forty subjects, each rating a total of 80 different combinations of the above connection parameters. The various network configurations were presented in randomized order with a different ordering used for each pair of subjects. The echo cancellers used in the study included both the AT&T EC32000 and the more recent AT&T Universal Services Echo Canceller (USEC).

The results from one representative experiment are summarized in Figures 1-3. The ordinate in each figure is the Mean Opinion Score (MOS) calculated from the voice quality ratings by first converting the categorical ratings to a 1-5 numeric scale (*excellent* = 5; *good* = 4; *fair* = 3; *poor* = 2; *unsatisfactory* = 1), then taking the arithmetic average of the transformed ratings. The MOS data are plotted as a function of EPD in the three figures, with Figure 1

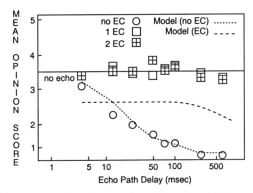

Figure 1:   Mean Opinion Scores for Echo Conditions with a Low Echo Path Loss (22 dB)

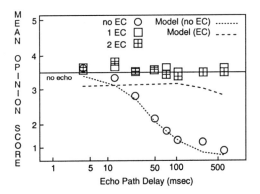

Figure 2:   Mean Opinion Scores for Echo Conditions with a Moderate Echo Path Loss (30 dB)

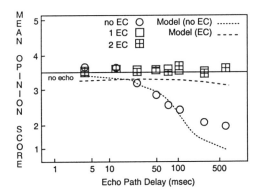

Figure 3:   Mean Opinion Scores for Echo Conditions with a High Echo Path Loss (38 dB)

showing the data corresponding to connections with a low EPL (22 dB), Figure 2 showing the data corresponding to connections with a moderate EPL (30 dB), and Figure 3 showing the data corresponding to connections with a high EPL (38 dB). In each figure, data are plotted separately for connections with no active echo canceller (open circles), with a single pair of active echo cancellers (open squares), and with a double pair of active echo cancellers (crossed squares). The MOS corresponding to an all-digital network control connection with absolutely no echo path (but with other connection parameters, such as end-to-end loss and noise, equivalent to the test connections) is shown in each figure as the solid horizontal line. Also plotted on each figure as dashed and dotted lines respectively, are the MOS values predicted by the current Grade-of-Service model for connections with and without echo cancellation devices (Cavanaugh et al., 1976; CCITT, 1990).

An examination of the data plotted in Figures 1-3 leads to the following conclusions:

- The perceived voice quality of a telephone connection with an electrical echo path but with no active echo control degrades significantly as EPD increases and as EPL decreases. At the lowest EPL tested (22 dB), even very short delay echoes (EPD = 4 msec) are noticeably degraded relative to a connection with no echo path. It should be noted that short delay echoes do not manifest themselves as echo *per se* but as an unusual telephone sidetone path. In such scenarios, customers might complain that the telephone connection sounds "hollow" or "like a rain barrel."

- Activating an echo canceller on connections with a linear, time-invariant echo path produces a level of voice performance essentially identical to that of connections with no echo path. This finding holds for all EPD/EPL combinations included in the experiment. Under these conditions, the cancellers can therefore be considered transparent (i.e., not introducing an impairment of their own) and effectively perfect at removing echo from the connection.

- Having dual tandemed pairs of cancellers activated on a connection did not degrade the voice quality relative to connections with single pairs of activated cancellers.

3.   Performance of Digital Circuit Multiplication Systems

Long-distance voice traffic in the United States is typically digitally encoded and transported using 64 kbit/s (μ-law Pulse Code Modulation (PCM).(Bellamy, 1982). PCM on a 1.544 Mbit/s DS1-level digital transmission facility (e.g., a T1 digital carrier system), for example, will accommodate the equivalent of 24 active voice trunks. To reduce transport costs, some private network applications and some international network applications utilize Digital Circuit Multiplication Systems (DCMS). DCMS are systems that employ various compression techniques to reduce the bandwidth required for the transport of voice information, thereby increasing the number of voice trunks that can be accommodated on a digital facility. Depending on (a) the type of DCMS deployed and, (b) the engineering guidelines used to configure the network, a DCMS could increase the voice carrying capacity of a digital facility by a factor of four or more. Going back to the example of the DS1-level transmission facility, it is possible that by deploying a DCMS, the voice capacity of that facility could be increased from the nominal 24 to as much as 100 active trunks with little impact on voice quality (Bowker & Dvorak, 1987; Bowker & Armitage, 1987; Karanam, et al., 1988).

Although there are a myriad of DCMS devices on the market today, they can all be placed into one of the following three categories:

> **Type I:** Systems that use some form of low bit-rate voice (LBRV) coding algorithm to increase capacity (LBRV defined as any coding rate less than that of the standard 64 kbit/s PCM codec);
>
> **Type II:** Systems that use Digital Speech Interpolation (DSI) algorithms to effectively allocate bandwidth during active speech periods but *not* during silence intervals;.
>
> **Type III:** Hybrid systems that use both LBRV and DSI.

Type II and Type III DCMS, given the nature of DSI multiplexing, tend to require higher bandwidth facilities (e.g., domestic T1 carrier systems at 1.544 Mbit/s or international carrier systems at 2.048 Mbit/s) to obtain their compression advantages. Most DCMS currently deployed on these higher bandwidth facilities fall into the third category. For smaller bandwidth applications (e.g., ISDN Basic Rate Interface facilities at 128 kbit/s), DSI multiplexing becomes far less effective and so Type I DCMS are generally used.

There are several important voice performance issues associated with DCMS that require thorough examination to ensure that telecommunications networks utilizing DCMS devices will provide good voice Grade-of-Service. First, for DCMS employing some form of LBRV coding (Types I and III), does the coding process produce any noticeable distortion of the voice signal? Does the degradation depend on the gender of the speaker? For Types II and III, does the DSI algorithm produce any clipping of the speech signal (i.e., misclassification of speech as non-speech)? Is the DSI algorithm negatively impacted by background noise or conversations? For Types II and III, does the voice quality of the DCMS vary with different network traffic loadings? For all types, what are the impacts of passing a voice signal through multiple tandemed DCMS? Finally, for all types, is there any transmission delay introduced by the system and, if so, what precautions are required to ensure adequate echo Grade-of-Service?

3.1 Voice Quality Associated with Low Bit-Rate Voice Compression

There are many different LBRV coding algorithms being used in commercially available DCMS and, unless the LBRV algorithm is one of the internationally recognized standards for voice coding, it is hard to predict *a priori* the performance of that DCMS. Formal evaluations are required to assess the voice quality provided by DCMS using non-standard coding since it has been widely demonstrated that certain LBRV algorithms degrade speech significantly more than others (Daumer, 1982; Hoyle & Falconer, 1987). We have frequently observed in our investigations that many of the non-standardized LBRV coding algorithms have a tendency to degrade female speech more than male speech. One must also worry about the encode/decode delay associated with the LBRV algorithms when dealing with telecommunications applications due to the potential for introducing echo impairments (Section 2).

Fortunately, many of the commercially available DCMS devices use LBRV algorithms that are internationally recognized standards. In such cases, the performance of the algorithms has been thoroughly examined and documented during the standardization process. Algorithms such as 32 kbit/s ADPCM (Adaptive Differential Pulse Code Modulation), as specified in CCITT Recommendation G.721, and 16 kbit/s LD-CELP (Low Delay-Code Excited Linear Prediction), which is being considered by CCITT for standardization, do not introduce significant encode/decode delays. These algorithms also produce essentially no perceptible distortion of voice for either males or females following a single encoding (Benvenuto et al., 1986; Chen et al., 1990).

Recently, higher and lower bit-rate variants of ADPCM have been standardized by the CCITT for special use in DCMS applications, particularly for DCMS of Type III. DSI compression, since it is statistical in nature, requires some means of accommodating momentary overloads in voice activity (i.e., when a statistically large number of the voice channels on a facility are active at one time). In several Type III DCMS, these statistical overloads are accommodated by using a lower bit-rate ADPCM to carry the voice signals on some of the channels for a few milliseconds at a time.

There are essentially two approaches to reducing the effective ADPCM bit-rate during momentary overloads. The first is to encode and decode the speech using ADPCM algorithms that are fixed at either 40, 32, or 24 kbit/s operation (the CCITT has recently standardized 40 kbit/s and 24 kbit/s extensions to the existing 32 kbit/s ADPCM standard). The second approach is to encode the speech with a special 40 kbit/s *embedded* ADPCM algorithm (recently standardized by the CCITT as Recommendation G.EMB) that can be decoded at either 40, 32, 24, or 16 kbit/s rates (Sherif, Bertocci, Bowker, Orford, and Mariano, 1990; Sherif, Bowker, Bertocci, Orford, and Mariano, 1990). In the first case, there must be a way for the transmitting DCMS terminal to communicate to the receiving DCMS terminal exactly which of the multiple ADPCM algorithms was used for each voice channel at each moment in time. If the wrong decoder was applied to a channel (e.g., if a voice channel was momentarily encoded at 24 kbit/s but the receiving terminal attempted to decode this speech at 32 kbit/s), the result would be garbled noise. In the case of embedded ADPCM, the receiving terminal always decodes the speech input using the same version of the algorithm with however many bits (2-5) it has available in the speech sample. The coordination between the transmitting and receiving DCMS terminals is therefore much less complicated. Another advantage to the embedded approach over the non-embedded approach is that, with embedded ADPCM, the bit-rate reduction can be made at any point in the network where congestion is encountered. With fixed rate (non-embedded) ADPCM, congestion can only be accommodated at the transmitting terminal before the speech is actually encoded. This approach, therefore, can really only be effectively used in point-to-point compression situations and can not be used in more complicated networking scenarios.

Voice quality rating data comparing the various standardized ADPCM algorithms were collected in a formal listening experiment. Forty-three people, recruited from outside of AT&T, rated the voice quality of segments of speech coded through several different versions of ADPCM. Participants

listened to the coded speech segments over calibrated telephone connections. The Mean Opinion Scores calculated from the participants' ratings

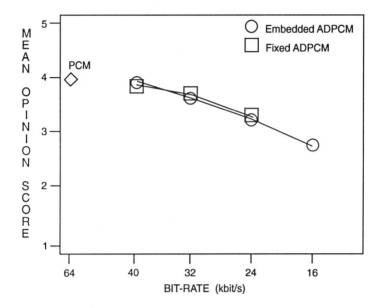

are plotted in Figure 4 as a function of bit-rate for the fixed (squares) and
embedded (circles) ADPCM algorithms. Also shown is the MOS for the 64
kbit/s PCM algorithm (diamond) which, again, is the algorithm most
commonly used in digital telephony. The rating data depicted in Figure 4
show that, at a given bit-rate, the embedded ADPCM algorithm performs
essentially the same as the corresponding fixed-rate ADPCM algorithms.

Figure 4:   Mean Opinion Scores versus Bit-Rate for Various CCITT
Standard Speech Coding Algorithms (Single Encoding)

3.2   Voice Quality Associated with Digital Speech Interpolation
Whereas there has been much standardization work surrounding the more
widely used LBRV algorithms, this has not been the case for DSI algorithms. DSI algorithms are almost always proprietary to the particular
DCMS vendor and there can be significant performance differences among
the implementations. Figure 5 plots the MOS values separately for each of
ten talkers across conditions in which the speech was not compressed ("DSI

OFF"), and in which speech was compressed using two different DSI algorithms ("DSI #1" and "DSI #2"). These data were collected in a listening test with forty-four participants recruited from outside of AT&T. Participants listened to triads of phonetically balanced sentences that had been passed through a simulated end-to-end telephone connection with an intervening DSI-based system. After each set of sentences, participants rated the voice quality of the passage on the standard five-point scale.

The rating data in Figure 5 clearly demonstrate the impact that different DSI algorithms can have on voice quality. The data also demonstrate that the impact of a particular DSI algorithm can vary greatly from talker to talker. In the case of the first DSI algorithm, the voice quality ratings were essentially unaffected for nine of the ten talkers. The tenth talker did suffer from some voice clipping impairments and this talker, in fact, has proven to be particularly susceptible to all DSI algorithms that we have examined. This talker happens to be a woman, but over the course of several performance evaluations of DSI that we have conducted, we have not observed significant gender effects attributable to DSI compression. The second DSI algorithm evaluated in the experiment was much worse than the first causing noticeable clipping impairments on eight of the ten talkers.

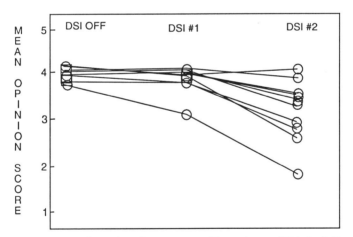

Figure 5: Mean Opinion Scores as a Function of Digital Speech Interpolation (DSI) for 10 Talkers

A voice performance issue intimately related to DSI is noise matching. In a DSI-based DCMS, the receiving terminal obtains, for each conversation, digital samples corresponding to active speech periods but does not obtain samples corresponding to the gaps between the active speech periods. What does the receiving terminal do during the inactive periods? If the receiving DCMS terminal outputs silence during the inactive periods, the person at the far-end of the telephone connection may often perceive discontinuities in the background noise-level of the connection. Some DCMS designs use an adaptive noise-matching technique to remove these discontinuities. The transmitting DCMS terminal makes a characterization of the background noise in the incoming conversation and then sends that characterization to the receiving DCMS terminal. The receiving terminal uses that information to reconstruct the conversation (active as well as inactive periods) as closely as possible. Formal voice quality evaluations conducted by the author have demonstrated adaptive noise matching techniques to provide significantly better voice performance than techniques using either fixed-level noise matching or no noise matching.

3.3 Voice Quality Associated with Hybrid Systems

As discussed above, most modern DCMS deployed on higher bandwidth facilities (1.544 Mbit/s and above) are Type III Hybrid systems using both LBRV and DSI techniques to obtain their compression advantages. At low facility loads, these DCMS will default to either 40 or 32 kbit/s ADPCM coding to transmit speech information. They will also use proprietary DSI and noise matching algorithms to allocate bandwidth only during active speech periods in a conversation. At moderate facility loads, due to the statistical nature of DSI compression, the DCMS will sometimes need to drop the effective ADPCM bit-rate below 32 kbit/s, resulting in some increase in quantization distortion on the connection. At higher facility loads, using lower bit-rate ADPCM algorithms will not always be sufficient to accommodate the momentary statistical overloads. When this occurs, the speech may be subjected to "freeze-out clipping" for short periods of time. Freeze-out occurs when the transmitting terminal literally has no bandwidth left on the outgoing facility to place the encoded speech information. Needless to say, this is a very disturbing impairment and is avoided at all costs.

Figure 6 depicts how voice quality varies with compression for three different commercial DCMS. The data shown are for conditions with a single DCMS encoding/decoding and with a nominal speech input level. For all DCMS evaluated in this experiment, voice quality ratings were relatively constant at low compression ratios and then dropped as the voice load on the systems was increased. Voice quality for all systems was essentially indistinguishable from uncompressed PCM network configurations at compressions up to 3:1. At higher loads, the performance of the three systems began to degrade with some variation in the rate of degradation observed across the systems.

In networks utilizing DCMS devices whose performance can vary significantly with load, safeguards must be put in place to ensure that the impinging loads never reach levels that would cause noticeable degradation of voice quality. Such systems generally allow for a configurable Dynamic Load Control (DLC) option that passes an overload signal back to the feeding network. Should the system performance begin to degrade with increasing load, the DCMS sets its DLC flag telling the feeding network to route traffic elsewhere until the load is relieved. Setting the DLC thresholds at conservative levels is effective at providing a good voice Grade-of-Service across facilities utilizing DCMS to reduce transport cost.

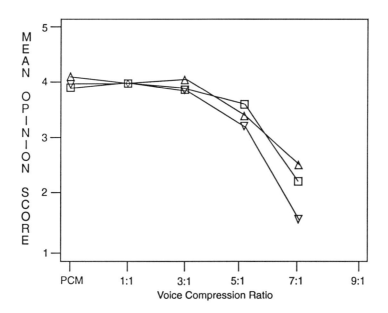

Figure 6:   Mean Opinion Scores for Three Commercial DCMS as a Function of Voice Compression (Single Encoding).

4. Concluding Remarks

The recent migration of telecommunications networks from analog transmission technologies to digital transmission technologies has not eliminated all of the Grade-of-Service issues associated with long-distance voice services. Certainly thermal noise impairments are not of concern in all-digital networks as they are in analog networks, but other impairments, such as echo and distortion, must still be controlled through careful network performance engineering. As has been discussed in the sections above, some digital network technologies are extremely complex from a speech processing perspective and therefore require thorough analysis and evaluation before they can be considered for widespread network deployment. Formal psychophysical customer-focused evaluations of speech transmission quality serve an important role in ensuring that a high level of voice performance is achieved in the process of telecommunications network design.

5. Acknowledgments

The author wishes to thank Cecilia Ward for conducting the voice performance evaluations described in this article. Thanks also to Vern Jensen and Ron Tegethoff for their assistance in installing and configuring the channel units and echo cancellers used in the echo experiments, and to Gonzalo Mariano, Ron Daggett, Cliff Sayre, Marco Bonomi, and Bill Daumer for their assistance with the equipment configurations used in the DCMS subjective tests.

6. References

Bellamy, J. C. (1982). *Digital Telephony.* New York: John Wiley and Sons.

Benvenuto, N., Bertocci, G., Daumer, W. R., & Sparrell, D. K. (1986). The 32-kb/s ADPCM Coding Standard. *AT&T Technical Journal, 65(5),* 12–22.

Bowker, D. O., & Armitage, C. B. (1987). Performance issues for packetized voice communications. *Proceedings of the National Communications Forum, 41(3),* 1087–1092.

Bowker, D. O., & Dvorak, C. A. (1987). Speech transmission quality of Wideband Packet Technology. *Proceedings of IEEE GLOBECOM '87,* 1887–1889.

Cavanaugh, J. R., Hatch, R. W., & Sullivan, J. L. (1976). Models for the subjective effects of loss, noise, and talker echo on telephone connection. *Bell System Technical Journal, 55(9),* 1319–1371.

CCITT. (1990). *Revisions of Supplement No. 3 of the P Series'*, *Contribution to Study Group XII on Question 7/ XII*, February.

Chen, J. H., Melchner, M. J., Cox, R. V., & Bowker, D. O. (1990). Real-time implementation and performance of a 16 Kb/s Low-Delay CELP speech coder. *Proceedings of ICASSP '90*.

Daumer, W. R. (1982). Subjective evaluation of several efficient speech coders. *IEEE Transactions on Communications, 30(4)*, 655–662.

Gayler, W. D. (1989). *Telephone Voice Transmission: Standards and Measurement*. Englewood Cliffs, NJ: Prentice Hall.

Hanson, B. L. (1983). A brief history of Applied Behavioral Science at Bell Laboratories. *Bell System Technical Journal*.

Hoyle, R. D., & Falconer, D. D. (1987). A comparison of digital speech coding methods for mobile radio systems. *IEEE Journal on Selected Areas in Communications, SAC-5(5)*, 915–920.

Karanam, V. R., Sriram, K., & Bowker, D. O. (1988). Performance evaluation of variable-bit-rate voice in packet-switched networks. *AT&T Technical Journal, B67(5)*, 57–71.

Sherif, M. H., Bertocci, G., Bowker, D. O., Orford, B. A., & Mariano, G. A. (1990). Overview of CCITT Draft Recommendation G. EMB. *Proceedings of ICC/SUPERCOMM '90*.

Sherif, M. H., Bowker, D. O., Bertocci, G., Orford, B. A., & Mariano, G. A. (in press). Performance of CCITT/ANSI Embedded ADPCM Algorithms. *IEEE Transactions on Communications*.

Chapter 16

Behavioral Aspects of Speech Technology: Industrial Systems

Jeremy Peckham[1]
Logica Cambridge

1. Introduction

Many of the first applications for speech recognition technology in the early 1970's were released in the manufacturing industry as part of the automation of the inspection process. Speech offered a potentially hands free method of data capture during routine inspection tasks undertaken as part of the quality control function. Falling hardware costs and improvements in the capability of speech recognition systems over the last ten years have now established this application area as both technically viable and cost effective.

This chapter provides an analysis of some human factors issues involved in the design of quality inspection systems using speech input and output. Many of the issues are of course not confined to these applications alone but have much wider implications for the general design of speech systems. Two specific industrial implementations of speech systems carried out by Logica for Jaguar Cars Ltd. and Caterpillar Tractor Ltd in the United Kingdom are discussed. The two implementations, although using the same technology, are different in scope and illustrate different aspects of the design process.

2. General Design Considerations

Many proponents of speech technology present it as the ideal human-computer interface. Designers of such interfaces, however, must look rather more closely at the proposed tasks before concluding that speech will be more efficient or simpler to use. We begin by reviewing some of the general characteristics of speech that may provide advantages in the human computer interface and conclude with some negative aspects of the use of speech.

[1]The work reported in this chapter was completed while the author was at Logica Cambridge Ltd., Cambridge, UK. Currently, J. Peckham works at Vocalis, Cambridge, UK.

The major benefits which speech may potentially bring in human-computer interaction are;

- reduced mental encoding

- faster transactions and text generation than keyboard as the information bandwidth increases

- possibility for more effective multiple task execution by combining verbal and manual tasks

Reduced mental encoding relates to the easier use of natural language than command languages and function key assignments, particularly for non-skilled or occasional users of a system. On the other hand, speech commands may run into a similar problem if the vocabulary of an application extends to a few hundred words and users forget which words are in the allowable vocabulary. This requires careful design of vocabularies in order that the advantage of speech in this area is not lost.

As far as transaction speed improvements are concerned, in applications where time is taken to verify each input, the transaction time for speech versus keyboard input will relate directly to the keyboard skills and talking rate of the operator and to the performance of the speech recognizer.

Apart from these advantages of speech as a method of input, there are certain types of applications in industry where speech can be justified by other criteria. They include situations where the user's hands or eyes are busy, where he or she needs to be mobile while using the system, or where he or she is remote from the system. Unlike keyboards, where the correct key must be located and then pushed, voice input does not involve the user of the hands or eyes, so the operator does not need to stop what he is doing while entering data or commands to a computer. This facility is most useful in applications where the user has objects, plans or drawings to inspect and handle, or equipment to control. Many successful applications of speech recognition have been found in parts inspection in quality control and the two applications cited in this chapter are of this type. In the Caterpillar application, significant gains in productivity have been reported by the company.

Even in hands- or eyes-busy applications, the high price of speech recognition equipment relative to keyboards and pointing devices means that a considerable reduction in transaction time may be needed to justify the cost. Welch (1980) describes a data entry application where the system operator was required to position an object in a measuring device and then enter the measurement by pushing the relevant button on the keyboard. Although the use of speech recognition dramatically reduced the time spent entering the measurement, the time spent on this part of the task was such a small fraction of the total that the overall reduction in the transaction time was not statistically significant.

The motivation for using speech to improve operator mobility is similar to that for hands- or eyes-busy operations. By using a head mounted microphone or radio the operator does not need to stop his or her principle task, for example inspecting a car for quality control, to find a terminal to enter data. Whether or not the transaction time is significantly reduced again depends on how much time the operator spends locating the terminal and entering data.

There are some disadvantages of speech as an input method compared to other means, however, and these should be considered before commencing a detailed design of a speech application.

One example can be illustrated from process control where traditional controls and status displays are usually discrete and grouped according to function. Experienced operators are generally able to quickly locate controls and scan displays and status indicators. The use of computer-based display technology may reduce the control panels to a few CRT's and limit the instantaneous information available, but it could prove less than optimal for the operator since information search and abnormal status detection time may be increased.

Pointing devices are much better suited than verbal commands for entering information on spatial location. This advantage may be combined with speech to good effect where there are a mixture of spatial location and selection tasks. An example in automated electronic circuit drawing is selection of standard circuit symbols from a library (using speech commands) and their placement in forming a circuit diagram by mouse.

One particular disadvantage of speech input over keyboards or pointing devices is the variability of speech production and the resulting speech signal. Keyboards have a standardizing effect on the input; as long as the appropriate command is used and there are no spelling mistakes, the system will know the user's intention. Any spelling or syntax errors are user initiated and can often be detected by the system. Speech is more like handwriting in that each person's is different, and occasionally unintelligible, even to the originator. Current speech recognition technology is limited in its ability to deal with variability and its performance under field conditions must be a matter of concern to system designers, particularly in respect to its impact on error rates.

Having briefly considered the advantages and disadvantages of speech in the human-computer interface we now consider the steps which should be taken in any design.

3.   Determining a Role for Speech Input

Aside from the potential advantages of speech in human-computer interaction, consideration should be given to the following factors when assessing the role of speech in any given application:

*   The *tasks* to be performed

*   The *users* of the system

*   The *environment* in which the tasks are carried out

*   Speech technology *capabilities*

3.1   Task Analysis

Assessing the potential benefits of speech as an input medium should first proceed from an analysis of the proposed changes to existing tasks. The analysis may proceed from the highest level, providing a specification of the system's objectives and functions, down to a detailed description of the smallest task and the relative priority and complexity of each interaction.

Figure 1 illustrates this process for a simple package sorting application using a single operator and a keyboard. In the case of an existing task or set of tasks this process can help in identifying improvements in task scheduling or where tasks may be removed by the use of alternative interface technology. In Figure 2 the potential saving in the number of tasks involved using speech instead of keyboard is shown. For this particular application (a sorting depot in the USA), use of a speech recognition improved the package thoughput by 30% and reduced errors from 4-5% to less than .05%.

3.2   Task loading

Task analysis may reveal potential for speech input to either reduce tasks as in the package sorting application, or allow tasks to be carried out concurrently. One of the main motivations for using speech has been in applications where the user's hands or eyes are already busy with another task. Parts inspection in the quality control function is an example.

The temptation to use speech as a method of input to allow task concurrency or reduce operator workload must be carefully evaluated. The experience

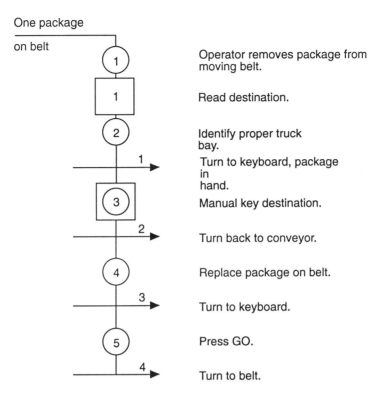

Figure 1: Flowchart of package handling, original method.

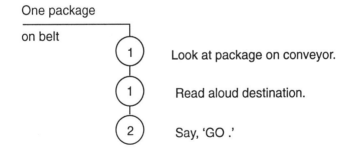

Figure 2: Flowchart of package handling, revised method.

of psychologists investigating the effects of dual tasking may prove useful in determining the requirements of systems used in this kind of high workload environment.

There are four main psychological theories attempting to explain how the brain's processing capabilities are organized (McLeod, 1977). The debate is over whether there are distinct processors for various channels of attention (motor, oral, etc.) or whether there is one single pool of processing capacity which must be shared by tasks.

The first model is the classic one developed by Broadbent in the late 1950s, which assumes that there is a single pool; allocating some capacity to one task means that there is less remaining for anything else. The second model is a variation of this, the difference being that the total pool of capacity is divided among different channels in fixed proportion. Like the first model, there is a decrease in performance when going from single to dual tasking, but unlike the first model, two tasks using different channels do not interfere with each other. The third model assumes that different channels are controlled by entirely independent processors, so there is no performance decrement due to dual tasking and also no interference between the tasks.

The final model has independent processors controlled by a higher level executive, which performs functions such as ensuring that two tasks do not interact. This means that, as in the second model, there will be an overall drop in performance when another task is introduced, but as there are independent processors no interference will take place.

McLeod (1977) carried out experiments with simultaneous tracking and identification tasks and a more difficult arithmetic and tracking problem. He compared manual and vocal responses to the identification task and two levels of difficulty in the arithmetic task. Both sets of experiments showed a single- to dual-task performance decrement and also that the two manual combination did not. McLeod claims that these results support the fourth model of independent processors with an executive controller.

The findings of Laycock and Peckham (1980) do not seem to follow the same pattern. In an experiment comparing vocal and manual data input during a manual tracking task, they found that the rate of degradation of the tracking task was the same for both manual and vocal input. The overall performance of the tracking task during voice input was superior only because of the reduced period of divided attention produced by faster entry times. However, the accuracy of the data entered was far superior with direct voice input than with keyboard input. This suggests that some advantage could be gained by pilots in a single-seater fighter required to enter or access information from an onboard computer. The primary task in a high-speed, low-level flight profile is controlling the aircraft. An interface technology that minimizes transaction time on interfacing with a secondary task may degrade overall performance less.

The relevance of this work lies not only in comparing the efficiency of manual and vocal input but also in showing that simultaneous tasking degrades the performance of both tasks.

3.3 User Population
The type of person using a system, frequent or casual, skilled or unskilled, is also an important factor to be evaluated in the design of an interface and its technology. This will be considered further under dialogue design. In using speech recognition devices, the accessibility of the user population for training the recogniser determines the viability of speaker-dependent systems. The user's level of motivation also plays an important role in achieving adequate accuracy with current technology.

3.4 The Environment
The environment in which the user is expected to operate can have an important impact on the choice and performance of the interface. A few examples illustrate the point: for a user who is required to wear protective clothing and gloves and finds keyboards difficult to use, speech may be an advantage. A noisy environment, however, may be detrimental to the accuracy of a speech recogniser, both from the point of view of noise added to the speech signal and changes in speech production (e.g., increased vocal effort).

3.5 Technology Capabilities
When assessing the potential of speech input, consideration must be given to the capabilities and the limitations of available recognition technology. Isolated utterance recognition will require slower input than connected and may require careful prompting to avoid utterances being joined together. Even connected word recognition technology does not completely solve the problem since some users may speak too rapidly. Various chapters in this book should give the reader a clear understanding of current technology capabilities.

4.   Optimizing System Design

Figure 3 shows a simple model of a human-computer interface using speech and the interaction of various factors and provides a focus for considering the optimization of system design.

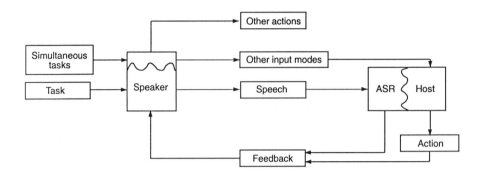

Figure 3:   A generic model of the human-computer interface using speech input illustrating the factors to be considered in optimizing design.

4.1   Transaction Time

In many human-computer interfaces, particularly where there is no concurrent task, the primary goal in interface design is to minimize the time taken to accomplish the user's goal. Achieving this requires more than just optimizing the processor power to minimize host response. We define transaction time here to be the time taken from the receipt of a stimulus to carry out a task or subtask, to the point at which the user is satisfied that the task is complete. This takes into account a number of factors in the transaction design such as the optimality of error correction strategies, dialogue design and feedback.

The choice of a suitable dialogue plays an important role in minimizing transaction time. Whether menus, commands or question answering is used depends largely on the type of use involved, and also to a certain extent upon any simultaneous tasks and the input mode (speech or manual) as discussed in the previous sections. Once the user has provided input for the computer, the system will respond in some way. The system may use primary feedback which means that it carries out the task immediately, or it may give the user a chance to verify that the input is correct by offering secondary feedback.

4.2 Dialogue Design

A dialogue that will minimize the transaction time must allow for the type of person who will be using the system and for any constraints imposed upon the user by the task environment. We now discuss the different devices used in dialogues, feedback and error correction and the situations in which one is more appropriate than another.

4.2.1 Dialogue Acts

Bunt *et al.* (1978) talk of man-machine interactions in terms of *dialogue acts* and draw a distinction between *goal-oriented acts*, which directly involve the communication of information needed to carry out a command, and *dialogue control acts*, which are more concerned with preventing and correcting errors in the dialogue.

The goal-oriented act is one in which the computer asks or is told what the user wants to do. The style chosen to convey this information should be the one which will result in the quickest and most error-free transaction, as a slightly longer, but more robust dialogue can save a great deal of time in correcting errors. For example, a naive or infrequent user will probably need a longer transaction time than a more experienced user, as it will be quicker in the long run to give the naive user as much information as is needed to provide correct input the first time. The experienced user, on the other hand, will want to bypass most help facilities and take the initiative to make the transaction as quickly as possible.

There are several established ways of conducting a transaction, including command languages, menus and question answering, or combinations of these. Experienced computer users usually prefer to use command languages; because they are familiar with the system they do not need to wait to be told what the options are.

Machine prompts such as menus and question-answering are slower but easier to use and so are more suitable for inexperienced users who will otherwise not know what information or commands to provide.

When speech is used as the input mode, a menu structure can improve the accuracy of a recognizer since accuracy is partly dependant upon the *branching factor* of the input, that is, the number of choices at any particular point. The branching factor is likely to be lower where questions or menus are used than when a whole range of commands are possible, with a resulting increase in accuracy. Consequently, in tasks where error costs are high or where recognizer performance is likely to be poor due to a large variety of speakers or a low quality communication channel, the speed of a command language will need to be sacrificed in favor of a system using prompts.

If the application dictates that any prompts must be aural rather than visual, further points must be considered. Menus of more than a few commands may be too much for the user to remember. Also if the the user is carrying out another task simultaneously his or her ability to concentrate on entering information is likely to vary according to the demands of the other task; the user may therefore prefer to take the initiative by using commands rather than having to respond to prompts. Finally, the constraints of short-term memory are such that if data are to be retained in working memory, it must be rehearsed constantly. Any aural prompts would interfere with rehearsal, whereas manual interaction would not. (No disadvantage has been found in using non-complimentary feedback, that is in using visual feedback with spoken input or voice feedback with manual input). In tasks where the oral/aural channel is the only one possible, some kind of "scratchpad" may be necessary for temporary data storage.

Just as goal-oriented acts can provide a naive user with details of the type of information needed, a dialogue control facility can help to describe how to use a system, the correct form of each command, or the way in which the user should speak for optimum performance.

Some applications may also require that the user confirm that the input has been correctly interpreted. This follows the pattern of human-to-human conversation, in which information is repeated back if the channel is poor (for example, over a telephone) or if the message is very important. Whether or not there is an opportunity for confirmation depends upon the type of feedback provided by the system.

4.2.2   Feedback

A system is described as having *primary* or *secondary* feedback, according to whether there is a confirmation phase in the dialogue.

Primary feedback occurs if a systems responds directly to the user's command. Situations where the action is invisible to the user, such as a database update, may involve the system telling the user what action has been performed, but this is not the same as letting the user check the input before anything happens.

Primary feedback is used in situations where errors are not critical, or where the time saved outweighs the cost of possible errors. In VDU control, for example, it is just as easy to correct a wrong display by repeating the command as it is to confirm an input before action is taken. Primary feedback also tends to be used in applications such as package sorting, where the small percentage of errors made does not warrant slowing down the whole process by introducing a verification phase.

Experiments by Schurick *et al.* (in press) on feedback for voice input shows that even in applications best suited to primary feedback it is worth having a "word confirmation dialogue" for cases where the recognizer cannot distinguish between two words. As the majority of inputs do not need this dialogue, there is no significant effect on the time taken to enter data, yet overall accuracy can be increased by about 5%.

With secondary feedback, the user has the opportunity to correct any errors before an action is performed, which can vastly improve accuracy. Applications that might need this facility include those that have permanent data capture (quality control, entry of co-ordinates in cockpits), or those where the cost of errors is high (industrial robot control).

The best way of providing secondary feedback depends on the user's environment and the type of data involved. Comparing visual and aural feedback of words and fields (groups of words), Schurick *et al* found that visual, word-by-word feedback with a history of the transaction proved optimal in terms of both time and accuracy. Where a large visual display is not available to show the history, for example in a cockpit, visual word or field feedback gives the best results. Some recognizers are used in an eyes-busy environment so that visual displays cannot be used at all; in this case, auditory word feedback is recommended as auditory field feedback takes much longer and is more likely to cause confusion.

4.2.3 Error Correction
The type of error correction that should be provided depends on the type of feedback used—word or field, aural or visual. Experiments to investigate the use of error correction commands in data entry were carried out by Schurick *et al.* (in press) for various feedback conditions, and by Spine *et al.* (1983) for auditory word feedback.

In Schurick's experiments the data was divided into fields and the words recognized were placed in an input buffer until a field was completed. The error correction commands available were "erase," which deleted the last word in the input buffer so that all data could be re-entered, and "verify" plus a field name, which allowed subjects to access and edit a previously entered field of data.

In visual field and word feedback and in auditory word feedback, subjects used the command "erase" much more frequently than "cancel." With auditory field feedback, "cancel" became the more popular command, which seems to show that auditory field feedback is more confusing, causing more subjects to cancel the whole input rather than try to edit it.

The verification command tended to be used as an editor for words in the input buffer and to help a subject determine where he or she was in the field. It is not surprising that verify was used more in field feedback than in word feedback.

As with goal-oriented acts, the initiative for error correction can be taken either by the system or by the user. The experiments by Spine *et al.* (1983) investigated both automatic and user-directed error correction techniques for auditory word feedback.

Subjects again had the option to erase or cancel and they could also request "runner-insertion," where the recognizer's second choice for a particular word was inserted in place of its first choice.

The erase command was again the most popular, closely followed by the runner-insertion. The cancel command was used infrequently, as subjects felt that it would "waste too much time." The use of error correction commands increased the number of messages correctly recognized from 63.52% to 89.29%.

The time taken to enter data also increased when error-correction was used, but the experiment shows that this time can be kept to a minimum by using smaller message lengths. The experiments also stress the notion that it is the total transaction time which is important: "time spent in correcting errors before transmission would be less time than the time spent in trying to regain control of the system had the errors been passed through to the host."

The utterances used were a set of simulated air traffic control messages, which had the advantage of conforming to a strict syntax and so allowing the user of a parser to correct errors automatically. Three approaches to automatic error correction were tried in the Spine experiments. The first method was to determine whether or not substitution of the second-choice word of the recogniser would result in a correctly parsed string. The second method determined whether or not there was only one possible word or class of words dictated by the syntax, regardless of what was recognized. The final method used truncating or deleting when extra words appeared in the message.

When automatic error correction alone was used, the percentage of correct messages improved from 63.52% to 82.91%. This shows that a significant proportion of error-riden messages can be corrected automatically so that much of the burden of error detection and correction can be removed from the human operator.

5.   Case Studies

5.1   Jaguar Cars

A complete quality surveillance system has been built by Logica for Jaguar Cars at the Browns Lane plant. The overall aims of the system were;

- identification of faults occurring in vehicle assemblies

- immediate feedback of this information to the assembly zones originating the fault

- management of fault rectification

- review of current and historical quality information

The options for data capture in such an application are hand-held terminals, static terminals or speech input with aural feedback and prompting. Speech input in this case provides greater mobility, hands- and eyes-free operation and greater flexibility that would have been the case with a hand-held terminal. The overall system architecture is shown in Figure 4. One in ten vehicles are taken from the production line for inspection and the audit requirements are to:

- perform explicit checks rather than free field

- identify the features and type of any faults

- indicate the severity of the fault

- identify the location of the fault if not incidental

The dialogue design was centered around achieving these objectives and resulted in a fairly large vocabulary of some 300 words with a total prompt list covering all variants of the vehicle of around 1500 items. For any one vehicle the number of prompt will be around 850. The initial aim had been to minimize the number of words in the vocabulary and to create a fairly simple dialogue structure with perhaps 30 to 40 words, thus making the training and the use of the system simple. It became clear fairly early in the detailed design that the audit objectives would not be fulfilled with such a restricted approach. The final dialogue design is shown in Figure 5.

One of the principal problems of such a structured design using speech prompting and input that covers a large list of items to be inspected is that users may not develop a good cognitive map of the checking process. A map will include such aspects as the items already inspected and those still to be inspected. With a visual system, either paper or terminal, such a map is much easier to form. In the speech system, navigation through the checks such as backtracking or skipping items could become cumbersome. In the Jaguar application provision is made for skipping items and also zones which include a number of items to be inspected.

The inspection proceeds with initial log-on and identification of the vehicle variant by bar code reader. Each vehicle is inspected by two inspectors covering different zones, and each receives a prompt over a radio link to a headset instructing him or her which part of the vehicle to check. If there is no fault the response "O.K." initiates the next prompt and the information is sent to the host computer and database. If a fault is found the word "fault" is spoken which loads a vocabulary of faults appropriate to the item or region of the vehicle being inspected. The feature of the item which is at fault may also be identified and the command feature loads a set of words appropriate to the item being inspected. The severity of the fault is finally identified and if above "incidental" is relayed to the trackside teletext displays.

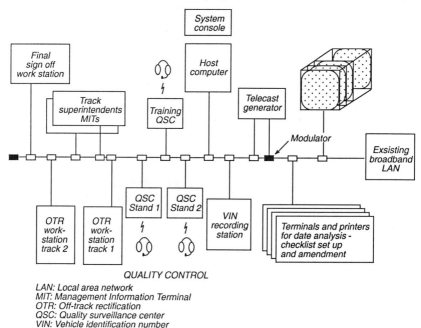

LAN: Local area network
MIT: Management Information Terminal
OTR: Off-track rectification
QSC: Quality surveillance center
VIN: Vehicle identification number

Figure 4: Block diagram of the Jaguar quality surveillance system.

A "help" command may be used to obtain more detailed instructions on the checks to be carried out. These are displayed on a large overhead display since lengthy help information is not ideally displayed aurally, and recall can be difficult. Since the dialogue is structured and the vocabulary limited the inspector may call up the allowable list of responses at any point in the dialogue, these are again displayed on the visual display.

Feedback and verification of the data was designed as a compromise between speed and accuracy. Normally the system will acknowledge an utterance with a "beep" except when the recognition score of the top scoring word is close to the second best choice. In this case explicit confirmation of the data entered is made, thus ensuring high reliability of data entered into the quality database. In practice the number of confirmatory dialogues is low.

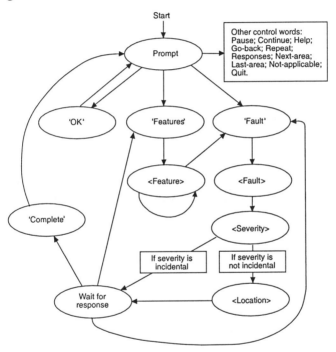

Figure 5: Dialogue design diagram for Jaguar Cars.

An important factor in achieving success with this and indeed any application of speech using such structured dialogues with users not familiar with the technology is training. The recognition system used was speaker-dependant, requiring multiple repetitions of each word to obtain high accuracy. A separate training package was created and a training system was provided off-line to introduce users to the technology and familiarize them with the training process and the vocabulary of the application. Users are able to build confidence in the system after training by checking recognition of each word and noting the score displayed as a red bar. The better the score the higher the bar moves, rather like a VU meter. Inspectors are able to experiment with voice changes and notice how tolerant the system is to such changes in pronunciation. Any poorly trained words are also identified in this way and can be retrained. After initial familiarization and training an inspector is then able to use the system on the inspection stand.

5.2   Caterpillar

A simpler shop floor data capture application than the one at Jaguar but in a more hostile environment is illustrated by a system installed by Logica in an acoustically sealed engine run-up booth at Caterpillar's Desford plant (Leicestershire, UK). The system records important information from an operator testing tractor engines when they are started up for the first time. During these tests the noise levels generated are so high that operators wear ear defenders, to protect their hearing. Prior to using the speech based data capture system, two operators were required to carry out the testing. One of the operators read off the engine revolutions and hydraulic pressures whilst the other operated the controls.

Caterpillar has derived real benefits since the system was installed as part of the production facility in September 1987 by doubling employee effectiveness. One operator now enters data about engine speed and oil and hydraulic pressure by voice input while adjusting the controls. All of the data required for future analysis can be captured using a vocabulary of around 20 words including the digits. (Figure 6). Previously this information had to be hand-written by one of the two operators onto a report card. Using speech input and output technology, eyes and hands are now free, and radio communication allows the operator to move easily around the vehicle while remaining in constant touch with the quality assurance computer.

The information to be entered in this application is very different from the Jaguar application, consisting mostly of numerical data from tachometer, temperature and pressure readings. For this reason feedback of each input field is provided to the operator using text to speech synthesis with a male voice and explicit confirmation of the correctness of the data is required. All other system prompts are provided at two levels, expert and novice.

The expert prompts are a shortened version of the full prompt and are appropriate for experienced users of the system who are familiar with all the checks to be carried out.

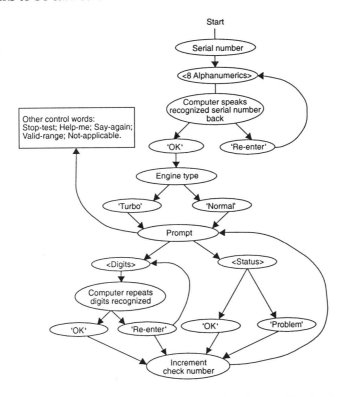

Figure 6: Dialogue design diagram for the Caterpillar backhoe loader

The system runs on an IBM-PC equipped with a speech interface board and a radio receiver. To overcome the severe noise problem a throat microphone is used and voice prompts are provided through a headset mounted in ear defenders. Data is accumulated, analyzed and presented graphically so that management may focus attention on key quality issues. At a cost of around £25,000 the system will have paid for itself in two years. Direct computer entry of the test data has improved accuracy as well as productivity, since the previous scheme gave rise to later transcription errors arising from the difficulty of reading some reports due to the working conditions under which they were generated.

6.   Conclusions

Speech technology is not a panacea for all human-computer interfaces; an understanding of some of the basic issues in design, particularly relevant to industrial applications, have been highlighted. The case studies cited in this chapter illustrate, however, that speech technology can be successfully applied and cost-justified in industrial applications. We have shown that the design of a speech-based human-computer interface requires care, and less than optimal design can still result, particularly when trying to converge application and commercial needs with technology limitations.

7.   References

Bunt, H.C., Leopold, F.F., Muller, H.F. and van Katwijk, A.F.V. (1978). "In search of pragmatic principles in man-machine dialogues." *IPO Annual Progress Report*, 13, p. 94–98.

Laycock, J. and Peckham, J.B. (1980). "Improved pivoting performance whilst using direct voice input." *Royal Aircraft Establishment Technical Report*, 80019.

McLoed, P., (1977). "A dual task response modality effect: Support for multiprocessor models of attention." Quarterly Journal of Experimental Psychology 29, 1977, p. 651–657.

Schurick, J.M. Willeges, B.H. and Maynard, J.F. (In press). *User Feedback Requirements with Automatic Speech Recognition.* Virginia: Virginia Polytechnic Institute.

Spine, T.M., Maynard, J.F. and Willeges, B.H. (1983). "Error correction strategies for voice recognition." *Proc Voice Data Entry Conference*, Chicago.

Welch, J.R. (1980). "Automatic Speech Recognition—Putting it to work in Industry." *Proc.*IEEE.

Chapter 17

Toys That Talk: Two Case Studies

Gene A. Frantz
Texas Instruments Incorporated

1. Introduction

I have been involved in two intriguing speech products in the last several years: The Speak & Spell from Texas Instruments Incorporated and the Julie Doll from Worlds of Wonder. They each required significant compromises between the state of the art of speech science and the product requirements. We will review these compromises along with an historical perspective of each of their developments.

2. Speak & Spell

During the latter part of 1976, Texas Instruments entered the educational products market with the introduction of the Li'l Professor learning aid. Sharing the same microprocessor technology used in hand-held calculators, the Li'l Professor taught children the basics of math—addition, subtraction, multiplication and division. The product's success indicated the existence of a large market for educational electronic learning aids. An evaluation of various product possibilities led to the suggestion that the next product thrust should be the subject of spelling. At the same time "brain storming" sessions were being held to find uses for a promising new technology, bubble memory. Paul Breedlove, my boss at the time, suggested that synthetic speech, with its large memory requirements, might make good use of bubble memories. The combination of large memories and a follow-on product for the Li'l Professor inspired the concept of the Speak & Spell.

The obvious way of presenting a spelling word without giving away the answer is to speak the word aloud, as is traditionally done for children when a cooperative friend or parent "calls out" spelling words. Using a picture to suggest the word might work for some nouns, but not for verbs or for abstract nouns such as "courage" or "jealous." Using scrambled letters could confuse the child, could be ambiguous, or could suggest an incorrect spelling. Having a synthetic speech device read the word aloud seems by far the most natural way to teach spelling.

2.1 Program Beginnings

Using speech to present spelling words posed a serious technical problem. The state of the art for solid state voice output was such that a typical system had a price tag of thousands of dollars and could not fit in a portable (or for that matter, desktop) product. Although this was discouraging, it clearly defined the necessary technological breakthrough: develop a low cost speech output capability for a handheld spelling product. The original design-to-cost goal is shown in Figure 1.

Programmable Products/Speech
Spelling Bee
Original 3Q78 Design-to-Cost Requirements

MOS

Control/Synthesizer Chip	2.00
ROM (200k bit)	2.50
Display (8 digit alphanumeric)	2.24
Keyboard (40 key x-y)	.55
PCB	.45
Plastics	.40
Discretes (module)	1.35
Speaker	.20
Packing	.25
Misc. (switch, batt, clip, overlay)	.40
Freight/Duty/Usage	.36
Subtotal	**10.70**
Labor	.60
MOH	.60
OOH	.70
Cost Adjustment	.05
Total Cost	**12.65**
AUP (35% GPM)	19.46
Retail (35% margin)	29.95

Figure 1   Design-to-Cost Model for the Speak & Spell

The speech system had to satisfy several requirements. The spoken spelling words had to be intelligible, even when spoken out of context. Memory usage had to be modest, and the product should be able to pronounce 200 spelling words and a few phrases using no more than 200K bits of low-cost read only memory (ROM). Finally, the speech generator had to be inexpensive, probably a single chip fabricated using a low cost semiconductor technology.

As originally proposed, we were unsure that the product was technically possible, or, if it could be built, that it would be commercially successful. The project was rejected under the normal Texas Instruments R&D system as too speculative. "Wild Hare," an alternative funding source for high-risk programs, also rejected it as too risky. The project was finally funded by IDEA, a program Texas Instruments established to fund the initial stages of very high risk projects.

In early December, the program began with a series of meetings attended by members of the Corporate Research Laboratories and of the Component Design Group of Consumer Products. The research staff was well aware of the problems to be solved. Waveform encoding techniques require an order of magnitude more memory than was available. Synthesizing compressed speech requires complex processors capable of a large number of arithmetic operations per second. If speech is compressed to data rates of less than 1800 bits per second, speech quality is a problem. However, compressed speech seemed the only feasible alternative since an order of magnitude breakthrough in memory was unlikely.

2.2 Alternatives
We first considered a synthesizer using stored phonemic descriptions with a set of rules for adding pitch inflection, stress and timing (See Syrdal, Chapter 3). Such a synthesizer can support a large vocabulary with modest amounts of memory. This approach was abandoned because the synthesizer could not be a simple digital circuit, and because we were concerned that the speech would not be clear enough to permit recognition of single words out of context.

Analysis-synthesis systems store representations of whole words, typically as formants or as linear predictive coding (LPC) parameters (see O'Shaugnessy, Chapter 2). We believed that such synthesizers would provide adequate voice quality and reasonable data rates and that the synthesis algorithm could be developed quickly. The LPC approach was chosen because of its proven high speech quality at low data rates, and because speech analysis routines were readily available.

2.3 Processing Architecture

LPC synthesizers require a large number of multiplies and adds for the digital filter. A two- multiply lattice filter was chosen because the computations could be done using fixed-point arithmetic and because it uses reflection coefficients directly (Itakura and Saito, 1971). This was considered important because the reflection coefficients are more suited for coding. At a 10 KHz sampling rate, however, the process would require 200,000 multiplies per second and a similar number of adds. By carefully sequencing and pipelining the arithmetic operations of the lattice filter, the speed and power constraints of P- channel MOS were met (PMOS was the least expensive integrated circuit technology at the time). This sequencing has been described in detail elsewhere (Wiggins and Brantingham, 1978 and Wiggins, 1980).

Besides the digital filter, the LPC synthesizer consists of a decoder, a parameter smoother, an excitation generator, and a D/A converter. Each of these functions required the development of specialized circuits to achieve the desired performance while minimizing the die area (Wiggins and Brantingham, 1980 and Puri et al., 1980). After only a few months, the basic processing architecture had been proposed and estimates of the required chip area had been completed. A complete 1200 bit per second speech synthesizer on a single chip now looked achievable.

2.4 Program Support

With several of the key technical problems solved, the next step was to sell the technology development program to management. We had a well-defined product that was aimed at a large-volume consumer market. Developing a custom integrated circuit would drive down the unit cost of the product which would in turn lead to large market demand. Nevertheless, there was some uncertainty that the speech technology would be successful. Funding for the development program was segmented so that money for the next segment was based on the successful completion of the previous segment. Obviously, as each milestone was reached, confidence increased, and funding was easier to obtain for larger portions of the program.

2.5 Market Assessments

In parallel with selling solid-state synthetic speech internally, we began laying the ground work for marketing the new talking learning aid to the consumer. We had hoped that the advantages of verbal interaction between the product and the student would be obvious. Unfortunately, they weren't. Most people had never heard synthetic speech, and assumed it would be a dull monotone, computer-like voice. Available talking children's products were pull string toys or analog tape recorders and the perceived capabilities, limitations and quality expectations for these toys also influenced the consumer's concept of a new talking product.

Focus groups were used to research the market for a spelling learning aid with speech output. The groups were composed of people chosen at random from the target market. There were six groups, one of fathers, three of mothers and two of teachers, all with children ages seven through 10. The concept of the talking product was introduced with the aid of posters and voice samples played on a cassette tape recorder. Several product concepts were presented to give the focus groups a feel for the product concept. These product concepts included the original Spelling Bee concept, a "Talking Typewriter," "Wordy Birdy," "Frankenspeller," and so on. Figure 2 shows drawings of a few of the concepts. Character voices for each concept were developed and used in the presentations. Unfortunately the visual and verbal techniques used to demonstrate the capabilities of the planned product reinforced existing prejudices about talking toys. The results were surprising and disappointing, although in retrospect they should not have been. The major concerns of the participants were:

1. A capacity of 250 words was not adequate.

2. Talking toys do not hold up.

3. The product would be another noise maker.

4. The pronunciation of words and accent would be "cold and computer-like."

5. The product would quickly become dull and the child would lose interest.

Although there were many negative comments by the participants, there were positive comments as well. A teacher remarked that using speech in a learning aid added an important dimension of listening and developing auditory perception. Most people said they liked the idea of a learning aid for spelling, although many didn't seem to think that speech was a necessary part of the product.

2.6 Product Design
Concern about word capacity was difficult to alleviate. The read-only memories (ROM's) that were being designed were the largest in the industry at the time with 131,072 bits of stored information. Even with this capacity, however, only 150 words could be stored in each ROM, and with two ROM's the product had a vocabulary of 300 words and phrases. But the

indications were that consumers believed this was inadequate. This per-ceived need for additional word capacity was solved to a large extent by providing plug-in speech modules that could be sold separately.

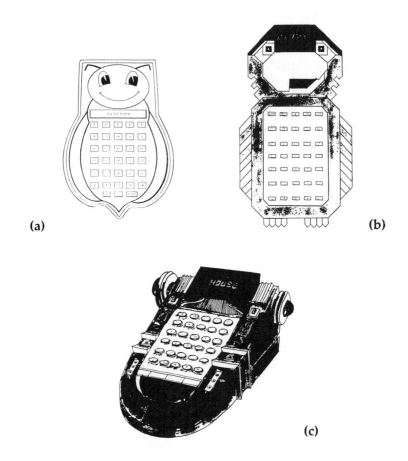

(a)   (b)

(c)

Figure 2   Early Speak & Spell concepts: a. Original product concept drawing used to get early IDEA funding,   b. "Wordy-birdy" concept drawing used in focus groups, and   c. "Talking Typewriter" concept drawing (all copyrighted by Texas Instruments Incorporated).

The second concern, that talking toys do not hold up, was probably well founded, since such toys were mechanical and used in a very abusive environment (i.e. small children). Speak & Spell had an advantage over existing talking toys because it had no moving parts. It would be important that the durability of Solid State Speech technology be stressed in the advertisement campaign.

The third point, that the talking product would be just another noisemaker, was a valid concern. A phrase that was exciting the first time would be annoying the tenth and unwanted noise the hundredth. The solution was to select multiple phrases for the responses, some randomized and some sequential. The result was a product that seemed to communicate in a human-like manner. The one constraint placed on the selection of phrases concerned the error messages. If the child missed a spelling, Speak & Spell used only one phrase for the first occurrence, "wrong try again," and a second single phrase for the second error, "That is incorrect, the correct spelling of ...... is ......" While we thought it would be fun to give the child raspberries, or a cat call, or some funny comment for a wrong spelling, we elected not to because we thought it important that the response for a wrong answer be less desirable than for a correct one. A spelling aid should not encourage incorrect spelling.

The next issue was the importance of word pronunciation and a correct accent. Picking the "correct" American dialect was not easy. However, the desire to have the product speak correctly eliminated some early suggestions for a "character voice." Instead, the emphasis was on finding a voice that would be compatible with the analysis-synthesis system, with an acceptable American accent.

Finally, "dull and boring" was a concern not only for the focus group but also for the design team. Perhaps it was assumed by the focus group that the product would be similar in operation to a tape recorder or that it would be a list giver with no interaction. For this reason, several word games were provided so that a child would have a variety of activities that were designed to build word skills.

In addition to using focus groups, leading educators in the field of teaching spelling were consulted. Some of their comments were not favorable. For instance, they recommended that the project be delayed until an appropriate display be developed with both upper- and lower-case letters. After careful consideration, this advice was ignored. In other cases, we adopted their recommendations. On the advice of educators, it was decided to use only words that did not follow the usual rules of spelling. These are the words that students must learn by rote and were therefore well-suited for teaching with the Speak & Spell learning aid. Future modules would contain words pointed toward teaching certain spelling principles or for certain grades.

2.7 Production Start-Up

Speak & Spell was announced in Chicago at the Consumer Electronics Show in June of 1978. The product was extremely well received and a success from the beginning. As the fall approached, it was clear that sales would be limited by production capabilities. Besides the success of the product itself, people were fascinated with the speech synthesis technology. Interacting with children by voice was even more successful than anticipated. Speak & Spell seemed to be holding children's attention for extended periods. The product seemed to assume its own personality, and that attracted children. The viability of educational toys based on solid state synthetic speech was firmly established.

With product acceptance in the market place, all that was left was to put it into production, which raised a whole new set of problems. The noise of the production line made it nearly impossible to test the product at various stages in the process. Would the people doing the tests need to be tested for hearing? Did we want people with exceptional hearing, average hearing, or poor hearing to do the testing? Should the testers speak English? How would we maintain consistency in testing between stations and over time? Without unnecessary details, I will give a few examples of how we answered some of these questions.

The noise problem was solved by building little "dog houses" for speech testers to sit in. The dog houses were three-sided insulated enclosures intended to reduce the noise level enough so the product could be heard. They were dubbed "dog houses" not because of their looks but because the individuals doing the testing were stuck in the enclosure and isolated from the rest of the production line: they were in the "dog house." During down times the insides of the dog houses were decorated with graffiti. It was not difficult to see the lack of love for this job assignment.

The need for hearing tests was brought to our attention in a memorable way. One day it was observed that many assemblies were making it through the test area with obvious speech problems. The problem was traced to one test station, and we discovered that the tester was hearing impaired. She didn't know the product talked.

Consistency of speech evaluation between test stations and final quality control was difficult. Daily meetings were held between various managers to separate "good" speech from "bad." Sample units were kept that were deemed to have minimally acceptable speech quality. During this process an interesting discovery was made. Evaluating speech quality was not like the evaluation of mechanical quality. If an inspector is looking for scratches on a plastic case, the learning process works in one's favor. The more plastic cases the inspector sees the more likely it is that a scratch will be noticed. But this is not so with synthetic speech. The more one hears synthetic speech the less critical he or she becomes of it. With some experience, grunts became intelligible.* We considered using "naive listeners", people unfamiliar with synthetic speech. However, we would soon run out of them unless we fired people when they became too familiar with synthetic speech.

2.8 Conclusions

In retrospect, the uncertainties associated with speech technology and product acceptance were unfounded. Nevertheless, there were times when advice had to be ignored, risks had to be taken, and compromises had to be made. But the nature of the product changed only slightly despite deviations from the original plan. Decisions were made on the basis of preserving the basic concept of the target product and of not delaying the planned release date. The time from the beginning of the program until the showing of the product was only 18 months. The program schedule was maintained throughout the effort.

One of the greatest difficulties in the program was to predict the consumer reaction to the product idea. This proved to be extremely difficult because the new technology involved in the product had not developed a base for consumer comparison.

The success of the effort is now apparent. The Speak & Spell product was pictured on the cover of Business Week in September of 1978. The product was selected by Industrial Research/Development as one of the 100 most significant new products of 1979, and was acclaimed by several PTA groups as one of the top 10 educational toys in 1979. It has now been in production for more than ten years with its original design—the best indication of the success of the Speak & Spell.

3. Julie Doll

Many years passed between the introduction of Speak & Spell and Julie Doll. Technology had progressed, but products since Speak & Spell were

---

*During this period of time there was a TV show called "Battle Star Galactica". Some of the characters in the show were called Silon warriors. They spoke with a terrible synthetic voice. I had become so used to synthetic speech that I was the interpreter for them at my house. I always declined to take part in the evaluation of speech quality.

not enjoying consumer acceptance. However, Texas Instruments had introduced a new line of Digital Signal Processors (DSPs) and associated software that could do speech synthesis and also vocoding and automatic speech recognition. The technology was available to support fully interactive speech-based toys, toys that could not only "speak," but also "listen."

This new technology had two serious problems. First, DSPs were expensive. When Texas Instruments introduced the TMS32010 DSP in 1982 it cost about $200.00. The TMS320C25 was introduced three years later at $500.00. We were, however, in the process of designing the TMS320C17, which we believed would have a combination of processing capacity and cost that would suit it for use in consumer products. Second, automatic speech recognition is an order of magnitude more expensive than a keyboard and an order of magnitude less accurate. When I gave talks on ASR, it was my custom to begin by saying, "There is no speech recognition system, at any cost, that meets the expectation of the user." While we were far from certain that the accuracy problem could be solved, we thought it might be possible to design a toy that would not frustrate or annoy the child with every misrecognition.

During the development of Speak & Spell, the product concept drove the technology development. At this point, we had promising technology, but no clearly defined product. Arrangements were made to present the available technology along with a set of example products to every major toy manufacturer in the United States. The hope was to find one company who could catch a vision of what might be possible. One of the companies visited was Worlds of Wonder (WoW). I met with them briefly in March. They were busy getting the Christmas product line into production and had no time for me. But when we met again later in the year they caught the vision and Julie was conceived.

3.1 Technology
As the product concept was being firmed up, we turned our attention to making sure that the technology that had excited WoW actually existed. The DSP that met the cost goals was still in design. The speech recognition algorithm existed, but not in the proper form. There was no speech synthesis algorithm but one could be developed by modifying a vocoding algorithm. The real difficulty was automatic speech recognition. TI had been licensing a speaker dependent speech recognition algorithm for several years as part of a IBM PC compatible speech board. However, that algorithm required 4K words of program memory, 16K words of data memory for templates and each template required about 250 words of

memory and would not fit into the TMS320C17. The speech research team at TI was given the product concept that WoW was considering and the device that it was to use. They were asked to make the existing speech recognition algorithm fit into the device while still leaving enough room for the synthesis and product algorithms. Their immediate reply was that this was impossible! They were being asked to reduce the size of the recognition algorithm, including enrollment, to less than 2K words and to reduce the total memory requirement for the templates to less than 256 words. They would need either more memory designed into the device or external memory. This was a reasonable request, but for cost reasons was unacceptable. So, we made a compromise. The research team would cut the ASR algorithm back to fit the size without regard to recognition accuracy.

The results were amazing—the revised code required 1.1K words of program and all 10 templates fit into 160 words of data space. And, it could actually recognize words: Later evaluation of the algorithm indicated that the recognition rate was about 80 to 90 percent. Because the templates had only one bit per feature, the enrollment procedure was limited to a single pass. A single pass enrollment procedure was considered easier to integrate into the product than a multi-pass one.

Speaker independent recognition would have eliminated the enrollment procedure completely and the templates could have been stored in ROM at a much lower system cost. We stayed with speaker dependent recognition for several reasons:

- Children of the age who would play with Julie were not consistent enough in their speech patterns for a simple speaker independent algorithm. This not only included variation from child to child within a region, but also variation from region to region.

- Worlds of Wonder was interested in an international market. Speaker independent recognition would make a worldwide fan-out more difficult.

3.2 Product Development
Product development was a joint effort of TI and WoW. TI would be responsible for the technology development (i.e., the device and speech algorithms) and WoW would be responsible for the system design. This division of responsibilities was necessary to assure that the system designer, Worlds of Wonder, would: 1) take ownership of the design and 2) learn the fundamentals of the technology for future product designs. The

position that we took was that if TI was going to do the system design then TI was going to sell the product. It was going to be the product design that sold Julie, not the technology. The system design included both the system hardware and system software design. WoW agreed that they needed to take ownership of the product and took on the product development task.

The development had three primary design goals. The first was to create a lifelike, interactive doll with a variety of play modes that could be guided by the child. Second, expansibility was required to allow not only increased vocabulary, but also new features such as interactive games and make-believe adventures. Third, several sensor inputs had to be integrated into the system in a functionally lifelike manner.

These goals were achieved with a combination of speech synthesis, speech recognition and a control algorithm managing speech and hardware sensor functions. These three routines comprised the application code executed by the DSP. Table I shows the utilization of the DSP.

Table 1:   DSP Utilization

Algorithm	Memory Pgm (KW)	Data (W)	CPU Utilize AVG/MAX
32kbps ADPCM (half-duplex)	0.45	95	40/42%
2.4kbps LPC Synthesis	1.3	105	60/82%
16W SD Speech Recognition	1.5	221	75/100%
Control Algorithm	0.75	35	<25%

The speech synthesis data and the play algorithm control instructions resided in external ROMs. Add-on modules could then replace or supplement the resident play algorithm. Sensor inputs included temperature, light, motion, low battery, "tickle" switch in the stomach, and a resistance-sensing probe in the doll's right hand to detect "magic spot" resistance patches in activity books.

Creating an effective play algorithm was difficult. The technology afforded so much flexibility that it was difficult to choose a consistent, smoothly flowing play strategy that included all of Julie's available features. Several play scenarios were created to be in the "core" algorithm. From these scenarios a list of words and sentences were generated for both synthesis and recognition.

It was understood from the beginning of the project that there would be significant problems recognizing a single word in a connected-speech sentence. Several strategies were used to overcome this problem. First, all of the recognition words were carefully evaluated to assure minimal errors. Second, the play algorithm took advantage of the error rate. Several key parts of the algorithm featured random selection independent of the response, which minimized the effect of the errors. Finally, certain control sequences were designed so that only a few of the sixteen words had to be searched for at once.

The synthesis algorithm was identical to standard speech synthesizers in the market. This made the development of the speech data relatively easy.

3.3 Product Integration
There were only three months from the start of design in November, 1986 until Julie was introduced at Toy Fair in February, 1987. Julie does some amazing things. She talks to you and expects you to answer.

She knows when its dark or light. She knows when it is cold or hot. And she knows when you are taking her somewhere. She is even ticklish. In short, she responds to aspects of her environment and to her friends much as a little girl would.

She is bright too; she can read a book. Speech synthesis and recognition are only a part of her capability. They are not a gimmick to sell the product but are necessary for a doll to take on a personality.

4. Conclusions
In both of these products the goal was to add speech to increase its value. In the case of the Speak & Spell, enough years have passed to show its success in the market. But not so with Julie. Just after Julie's introduction, Worlds of Wonder found itself in financial difficulty and declared bankruptcy. Production of Julie was stopped and as of this writing has not been restarted. Those who had an opportunity to play with her loved her. But success still cannot be declared.

It was the purpose of these case studies to discuss the system level considerations of adding speech to a toy. If you would like to read further, these case studies are based on several articles listed in the reference section.

5. References

Frantz, G., Reimer, J., & Wotiz, R. (1988). Julie: The Application of DSP to a Consumer Product. *Speech Technology, 9/10,* 83f.

Frantz, G., & Wiggins, R. (1981). The Development of 'Solid State Speech' Technology at Texas Instruments. *ASSP Newsletter, 3,* 34.

Frantz, G., & Wiggins, R. (1982). Speak & Spell: A Case Study. *IEEE Spectrum, 2.*

Harvard University. (1982). *Texas Instruments, Inc.—Educational Products.*

Industrial Research/Development.(1979). *IR 100 Award Winning Products.*

Itakura, F., & Saito, S. (1971). Digital Filtering Techniques for Speech Analysis and Synthesis. *Seventh International Congress on Acoustics, Budapest, Paper 25C1,* 261–264.

Puri, A., Caruso, M., Dennison, S., & Brown, J. (1980). *MOS Digital to Analog Converter Employing Scaled Field Effect Devices.* U. S. Patent 4,209,781, June 24.

Staff. (1978). Special Report: Texas Instruments Shows U. S. Business How to Survive in the 1980's. *Business Week, Sept. 18,* 84.

Wiggins, R. (1980). An Integrated Circuit for Speech Synthesis. *Proc. 1980 IEEE Conf. on Acous., Speech and Signal Proc., Denver, CO.*

Wiggins, R., & Brantingham, L. (1978). Three Chip System Synthesizes Human Speech. *Electronics, 50(18).*

Wiggins, R., & Brantingham, L. (1980). *Speech Synthesis Integrated Circuit Device.* U. S. Patent No. 4,309,836, June 24.

Whalen, D. H., Wiley, E. R., Rubin, P., & Cooper, F. S. (1990). *The Haskins Laboratories' Pulse Code Modulation (PMC) System.* Haskins Laboratories internal documentation note.

Zue, V. W., Cypers, D. S., Kassel, R. H., Kaufman, D. H., Leung, H. C., Randolph, M., Seneff, S., Unverferth, J. E. III, & Wilson, T. (1986). The Development of the MIT LISP-Machine Based Speech Research Workstation. *Proceedings of the ICASSP 86, International Conference on Acoustics, Speech, and Signal Processing, held in Tokyo, Japan, April 8–11,* 329–332.

Chapter 18

HADES: A Case Study of the Development of a Signal Analysis System[1]

Philip E. Rubin
Haskins Laboratory

1. Introduction

Research on speech and language, and the development of useful technology based on this research, depends on increasingly sophisticated tools, and most particularly on signal analysis systems. We are using ever more powerful tools to display, measure, edit and analyze time domain signals including both acoustic productions and physiological activity. The evolution of speech and signal analysis systems at Haskins Laboratories over the past 15 years will be described. The details of our systems are dependant on our particular computing environment, but many of the issues that are discussed are quite general and likely arise in some form whenever an attempt is made to create research tools for general use.

2. Background

The development of speech analysis systems at Haskins Laboratories has been influenced by the nature of the institution, the interests and needs of the researchers associated with it, and the available hardware. Haskins is a non-profit research institution affiliated with academic institutions in the Northeast and internationally, including Yale University, the University of Connecticut, City College of New York, Wesleyan University, Wellesley College, and the Hebrew University. The Laboratories provide a central facilities resource for research in areas related to speech and language,

---

[1] The development of many of the systems mentioned in this paper and the preparation of this document were supported, in part, by a variety of grants and contracts to Haskins Laboratories including NIH Grants HD-01994, MS-13870, NS-13617, and NIH Contract N01-HD-5-2910.

including speech perception, speech production, phonetics, phonology, reading, motor behavior, and cognitive and ecological psychology. The Laboratories serve a small group of full-time research and technical support staff and a larger group of part-time researchers, graduate students, undergraduates, and postdoctoral students from many institutions.

Since the mid-1970s software efforts have concentrated on the development of special-purpose tools for a VAX -11/780, and more recently the associated VAX minicomputers that are part of our local area VAX cluster. A major goal of new software development has been to exploit the power of the VAXstation workstations while ensuring that new tools are integrated with our day-to-day computing environment. In addition, our systems must provide the power, consistency, features, and speed demanded by long-term users, while still being accessible to visitors who need to get their work done quickly and with minimal support from the relatively small technical staff.

3. Early Developments—WENDY and SPA

The design of new display and analysis systems has been influenced by systems that were developed in the early 1970s, many of which are still in use at Haskins and other institutions. One of the most influential programs, still in daily use, is the Waveform Editor aNd DisplaY program (WENDY). The program is used to edit 12-bit sampled data (PCM)[2] files (see O'Shaugnessy, Chapter 2, and Gopal, Chapter 8) that conform to a local standard. While the system is most commonly used for speech signals, it is readily adapted to physiological records, model-generated data, or the

---

[2] Haskins Laboratories uses the Pulse Code Modulation (PCM) method of digitizing analog signals, which consists of taking amplitude samples at frequent, regular intervals, and representing the continuously varying signal as binary digital numbers (Whalen, *et al.*, 1990). The number of intervals per unit of time is known as the sampling rate. At Haskins, sampling rates of 10,000 and 20,000 Hz (samples per second) are used for speech data, while physiological signals are samples at a wide variety of rates, including non-integer sampling rates. The resolution within the voltages that the system can encompass (known as the dynamic range) is specified by the number of bits used for the encoding. In the case of the Haskins system, the approximate range of -10V to +10V is coded into 12 bits. The Haskins systems, like many others, avoids having a sign bit by adding a dc offset half as large at the dynamic range. For a 12 bit system, the original values (-02048 to +2047) are internally stored as values in the range of 0-4095; the Haskins systems represents these values as 16-bit two's complement numbers with the highest four bits reserved as a control field. The Haskins PCM file format saves sampled data in a binary file (64 words per record), with a 4-record header block that supplies additional information about the file (Whalen, *et al.*, 1990). Segment labels can either be stored in trailer blocks (old label format) or as separate ASCII files (new label format).

output of synthesizers. Signals can be displayed as waveforms, amplitude and duration measurements can be made, and signals can be combined or edited as needed. The program also includes a procedural language for performing iterative operations and defining macros to repeat complex or frequently used operations. WENDY was designed to run on a single central CPU (originally a PDP 11/45 and later a VAX 11/780) that supported a number of Tektronix 4010/4014 compatible display terminals.

Figure 1 shows a typical display from the program. In the top panel is the amplitude waveform of an adult male saying "The cow chewed its cud." The bottom panel is an expanded section of a portion of this signal. Amplitude waveforms are shown in "display ports"; WENDY can accommodate up to eight simultaneous display ports.

WENDY is well adapted to performing its main function: displaying and editing signal waveforms. It can handle multiple signals, and the internal procedural language provides considerable flexibility for the manipulation of these signals. The program can be run from a variety of Tektronix-compatible terminals, including Digital VT240, GraphOn, and microcomputer-based Tektronix emulators. However, the program is not easy to learn. The command set is unique to this program, and is not self-documenting, and the functions of many commands are not intuitively obvious. The LISP-like procedural language is powerful and flexible once mastered, but is sufficiently difficult to learn that many users never take full advantage of it. The storage-mode display technology results in long display times, with many total screen redisplays. The program is also not well integrated with other forms of signal analysis used at the Laboratories.[3]

Shortly after the development of WENDY, a program called SPA (SPectral Analysis) was designed to provide FFT-based spectral analysis (see O'Shaugnessy, Chapter 2). SPA was intended to supplement ILS (Interactive Laboratory System), a commercial package from Signal Technology Incorporated of LPC-based analysis and filtering routines. SPA is a menu-driven program using the standard IEEE routines (IEEE, 1979) that is powerful, and much more accessible to the occasional user than ILS. Table 1 illustrates the SPA command menu (which is based on a Laboratory-wide applications interface shell called HUI—Haskins User Interface). Sampled

---

[3] An exception to this is *WES*, which is a modifies version of *WENDY* that runs as an integrated component of our *PSP* Physiological Signal Processing system, allowing display, edition and measurement of waveforms from within *PSP*.

data files can be analyzed, displayed, and saved in a Discrete Fourier Transform (DFT) format. Graphical interactions with the spectral data are, once again, limited by the inadequacies of the storage mode displays.

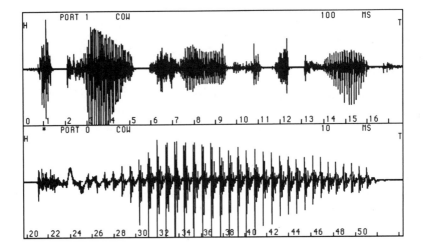

Figure 1: *WENDY* waveform display. Top panel—the utterance "The cow chewed its cud." Bottom panel—expanded view of the portion of the waveform that contains the word "cow."

Table 1: Menu of *SPA* commands.

MENU OF SPA COMMANDS:

SPE	SPEctral analysis
DIS	DISplay spectrogram
DSP	Display SPectral Cross-section
PRI	PRInt spectral values
AVE	AVErage magnitude spectra
RATE	decimation and interpolation (rate)
RMS	RMS signal energy
S3D	diSplay 3-Dim. spectrum
WAVE	WAVEform display
SET	SET variables, flags
SHOW	SHOW variables, flags
VAX	VAX DCL command
MACRO	MACRO definition
SUM	SUMmary of SPA
HELP	HELP
MENU	MENU of SPA commands
EXIT	EXIT SPA

Figure 2 shows a pseudo-spectrogram of the first 275 msec. of the utterance, "The cow chewed its cud." The figure is of low quality because spectrogram displays require gray-level representation: time is on the horizontal axis, frequency on the vertical, and intensity is represented by darkness. Figure 2 represents the best that can be done on a monochrome display without resorting to simulating a grey-scale using custom dot patterns. Even such a crude display is often useful (e.g., choosing points for drawing spectral cross-section information), and when additional resolution is needed the user can always use an analog spectrograph.

4. HUI—The Haskins User Interface Shell

During the mid-1970s, a wide variety of application programs were developed at the Laboratories. There were PCM file format support programs such as AFM (Arithmetic File Manipulation), CPC (viewing PCM data), INPUT (converting analog signals to PCM), and OUTPUT (PCM to analog). There were also programs to synthesize speech and other sounds, including SYN (acoustic synthesis and synthesis-by-rule), ASY (articulatory synthesis), and SWS (sinewave synthesis). PSP (Physiological Signal Processing), ACT and ACE were developed to display and analyze physiologi-

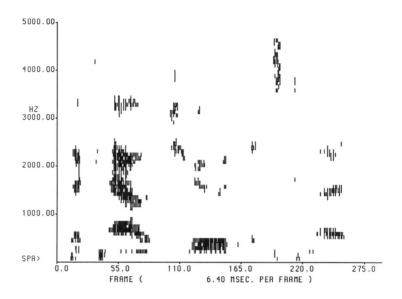

Figure 2: *SPA* pseudo-spectrogram.

cal time domain data. Because the user population was large and varied, and the number of application programs was growing quickly, we decided to create a simple, generic application shell that we called the Haskins User Interface, or HUI. HUI provides a flexible and consistent user interface, and gives programmers a framework and collection of tools for developing new applications. The basic HUI commands, those common to all applications, are shown in Table 2. HUI also supports a standard command-line parser to ensure commonality of command format. Except for enhancements to the MACRO function, HUI has been stable for many years.

Table 2: Menu of basic HUI commands.

MENU OF HUI COMMANDS:

EXIT	Exit from program
HELP	Display help for commands
MACRO	Define a macro
MENU	Display a list of commands
NEWS	Display the latest program news
SET	Set program flags
SHOW	Show program flags
VAX	Execute a DCL command

5. A New Approach to System Development

The design of speech and signal analysis systems at Haskins, and at many other institutions, has changed radically in recent years because of the ready availability of powerful engineering workstations and raster graphics displays. Our earlier systems were severely restricted by relatively scarce and expensive processing capacity and by the limitations of storage mode graphics. During the latter half of the 1970s we expended considerable effort in creating our own workstation, known as the Digital Pattern Playback(DPP) (Nye, *et al.*, 1975, Nye, *et al.*, 1977). This system combined custom-designed software with special-purpose hardware including a DEC GT40 display processor connected to a PDP 11/45 minicomputer, a Hewlett Packard gray-scale raster display screen, RAM accessible to both processors via a bus window, a hardware spectrum analyzer, a 40-channel speech vocoder, potentiometer input control devices, a GT40 lightpen, and a Summagraphics writing tablet.

The user interface was based on a primitive windowing system with lightpen-controlled menus. Speech could be input directly or from disk files, a scrolling waveform could be displayed on the GT40, frequency-band analysis was done by hardware, and one or two gray-scale spectrograms could be displayed on the HP screen. The user could make a variety of waveform and spectral measurements and do spectral editing with subsequent vocoder resynthesis. This system had many of the features that are common today, including using special-purpose hardware to relieve the CPU of processing-intensive tasks, and a windowing system that supported both gray-scale and vector graphics. However, the system was complex, very specialized, and difficult to maintain. The Digital Pattern Playback foreshadowed many features that have now become commonplace, and was an important step from time-sharing systems to modern distributed workstations.

The desire to modernize our approach to signal display and analysis has been spurred by a variety of factors. These include a change in the mid-80s to a distributed processing workstation computing environment (Talkin, 1989), the availability of affordable new display technologies, and the rapid development and acceptance of graphical user interfaces (GUIs such as the operating environments on the Xerox Star, the Apple Lisa and Macintosh, Suns, etc., and more recently, *Windows, Open Look and Motif*). While our newest systems are a logical continuation of what we tried to do with DPP, we have profited from such pioneering systems as enthusiasm and excitement generated by low-end solutions such as the *MacRecorder/Sound Edit* system on the Macintosh (Farallon, 1989).

A number of considerations influenced the direction of our newest systems. Of most importance, we needed the power of a VAX or a Sun workstation combined with a graphical user interface. The complexity and sheer number of applications made the consistency and ease of use of GUIs imperative, but at the time micro-computer based applications lacked the support, hardware integration, and raw processing power necessary for modern signal-processing tasks.

The need for VAX compatibility precluded the use of products from other workstation vendors such as Sun, Apollo, MASSCOMP, or Lisp Machine. We were also faced with a proliferation of new types of data (e.g., magnetic resonance images, microbeam and X-ray data, model-generated values) that made it necessary to display significantly more data channels than we previously had, and to maintain internal consistency between applications and Haskins-specific data types. Finally, since we have formal and informal ties to many institutions, it was essential to both generalize and standardize our data types to facilitate file interchanges with individuals and laboratories world-wide.

As is true for any institution, we had to work within our own limitations. Haskins is not a software company—our primary mission is research—and we generally cannot support speculative projects; nor can we afford to do system development just because "someone should do this." However, the arrival of our first VAXstation II/GPX system in 1986 forced us to embark on some pioneering efforts, largely because the graphics windowing software system (VWS) was new to us and to DEC. While we realized that our initial efforts might not result in a completely successful system, we believed that we would gain essential knowledge and hoped to develop a set of software tools that future applications could use.

6.   Initial Steps to a Modern Design: *SPEED*

SPEED was conceived as a prototype signal processing, display, and editing program that, while limited in functionality, would be easy to learn and to use. Our initial requirements for the user interface included:

- Simplified command set
- Integration of waveform and spectral functions
- Graphical User Interface (GUI)
     Menu Bar with command-key equivalents
     Windows for displays
     Mouse control

Widgets: close and resize boxes, options; elevators and scroll bars, on-screen tools
Control Panel (toolbox with icons)
Dialog boxes for options
File finder

- Advanced Graphics features
    Scrolling waveform displays
    On-screen readouts
    On-screen option selection
    On-screen cursors for measurement
    Graphical text editor
- Cut-and-paste editing of signal sections
- Beginnings of limited analysis and modification primitives

SPEED is currently in use at a number of sites around the world. The most recent version provides simple waveform editing, display, and measurement, and limited spectral analysis, in a modern GUI environment of menu bars, pop-up menus, windows, icons, and dialog boxes. The program displays data in the Haskins PCM format, and performs Discrete Fourier Transform analyses of the data. Up to four PCM files can be displayed at once, each in a "main" and an optional "scrolling" window. Basic waveform editing operations are available, including cut, copy, paste, save section, invert, rectify, set to silence, reverse, etc. Only one DFT file can be displayed, but several views are possible: the main spectrogram; up to four spectral cross-sections, providing a frequency-magnitude plot at a given time frame; and a "waterfall" spectrogram with overlapping cross-sections for a series of frames.

Figure 3 shows an example of the basic SPEED displays. The menu bar is at the top of the screen, with individual commands accessed using pull down menus. The menu structure is simple:

SPEED	Help, Quit
Display	Wave, Display DFT
Analysis	Spectral
Windows	Free, Aligned, Hard Copy, TIFF (Tag Image Format)

The "Display Wave" command invokes a "file finder" dialog box that the user can use to locate a file by entering a name or selecting a name from a list. Once selected, the file is opened and displayed in a waveform window that has a graphical display of the waveform and an array of numerical

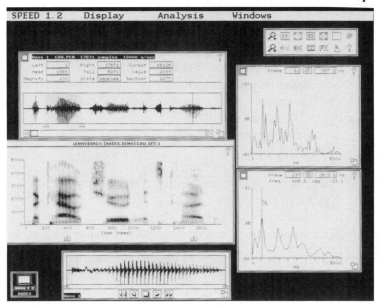

Figure 3:   *SPEED* displays

values for the various display and editing parameters. *Left* and *Right* show the start and end of the waveform displayed, and *Head* and *Tail* point to a marked *Section*, which is the part of the waveform to which all editing commands are applied. *Cursor* shows the position of the graphics cursor, and *Value* shows the magnitude of the wave at the cursor position. Values can be changed by typing into fields or by graphical operations: placing the cursor by clicking on the waveform rectangle, moving the head by dragging a handle (a small triangle at the bottom of the display), and so on.

At the top right in Figure 3 is the control panel, a small window with two rows of icons, which is similar in function to the tool palette in programs like MacPaint. The controls affect the active waveform window. From left to right the icons are:

Top row: magnification increase; zoom-in display; zoom-out display; zoom-in section display; zoom-out section display; section control; open/ close scrolling section window.

Bottom row: magnification decrease; play entire file; play section; cut-and-paste editing functions; special effects such as reverse, set to silence, rectification; labeling options dialog; general options dialog.

The waveform at the bottom of Figure 3 is a scrolling window that displays the section marked in the waveform window. The scrolling window has tape-recorder-like controls that provide a convenient way of tracking an enlarged portion of the master file or for making fine adjustments in section size and location.

Spectrograms (the middle window in Figure 3) are generated by Discrete Fourier Transform analysis of the sampled data files using the IEEE package of signal processing routines (IEEE, 1979). A dialog box guides the user through the selection of such analysis options as source data file, analysis type, window type and size, starting and ending portions of the waveform, and so on. Up to four spectral cross-section windows are visible at a time, two are shown on the right-hand side of Figure 3. Spectral cross-sections show frequency-magnitude information for a single frame that can be moved by dragging markers (the "houses" labelled "1" and "2" at the bottom of the Spectrogram window) or by entering a time value in the cross-section window. Although not illustrated, part or all of the spectrogram can be displayed in "Waterfall" form, a projection of a three-dimensional plot of successive cross sections.

Dialog boxes proved to be an essential tool for the SPEED interface, and contribute greatly both to the power and ease-of-use of the system. A judicious use of dialog boxes makes the system nearly self-documenting, provides useful default values for novice users, and imposes negligible time penalties on experienced users. We have also found it useful to include buttons that set values for a group of choices. For example, the Wide Band and Narrow Band buttons will set the Window Width, Skip Between Frames, and # Spectral Values variables to values appropriate for wide and narrow band spectral analyses.

7. The HADES Prototype: An Advanced Design

SPEED was intended to provide a low-end VAXstation speech analysis and display system that used the full power of VAX workstations. It was, however, conceived as a prototype and never intended to be a large-scale system. Our next step was to be a system that had an extensible programming language with flexible signal processing primitives, and that was fully integrated with other Haskins software tools. The Haskins Analysis Display and Experiment System (HADES) would provide a vehicle for standardizing and consolidating many of the signal processing tools (e.g., PSP, ACT, ACE) that had been developed at the Laboratory over the years. Our initial design requirements included:

- The development of a single system to handle data acquisition, in an experimental context, with subsequent display and analysis.

- Multiple waveforms in multi-panel windows, for manipulation of multi-channel data (e.g. physiological measurements, dichotic speech).

- A display primitive for multiple waveforms within a single window, using different colors or line types to differentiate the individual signals.

- The implementation of a procedural programming language within the program.

- Consolidation of a variety of signal-processing tools from other programs.

- A command window for entering text commands and/or command strings.

- Handling both existing Haskins label structures and the new Haskins label structure.

- Improvements in the quality of the spectrographic display.

- Redesign of the spectral analysis section so that:

  a. Analysis is performed on signals or signal sections.

  b. Analysis results can be stored in a buffer instead of in a file.

- A journaling feature for recording data readings, such as spectral peaks, duration measurements, etc.

- Spectral averaging: both non-destructive display (like cross-section) and actual data averaging.

- Specialized display primitives for frequently occurring activities and for new data types (such as images).

At the heart of HADES are three functions: acquisition, display, and analysis.The proposed final system will include acquisition of multiple streams of data in real-time, experimental set-up and interactive control of experimental conditions and peripheral devices, standardized data-conditioning and signal-processing routines, multiple display tools for qualitative data exploration, and general-purpose analysis procedures. The internal procedural language (SPIEL) supports the creation of specialized analysis macros that can be stored and manipulated as text files or executed from a command-line entry. All data displayed by or stored in HADES are accessible to SPIEL as variables, and all operations are available as commands.

A typical HADES display is shown in Table 3. The menu bar commands are substantially more elaborate than in SPEED and in particular the Display options are greatly augmented:

WAVE   sampled data format multi-panel waveform display

OVERLAY   multiple overlaid waveform display

LISSAJOUS   plot X (horizontal axis) versus Y (vertical axis)

PHASE PLOT   phase plane: value on X versus delta value on Y

TIFF   tag image file format for raster images

SPECTROGRAM   gray-scale spectrogram

CROSS SECTION   spectral cross-section

3D   3D waterfall spectral display

Table 3: *HADES 0.1* menu structure.

Hades 0.1		Data		Display		Analysis	Misc.
Flags	•F	Acquire	•F	Wave	•W	Spectral	Show Journal
Edit	•E	Save	•E	Overlay			Save Journal
Show control panel	•I	List	•I	Lissajous			Experiment
Hardcopy		Open	•O	Phase plot			Layout
News		Play	•P	TIFF			
Help	•?	Spectrogram					
Quit	•Q	Cross section					
		3-D spectrogram					
		FBA					

The HADES control panel (bottom of Figure 4) has 21 icons and permits much greater control over multiple window displays and reduces the number of mouse movements needed to set values. The spectrographic display is much better than that provided by SPEED (compare Figure 3). Examples of some of the additional display tools can be seen in Figures 5 and 6. A multiple waveform display window; with two panels is shown at the top of Figure 5. The top panel (PXLA) is a model-generated signal showing values of lip aperture; the bottom panel (PXLH) shows lip height. The small window at the bottom left is a phase display for the PXLA data. The small window at the bottom right plots PXLA data on the horizontal axis and PXLH data on the vertical axis (a LISSAJOUS display). An additional display type can be seen in Figure 6. At the top are waveforms representing speech and physiological records of the positions of speech articulators derived from microbeam analysis. Below the waveforms are two windows containing gray-scale images. At the right is a midsagittal MRI view of a head, showing a portion of the vocal tract. The program can display and save files in TIFF format (Davenport and Vellon, 1987). Using a public-domain format for digital images allows free interchange between Macintosh, AT-compatible, and VAXstation-based programs.

The text window at the bottom of Figure 5 is the HADES command window. This feature is a significant departure from SPEED, and was included to allow for preferred user workstyles. Different interface designs are needed for users who need easy access to program tools with minimal training and users who wish to bypass the graphical interface to get at the raw processing power of the system. The command window also lets users run non-graphics HADES commands from text only terminals.

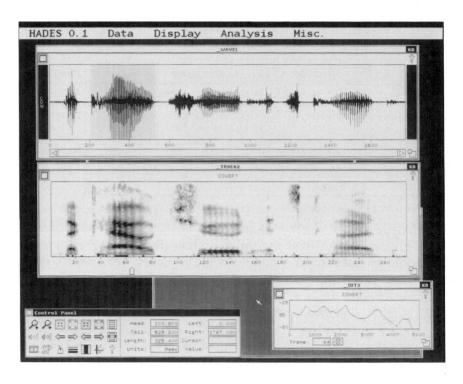

Figure 4:   *HADES 0.1* displays.

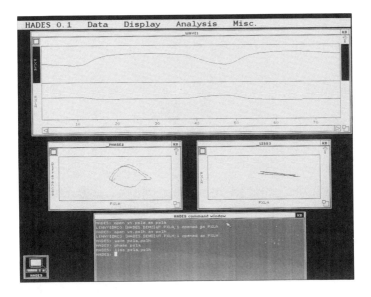

Figure 5: Additional *HADES 0.1* displays.

8. HADES 0.8: The Beta Version

As is typically the case when moving from a conceptual prototype to a release version, many of the low level routines were redesigned to increase robustness, system performance, ease of maintenance, and extensibility. Improvements in system functionality are readily seen by looking at the menu structure summarized in Figure 7. The new structure includes hierarchical menus, EDIT and PLAY functions as menu selections with command key equivalents, and additional FLAG, DATA, and LABEL options. We also eliminated the control panel, some of its functionality has been incorporated in the main menu while other tools appear at the bottom of the temporal displays (see Figure 8). Breaking with the Macintosh tradition, all three buttons of the VAXstation mouse are used. For example, clicking on the Selection Zoom icon with the right button increases the selection size, pressing the left button decreases it, and clicking with the center button selects the entire display. The readout portion of what was the control panel has been enhanced and is shown in its new form at the bottom of Figure 8. The readout panel now contains information about signal values (minimum and maximum values) and, on occasion, analysis results.

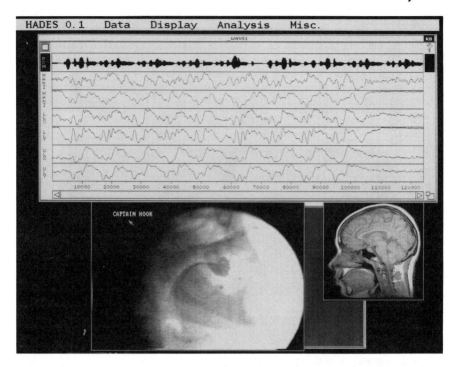

Figure 6:   *HADES 0.1* multiple waveform and TIFF displays.

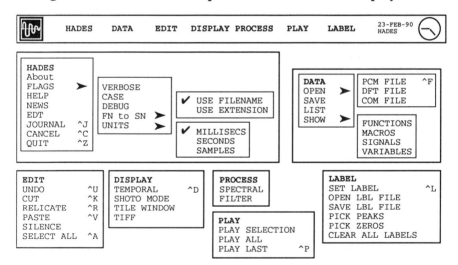

Figure 7:   *HADES 0.8* menu

What was formerly considered to be a waveform display window has been reconceptualized as a temporal display window. This reformulation provides for easier synchronization of data, as shown by the waveform and related spectrogram in Figure 8. Time domain waveforms have also been integrated and simplified as is shown in Figure 9, in which the two panels of WINDOW1 have been combined into a single panel in WINDOW2 by using the OVERLAY option. The VERTICAL DISPLACEMENT icon could be used to reposition the panels for comparison purposes. Many other small changes in the interface have been made in response to user testing or user requests.

9. Moving to Release

Few interface changes are planned as we move from Beta test to the release version of HADES. It is, however, anticipated that the signal processing portion of SPIEL will be enhanced and refinements will be made in the facilities it provides for designing and conducting experiments. Considerable care was taken to maintain a high level of modularity in the design, and many new primitives will be imported from existing programs. In future releases of HADES we expect to pay particular attention to the issues associated with file interchanges both between other Haskins applications and systems at other institutions (see Mertus, 1989, for a discussion of the issues associated with standardization of file formats). We are also evaluating the possibility of migrating our system to the DECwindows (or MOTIF) implementation of the X windows systems (Nye, 1988).

10. Conclusion

The evolution of the signal processing environment at Haskins is a good example of the many influences including political, scientific, academic, human, and technological that contribute to final system design. Developing a powerful but accessible signal processing system has forced us to balance what often appear to be conflicting design requirements. Our systems must always meet the needs of a diverse user population so we must constantly be aware of the subtle interplay between power and ease of use. While we try to build on the work of others, Haskins is unique and new tools must be integrated into our environment. User interfaces should simplify the user's task, but can also enrich their understanding of the problem domain and provide ever more sophisticated and powerful tools. While we need to provide continuity, speech research is a dynamic, rapidly changing field and we must provide flexible open-ended systems that gracefully respond to changing user needs. We need to be constantly aware of "real-world" constraints on our development projects

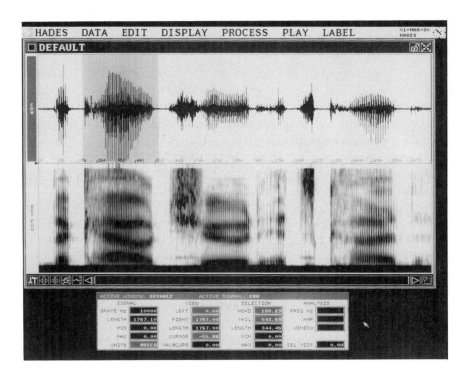

Figure 8: *HADES 0.8* waveform and spectrogram

including not only resource limitations, but also changes in user workstyles, the need to maintain continuity despite changes in programming staff, and institutional decisions such as funding, changes in priorities, and delays due to competing obligations. Finally, we must contend with a need to support projects that are likely to have immediate benefits, while still reserving resources for exploratory work so we will be prepared to take advantage of technological and scientific innovations.

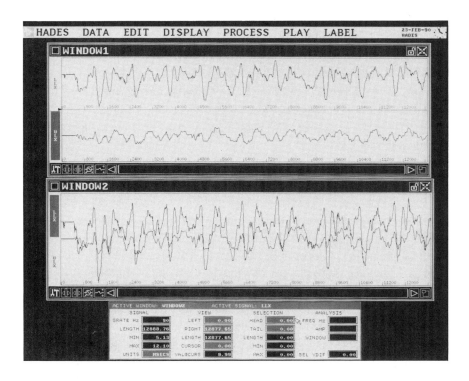

Figure 9: *HADES 0.8* multiple waveform and display comparison.

11. References

Cyphers, D. S. (1985). *Spire: A Speech Research Tool.* S. M. Thesis, Massachusetts Institute of Technology.

Davenport, T., & Vellon, M. (1987). Tag Image File Format—Rev. 4.0. *Aldus/Microsoft Technical Memorandum,* 4–31.

Farallon Computing, Inc.(1987). *MacRecorder User's Guide.* Berkeley, CA: Farallon Computing, Inc.

Gayvert, R. T., Biles, J. A., Rhody, H., & Hillenbrand, J. (1989). ESPRIT: A signal processing environment with a visual programming interface. *Journal of the Acoustical Society of America, 85(Sup1),* S57.

Hancock, B. (1989). DECwindows: X'ing with a vengeance. *DEC Professional, 8(2),* 70–84.

Henke, W. L. (1987). MITSYN Languages: A Coherent Family of High-Level Languages for Time Signal Processing. *Language Reference Manual, V6.0.* Belmont, MA: WLH.

IEEE Acoustics, Speech, and Signal Processing Society (1979). *Programs for Digital Signal Processing.* New York: IEEE Press.

Jamieson, D. G., Nearey, T. M., & Ramji, K. (1989). CSRE: A Speech Research Environment. *Canadian Acoustics / Acoustique Canadienne, 17(4),* 23–35.

Maverick, V., & Rubin, P. (1988). *SPEED—Signal processing, editing and display.* Internal Haskins Laboratories documentation note.

Mertus, J. (1989). Standards of PCM Files. *Behavior Research Methods, Instruments, & Computers, V21(2),* 126–129.

Nye, A. (1988). *Xlib Programming Manual Volume One.* MA: O'Rielly & Associates, Inc.

Nye, P. W., Cooper, F. S., & Mermelstein, P. (1977). Interactive Experiments with a Digital Pattern Playback. *Haskins Laboratories Status Report on Speech Research, SR-49,* 86–96.

Nye, P. W., Reiss, L. J., Cooper, F. S., McGuire, R. M., Mermelstein, P., & Montlick, T. (1975). A Digital Pattern Playback for the Analysis and Manipulation of Speech Signals. *Haskins Laboratories Status Report on Speech Research, SR-44,* 95–107.

Scully, W. (1988). *User's Guide to the HUI system (Haskins User Interface, V 2.0).* Haskins Laboratories internal documentation note.

Szubowcz, L. S. (1982). *WENDY Version 1.6 Reference Manual.* Haskins Laboratories internal documentation note.

Talkin, D. (1989). Looking at Speech. *Speech Technology, V4(4),* 74–77.

Whalen, D. H., Wiley, E. R., Rubin, P., & Cooper, F. S. (1990). The Haskins Laboratories' Pulse Code Modulation (PCM) System. Haskins Laboratories internal documentation note.

Zue, V. W., Cyphers, D. S., Kassel, R. H., Kaufman, D. H., Leung, H. C., Randolph, M., Seneff, S., Unverferth, J. E. III, & Wilson, T. (1986). The Development of the MIT LISP-Machine Based Speech Research Workstation. Proceedings of the ICASSP 86, International Conference on Acoustics, Speech, and Signal Processing, held in Tokyo, Japan, April 8 – 11, 329–332.

12. Acknowledgments

The systems described in this paper have been worked on by a large number of individuals at Haskins laboratories over a period of 15 years. There is not room to give proper credit to everyone involved with these projects, however, I would like to give special thanks to the following individuals: Leonard Szubowicz, Patrick Nye, Marion MacEachron, Mark Tiede, Vance Maverick, Michael D'Angelo, Vincent Gulisano, William Scully and Ed Wiley.

Chapter 19

The Perceptual and Acoustic Assessment of the Speech of Hearing-Impaired Talkers

Richard Goldhor
Massachusetts Institute of Technology

1. Abstract

Recorded speech from 29 hearing-impaired and four normal-hearing speakers was subjected to perceptual and acoustic analysis. Two listeners (trained phoneticians) judged selected segments of the recorded speech according to 14 phonetic attributes, such as consonant manner and place, vowel fronting, and breathiness. Independently, approximately 20 measures of acoustic properties were extracted automatically from the digitized and hand-segmented speech waveforms. These properties included fundamental frequency, formant locations and bandwidths, and energy within various frequency bands. Analysis of the relationship between measures of speaker intelligibility, perceived phonetic accuracy, and agreement between the perceptual judgments of the expert listeners reveals a strong relationship between intelligibility and phonetic accuracy, and a similar relationship between intelligibility and perceptual agreement. Useful acoustic predictors of phonetic judgments were established for the attributes of vowel fronting, stridency, nasal manner, and pitch. Small but statistically significant correlations were discovered between acoustic properties and breathiness judgments.

2. Introduction

The assessment of impaired speech based on the perceptual judgments of phonetically trained speech scientists and clinicians is a widely accepted technique used to determine the nature of speech and voice impairments and to establish corrective therapy (Ling, 1976; Subtelny, 1980). However, such perceptual assessments are time consuming, difficult, and prone to error (Bassich and Ludlow, 1986; McGarr, 1983; Samar and Metz, 1988). The validity of this practice depends on the ability of the clinician or researcher to accurately recognize problems in speech production based on phonetic judgments of the sounds produced, even though the sounds may differ substantially from normal speech in a number of dimensions and are often produced in environments not conducive to reliable perception (e.g., poor signal to noise ratio).

Conceivably the use of perceptual judgments for assessing impaired speech could be supplemented or in certain cases replaced with an analysis of the acoustic properties of the speech. In order to make use of such an analysis it must be possible to establish a relationship between acoustic properties that can be reliably extracted from speech waveforms using automatic or semi-automatic methods, and the underlying voice or speech production impairments and deficiencies. Because the use of perceptual judgments is standard clinical practice, the demonstration of a relationship between acoustic properties and perceptual judgments would be most persuasive. The ability to reliably predict of perceptual judgments of phonetic attributes in impaired speech from acoustic properties of the speech waveforms would indicate that impaired speech could be objectively assessed on acoustic grounds as well as by trained human listeners.

The intent of this study was to examine the nature of phonetic judgments of impaired speech, and the relationship between those judgments and acoustic properties that could be extracted automatically or semi-automatically from the same speech. Table 1 lists the phonetic attributes for which we collected judgments. A secondary goal of the study was the development of a database of phonetic judgments for a substantial corpus of normal and impaired speech, and a parallel database of acoustic properties extracted from the same corpus, which together could be used for further studies of impaired speech assessment, such as acoustic contributions to speech intelligibility.

Considering, first the character of phonetic judgments, we were interested in learning what the relationship was between overall intelligibility and the judgment of phonetic "accuracy" (i.e., the judgment that a particular phonetic attribute such as stridency had the desired value). We were also curious about the degree of consensus between trained listeners in their perception of phonetic attributes, and the effect that intelligibility might have on such agreement. In other words, we wondered whether phonetic judgments might become increasingly unreliable as the overall quality of the speech deteriorated.

Table 1: Phonetic attributes for which judgments were collected.

Manner Attributes	*Place attributes*
Stop Manner	Stop Place
Stridency	Fricative Place
Nasal Manner	Vowel Fronting
	Vowel Offglide
Voicing Attributes	*Suprasegmental Attributes*
Stop Voicing	Stress
Nasality	Extra Syllables
Breathiness	
Pitch	
Pitch Contour	

The goal of our acoustic analysis was to discover whether the judgments of specific phonetic attributes by trained listeners could be predicted from acoustic parameters that we can currently extract automatically from the speech waveform. In this initial study we attempted to predict judgments of vowel fronting, stridency, pitch, nasal manner in consonants, and breathiness.

3. Methods

3.1 Subjects

The speakers in this study included 29 hearing-impaired subjects and four normal-hearing subjects. Recordings of hearing-impaired subjects were made in June of 1977 for an unrelated project (Nickerson, 1979; Stevens, 1978). These subjects were between 11 and 17 years old at the time of the recordings. Fifteen of the speakers are female, fourteen are male. No information was available to the present authors regarding the degree or origin of hearing impairment. The intelligibility of these subjects' speech had been measured approximately three months before the recording session using a Magner intelligibility test (Magner, 1972). As shown in Figure 1, these scores range from the 40s to the 90s (out of a possible range of 0 to 100), except for one speaker with a score in the mid 20s.

Four normal-hearing subjects were recorded for the purposes of the present study. These subjects ranged in age from 13 to 15 years. Two were female, two male. No detailed audiological or speech intelligibility tests were performed. The subjects appeared to speak entirely normally, and when questioned reported no hearing impairment.

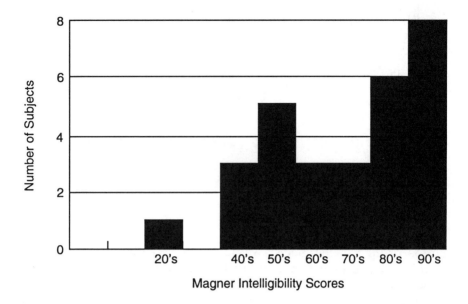

Figure 1 Distribution of Magner Intelligibility Scores for Hearing-Impaired Subjects

3.2   Material

The material produced by the hearing-impaired subjects consisted of 104 short phrases and sentences, such as "he cut up the apple" and "she went to the party." Not all speakers read the same material. On average, each subject spoke less than one dozen phrases. For the purposes of this study 94 words in the corpus were selected for analysis. These words, and the phrases in which they are embedded, are shown in Appendix A. In order to increase the number of multi-syllable items available for pitch contour studies, a number of analysis "words" actually consist of two-syllable article-noun phrases, such as "A-DIME" in sentence 2. These phrases are identified with a hyphen in Appendix A. In all of our analyses, and all of the discussions in this paper, such phrases are treated as a single word. We selected for analysis those words and phrases from the corpus which provided the phonetic contrasts implied by the attributes listed in Table 1, and for which we had recorded utterances by a substantial number of hearing-impaired speakers. In all, 713 words from 243 utterances elicited from impaired-hearing subjects were analyzed.

Each normal-hearing subject spoke all of the starred sentences in Appendix A. Spell out 59 words were selected from these starred sentences for detailed analysis. In all, 236 words were analyzed from the 160 utterances elicited from the normal-hearing subjects. The final speech database consisted of 402 sentences, within which 944 words received detailed analysis.

3.3 Recording Conditions

The original impaired speech data was recorded with a head-mounted close-talking microphone and a nasal accelerometer. The speakers were closely monitored and prompted by the experimenters. Procedural errors and gross failures in speaking were corrected under the guidance of the experimenters. The original speech had been recorded on 7-inch audio tape. Because the original tape had suffered substantial degradation, the tapes were copied onto audio cassettes at the beginning of the current study. No print-through was evident on the original or the copy, and spectral levels of, for example, vowel and burst formants of some normal speech on the tape were roughly as expected. The accelerometer track was not copied.

The normal-hearing subjects were recorded in a sound-proof room using a ceiling-hung microphone positioned three inches from the speaker's mouth. Their speech was recorded directly onto audio cassettes.

3.4 Digitization and Phonetic Judgment

Each utterance containing a word to be analyzed for phonetic content ("target word") was digitized at 16 kHz and stored in a computer file. Using waveform inspection and listening, approximate word boundaries were located around each target word. A program was developed that allowed any target word as spoken by any subject to be selected at random, and the word itself, or its containing sentence, to be played out through headphones.

A database program was also written that displayed a data collection form for each target word. This form specified exactly which phonetic attributes from Table 1 were to be judged for that word. Forms could be called up at random for any target word as spoken by any subject.

Phonetic judgments were supplied by two listeners. Each listener was a trained phonetician. One of the judges has extensive experience with assessing impaired speech, both in clinical and research settings.

The listeners judged the values of selected attributes of the target words. Not all attributes were judged for all target words. Table 2 shows the possible responses for each of the phonetic attributes judged, and the number of such judgments made for that attribute.

Table 2:   Phonetic attributes judged, possible judgment values, and number of judgments collected per attribute.

Attribute	Possible Values	Judgments
Stop Manner	Yes/No	1908
Nasal Manner	Yes/No	964
Stridency	Yes/No	980
Stop Place	Labial/Alveolar/Velar/Glottal/Other	1908
Fricative Place	Labial/Dental/Alveolar/Palatal/Other	980
Vowel Fronting	Front/Back/Other	1538
Vowel Offglide	w-like/y-like/u-like/none	1538
Stop Voicing	Yes/No	1908
Nasality	9 point scale: 9 = very nasal	1568
Breathiness	9 point scale: 9 = very breathy	1558
Pitch	High/Mid/Low 1200	
Pitch Contour	Falling/Rising/Other	1354
Stress	Primary/Secondary/Other	494
Extra Syllables	Yes/No	1880

Other Judgment Values	X: Segment doesn't exist
	O: Phonetic Evidence ambiguous

Total judgments collected: 19778

For each attribute, judgments were made as to the value of the attribute for a target word, not the appropriateness of the attribute. Thus for the attribute STRIDENCY, a YES judgment meant that the corresponding phoneme sounded strident, regardless of whether the correct pronunciation was /s,i/ (strident) or /hi/ (nonstrident). The listeners knew the correct pronunciation of the target words from the collection form, and had been carefully taught within which segment in the (correctly pronounced) target word the selected attribute was to be judged.

The listeners were allowed to judge the material in any order. They could listen to individual words or entire sentences as many times as desired, and they could revise their judgments as many times as desired. However, they could only listen to the material and look at the database forms to determine the target pronunciation. They had no access to any spectrographic, waveform, or other acoustic displays.

Initially, the judges listened to some of the material together, discussed perceptions, and compared judgments. Each judge then analyzed all of the material individually, evaluating nearly 10,000 specific attributes. The listeners reported that many of the judgments were quite difficult to make.

Each listener required approximately 50 hours to judge all the material, which corresponds to about three judgments per minute.

The completed sets of preliminary judgments were scanned by a computer program which identified specific target word utterances and attributes for which a substantial disagreement existed between the judgments of the two listeners. Each of these words was reviewed by the two listeners working together. As a result of this review, some judgments were modified. In other cases, the judges continued to disagree, and the existing responses were left unchanged.

A phonetic distance metric was defined in order to permit comparisons between phonetic attribute values. A distance of 0 indicates the two values are identical. A distance of 1 indicates a minor difference. A distance of 2 represents a major difference. The metric was defined for each of the phonetic attributes listed in Table 1. Differences in attributes having binary values (e.g., vowel fronting) were considered major (D=2). "Can't judge" and "segment not present" judgments were considered to differ in a major way (D=2) from other judgments. Adjacent place judgments were considered to differ in a minor way (D=1), with the glottal place of articulation treated as not adjacent to any other place. The breathiness and nasality judgments of the two listeners were normalized using a linear regression analysis. A difference of two points (out of 9) on the resulting normalized scale was considered a minor difference (D=1), and 4 or more points was considered a major difference (D=2).

3.5   Acoustic Analysis

An acoustic analysis of the recorded speech was carried out in order to relate acoustic properties to phonetic judgments. The acoustic analysis measured the value of acoustic properties within sublexical segments of the target words. The analysis process consisted of the following steps: 1) creation of a lexical database specifying the phonetic structure of each target word; 2) location "by eye" of approximate segment boundaries in the recorded speech; 3) automatic adjustment of segment boundaries according to acoustic criteria; 4) measurement of acoustic properties within time windows relative to the segment boundaries.

A computerized dictionary was created which specified the transcription, or correct pronunciation, of each target word as a sequence of sublexical segments. Each segment was identified as belonging to a particular acoustic-phonetic class. The location (corresponding segment) was specified for each phonetic attribute evaluated for that word. Table 3 shows the segment classes specified in this dictionary.

A rough segmentation of the recorded speech signals was then carried out manually. The goal of this procedure was to locate the approximate beginning and end of each segment that had any perceptual attribute associated with it in the lexicon. The segmentation was performed by examining waveform and spectrographic displays of each utterance in the database, using the Waves+[1] signal display package (Shore, 1988). It should be noted that because of speech errors, many target words were missing segments that should have contained attributes to be judged.

Table 3: List of segment classes used in dictionary

Symbol	Class	Symbol	Class
c	Stop Closure	V	Stressed Vowel
s	Stop Release	v	Unstressed Vowel
a	Affricate Release		
		r	article
f	Fricative	{ }	Sentence Boundary
h	/h/	[ ]	Word Boundary
		I	Segment Boundary
n	Nasal		
g	Glide		
l	Liquid		

The manually located approximate segment boundaries were then automatically adjusted based upon a set of frequency-limited segment energy profiles. Log power values within five frequency bands were calculated for all speech signals. The frequency bands were 120 to 750 Hz, 750 to 2250 Hz, 2250 to 4000

---

[1] Wavest is a product of Entropic Research Laboratory, Inc.

Hz, 3 to 8 kHz, and 120 Hz to 8 kHz. Table 4 indicates the relevant frequency bands, and expected energy profiles, for the various segment classes.

Table 4: Frequency band used to adjust segment boundaries, and relative energy expected in that band, for each segment class.

Segment Class	Frequency Band Examined	Expected Energy
Vowels	750 to 2250	High
Liquids	"	High
Glides	"	High
Closures	"	Low
/h/	"	Low
Nasals	2250 to 4000	Low
Fricatives	3000 to 8000	High
Affricates	"	High
Stop Bursts	"	High

(This process of specifying rough segment boundaries by hand and then automatically adjusting them using energy profiles can be regarded as a simulation of the effect of a more sophisticated automatic segmentation algorithm. The reliability of the actual segmentation is uncertain, because the speech of the hearing-impaired subjects often did not exhibit clear segment boundaries. However, in considering the extension of this study to fully automatic techniques, it would be well to keep in mind the possibility that the segmentation process described above might yield better results than any that could be achieved with an entirely automatic segmentation.)

Segment onset, midpoint, and offset locations were identified within the adjusted boundaries of each segment. The intent was to place these locations at points in the signal where the acoustic properties of the segment were well established. The technique used to accomplish this goal was as follows. The midpoint was placed at the center of gravity of the energy profile for the segment. The onset was located by scanning forward from the initial segment boundary toward the segment midpoint, until the energy profile rose (or fell) to within 10 percent of its average value in the segment. The onset was placed 10 msecs later. The offset was positioned using a similar strategy: The energy profile was scanned from the final segment boundary backwards toward the midpoint until the energy profile rose or fell to within 10 percent of its average value, and the offset was placed 10 msecs earlier.

Each segment was then processed to extract information about the average value of certain acoustic properties over the duration of the segment, and the instantaneous value of certain other properties at the onset, midpoint, and offset of the segment. Pitch and voicing probability values were calculated using an algorithm developed by Secrest and Doddington (1983). This algorithm uses a dynamic programming technique to smooth candidate pitch values derived from a correlation function applied to an LPC prediction residual. (See O'Shaughnessey, Chapter 2.) Formant values were calculated using a technique described by Dupree (1984) and developed by Talkin (1990). Once again, candidate formant frequencies derived from an LPC analysis of the waveform were smoothed using a dynamic programming technique to derive optimal formant trajectories.

The acoustic information and corresponding perceptual, subject, and corpus information were combined to form two parallel databases: a perceptual database containing information on 20,000 perceptual judgments; and an acoustic database containing information on 6,000 acoustic segments. The information contained within each record in this database is listed in Table 5.

4.   Results

4.1   Intelligibility, Perceptual Consensus, and Phonetic Distortion
The overall degree of consensus in phonetic judgments between the two listeners was estimated by calculating the average difference between their judgments for each attribute, as measured using the phonetic distance metric discussed above. The combined results for hearing impaired and normal hearing speakers are presented in Table 6. As can be seen, the attributes within a particular class, such as manner judgments, tend to have similar average differences. The high degree of consensus for "extra syllable" judgment is perhaps due to the fact that very few words were judged to have been pronounced with an extra syllable. The next highest degree of consensus was achieved for manner attributes, and the lowest for voicing attributes. Figure 2 shows how the average difference in listeners' judgments varies as a function of both attribute class and intelligibility level.

In order to measure the success with which a speaker uttered each target word, a rough measure of phonetic distortion was constructed. The segmental information stored in the dictionary described above was used to determine the appropriate value of each phonetic attribute that the listeners judged. A distortion value was determined for each such attribute in a word, and the average distortion value used as a measure of how well the word was pronounced. (Appropriate values for the voice quality attributes were assigned as follows: "1" for breathiness; "1" for nasality in non-nasal contexts and "5" for nasal contexts; "MID" pitch values; "*" for pitch contour, indicating that any contour is acceptable. Appropriate values for

Table 5: Contents of perceptual and acoustic databases.

Judgment Database	Acoustic Property Database
Subject ID	Speaker ID
Gender	Gender
Intelligibility Score	Intelligibility Score
Sentence Number	Sentence Number
Spelling and Transliteration of Word	Spelling and Transliteration of Word
Initial Segment Number	Segment Symbol
Final Segment Number	Segment Number in Word
Reference Segment Number	Segment Count
Attribute Code	Segment Onset, Center, and Offset Times
Appropriate Value of Attribute	Segment Span and Duration
Attribute Judgment: Listener 1	Average Log Power in Five Frequency Bands
Attribute Judgment: Listener 2	Average Pitch
Attribute Distortion Index	Average Voicing Probability
Judgment Similarity	Average F1 F2 F3 F4
	Average B1 B2 B3 B4

For each of the Onset, Offset, and Midpoint Locations:

Log Power in 5 Bands
Pitch
Voicing Probability
F1 F2 F3 F4
B1 B2 B3 B4
Frequency of H1 . . . H7
Amplitude of H1 . . . H7
Log Magnitude Spectrum

Table 6:   Consensus in judgments between the two listeners.

Attribute Class	Attribute Name	Average Attribute Difference
Syllabic	Extra Syllable	0.06
Manner	Nasal Manner	0.10
	Stridency	0.11
	Stop Manner	0.11
Stress	Stress	0.14
Place	Fricative Place	0.20
	Vowel Fronting	0.21
	Stop Place	0.22
	Offglide	0.30
Voicing	Pitch	0.26
	Pitch Contour	0.31
	Stop Voicing	0.39
	Nasality	0.48
	Breathiness	0.52

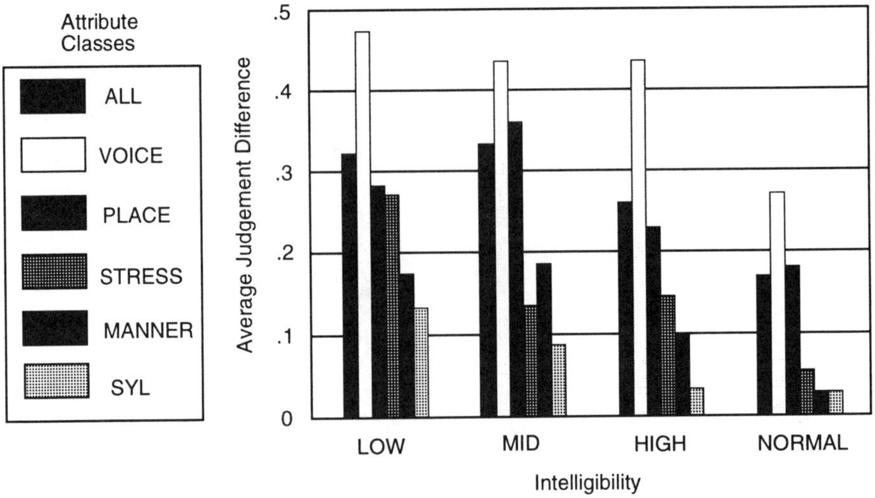

Figure 2   Judgment Differences By Attribute Class and Speaker Intelligibility

place and manner features are implicit in the pronunciation of the target word.)

Differences between the appropriate and perceived attribute values were considered to represent phonetic errors, or phonetic distortion, in the recorded speech. Average distortion values were calculated for each attribute by averaging differences across all word contexts and both judges. Figure 3 shows the relationship between intelligibility and perceived phonetic errors for attributes in different classes. An average distortion value was also calculated for each speaker, using the distance metric described above. This average distortion value improves on the Magner intelligibility scores by providing a measure of speech quality for each subject based on the speech in this corpus. It is reassuring to see (in Figure 4) that a strong relation exists between speaker intelligibility and average phonetic distortion: the Pearson Product-Moment Correlation value is -.83, which is statistically highly significant for N=33. (Note that the normal hearing speakers were assigned an intelligibility level of 100 for the

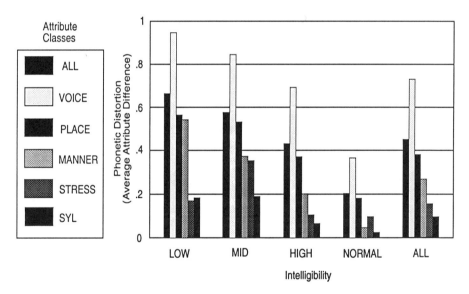

Figure 3   Phonetic distortion by attribute class and speaker intelligibility. An average attribute difference of 0.0 would represent completely appropriate values for that attribute class in all words. An average attribute difference of 2.0 would represent completely inappropriate values for that attribute class in all words.

purposes of this analysis. None of the hearing-impaired speakers had an intelligibility score of 100.)

Figure 2 indicates that a relation exists between speech quality and listener consensus: the listeners' judgments were more apt to disagree for low-intelligibility speakers than for high-intelligibility speakers. Figure 5 demonstrates that a similar relationship holds between average distortion and

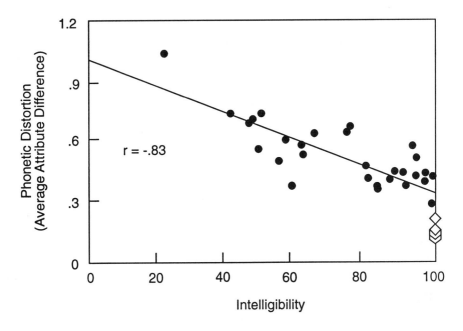

Figure 4: Relationship Between Speaker Intelligibility and Phonetic Distortion

average judgment difference for each speaker. The Pearson Product-Moment Correlation for this relationship is .77, also statistically highly significant.

4.2   Acoustic Properties and Perceptual Judgments
A major goal of the study was a preliminary investigation of the utility of acoustic properties in predicting perceptual judgments of phonetic attributes. We report here on the results of five potential acoustic predictors.

4.2.1 Vowel Fronting

It is commonly known that the FRONT/BACK distinction in vowels in normal speech is related to the relative positions of the first three formants (Pickett, 1980). Figure 6 shows the relation between an acoustic predictor constructed from the ratio of the $F2-F1$ and $F3-F1$ distances and corresponding perceptual judgments for both normal and impaired speech. The following procedure was used to construct this and succeeding figures: the value of the acoustic predictor was calculated for each segment for which

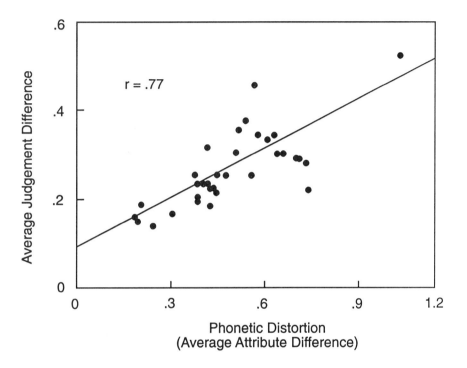

Figure 5: Relationship Between Phonetic Distortion and Differences in Judgment (for both hearing-impaired and normal-hearing subjects)

the relevant phonetic judgment was made. All of the selected segments were then sorted according to the value of the acoustic predictor. The sorted segments were then grouped. The size of the groups is specified in each figure. Finally, the average perceptual judgment within each group was calculated and plotted against the value of the acoustic predictor, as indicated in the figures.

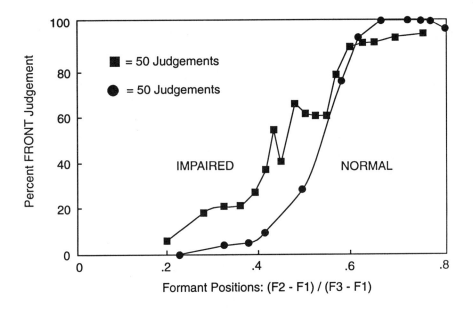

Figure 6: Relationship Between F2 Ratio and Front Judgments

4.2.2 Stridency

The perception of the phonetic attribute STRIDENT is known to be related to the amount of high frequency energy in the speech signal (Strevens, 1960). We used an acoustic predictor consisting of the increment in the log of the power between 3 kHz and 8 kHz in a consonant over the log of the power in the same frequency band in the vowel of the same syllable to predict stridency judgments. The results are shown in Figure 7 for both normal and impaired speech.

4.2.3 Nasal Manner

The predictor used for judgments of nasal manner in consonants was constructed as follows: the duration of the consonant was measured, and a factor D assigned one of the following values:

> 0 if the segment duration was less than 10 msecs;
> 2 if the segment duration was greater than 40 msecs;
> 1 + (segment duration - 25 msecs)/30 msecs otherwise.

The difference was calculated between the total log power in the consonant and the log power below 750 Hz. A factor L was assigned one of the following values:

0 if the log power difference was greater than 10.0 dB;
1.5 - log power difference in dB otherwise.

The difference was calculated between the log power below 750 Hz in the consonant and the same power in the vowel of the same syllable. A factor R was assigned one of the following values:

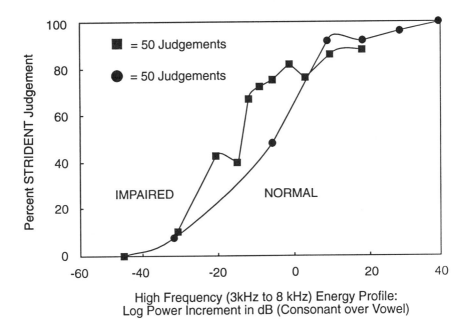

Figure 7: Relationship Between High Frequency Power Increment and Stridency Judgments

0 if the log power difference was less than -25 dB;
2 if the log power difference was greater than -5 dB;
2.5 + 0.1 * log power difference in dB otherwise.

The nasal manner predictor was then calculated using the formula

Predictor = cuberoot(D*L*R) - 1.0

This predictor has a range between -1.0 and +1.0. The relationship between the predictor and the corresponding NASAL manner judgments is shown in Figure 8. The data for normal and impaired speech are combined in this figure.

4.2.4   Fundamental Frequency

Figure 9 shows the relationship between f0 estimates extracted from vocalic segments of the speech corpus and corresponding pitch judgments by the listeners. The curves relating LOW, MID, and HIGH pitch judgments to estimated f0 generally have the expected shapes, except for anomalies around 160 Hertz, which might be due in part to inadvertent "pitch-doubling" and "pitch-halving" errors by the estimating algorithm.

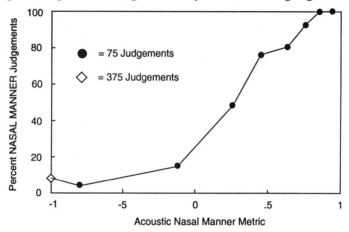

Figure 8:   Relationship Between Acoustic Nasal Manner Metric and Nasal Manner Judgments (for both hearing-impaired and normal-hearing subjects)

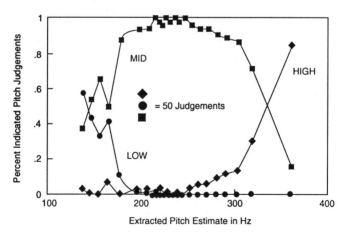

Figure 9:   Relationship Between Pitch Estimate and Pitch Judgments (Each data point = 50 judgments)

4.2.5 Breathiness and Nasality

Appendix B shows the results of a multiple regression analysis between breathiness judgments, nasality judgments, and three acoustic measures. These measures are F0, the pitch estimate for the syllable in question, H1, the log amplitude of the first harmonic minus the log amplitude of the second harmonic, andhigh-frequency noise (HFN), the average peak-to-value depth in the log magnitude spectrum of the syllabic nucleus between the frequencies of 3500 and 5000 Hz. HFN was taken to be an estimate of the ratio of harmonic to turbulent energy in the syllabic nucleus.

5. Discussion

It is clear from Figure 2 that consensus in phonetic judgment is a function both of the particular attribute being judged and of overall speech quality. Consonant manner judgments such as nasal or stop manner and stridency can be made with the greatest degree of consensus. Voice quality judgments such as breathiness and nasality, on the other hand, result much more frequently in disagreements. And consensus deteriorates for all types of attributes as intelligibility deteriorates, with only minor exceptions. (It might be argued that these results are most simply explained by the fact that voice quality judgments are non-phonemic in American English and non-categorical. However, judgments of stop voicing, which is both phonemic and categorical, achieved the third lowest level of consensus of the 14 attributes measured.)

An interesting conclusion that emerges from Figure 2 is that consensus in phonetic judgment of normal speech is not qualitatively different from consensus in judgment of impaired speech. The relative frequency of consensus for different classes of attributes appears quite similar, with obvious differences only for stress judgments. The most striking difference in the consensus data for normal speech is that overall rates of disagreement are lower than for impaired speech. Normal speech behaves, at least by this measure, as simply an asymptotic result of improving the intelligibility of impaired speech.

One would expect a strong relationship to exist between overall measures of speech intelligibility and the frequency of errors in producing specific phonetic attributes. This hypothesis is supported by the data in Figure 3. Although there are substantial differences in the overall error rates of particular attribute classes (as measured by average distortion values), error rates for all classes increase as speaker intelligibility decreases. The only exception to this is a substantial decrease in the rate of stress-related errors measured for low-compared with mid-intelligibility speakers. The reason for this reduction is not known. Figure 4 demonstrates yet again that phonetic distortion and speaker intelligibility are intimately connected. It would be reasonable to conclude that the mechanisms employed in lexical access (the basis for speech intelligibility as measured by the Magner score) and the mechanisms employed in judgments of phonetic attributes have much in common.

These relationships between intelligibility, consensus, and distortion lead to the important relationship displayed in Figure 5: the deterioration in consensus of phonetic judgment with increasing phonetic distortion. The conclusion implicit in this figure is that the ability of human listeners to make reliable phonetic judgments decreases as segmental and suprasegmental phonetic attributes of the speech become increasingly inappropriate.

Turning now to the acoustic prediction of phonetic judgments, Figure 6 demonstrates that a simple acoustic measure can do a reasonable job of predicting vowel FRONT/BACK judgments. The data for normal speech displays the S-shaped curve typical of categorical judgments. That overall shape is also apparent in the curve on impaired speech, but several differences can be noted. First, the impaired speech data does not saturate at 0 and 100% FRONT judgments for extreme values of the acoustic predictor, in contrast to the normal speech data. Second, the transition range is approximately twice as wide for the impaired speech data as for the normal data. These differences suggest that listeners may appeal to some property of the impaired speech other than formant position when asked to make FRONT/BACK judgments.

An interesting variation of this situation exists for acoustic prediction of stridency judgments. It can be seen from Figure 7 that the particular acoustic predictor we have constructed results in a sharper transition zone for impaired than for normal speech, with better saturation at the STRIDENT end of the scale for normal speech and better saturation at the NONSTRI-DENT end of the scale for impaired speech.

The prediction of breathiness judgments from acoustic information is much more problematical, as shown by the multiple regression analysis in Appendix B. The results of this analysis can be summarized by saying that the factors tested (estimated pitch, amplitude increment of the first minus the second harmonic, average peak-to-valley depth of log magnitude spectrum in mid-frequency range, and the perceived nasality of the same syllable) were each significantly correlated with breathiness, but individually and collectively account for only a small fraction of the variation in breathiness judgments. This seemingly paradoxical effect is possible because of the amount of data analyzed. The practical consequence is that no useful predictor of the per-ception of breathiness has been identified for this set of data. Based on informal observations and impressions, a partial explanation for this failure is that breathiness judgments may depend in complex ways on the acoustic properties of segments surrounding the syllabic nucleus, as well as the acoustics of the nucleus itself. It is also possible that more sophisticated measures of the harmonic to turbulent energy in the speech signals, such as those described by Cox et al. (1989), may be better predictors of breathiness judgments.

6. Conclusion

It is apparent that listener consensus is a function both of the phonetic attribute to be judged and of the intelligibility of the speech. Consensus is greatest for manner judgments of clear speech. Substantially less consensus can be expected for voice quality judgments, such as breathiness and nasality. Most importantly, consensus in phonetic judgments of all types decreases as speech intelligibility decreases. The implication is that clinical assessment of impaired speech might be expected to be least reliable for speakers with the greatest impairments.

Speech intelligibility appears to be strongly linked to phonetic distortion, as one would expect. As with intelligibility, consensus in phonetic judgments decreases as phonetic distortion increases.

The clear relationships between acoustic predictors and judgments of the phonetic attributes of pitch, vowel fronting, stridency, and nasal manner in consonants can at best be considered encouragement for further work. The failure to identify a similarly robust acoustic predictor for the attribute of breathiness may be considered a warning that substantial progress will be required before automatic or semi-automatic acoustic analysis systems will do as well as trained human listeners.

7. Acknowledgements

This study was conceived and proposed by Robert Berkovitz, Kenneth Stevens, and Nathaniel Durlach. Partial support was provided by an SBIR grant from the National Institutes of Health to Sensimetrics, Inc. The hearing-impaired speakers were originally recorded by Ann Rollins. Corine Bickley and Sharon Manuel provided valuable assistance with corpus selection and phonetic judgments. The author is grateful to the MIT Speech Communication Group for access to laboratory facilities and research support.

8.   References

Bassich, C.J. and Ludlow, C.L. (1986). "The Use of Perceptual Methods by New Clinicians for Assessing Voice Quality," *Journal of Speech and Hearing Research*, **51**, 125–133.

Cox, N.B., Ito M.R. , and Morrison, M.D. (1989). "Technical Considerations in Computation of Spectral Harmonics-to-Noise Ratios for Sustained Vowels," *Journal of Speech and Hearing Research*, **32**, 203–218.

Dupree, B.C. (1984). "Formant Coding of Speech Using Dynamic Programming," *Electronic Letters*, **20**, 279–280.

Ling, D. (1976). *Speech and the Hearing-Impaired Child: Theory and Practice.* WA: The Alexander Graham Bell Association for the Deaf, Inc.

Magner, M.E. (1972). *A Speech Intelligibility Test for Deaf Children.* Northampton, MA: Clarke School for the Deaf.

McGarr, N.S. (1983). "The Intelligibility of Deaf Speech to Experienced and Inexperienced Listeners," *Journal of Speech and Hearing Research*, **26**, 451–458.

Nickerson, R.S., Stevens, K.N. and Rollins A.M. (1979). "Research on Computer Based Speech Diagnosis and Speech Training Aids for the Deaf," Report No. 4029, Cambridge, MA: Bolt Beranek and Newman, Inc.

Pickett, J.M. (1980). *The Sounds of Speech Communication.* Austin, TX: Pro-Ed.

Samar, V.J. and Metz, D.E. (1988). "Criterion Validity of Speech Intelligibility Rating-Scale Procedures for the Hearing-Impaired Population," *Journal of Speech and Hearing Research*, **31**, 307–316.

Secrest, B.G., and Doddington, G.R. (1983). "An Integrated Pitch Tracking Algorithm for Speech Systems," Boston, MA: *Proc. Intl. Conf. Acous., Speech and Signal Proc.*

Shore, J. (1988). "Interactive Signal Processing with UNIX," *Speech Technology*, **v. 4, # 2**, 70–79.

Stevens, K.N., Nickerson, R.S. and Rollins, A.M. (1978). "On Describing the Suprasegmental Properties of the Speech of Deaf Children," Report No. 3955, Cambridge, MA. Bolt Beranek and Newman, Inc.

Strevens, P. (1960). "Spectra of Fricative Noise in Human Speech," *Language and Speech*, **3**, 32–49.

Subtelny, J.D. (1980). *Speech Assessment and Speech Improvement for the Hearing Impaired*. Washington: The Alexander Graham Bell Association for the Deaf, Inc.

Talkin, D. (1990). "Formant Trajectory Estimation Using Dynamic Programming with Modulated Transition Costs," personal communication.

Appendix A: Corpus of Utterances

In the list below, capitalized words represent words for which one or more phonetic judgments were requested. Hyphenated phrases were treated as single words. Starred items were spoken by all of the normal-hearing speakers.

* 1. a BLACK DOG
  2. A-DIME
* 3. at THE-GAME
  4. BIG RABBITS
  5. BILL PLAYED in the WATER
* 6. BILL SLEEPS in a BIG BED
* 7. BLUE CURTAINS
* 8. BOB RAN with HIS FATHER
* 9. BOB WORKED on a LARGE FARM
* 10. FIND THE-BOOK
* 11. FIVE BOYS CLIMBED UP THE-HILL
* 12. FOUR BOYS RAN in THE-RACE
  13. FOUR TALL TREES
* 14. HE CUT UP the APPLE
* 15. HE GAVE BREAD to THE-BIRDS
* 16. HE SAT at the TABLE
* 17. HE SAW BIRDS in THE-PARK
* 18. in A-BOOK
* 19. JACK LIKES DOGS
* 20. JEAN SAT on the BIG CHAIR
  21. JEAN wore a BIG RED HAT
* 22. JOHN FOLDED the PAPER

* 23.   LARGE CAGES
* 24.   PAPER
* 25.   RED PENCIL
* 26.   RUN FIVE LAPS
  27.   RUN THE-RACE
* 28.   SAM TURNED on the RED LIGHT
* 29.   SAM WENT to the MOVIE
* 30.   SHE JUMPED in the WATER
* 31.   SHE PUT TOYS on THE-BED
* 32.   SHE WENT to the PARTY
* 33.   SHE WROTE on the PAPER
* 34.   the BIG BOY
  35.   the BLUE SOCKS
* 36.   the BOY HAD a NEW BOOK
* 37.   THE-GAME
* 38.   the GIRL MADE a RED DRESS
  39.   the MAN HAS a BLUE CAR
* 40.   the PAPER
* 41.   the TALL CHURCH
  42.   the WATER
* 43.   TWO BAD BOYS
  44.   TWO BIRDS FLEW in THE-SKY
* 45.   TWO BOYS GAVE US A-DIME
* 46.   TWO DOGS RAN to THE-SCHOOL
* 47.   WE CUT BREAD with A-KNIFE
* 48.   WE MADE a CAKE at SCHOOL
* 49.   WE RAN the RACE TODAY
* 50.   WHITE PAPER

Appendix B: Multiple Linear Correlation and Regression Analysis of Factors Influencing BREATHINESS Judgments

Factors: BR: Breathiness judgment
                      NA: Nasality judgment (by same listener)
                      F0:   Acoustic pitch estimate
                      H1:   Amplitude of H1 minus amplitude of H2
                      HFN: Ave peak-to-valley depth of log magni
                             tude spectrum in 3500 to 5000 Hz range.

Correlation Matrix:

	BR	NA	F0	H1	HFN
BR	1.0000				
NA	0.1861	1.0000			
F0	0.1095	0.1799	1.0000		
H1	0.1702	0.0736	0.1434	1.0000	
HFN	-0.0597	0.1877	0.6932	-0.0657	1.0000
Variable	BR	NA	F0	H1	HFN

Regression Equation for BR:

BR = 0.1864 NA + 0.0061 F0 + 0.0256 H1 + -0.0669 HFN + 3.70547

Significance test for prediction of BR

Mult-R	R-Squared	SEest	F(4,1497)	prob (F)
0.3045	0.0927	1.4471	38.2563	0.0000

Significance test(s) for predictor(s) of BR

Predictor	beta	b	Rsq	se	t(1497)
NA	0.1829	0.1864	0.0450	0.0257	7.2611
F0	0.2341	0.0061	0.5175	0.0009	6.6058
H1	0.1068	0.0256	0.0779	0.0061	4.1654
HFN	-0.2493	-0.0669	0.5136	0.0095	7.0631

Chapter 20

The Development of Text-To-Speech Technology For Use In Communication Aids

Sheri Hunnicutt
Royal Institute of Technology
Stockholm, Sweden

1.   Introduction

During development of the multi-language text-to-speech system at the Royal Institute of Technology in Stockholm, special attention has been paid to preparing for its use as a communication aid. The earliest prototypes were made available for trial by disabled users, and high priority was given to interaction with these users and their audiences to see that desired features were included. A number of technical aids, based on this text-to-speech system, have been developed as well. These include a portable communication aid, a symbol-to-speech system, word predictors, talking terminals and a daily newspaper. Recently, speech recognition has also been used in a communication and environmental control aid.

2.   The Multi-Language Text-To-Speech System

Versions of the text-to-speech program are presently available in nine languages (or dialects): American and British English, German, French, Italian, Spanish, Norwegian, Danish and Swedish (Granström and Gustafson, 1986; Bladon et al., 1987; Granström et al., 1987; Barber et al., 1987; Kohler, 1988; Carlson et al., 1988). The language-specific parts of the program are formulated in a notation close to that used in generative phonology. This notation is familiar to most speech and language researchers; thus cooperation with experts in the various languages has been much facilitated.

This language-specific knowledge is expressed in several components. A first set of components produces a phonetic text from the orthographic text. The phonetic text is produced by a set of grapheme-to-phoneme rules for regular pronunciations and a lexicon for irregular pronunciations. A user lexicon is also available for special user-specified pronunciations. Special number rules convert digit sequences to phonetic text. An additional component is the set of phonetic rules that create appropriate allophones by adjusting formant frequencies, aspiration and transition timing, and determine phoneme duration and utterance fundamental frequency depending on context. This information is stored in parameters that are sent to the digital speech synthesizer each 10 msec. This synthesizer has a combined parallel/ cascade filter structure and can use either voiced (pulses) and/or unvoiced (noise) excitation. The synthesis hardware is based on a Motorola 68000 and a NEC7720 speech processing chip.

3.   Special Features for Applications

The text-to-speech system has been programmed with special features as needs have arisen in applications work. These features include reading tempo and mode and the ability to make and save various changes in the pronunciations, voice quality and prosodics. It is also possible to index the text for graphic insertions and to use several languages.

3.1   Reading Mode

Several reading modes are available. Continuous reading of a text can be helpful to a blind user or to a non-speaking person preparing an extensive verbal contribution to a meeting. When reading continuously, output from the synthesizer can be stopped and continued again as desired. Reading of sentences is useful in conversation for non-speaking persons, in inspection of text for blind persons, and in various types of training for the motorically disabled. Line mode reading was requested for blind computer programmers and is also useful for reading hierarchical charts and material organized in columns. Training programs for persons with reading and writing problems and screen reading programs for blind persons may take advantage of both word and spelling modes as well.

3.2   Speech Tempo and Loudness

Speech tempo and loudness are both adjustable, either in a number of steps given by a command, or continuously with a knob. Slow tempos may be chosen in phonetic training for non-speaking persons and in repetition of words or sentences not understood at first by a listener. Fast tempos are desirable for blind persons listening to a text. Normal speaking rate is often estimated to be around 150 words per minute, but the demand from the blind is to obtain speaking rates of around 500 words per minute to approximate fast silent reading by sighted persons. In order for speech to be both possible and acceptable at such a fast rate, the phonetic component of the text-to-speech system has been modified. Prosodic rules have been simplified, mean pitch increased, and a new set of inherent durations has been developed.

3.3 Variation in Voices

Voice parameters may be set to individualize the voice output. Four standard voices are included — a standard man's voice, a deep man's voice and voices that approximate those of a woman and a child. In these voices, pitch level, formant frequency scaling, varied dynamic range and breathiness are used to create the voice effects. Users may begin with one of these four voices and change the pitch level, dynamic range and breathiness to their own specifications. The dynamic range allows a voice to take on characteristics from monotone to very expressive. Of the standard voices, the standard male voice has the least pitch dynamics, followed by the deep male voice, the "light" voice (female) and the "very light" voice (child). Small amounts of breathiness are useful in making a voice sound more woman-like or child-like. Maximum breathiness produces a whispered voice. Voice types may be stored and retrieved during any single session.

It has been reported frequently that some users find difficulty in identifying with voices that one could not imagine being their own. In particular, it is often mentioned that one cannot expect a woman or child to use a male voice. In our own experience of introducing communication aids, however, we have not often heard such comments from users themselves. Children, epecially, seem to treat the communication aid as a computer with its own voice rather than identifying the voice as their own. One woman said she preferred the male voice, expecting that she would command more authority with it. There was one complaint: a young woman preferred not to talk to her boyfriend over the telephone with the male voices, and felt that the "woman" and "child" voices were not sufficiently intelligible or natural.

3.4 A New Voice Source

A more realistic voice source is now being included in the text-to-speech development system which will make all voices more natural-sounding, but will make the most noticeable improvement in the woman and child voices (Fant et al., 1985, 1987; Gobl, 1988; Karlsson, 1988). Rules for contextual variations, segmental assimilations and prosodic categories as well as interactions between the voice source parameters and parameters of the vocal tract will be handled by rule.

3.5 Modeling Style

An initial attempt has been made to model "style" in British English by providing a "style variable," a user-set range of ten values (Bladon et al.,

1987). In this scheme, a low style variable indicates casual speech, whereas a high style variable indicates formal speech. Areas that have been explored are various degrees of affrication and various versions of function words.

3.6   Controlling Emphasis

It is also possible to control emphasis. By adding a number before a word (or words) in a sentence, one can vary the prosody to achieve a particular effect of emphasis. In this way, it is possible to overrule default sentence stress assignment and function word reduction, and to force different degrees of emphasis on particular words. This facility is particularly useful in conversations, but can also be useful in reading of prepared texts.

3.7   Saving Sentences

One may also save a number of sentences and read them out later at a listener's convenience. This facility is very useful for nonspeaking persons with slow text input abilities. It has been incorporated in both the communication aid and the symbol-to-speech system, and is used in preparing for conversations both in person and by telephone. Demonstrations of communication aids by non-speaking motorically disabled persons have benefitted from this feature as well.

3.8   User-Defined Pronunciations

A user lexicon is provided in which user-specified pronunciations may be stored. These can be words or names that would otherwise be pronounced incorrectly or inappropriately, and can also be user-defined abbreviations. Since recursion is allowed in this lexicon, efficient abbreviation systems can be created by the user. This facility is, of course, very useful to persons with motoric disabilities.

An additional feature is the ability to have multiple user lexicons for special applications. This feature was primarily conceived for use in professional areas requiring special terminology or sets of terminologies. It has also found an application in communication aids for choosing an additional lexicon for various physical environments and areas of personal interest. The same spelling may then have different pronunciations in different user lexicons, and, more importantly, the same abbreviation may have different expansions.

If there is not enough motivation for a word with special pronunciation to be saved in the user lexicon, its pronunciation may be entered directly within the orthographic text by prefacing its phonetic representation with a special symbol.

3.9 Indexing

There is an indexing facility that is intended for programmers writing applications with text-to-speech. Indexing allows the programmer to time the synthetic speech to coincide with another event, e.g., showing a particular graphics display. This facility would also be useful to a non-speaking person preparing a presentation that includes graphic material to be displayed on the computer screen.

3.10 Changing Language

Another possibility is to change among several languages. The situation in Europe is such that having access to several languages is not a luxury. With the opening of borders in Europe, more and more people, including employed disabled persons, will use several languages on an almost daily basis. Already, 25% of our systems are being ordered with more than one language.

4. Text-To-Speech In Voice Prosthesis

The first use of the Swedish text-to-speech system as a communication aid was in 1978. This early system was based on a minicomputer and could be moved around on wheels. A teenager, diagnosed as suffering from cerebral palsy, used the system for several years before beginning to use one of the newer variety. Writing on the keyboard using a mouthstick, he used the system in school for about a year, and then in job training. It was apparent that the system increased his ability to communicate and his linguistic competence. At the same time, it increased his general motivation in other areas of his schoolwork as well. The results were quite encouraging, and valuable information was gained regarding psychological and social factors as well as regarding the functional design of aids with synthetic speech (Carlson et al., 1980). At the beginning, when he first started training sessions together with the therapist, he had difficulty thinking of something to write. However, as he continued to train, the sessions became more and more like an ordinary conversation. He began using these opportunities to initiate communication in explaining his own points of view, in asking questions, and in asking for help as well as to engage in the more passive activities of answering questions and making responses.

He felt that the communication aid would be particularly helpful in several areas. Speaking with children had often been a problem for him. Children he did not know would sometimes become aggressive or tease him when he did not answer them. And even children he did know, if they could not read, could not be communicated with except by gestures. Synthetic speech was a good solution. He also felt that being able to use the telephone would lead to much more independent living. Situations he foresaw for telephone use were calling friends and family, calling a taxi, calling for help, and leaving messages. He also looked forward to being able to participate more in group discussions and other group activities.

It was also important to him that non-speaking small children be introduced to synthetic speech as early as possible, perhaps with pictures or symbols as input. He felt that his own development in learning to read and write would have been much facilitated by earlier exposure to synthetic speech (if it had been available) and that it would have reduced his general dependence on others. He felt that this dependence made non-speakers passive; he found it especially difficult if his assistant did not transmit his entire message, which sometimes happened with emotional expressions.

The emotional expressions he refers to may have been anger and frustration. It has been observed that those who choose symbols and words for non-speaking persons have often selected more polite terms and subjects than the non-speaking person would have chosen. With the advent of the first spoken words, one cannot always expect that gratitude will be the first feeling expressed. After many years of silence and kindly intended, but nevertheless imposed, choice of expression by others, anger and frustration may rank higher on the list of first expressions.

The first functional change in the system was made after noticing that both mistakes and waiting time for the conversational partner caused particular concern or frustration. This led to the added feature that each word, when first typed, could be pronounced with prosodic rules for an isolated word. The user could then listen to each word and change it if it was incorrect. Furthermore, the listener was able to maintain interest during the formation of the sentence. The entire sentence, when complete, was then read out with appropriate sentence-level prosodic rules.

The user also felt that the aid should be fast and that it sould be portable. It should have as optional features both a print-out and a display and should be useable in the dark. ("I've never been able to talk in the dark," he once said.) And a memory for longer messages was also desirable.

Due to advances in integrated circuit technology, a prototype portable device was soon available that was fast and had a larger memory. A special light was attached to the display so that one could indeed "talk in the dark." Soon thereafter, a synthesis card for personal computers was made commercially available. Faster input has been facilitated on such systems by using algorithms for word prediction. A product called Multi-Talk, using an Epson computer and designed specifically as a communication aid, was also developed. It is more easily portable and has both print-out and display capabilities as well as functions for storing partial or complete utterances. And a communication aid for small children with symbol input, called Blisstalk, has also been developed. These methods and devices will be discussed in more detail below.

In the years following the appearance of the first portable prototype, when the new systems containing microcomputers with signal processing chips became available, a number of other persons with various needs began to use them for verbal communication. Some examples from a study by the Swedish Institute for the Handicapped follow (Schildt and Sterner, 1986):

One man, who has had both a laryngectomy and a glossectomy uses the system quite flexibly. He types quickly, and, particularly with the abbreviations possible in the user lexicon, can carry on a conversation in near normal time. He finds speech a much more natural way to communicate than writing, and uses it in conversations with his family. Telephone conversations have also become a possibility once again. This seems to be a very important use for others, as well, since it gives a great deal more independence and privacy. Another man, left without speech after a stroke, began to use the system while still in a hospital. He later moved to a service apartment where he lives independently, having the help of an electric wheelchair, a personal computer and his speech synthesis device.

The device has also been used frequently for training reading and writing, particularly for practicing spelling. One non-speaking boy who seemed not to be able to learn to write more than a few short words, learned easily with the speech synthesis device. Using a "sounding out" mode, he listened to the sound of each letter until he could begin to write words. Another child, who has a brain injury and autism, was able to immediately transfer his experience with a communicator, and began writing right away. He was further motivated by the device and greatly enjoyed hearing words with particular meaning for him. A group of non-speaking students has used it for reading a theatre play together. The play was typed in a file in the computer. When a particular actor's turn came, only his/her keyboard would trigger the reading of that part.

5.   Multi-Talk

The speech synthesis device has been packaged in an attache case as a special-purpose communication aid called Multi-Talk (Galyas and Rosengren, 1989). To use it, one simply lifts the, turns on the device, and begins to type on the Epson keyboard. It runs on either rechargeable batteries or a built-in AC adapter. Multi-Talk comes equipped with up to four of the available languages; a language can be chosen by simply pushing a function key. (See Photo 1.)

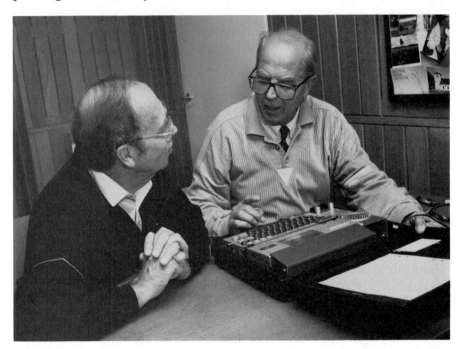

Photo 1:   Multi-Talk (Photo by Björn Lind)

In addition to the usual text-to-speech features such as abbreviation and control of voice quality, Multi-Talk includes several features specially designed to aid communication. There is a contrast-adjustable screen to see what is being written, and a function key to hear what has already been written in the current sentence. The last sentence can be repeated, even in the middle of the following sentence, and can be repeated word by word if desired. Any word can even be spelled out if it has not been understood. The printer included in the Epson can always be used to print out the text that is visible on the screen.

The speed of communication can be greatly increased by the availability of two "higher levels." One higher level allows the user to access stored messages with any single key. This level can be accessed for saying a message without disturbing work in progress at the base level. The other higher level also allows the user single-key access to messages. These messages, however, can be completed with further typed text, or can be copied into the sentence in progress on the base level.

In early trials with Multi-Talk, it was observed that young school children became more interested in practicing reading and writing when speech output was provided to them. This led to the design of a series of computer programs for developing phonological awareness (Dahl and Galyas, 1989). These programs include practice in sound discrimination, phoneme identification, letter and phoneme relationships and spelling. While constructing a sentence, the pupil may listen to phonemes, syllables, words and sentences. Listening augments the ability to detect spelling errors such as omitted letters, reversed words, and missing words. The student's activities are logged continuously, providing the teacher with information about his/her progress. The most apparent effect of working with these programs has been the high level of motivation. An increase in the pupil's self esteem has also been observed in many cases.

Controlled experiments and case studies have shown unexpectedly large improvements. A study in which 87 second-grade pupils were tested for spelling is an example. In this study, the pupils were presented with three lists of twenty equally difficult words each, and were to spell them in three different conditions: (1) with paper and pencil (2) on a computer keyboard, and (3) on a computer keyboard with speech feedback, i.e., phoneme sounds for each letter as well as pronunciation of each spelled word. Unlimited corrections were allowed. There was no significant difference between the mean values for correct answers in the first two conditions. However, an improvement of 25% was evidenced with synthetic speech feedback in the third condition. Taking as a special group the "under-achievers," i.e., those students who had a score of six or less words correct when using paper and pencil (condition 1), the test showed a dramatic improvement: their mean rose from 4.07 correct answers with paper and pencil to 13.50 correct answers on the computer with synthetic-speech feedback. It was also observed that pupils spent much more time spelling a word with speech feedback, taking the time to try and listen to various phonemes and phonene combinations, thus giving themselves valuable experience in phonological awareness.

6. Blisstalk

The symbol system that is now referred to as Blissymbolics was first developed by Karl Blitz in the 1940s. He was deeply impressed by difficulties in communication among people who spoke different languages, or even the same language with different intentions, and was inspired by the Chinese ideographs to develop his own set of characters. He hoped they could be used as the basis of a system of world-wide commonality of expression and understanding (McDonald, 1980). This system was set forth in his nearly 1,000-page work, *Semantography* (Bliss, 1965).

The use of Blissymbols for young non-speaking children in Sweden began in 1976 at two regional habilitation centers. Since then, their use has spread widely in Scandinavia. Because of this wide interest, another device containing speech synthesis and taking Blissymbol input was developed. It is an electronic communication board called Blisstalk (Hunnicutt,1986) which was first built and tested in 1981. As a symbol board with a "voice," it makes its users heard. Communication is not so highly dependent upon the willingness of a "listener" to watch and to interpret the symbols. (See Photo 2.)

Blisstalk is now being produced by a Swedish company. On it are up to 500 Blissymbols that are selected by a magnet or by scanning. The board can

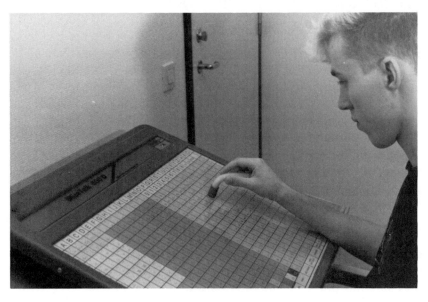

Photo 2: Blisstalk

be reprogrammed with any of 1400 available symbols: a few large symbols may be chosen for a beginner, and more can be added as the user progresses. Each symbol is represented in a lexicon by one or two corresponding words, their pronunciation and grammatical categories. Some symbols have grammatical functions themselves, e.g., plural, verb tenses, possessive. Blisstalk also contains a special phrase-structure grammar that takes account of word order, phrase order and grammatical information in the lexicon to produce well-formed sentences.

Besides this sentence mode are also a word-by-word mode, which does not access the grammar, and a character mode for pronouncing numeral and letter names. A sentence or other completed expression may be repeated, and up to 10 sentences may also be temporarily stored and quickly retrieved. The letters may be used to supplement the symbols by spelling out words, just as in the usual text-to-speech system. This facility has perhaps contributed to the fact that this system has been sold not only for young children, but for young adults who have "grown up" with Blissymbols and are learning to write words and sentences while still using the familiar symbols to which they have become accustomed.

Systems for Swedish, English and French have been distributed. A system for Spanish is also ready for use.

7. Word Prediction

An adaptive word prediction scheme was developed several years ago to be used in conjunction with our speech synthesizer (Hunnicutt, 1987). It was developed in response to the need of a non-vocal user of the synthesizer who found that her listeners were guessing the word she was typing before she finished. In order for the word to be synthesized and pronounced correctly, however, it was necessary for her to finish typing it. It seemed that a word prediction scheme, based on a frequency-sorted lexicon, could be a decided help.

Given an initial letter by the user, a word is predicted based on word frequency and recency of use, and optionally, on a simple phrase structure grammar. A semantic component is currently being developed, as well. Typing the first letter of a word results in accessing the most frequent word beginning with that letter. It is also possible to input letters by using speech recognition. Successive predictions are made from a large lexicon and from a lexicon that stores new typed words. A lexicon containing word pairs is consulted when a word is terminated. If found, the word following it is automatically predicted without its initial letter being typed. The program has recently been modified to serve as part of a word processing system; a memory-resident version is under development.

Another word prediction program has been developed for use with aphasics and children learning to spell. It also provides word prediction to aid in easier message construction. However, it does not presuppose the ability to spell a word. The goal is to use any information that the person has about a word, such as any letter it contains, the number of syllables it has or the word class to which it belongs, to access it. The word, or a list of word predictions, can then be synthesized for the user to hear and to choose among. An investigation is now underway to determine whether approximate word length and an indication of initial or non-initial primary stress would also be usable input options.

Emphasis has been placed on the use of substantial linguistic support to make the programs give reasonably expected choices. Psycholinguistic literature on the topic of "lexical access" was also of primary importance in forming these prediction schemes. For example, frequency and recency of word use are designed to be deciding factors. Support for this decision can be found in Broadbent's (1967) hypothesis that a person's mental lexicon is, in some sense, frequency-weighted. For example, the more frequent a (content) word in a language, the faster the reaction time of a person hearing that word in classifying it as a word of the language (Bradley, 1978). The main lexicon in the word prediction programs is a frequency-ordered lexicon that may contain up to 10,000 words. A lexicon that collects all except the most frequently used words is consulted as if its contents followed the 200 most frequent words in the main lexicon. This provision allows the 200 most frequent words, most of which are function words, and which can be expected to make up over 50% of a text (Kucera and Francis, 1967), to precede these recently-used words.

The program developed for use by aphasics and children learning to spell benefits from studies showing, for example, that the initial sounds and the initial letter(s) of a word are "access points." That is, a person can guess a word faster given its initial letter(s) than given medial or final letters (Marslen-Wilson and Welsh, 1978, Jakimik and Cole, 1985). Many other psycholinguistic studies concerning grammar and semantics in word recognition have also been useful in building a foundation upon which to write word prediction programs.

8.   Talking Terminals

The most widespread use of the speech synthesis system as a technical aid at this time is as a "talking terminal." In this application, information that is printed on a computer screen is read by the device. Over 300 systems have already been installed as talking terminals. This technique is most used by blind persons and persons with poor vision, and has been implemented in a number of work stations in Sweden. These work stations are typically built around a personal computer, and include a Braille display and printer as well as a speech synthesis device. The results have been quite promising, particularly in several office applications such as word processing, register handling and local switchboard operation.

There are also several distributors of screen-reading programs, for ABC80, ABC800, IBM-PC and VT100 terminals. These programs detect certain commands from normal text input such as "Read current line," "Give cursor position" or "Read word by word" which are interpreted in special routines. These routines access the appropriate text and send it to the synthesis device to be read.

9.   Daily Newspapers

Another application of speech synthesis for the visually handicapped is in the area of reading text that has been typeset by computer—a common practice in printing offices nowadays. A project that has continued for several years in Sweden is to make daily newspapers available to persons with visual disabilities (Carlson and Granström, 1986). At present, newspaper text is broadcast digitally to the homes of about 30 blind subscribers where it is stored on a magnetic disk during the night. The user can then, at leisure, search the material for sections, headlines, or particular words with the help of a small microcomputer. The selected text can then be presented as synthetic speech. (See Photo 3.)

10.   Public Applications

Speech technology currently used in services for the general public could be equally interesting for blind persons. Typical examples are information services in the telephone network. Coded natural speech is typically used in these applications, but one application has been developed with our text-to-speech system: an automatic stock exchange information service. Telephone access to electronic mail is an important potential application, but electronic mail is still rather limited in Sweden.

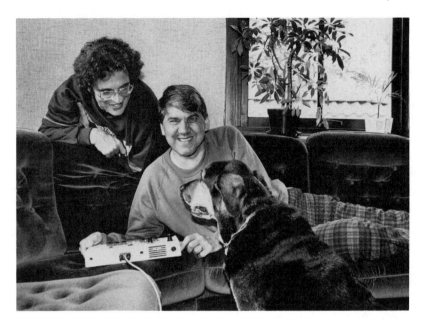

Photo 3:   Daily Newspaper via Text-to-Speech (Photo by Pelle Lund)

11.   Speech Recognition

Although it has not been the major emphasis of this discussion, an area that will be increasingly useful in technical aids in the future is speech recognition. The system developed at the Royal Institute of Technology in Stockholm is a pattern-matching system (Elenius and Blomberg, 1986). The system digitally implements a 16-channel filter bank. This filter bank covers frequencies from 200 to 5000 Hertz in bands spaced according to the critical band scale, which represents the frequency characteristics of the human auditory system. (See Marcus and Syrdal, Chapter 1.) Thirty-two sample points derived from this information are matched with the stored reference patterns by dynamic programming time alignment. Speech analysis and dynamic programming are accomplished using a NEC7720 signal-processing chip. Control of the recognition process and storage of the reference vocabulary are handled in the microprocessor and memory of the PC.

There are several ways in which the recognition system can be used as a technical aid. It may be used as a stand-alone unit to voice-control another device connected to an I/O-port of the PC. Such an application would be voice control of an environmental control device. It may also be used to add speech control to any already existing program. After speech input is initialized, the response strings of recognized utterances look like keyboard entries to the program to be run. A motorically disabled person capable of producing different (but consistent) utterances for each key on the keyboard would thereby have full control of any user program. One particularly useful application is word processing in which utterances would access both keys and editing commands. Another use would be to fully integrate speech control into an applications program with calls to the recognizer's special functions. This could be an especially useful tool for a disabled programmer.

A system using speech recognition has been developed as an alternative for environmental control for a motorically handicapped person who has full use of his head and neck. With his previous sip-and-puff device he could switch on the radio, TV and lights. He could also open the door to his apartment and make telephone calls. These functions were controlled through infrared light. The system has now been augmented by a personal computer with speech recognition connected to a a programmable remote control. With the new system he can control, by speech, all the old devices and also get the full use of all the functions on standard consumer electronic devices such as TV, VCR and radio. Software on the PC gives the appropriate feedback such as selections from the telephone list. Now he can also use the PC for tasks such as creating and editing messages. It is planned to include the previously described word predictor to allow faster input of text while giving oral typing commands.

12. Conclusions

It is now possible for both speech synthesis and speech recognition to be used in technical aids for disabled persons. Special features for these applications have been included in the text-to-speech system developed at the Royal Institute of Technology. These features and their uses for disabled persons were discussed, aids which have been developed at RIT were described and ongoing work reported. Included were word predictors, the use of text-to-speech as a voice prosthesis, a specialized communication aid called Multitalk, a Blissymbol-to-speech system called Blisstalk, talking terminals, a daily newspaper source for the blind, a public application of the text-to-speech system useful for the blind, and a communication system that includes speech recognition.

A major portion of this chapter was previously published in the Proceedings of the Second Australian International Conference on Speech Science and Technology, Sydney, November 1988.

13.   References

Barber, S., Granström,B. & Touati,P. (1988). "French prosody in a rule-based text-to-speech system," Proceedings of Speech '88, 7th FASE symposium, Edinburgh, Scotland.

Bladon,A., Carlson, R., Granström, B. Hunnicutt, S. & Karlsson, I. (1987). "Text-to-speech system for British English, and issues of dialect and style," European Conference on Speech Technology, vol. 1, Edinburgh, Scotland.

Bliss, C.K. (1965). *Semantography*, Semantography Blissymbolics Publications. 2nd Edition. Sydney, Australia.

Bradley, D. (1978). "Computational Distinctions of Vocabulary Type," doctoral thesis, Dept. of Psychology, M.I.T., Cambridge, Massachusetts.

Broadbent, D.E. (1967). "Word-Frequency Effect and Response Bias." Psychological Review, 74, pp. 1–15.

Carlson, R. Galyas, K., Granström, B., Pettersson, M. & Zachrisson,G. (1980). "Speech Synthesis for the Non-Vocal in Training and Communication," STL-QPSR, Vol 4.

Carlson, R. & Granström, B. (1986). "Applications of a Multi-Lingual Text-to-Speech System for the Visually Impaired," in *Development of Electronic Aids for the Visually Impaired*, P.L. Emiliani, ed., Martinus Nijhoff/Dr W. Junk Publishers, Dordrecht.

Carlson, R., Granström, B. & Hunnicutt, S. (1988). "Rulsys - The Swedish Multilingual Text-to-Speech Approach," SST-88.

Dahl, I & Galyas, K. (1989). "Computer Programs with Speech Output in Teaching Reading and Writing—Experiences and Results," Speech Research '89, Budapest, pp. 41–44.

Elenius, Kj. & Blomberg, M. (1986). "Voice Input for Personal Computers," in *Electronic Speech Recognition*, Geoff Bristow, ed., Collins Professional and Technical Books, London.

Fant, G., Liljencrants, J. & Lin,Q. (1985). "A four-parameter model of glottal flow," STL-QPSR 4/1985.

Fant, G., Gobl, C., Karlsson, I. & Lin, Q. (1987). "The female voice—Experiments and overviews," J. Acoust. Soc. Am., 82, S90(Abstract).

Galyas, K. and Rosengren, E. (1989). "Synthetic Speech in Communication Aids: Experiences in Sweden," Speech Research '89, pp. 163–165.

Gobl,C. (1988). "Voice source dynamics in connected speech," STL-QPSR 1/1988.

Granström, B. (1987). "Speech technology for the visually impaired—the Swedish perspective," STL-QPSR 1/1987, pp. 29–38.

Granström, B. & Gustafson, K. (1986). "Toneme 1 1/2 in a Norwegian text-to-speech system," Nordisk Prosodi IV, Odense.

Granström, B., Molbaek Hansen, P. & Grönnum Thorsen, N. (1987). "A Danish text-to-speech system using a text normalizer based on morph analysis," European Conference on Speech Technology, vol. 1, Edinburgh, Scotland.

Hunnicutt, S. (1986). "Bliss Symbol-to-Speech Conversion: 'Blisstalk'," Journal of the American Voice I/O Society, Vol. 3.

Hunnicutt, S. (1987). "Input and Output Alternatives in Word Prediction," STL/QPRS 2–3, 19–29.

Jakimik, J. and Cole, R. (1985). "Sound and Spelling in Spoken Word Recognition," unpublished manuscript.

Karlsson, I. (1988). "Glottal waveform parameters for different speaker types," Proceedings of Speech '88, 7th FASE symposium, Edinburgh, Scotland.

Kohler, K. (1988). "An intonation model for a German text-to-speech system," Proceedings of Speech '88, 7th FASE symposium, Edinburgh, Scotland.

Kucera, H. & Francis, W.N. (1967). *Computational Analysis of Present-Day American English*, Brown University Press, Providence, Rhode Island.

Marslen-Wilson, W. & Welsh, A. (1978). Processing Interactions and Lexical Access during Word Recognition in Continuous Speech," Cognitive Psychology, 10, pp. 29–63.

McDonald, E. (1980). *Teaching and Using Blissymbolics*, Blissymbolics Communication Institute, Toronto.

Schildt, A. & Sterner, M. (1986). *Talsyntes som Talhjälpmedel*, Swedish Institute for the Handicapped, Bromma, Sweden.

Chapter 21

Computer Assisted Speech Training: Practical Considerations

Diane Kewley-Port and Charles S. Watson
Indiana University

1. Introduction

The problems discussed in this paper were formulated during five years of collaboration by an interdisciplinary group, whose goal was the development of a computer-based speech training aid. The short-term goal was to extend the use of a computer-based, speaker-dependent speech recognizer, originally applied to speech training at the Boy's Town National Research Hospital (Lippmann and Watson, 1970), and to implement it on an IBM PC. The resulting system, the Indiana Speech Training Aid (ISTRA), was developed to provide independent speech drill for a variety of speech-disordered children and adults (Kewley-Port et al., 1987). The ISTRA system, however, is not the primary focus. Our own research, together with that of several other groups in this country (Fletcher, 1989 and Bernstein et al., 1988) and abroad (Watanabe et al., 1985; Yamada et al., 1988; Povel and Wansink, 1986), provides convincing evidence that computer-assisted speech training can become an efficient, common-place instructional mode within ten to fifteen years. This paper highlights certain requirements that must be met by the developers and evaluators of these systems if this goal is to be achieved.

In particular, the discussion that follows will focus on four topics. The first is a generic description of computer-assisted speech trainers, followed by a brief description of the ISTRA system which serves as an example in this paper. Second, we discuss the central aspect of speech trainers, namely the nature and source of the feedback presented to the client. A taxomony for describing feedback is discussed with reference to how specific types of feedback must be calibrated and validated for the purposes of speech training. Third, we show how computers can enhance speech training provided by a human speech pathologist. It is argued that the developer of a computer-based trainer must be responsible for creating speech training curricula that can guide the speech pathologist to make effective use of the trainer in speech therapy. The final topic discusses the most critical step in the development of speech training systems, namely the demonstration in actual clinical trials that the speech of clients improves as a result of computer-assisted training. Four levels of clinical evaluation are discussed.

2. Computer-Based SpeechTraining (CBST) Systems

A computer-based speech training (CBST) system is programmed to process one or more signals (acoustic, articulatory movement, electrophysiological, etc.), derived from the speech of a client, for the purpose of providing feedback about the utterances. This may be contrasted with some commercially available systems that prompt a client to speak, but do not provide feedback. A CBST should be able to keep detailed records of the course of speech training. CBST systems, now and in the foreseeable future, should be designed as *training aids* which supplement and presumably enhance speech training under the guidance of a human speech pathologist or teacher. While some systems may be suitable for providing speech drill conducted independently by the client, the general use of the CBST system should be considered in relation to the tasks that will be conducted by the human teacher or clinician. This relation between human and computer is not often explicitly considered (see Training Curriculum section below), but it is an essential factor in the use and potential success of computers in speech training.

The ISTRA system is the product of ten years of research and development and is therefore a moderately advanced example of CBSTs. (For reviews of other CBST systems, see Bernstein et al., 1988; Braeges and Houde, 1982; and Lippmann, 1982.) ISTRA is implemented on a PC-type microcomputer equipped with a speaker-dependent speech recognition board (Interstate Voice Products, Inc.). Feedback on the quality of speech production is derived from a goodness-of-fit metric. This metric is an estimate of the similarity between a new utterance and a stored template representing the best recent effort to produce those same utterances. Syllables or words used to form the templates are periodically updated as speech intelligibility improves. Speech pathologists use standard diagnostic and treatment methods to implement ISTRA speech drill as outlined in a speech training curriculum. The speech drill is presented to the client in the form of video games, with nine games currently available at different training levels.

Records of all training for a given client are stored on floppy disk and can be easily reviewed by the speech pathologist in printed or graphic form.

The development of CBST systems is often driven by available technology rather than by more theoretically based considerations that might focus on the global relationship between technology and speech training. Two recent articles in Volta Review have examined several theoretical issues underlying the development of CBST systems (Bernstein, 1989; Watson and Kewley-Port, 1989). As background for our Volta Review article, we reviewed 28 CBST systems existing at that time in laboratories or as commercial products. We can add to those several more described in published literature and some more recently marketed systems. It appears to us that, possibly because computer assisted speech training is still a young research area, there are several practical considerations frequently neglected during the development of CBST systems. This paper will discuss three of these considerations: (1) the design and validation of the feedback to be presented to the client; (2) the development of a speech training curriculum integrated with the technical requirements and advantages of CBST technology; and (3) the selection of appropriate levels of clinical evaluation of CBST systems.

3. Design Considerations for Speech Feedback

Watson and Kewley-Port (1989) provided a theoretically motivated description of the nature of feedback in speech training. Here we extend that earlier discussion to include validation of the feedback that has (presumably) been selected on theoretical grounds. Feedback is often presented in a video-game format, and the relation between a monkey climbing a palm tree and throwing coconuts (from IBM SpeechViewer, see Ryalls, 1989) and either the speech parameters represented in the graphics or the expected aspect of speech to be learned by the client may be very complicated. Moreover, the optimal form of feedback in speech training may be different for different speech disorders. In the case of a hearing-impaired individual, the feedback should probably serve as a *substitute* for feedback (sidetone) in the auditory channel. For normal-hearing, misarticulating persons, feedback should probably provide information to *augment* that derived from the auditory channel.

A general taxonomy for describing feedback has been proposed by Watson and Kewley-Port (1989). Types of feedback are described by three discrete dimensions, or *properties* as illustrated by the cube in Figure 1. The first property is the **physical measurement** on which the feedback is based.

Three possible measures of the spoken response were specified, electro-physiological, articulatory movement and acoustic.

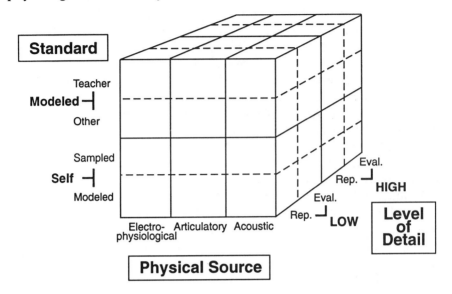

Figure 1:   Feedback in Speech Training

The second property of feedback in the taxonomy is the **standard** of speech performance in relation to which the measured speech production is evaluated. One standard is a normative sample, one that is representative of normal speech produced by the speech teacher. The second standard, which is also normative, is previously stored in the CBST system as a representation of normal production (for example, a point in normalized vowel space (Povel and Wansink, 1987)). The third standard uses a sample of speech from the individual in training, to represent a "personal goal." When the stored sample represents the current best utterances, this type of standard is a *model* of high quality productions derived from the individual's previous productions.

The third property of feedback is the level of **detail** that is presented to the trainee. A high level of detail is provided by a spectrogram while a single acoustic dimension, like pitch, provides a low level of detail. Feedback may be a direct *representation* of the source speech signal or a comparison of the utterance against a standard in terms or "speech quality." The difference is whether the client observes a spectrogram (for example) of his or her utterance and must learn how to determine if that particular spectrogram means a good or a poor production, versus having a computer algorithm *evaluate* speech quality and provide feedback using words or graphic displays to indicate "excellent," "good job" or "poor—try again."

In the three-dimensional cube, the various combinations of properties represent 48 possible choices for speech feedback. Considering the 30+ CBST systems that have been developed, less than a quarter of the possible feedback options have been tried. We do not suggest that all 48 options need to be systematically investigated. However, we believe that an awareness of the alternatives might lead to the development of important new techniques in speech training. In particular, since systems that provide evaluative feedback, such as ISTRA, are in the minority, some thought should be given to the reason for this. Is it because it is difficult to develop algorithms to make a valid evaluation between a standard and a new utterance? Or is it because clients might make use of nearly any portion of feedback that is rich in information, compared to the drastically reduced information contained in a positive or negative evaluation?

Consideration of this taxonomy for speech feedback may suggest some general principles for the evaluation of a CBST systems. For example, what documentation *should be required* of the producer of a CBST system as evidence that the feedback presented is valid for speech training purposes? Depending on the physical source from which the feedback is derived, specific standard verification and calibration procedures should be performed on the transducers. If the standard against which new utterances are evaluated is sampled, then the coding algorithms should be described. If the standard is normative, then the normalization procedures and statistical verification of the success of the normalization should be provided. If the standard is modeled from the client, again the model should be described and its applicability to various talkers should be documented.

Finally, if the feedback presented is representative of the physical source, verification of the accuracy of the information represented *in the feedback display* must be provided. For example, SpeechViewer (Friedman, 1989; Ryalls, 1989) has numerous graphic displays of pitch, from thermometers to camels finding water holes, but the relationship of the graphics to the control of pitch over time is not specified. On the other hand, if the feedback is evaluative, then the quality metric itself must be validated. At this time, the only suitable metric of speech quality, especially for disordered speech, is the judgment of the human listener. Therefore, this validation requires a correlation between the quality metric calculated and the quality ratings of these same utterances by human listeners (for example, see Watson et al., 1989).

4. Speech Training Curriculum

It seems obvious that part of CBST development should include consideration of the specific ways in which speech training methods used by a speech pathologist might be enhanced by the addition of the speech training aid. Unfortunately, this is rarely done. For example, one approach, common in advertising brochures, is to assert that CBST systems offer such a wonderful bag of tricks that, after investing in one, any speech pathologist will surely discover a variety of ways to use this new technology. A variant of this approach, apparently used by IBM for SpeechViewer[1], is to distribute a number of free systems and then report what speech pathologists thought were appropriate and successful clinical uses.

If clinicians or teachers are to use CBST systems successfully it is important that *training curricula* for their use be developed hand-in-hand with the systems. This same point was underscored in research conducted by McGarr et al. (1989). They compared training methods for voiced pitch remediation for the hearing-impaired including standard (auditory) training, training with a CBST system, and training with a tactile aid. While the comparison would not have been possible without a suitable curriculum that could be used for all three training methods, the study emphasizes the need for curricula for training methods.

It is unreasonable for the developers of CBST systems to expect each teacher to adapt the new technology to their standard training methods. Similarly, computers installed in normal classrooms are of little educational value without appropriate Computer-aided instruction (CAI) packages integrated into a regular curriculum. One possible exception for CBST systems might be those with very simple feedback, such as a single-dimensional representation of pitch or loudness. Nonetheless, the introduction of the technology without a curriculum is still a burden for the speech pathologist using it with a particular client. Developers of more sophisticated speech technologies, like the glossometer (Fletcher, 1989) or the ISTRA system, are clearly obliged to develop a curriculum along with the technology.

The ISTRA training curriculum provides an example of how to integrate standard procedures used by a speech pathologist with the use of a CBST system. The special advantage of ISTRA is that it has speech-drill programs that most clients can use with little direct supervision. The ISTRA curriculum

---

[1] "SpeechViewer. A Guide to Clinical and Educational Application." Available through IBM in November, 1989.

includes the tasks needed before drill, especially template making, and four levels of speech drill, each providing a different type of feedback.

Stages of speech training in the ISTRA curriculum, outlined in Figures 2 through 5, are based on the traditional articulation therapy methods most often used in the Indiana University Speech and Hearing Clinic. In these figures the first column shows the stages of speech training; the second column lists the tasks conducted by the speech pathologist; the third column lists the names and descriptions of the software developed for ISTRA; and the fourth column lists related programs that come with ISTRA, but do not use the speech training templates.

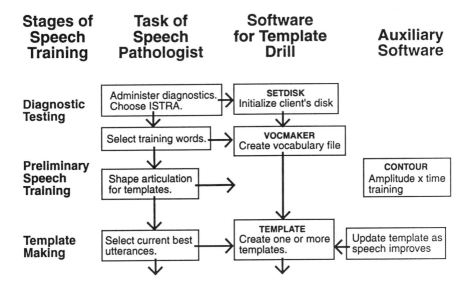

Figure 2:   ISTRA Training Curriculum

The tasks shown in Figure 2 are conducted before speech drill. First, standard diagnostic tests for articulation disorders are administered. The training curriculum at this point should assist the speech pathologist in determining whether a particular type of computer-based training is appropriate for given disorders and clients (i.e. age, multiple-handicaps, etc.). If a CBST system is used, then selection guidelines for the speech errors that can be corrected should be provided (making the reasonable assumption that not *all* speech errors can be corrected on a single system). Unfortunately, reasonably accurate guidelines as to which errors can be successfully corrected require a program of clinical research that is not easily accomplished (see below). Nonetheless, it should *not* be left to trial and error by the speech pathologist to obtain this information.

In standard articulation training, the next step (following the selection of particular sounds to be trained) is the "shaping" of the target sound. Shaping methods help change an incorrect speech production into a correct one. In ISTRA, this stage of training is incorporated by a speech pathologist into the template-making procedure. When a speech pathologist makes templates, the goal is to encourage the client to produce the best possible utterances that are subsequently captured for use as short-term training standards. The shaping methods employed are basically the same as those commonly used in most clinics except that the speech pathologist is asked to rate each utterance on a one-to-nine scale of overall quality. The three utterances receiving the highest ratings are used by the speech recognizer to form the template.

Many CBST systems are more useful for shaping than for providing quantities of speech drill. For example, aids that use feedback based on physiological measures provide information to the client about how to modify an incorrect articulation, information that might otherwise be unavailable. However, in most cases, little is known about how a correct production of a sound is specified in terms of, say, a glossometric representation (Fletcher, 1989). As noted earlier, the final judgment of a correct production is made by humans, based on the *acoustic* signal. Thus, the use of physiological feedback for speech drill requires that the relation between the physiological response and the perceptual quality of utterances be known by at least the speech pathologist. This relation would in most cases be a challenging one to experimentally validate. Thus, acoustic-based feedback may provide a more direct correlation with speech quality (see Watson et al., 1989) and is probably a better choice for speech drill. This conclusion, however, requires additional experimental support. One might envision that in the future hybrid computer-based training aids could incorporate different types of feedback, acoustic or physiological, for articulatory shaping prior to repetitive, acoustic based drills, similar to those of ISTRA.

ISTRA currently includes one auxiliary program, Contour, used in shaping. Contour presents a typical amplitude-by-time display for whole words, and is useful since it provides a visual representation of the differences between hard (stop consonant) and soft (fricative) onsets of words, deletion or insertion of sounds, etc.

The ISTRA system provides four levels of speech drill that vary primarily in the type of feedback. The feedback is generally evaluative and indicates speech quality, in terms of how well a new utterance matches a stored template. The first stage of drill (Figure 3) provides feedback that represents this evaluation in one of several graphics displays. The basic feedback is a bar graph with higher bars indicating better speech quality. A second display is a bull's-eye target where greater distance from the bull's-eye indicates poorer speech quality. Feedback is given rapidly after every utterance, and a summary of performance over every 20 utterances is automatically generated. This use of feedback is loosely based on principals of learning (operant conditioning) that suggest that in early stages of training, when the errors are far from the targets, frequent and carefully graded evaluations of performance are needed to move the client toward improved productions.

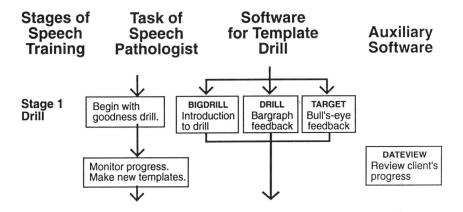

Figure 3: ISTRA Training Curriculum

The next stage of drill is appropriate for clients who have achieved a reasonably consistent and higher quality production of the target utterance. At this point, feedback based on the goodness metric from the recognizer will have only a limited range of values, and graphic representations of these small differences are not particularly noticeable. Following common practice in speech therapy, the second level of ISTRA drill uses a criterion or threshold below which no feedback is given. The feedback threshold is made additionally effective by using an algorithm so that the threshold "floats" depending on the client's performance. Better productions cause the threshold to rise, while poorer productions cause it to fall.

(The threshold-tracking algorithms are based on procedures described by Levitt, 1971.) This stage of drill is therefore referred to as a *variable criterion drill.* Two different graphic formats are used. The first is a "baseball" game in which the goodness scale above the threshold is divided into levels representing singles, doubles, triples and home runs, while subthreshold responses yield an "out." This is the most popular of the ISTRA drills. The second format is a footrace, in which different training words are represented by different runners.

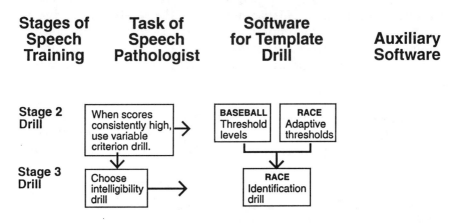

Figure 4:   ISTRA Training Curriculum

The third-level drill, identification drill, is primarily for the hearing-impaired. It is also a criterion-based drill and is a variant of RACE but with a slightly different goal. In identification drill, speech produced above the criterion is used to identify one word among several selected. Identification drill is intended to encourage the client to speak intelligibly, and to demonstrate to him or her that their own selected utterances are recognizable.

Operant-conditioning research (Ferster and Skinner, 1957) suggests that as training progresses, feedback should not be administered on every trial. Rather clients should gradually internalize a standard of goodness against which they evaluate the quality of their own productions, a process that occurs more rapidly when external feedback is given less frequently. Stage 4 of the ISTRA drill includes *fixed-ratio-reinforcement-schedule* feedback in a program called MOONRIDE. This program allows the speech pathologist to choose a reinforcement schedule in which feedback is given once out of every N times that the goodness score exceeds a threshold, for each prompted word. The threshold is automatically increased or decreased, based on the client's performance after the rocket is launched toward the moon.

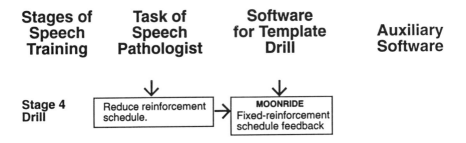

Stages of Speech Training	Task of Speech Pathologist	Software for Template Drill	Auxiliary Software
Stage 4 Drill	Reduce reinforcement schedule.	MOONRIDE Fixed-reinforcement schedule feedback	

Figure 5: ISTRA Training Curriculum

The ISTRA training curriculum provides good examples of how technology can enhance the speech training capabilities of the speech pathologist. The concepts of criterion-based drills and reduced-reinforcement schedules come directly from research on human and animal learning and can be implemented in systematic ways on the computer. Moreover, feedback given in video-game format seems to be more interesting to clients, particularly children, than other forms of drill. Highly repetitive drill is the only known route to accurate speech production. Conducting repetitious drill is time-consuming for the speech pathologist and does not use the full range of human skills and knowledge; therefore, it is a task well-suited to computers. In particular, computer-based drill can remain interesting and challenging even at later stages of training by carefully integrating the training tasks with varied forms of graphic feedback.

5. Role of Clinical Evaluation

The ultimate test of the success of a computer-based speech training system is verification that the disordered speech of an individual improves with training. While many developers of CBST systems and speech pathologists will probably agree on the importance of clinical evaluation, arguments abound over how, when and by whom the clinical test should be conducted. Because CBST technology is new, developers find the burden of solving the engineering and software issues difficult and time consuming. At the end of system development, it seems unfair that another project, clinical evaluation, that is also costly and time consuming, needs to be done before the system can be generally distributed, much less sold. Clinical evaluation also involves a set of skills not usually well-represented (if at all) on the team of CBST developers. Thus, new staff and frequently new testing sites are needed. Even if significant commitment to clinical evaluation is made by the developers, there is little in the published literature on how such evaluations should be done.

The role of clinical evaluation in the development of CBST systems may be systematized by identifying four reasonably distinct levels of evaluation: (1) Tests of the **acceptability** of the system by clients and speech teachers; (2) Tests of the clinical **effectiveness** of the device to improve speech ; (3) **Independent verification** of clinical effectiveness. (4) **Beta-test** evaluations at off-site locations; and These levels are discussed below, based on experience gained in the evaluation of speech training on ISTRA with approximately 50 clients in three clinical settings (for an early report, see Kewley-Port et al., 1991).

5.1   Acceptability Evaluations.

The first level of evaluation involving clients and teachers is the study of how acceptable the CBST system is for speech training. Evaluations are based on observations or discussions with the clinical users about the appropriateness of the feedback displays for age or type of client, choice of microphone, etc. The needs of the speech pathologist, in terms of the suitability of a drill to a particular type of therapy or the flexibility of training for a particular client, are also evaluated. As wide a variety of clients and clinical settings as possible should be included. Note that the data collected in this type of evaluation is primarily *testimonial*. During early evaluations of systems, these observations usually result in frequent changes in the system as developers fine-tune the software.

In later stages (which may be part of beta-tests), training logs or questionnaires may be used to collect the testimonials in a more systematic way. In a recent example, IBM undertook a large acceptability study of SpeechViewer by placing systems in clinics in 29 countries (Ryalls, 1989). Testimonials collected in such studies should not, however be regarded as adequate substitutes for clinical evaluations involving control groups and vigorous testing methods to demonstrate actual speech improvement, which is the goal of the next level of evaluation.

5.2   Clinical Effectiveness

Speech pathologists are interested in research methods that can demonstrate that a client improved (or failed to improve) as a result of a particular training method. Because clients in need of similar speech therapy frequently differ in terms of age, education, etiology, presence of multiple disabilities, etc., studies using experimental and control groups are rarely used (but see McGarr et al.,

1989). Recently, many studies of clinical effectiveness have used *single-subject designs* (McReynolds and Thompson, 1986). In this type of study, several different speech errors may be present. Treatment (training) is introduced for one error at a time, while performance on each of the speech errors is monitored during each session. If the treated error improves, while performance on all others remains constant, this is support for the causal relation of the treatment to the improvement in performance.

In any case, studies of the clinical effectiveness of speech therapy require a great deal of time and effort. It is therefore not at all surprising that many developers of CBST systems have not conducted evaluations of clinical effectiveness, and have instead sometimes presented only the results of acceptability evaluations in their place. There is almost certainly a positive correlation between high ratings on acceptability evaluations by speech pathologists and clinical effectiveness. However, it should be stressed that these are distinctly different types of evaluation, and that the clinical literature contains many cases of apparently "acceptable" treatments that were later shown to fail tests of clinical effectiveness.

Let's consider further the nature of the data collected in single-subject designs. Correct production of an utterance is usually judged by the speech pathologist, who is also the person conducting the speech therapy. On some occasions, an independent judge makes an additional evaluation. Lists of words containing the speech errors are spoken by the client, either every treatment session, or more commonly, every second or third session. Each word is judged as correct or incorrect, and a percent of words correctly produced is calculated over the whole word list. The percent correct values for a speech error are then plotted on a time axis, thereby tracking correct speech production over the course of therapy. However, since the speech pathologist is the person most closely working with the client, these time-line analyses are potentially biased towards demonstrating improvement in speech production. (Unfortunately, this bias might be even stronger if the speech pathologist is being paid by a CBST developer to clinically evaluate the devices.)

We prefer to think of the judgments of correct production made by the speech pathologist as presenting the *clinical record* of treatment progress. The independent verification of that record still needs to be done, as discussed in the next level of evaluations. Even if there is an inherent bias in studies of clinical effectiveness done or directed by the developers, such studies ought to be done, *at a minimum*, before any CBST system is marketed. These studies would at least assure a potential user of the system that it did improve the speech of a certain number and type of client, within the limitations of the studies. Without such minimal evidence there is clearly considerable ethical uncertainty surrounding the use of the device on clients except for research. In a survey of CBST systems (Watson and Kewley-Port, 1989) only one-third collected and reported data at even this minimal level of clinical evaluation.

5.3 Independent Verification of Clinical Effectiveness

It seems obvious that studies conducted by persons not associated with the developers would have less potential experimenter bias than those directed by the developers. While this is true, we still need to consider how data collected in speech therapy can be assessed without relying on judgments of the speech pathologist conducting the therapy. Several methods have been proposed (McReynolds and Kearns, Chapter 5, 1983) to provide a second independent judgment of the clinical record data. For example, a second clinician could listen to a tape recording of the word lists every third time, and then resolve differences with the correct/incorrect scoring done on-line by the speech pathologist.

In our opinion, truly independent verification of the clinical scoring is best done by listener juries who are "blind" to the purposes of the project. Word lists can be collected before, during and after therapy, randomized and presented to listeners for evaluation. We have followed this procedure in the ISTRA project, but these listening studies are time-consuming, mostly because the randomization requires digitization and computer editing of many tape recordings. Out of 11 single-subject studies for ISTRA, independent jury evaluations were completed for only three of them.

The results of the correspondence between our jury-listening data and the time-line presentation of percent correct production (judged by speech pathologists) underscores the point we are trying to make here. One of the jury-listening tasks was to rate the intelligibility of the word spoken on a five-point scale (from 1 = "unintelligible" to 5 = "normal"). Three speech errors were trained in each of the three single-subject studies, so there are nine sets of data to compare. For six of the nine comparisons, a good replication of the clinical measure was obtained for the average jury ratings. However, we were surprised by the lack of correspondence in the other three cases. Further examination indicated that the source of the problem was different in each case. For example, in one case the jury of certified speech pathologists did not consistently rate the "th" sound (in "think") from audio recordings. While judgment of the improvement of speech must be done by persons other than the speech pathologists who conducted the therapy, not enough information is available on what methodology should be followed in obtain reliable measures of improvement.

5.3 Beta-test Evaluations

Off-site evaluations of computer-based speech trainers can begin early in development. In fact, developers are often forced to begin acceptability evaluations off-site because they have no on-site access to clients. In this discussion, however, off-site testing for any of three types of clinical evaluation described above are to be distinguished from beta-test evaluations that are conducting just prior to general distribution (or sale) of a system. Beta-test evaluations are used to *fine-tune* the device to speech-training tasks in environments in which it will most frequently be used. They are also used to improve the general robustness of the system when the developers may not be readily available to assist the user. General performance of the hardware, the user-friendliness of the software, and the effectiveness of the documentation are all considered in beta-test evaluations.

Beta-test site evaluations of CBST begin near the end of product development. In order to determine how the systems will perform in actual clinical use, the speech pathologists participating in these evaluations should operate as independently as possible from the developers. Feedback given to the developers is usually testimonial from survey or from logs.

Naturally, developers are frequently anxious to collect clinical evaluation data during beta-testing. If the CBST system can store and retrieve records on the use of the system, then at least simple statistics can be generated from these data concerning the number of clients, the hours spent in each training stage, etc. (A surprising number of systems being marketed do not store such information.) To go beyond usage, testimonial information about the clinical effectiveness of the system can be elicited. However, it is difficult to collect data that can actually document speech improvement. Since the CBST system at the beta-test site is intentionally not under the control of the developers, speech training is not likely to be as systematically conducted as is required for research purposes. For example, the ISTRA project has attempted to record word lists produced several months apart at two beta-test sites to be evaluated by listener judgments later in the laboratory. An overall improvement in percent correct productions of 12% was observed for the final versus initial recording of the 16 clients at one site. However, listeners judged the productions of four clients above 96% correct on the initial recording, which is certainly not a desirable situation because there is little room for improvement.

A different approach for establishing a beta-test site is to form a consortium of the research group and the developers to conduct clinical evaluations. Such arrangements are not uncommon for evaluating medical treatments.

The voice remediation study by McGarr et al. (1989) might be considered an example of this type of evaluation of CBST systems, but was in fact a very extensive control study, one whose cost and effort make it unlikely that similar studies will be undertaken frequently.

6. Summary

We have discussed several problems related to the development of computer-based speech trainers that are often not given enough attention during system development. Three of these problems can only be addressed by carefully conducted research. First, the feedback to the client must be calibrated and validated for the purpose of providing suitable information to improve disordered speech. Second, a speech training curriculum that can enhance the delivery of speech therapy by the human speech pathologist must be created and tested, probably by the developers of the computer speech trainers themselves. Third, clinical evaluations that go beyond acceptability testing ("testimonials") and demonstrate some level of clinical effectiveness for the speech trainer must be provided before the system is generally distributed. While the time and expense to conduct this research may seem a deterrent to the development of computer-based speech trainers, it is the only ethical way that new methods of speech therapy can be promoted for general use with clients. We hope that the discussion of these three topics will help developers of computer-based speech trainers understand what needs to be done, and also help the potential purchasers of those systems develop their own selection criteria.

7. References

Bernstein, L., Goldstein, M. and Mahshie, J. (1988). "Speech training aids for profoundly deaf children I: Overview and aims," *J. Rehabilitation Res. and Development*, 25 (4).

Bernstein, L. (1989). "Computer-based speech training for profoundly hearing-impaired children: Some design considerations," in *Research on the Use of Sensory Aids for Hearing-Impaired Persons*, N. McGorr (Ed.), *Volta Review*, 91(5), 19–28.

de Bot, K. (1983). "Visual feedback of intonation I: Effectiveness and induced practice behavior," *Language and Speech, 26*, 331–350.

Braeges, J., and Houde, R. (1982). "Use of speech training aids," in D. Sims, G. Walter, and R. Whitehear (Eds.), *Deafness and Communication: Assessment and Training*, Baltimore: Williams and Wilkins.

Ferguson, J. B., Bernstein, L.E., and Goldstein, M.H. (1988). "Speech training aids for hearing-impaired individuals, II: Configuration of the Johns Hopkins aids." *Journal of Rehabilitation Research and Development*, 25.

Ferster, C. B. and Skinner, B.F. (1957). *Schedule of Reinforcement*. New York, N.Y.: Appleton-Century-Crofts.

Friedman, S. (1989). "SpeechViewer," Review Supplement, *ASHA 31*, 45.

Fletcher, S. G. (1989). "Visual articulatory training through dynamic orometry," *Volta Review*, 91(5), 47–64.

Kewley-Port, D., Watson, C.S., Maki, D. and Reed, D. (1987). "Speaker-Dependent Speech Recognition as the Basis for a Speech Training Aid." Proc. 1987 IEEE Int. *Conf. Acoustics, Speech and Signal Processing*, Dallas, Texas, 372–375.

Kewley-Port, D., Watson, C.S., Elbert, M., Maki, K., and Reed, D. (1991). "The Indiana Speech Training Aid (ISTRA) II: Training curriculum and selected case studies," *Clinical Linguistics and Phonetics*, 5, 13–38.

Levitt, H. (1971). "Transformed up-down methods in psychoacoustics," *J. Acoust. soc. Am.*, 49, 467–477.

Lippmann, R.P. and Watson, C.S. (1979). "New computer-based speech training aid for the deaf," *J. Acoust. Soc. Am.*, 66, S13.

Lippmann, R.P. (1982). A review of research on speech training aids for the deaf. In N.J. Lass (Ed.), *Speech and language: Advances in basic research and practice*, 7, 105–133. New York; Academic Press.

McGarr, N. S., Youdelman, K. and Head, J. (1989). "Remediation of phonation problems in hearing-impaired children: Speech training and sensory aids," *Volta Review;* in *Research on the Use of Sensory Aid for Hearing Impaired Persons*, N. McGarr (ed.), 91(5), 7–17.

McReynold, L. V. and Kearns, K. P. (1983). *Single-Subject Experimental Designs in Communicative Disorders*. Baltimore: University Park Press.

McReynolds, L. V. and Thompson, C. K. (1986). Flexibility of single-subject experimental designs. Part I: Review of the basics of single-subject designs. *Journal of Speech and Hearing Disorder*, 51, 194–203.

Povel, D. J., and Wansink, M. (1986). "A computer-controlled vowel corrector for the hearing-impaired, "*Journal of Speech and Hearing Research*, 29, 99–105.

Ryalls, J. (1989). "Comparison of two computerized speech training systems: SpeechViewer and ISTRA," *Journal of Speech-Language Pathology and Audiology*, 13(3), 53–56.

Watanabe, A., Ueda, Y. and Shigenaga, A. (1985). "Color display system for connected speech to be used for the hearing impaired," IEEE Trans. Acoustics, Speech and Signal Processing, ASSP-33,164–173.

Watson, C. S., Reed, D., Kewley-Port, D. and Maki, D. (1989). "The Indiana Speech Training Aid (ISTRA) I: Comparisons between human and computer-based evaluation of speech quality," *Journal of Speech and Hearing Research*, 32, 245–251.

Watson, C. S. and Kewley-Port, D. (1989). Computer-based speech training (CBST): Current status and prospects for the future, in *Research on the Use of Sensory Aids for Hearing-Impaired Persons*, N. McGarr (ed.), *Volta Review*, 91(5), 29–45.

Yamada, Y., Murata, N. and Oka, T. (1988). "A new speech training system for profoundly deaf children." *Journal of the Acoustical Society of America*, 84 (Suppl. 1), S43. (Abstract)

8.   Acknowledgments

Our collaborators on the ISTRA project have contributed extensively to the research discussed in this manuscript. The special contributions of Dr. Mary Elbert (Speech Pathology), Dr. Daniel Maki (Mathematics), Patricia Cromer (CCC-SLP, CED), Daniel Reed (M.A., Linguistics) and Ric Houghton (B.S., Computer Sciences) are gratefully acknowledged. Some of this material was presented at the 1989 Annual Meeting of The American Speech-Language Hearing Association, St. Louis, Missouri.

Chapter 22

What Computerized Speech
Can Add to Remedial Reading

Barbara W. Wise and Richard K. Olson
University of Colorado

1. Introduction

Synthetic and digitized speech capabilities for microcomputers have enabled powerful new techniques to be developed for the remediation of reading disabilities. Computer programs can be easily individualized for different children's abilities and interests, can respond with immediate feedback for errors, and are highly motivating to many children. Computers linked to digitized or synthetic speech can have additional benefits for poor readers. They can provide speech support for unknown words, or directions so that disabled readers can enjoy more advanced texts than they could read independently. More importantly, speech support can help remediate the deficits underlying reading disabilities. After a brief discussion of the deficits producing reading disabilities, we will discuss the advantages and disadvantages of different types of computer speech for conducting research about reading disabilities and their remediation. We will conclude with reports of our own ongoing research in this area using synthetic speech linked to microcomputers.

2. What is the Deficit Underlying Reading Disabilities?

Reading disabled children, by definition, have normal intelligence, sensory abilities, and educational background, yet still have difficulty reading. The primary deficit underlying reading disabilities is a subtle and heritable language deficit (Olson et al., 1989; Snowling, 1981) that interferes with the ability to segment speech below the syllable level, making the learning of alphabetic print-to-sound associations difficult. Disabled readers experience problems in segmenting and blending spoken language, in repeating nonsense words aloud, and in reading decodable nonsense words. Older disabled readers are less capable at these tasks than younger normal children matched for ability to read real words (Olson et al., 1989). Prereaders' skill in phonemic segmentation is the strongest predictor of later reading success (Bradley and Bryant, 1983; Lundberg et al., 1980), and this ability correlates with reading performance through twelfth grade (Calfee et al., 1973).

Disabled readers' poor word-decoding skills make most of them dependent on *context* for word identification. Stanovich, (1986) has shown that most disabled readers rely more on context for word identification than good readers do, but they do so with less success. Guessing too much and too inaccurately from context leads them to accept many misread words as if correct. Orthographic segments can then be inappropriately and inconsistently associated with phonologic segments, further depressing phonological skills. For example, a reader who confuses *never, ever, very, even,* and *ever* demonstrates poor print-to-sound associations and also increases the inconsistency of these associations with every misreading. Poor word decoding impedes reading comprehension directly, due to mistakes in the identification of words. It also impedes comprehension indirectly, by demanding so much attention that few resources remain available for comprehension processes.

Training in phonemic segmentation and blending can benefit reading, at least for some children with poor phonological coding skills. Successful outcomes have been found in school-aged readers from preschool training (Bryant and Bradley, 1983; Lundberg, et al., 1988), and from field and experimental interventions after the children have begun reading (Cunningham, 1989; Williams, 1980). Researchers are exploring and comparing different methods of improving phonemic segmentation and blending skills prior to and concurrent with reading instruction, and some of this research uses computers with speech support.

Computers can provide a powerful research tool for comparing instructional methodologies, since they consistently present whatever method has been programmed. Findings from computerized research must be balanced against research with human teachers for generalizability, but comparisons within the computerized methodology should be relatively unconfounded. Computers with speech support can also supply an important instructional methodology, since problems with print-to-sound associations are so central in reading disabilities. Having highly intelligible speech is obviously important, since disabled readers' phonological problems hamper their ability to repeat unfamiliar utterances. Intelligible digitized or synthetic speech can be used to support word recognition in text-reading, freeing attentional resources for higher level skills. Computers that talk can also highlight the relationships between speech segments and consistent printed letter patterns (orthographic segments), and may improve deficient phonological coding skills.

3.   What Digitized Speech Allows

The main advantage of digitized speech over synthetic speech is its high intelligibility. Its disadvantages include high storage requirements and a lack of flexibility. A program with digitized speech must store pronunciations for instructions and for predefined sets of words that developers expect to be difficult. The limitations of storage requirements can be ameliorated by using compressed speech. As storage becomes cheaper, programs will be able to store more speech at a reasonable cost. But the other limitation of digitized speech seems fixed: it can only speak previously pronounced items, making it less flexible. Programs with digitized speech cannot pronounce children's typed in names, nor can they permit interactive writing and hearing of print-to-sound relations with novel or misspelled input. Thus digitized speech may be adequate for providing whole-word speech support for unknown words, enabling poor readers to read age-appropriate amterials accurately and with more resources available for comprehension. However, digitized speech may be less useful for improving decoding skills.

Houghton-Mifflin's commercially available Reading Comprehension series exemplifies the efficient use of digitized speech, delivered through various models of ECHO speech synthesizers. This program provides stories at first- second- and third-grade levels for children to read on Apple and IBM-PC computers. The program provides whole-word support and even definitions for some difficult words, but does not attempt to improve decoding skills. The goal is to free resources for comprehension. However, the program can be frustrating for severely disabled readers, because many words do not have speech support available. If the child requests help on any of these, the program advises, "Please use the context," not always a helpful strategy with words like "someone" and "through." Yet for the child with some, but limited, decoding abilities, this program can provide hours of "independent," speech-supported reading experience.

Some programs use digitized speech to attempt to improve fluency or automaticity in sight word recognition using games (e.g., Hint and Hunt, developed by Roth and Beck, 1987, and available through Developmental Learning Materials, DLM). Roth and Beck also helped develop one of the few programs using digitized speech that does attempt to improve phonological skills. The program uses preprogrammed word segments, and children try to construct as many isolated words as they can within constantly decreasing time limits. Experimental evidence shows that Roth and Beck's programs benefit word recognition and decoding skills among poor readers (Roth and Beck, 1987). Weaknesses of the programs might include that the words are isolated from *context*, and a lack of flexibility since the programs must use prescribed sets of words. Certainly these programs would be inadequate as a total reading curriculum, but that is not their purpose. Instead, they provide good practice in recognizing whole words automatically and in blending word segments.

Important advantages of synthesized over digitized speech for remedial reading programs include its circumvention of storage problems and its greatly increased flexibility, since a speech synthesizer can produce rule-based pronunciations for any letter-string provided by the child or the text. The disadvantage of synthetic speech is lessened intelligibility. The ECHO, for example, is quite intelligible with digitized speech but is painfully unintelligible in its synthetic mode (see below). The creative "Talking Text-Writer" program by Scholastic uses the flexibility of ECHO's synthetic speech to allow children to hear what they are typing in a word-processing program. However, ECHO's poor intelligibility in its synthetic mode makes the program frustrating and inappropriate for disabled readers.

We conducted our own intelligibility tests of speech synthesizers. Greene and Pisoni (1986) reviewed studies of the intelligibility of several text-to-speech synthesizers as compared to natural human speech. They concluded that DECtalk's[1] "Perfect Paul" provided the most intelligible synthetic speech, so we chose to compare that voice to others in our investigations. DECtalk is programmed with correct pronunciations of some 4000 common and exception words. It can also apply text-to-speech phonologic rules to "sound-out" unknown letter strings, and it has its own phonemic code that can be used to code words and word segments phonemically.

Half of our subjects tried to identify Perfect Paul's renditions of isolated words from a list of 96 randomly ordered words, derived from the eighth grade level Spache Oral Reading paragraphs. Half heard the same list pronounced by tape-recorded natural speech (Olson et al., 1986). Adults could identify as many words pronounced by DECtalk (95.8%) as by natural recorded speech (96.1%). Nine disabled readers between eight and

---

[1] DECtalk is a product of Digital Equipment Corporation.

twelve years of age identified slightly fewer of the items pronounced by DECtalk (94.5%) than natural speech (98.4%). It is important to note that the disabled readers' recognition rate for DECtalk was nearly the same as adults'; the significant difference between synthetic and natural speech was because disabled readers did better on natural speech than unimpaired adults did. One could expect even higher identification of words by both groups if identification were aided by spoken or written context.

Subsequently, we used the same paradigm and stimuli to test two other less expensive speech synthesizers, the ECHO-II by Street Electronics and the Smoothtalker by First Byte (Wise et al.,1989). We first tested these with 10 adult subjects, five on each system. Subjects correctly identified only 46% of ECHO-II's and 48% of Smoothtalker's pronunciations of the 96 items. These percentages translate to error rates of 54% and 52%, not significantly different from each other, but more than ten times the 4% error rates with DECtalk. These extremely high error rates led to our decision not to test these systems further with children, nor to use them in our research.

3.1 Short-term Studies with DECtalk Speech Synthesizer

DECtalk's intelligibility, low storage demands, and flexibility make it an ideal tool for studying ways to improve disabled readers' phonological coding and word recognition skills. DECtalk's phonemic coding system has allowed us to present word segments as a "phonics" robot teacher might pronounce them, as in "puh" "ig" = pig. We have examined learning effects from different types of orthographic and speech feedback units, so we have called our system ROSS, for Reading with Orthographic and Speech Segmentation.

DECtalk's ability to present phonemic segments has been used in short-term studies comparing young children's learning of isolated words by whole words or segmented feedback, segmented into syllables, "onset-rhyme" subsyllables, and single phoneme units (e.g., resting, rest/ing, r/est/ing, r/e/s/t/i/ng) (Wise, 1987; Wise, submitted; and see Wise, Olson and Treiman, 1990, for studies comparing different subsyllabic units. See Marcus and Syrdal, Chapter 1 for a discussion of these linguistic units.) Not surprisingly, the children fared by far the worst with the presentation of single phonemes, having difficulty remembering and blending so many segments. The other levels of feedback were roughly equivalent for the children, except that the lowest first-grade readers learned fewer *multisyllabic* words by subsyllables than by presentations of larger units.

We elected to compare the three larger segments in another short-term study where reading-disabled children received feedback for words in the context of meaningful paragraphs (Olson et al., 1986). The children showed significant and approximately equal learning of the words whether they were given whole word, syllable, or subsyllable feedback. Although the benefits of the different feedback conditions were not significantly different in this short-term study, we hypothesized that differences might emerge in a long-term training study, particularly for the development of generalizable phonological coding skills.

3.2 Long-term Studies with ROSS

In our ongoing long-term study, reading-disabled children read stories of interest to them on the computer, asking for speech feedback on difficult words by pointing at the word with a mouse (Wise et al., 1989) The low storage requirements of synthetic speech have allowed us to provide pronunciations, by whole words and by syllables and subsyllables, for every word in a corpus of ten directories of books and stories, with more than 25 stories or books per directory.

Stories were assigned directories from primer through sixth-grade reading levels. Directory placement has been determined mainly by average word length and secondarily by sentence length and story structure considerations, since disabled readers' reading is limited primarily by poor word recognition. After stories were typed in, our staff prepared comprehension questions to be presented every 4-8 pages and coded all new words for segmentation and pronunciation at all levels. This information was stored in a dictionary, so each word was coded only once (Wise et al., 1989). Our dictionary now contains segmentation and pronunciation information for more than 20,000 words.

In the first semester of the project, 48 third- to sixth-grade reading disabled children spent two weeks taking pretests and training on the use of the ROSS system. They then read on the computer 25 minutes a day, 4 or 5 days a week, for eight to nine weeks before taking posttests. They read with the computer during time they would otherwise have spent on reading and language arts instruction. After the training period, the tester returned once a week to monitor progress and change story directory assignments to ensure targeting rates of 1% to 5% of the words. Training and monitoring concentrated on getting the children to ask for help on all missed words, and to pay attention to the presented segments.

When children targeted a word with the mouse, the computer highlighted and then simultaneously highlighted and pronounced the word or its ordered segments. The children were assigned to whole word, syllable, subsyllable, or a combination of subsyllable and syllable feedback conditions. A group of eleven comparison control children were pre- and post-tested, but received only their normal classroom reading and language arts instruction.

The children targeted words 80% as frequently when reading independently as when reading monitored by testers, and they scored only 6% less on computer-scored measures of comprehension. Students, teachers, and parents of trained children overwhelmingly reported positive changes in reading behavior and attitudes about reading. All groups of trained children also made significantly greater gains than the control children on measures of word recognition and phonological coding (at least twice the gain). Students receiving subsyllabic feedback also made significant improvements in nonword reading over the other feedback conditions. This result intrigued us because it suggested that presenting words in segments might specifically benefit phonological coding skills.

In our second phase of the study we eliminated the combination condition, because children did not seem to pay attention to the second pronunciation by syllabic feedback, and thus were spending less time studying each word (Wise and Olson, 1991). We trained 117 students and also tested 38 controls, with the same number of testers. This necessitated a reduction in training and monitoring time, and students' independent performance with the system suffered. Subjects now requested computer-speech feedback only about 40% as often on independent days as on monitored days. The previous intriguing and significant nonword-reading advantage for subsyllabic over other types of feedback was not replicated. However, children who read with the computer still averaged twice the gains of control subjects on measures of word recognition, nonword reading, and comprehension. The second study's lack of a segmentation effect suggests that much of this progress was related to factors common to all trained conditions. Thus, the immediacy of pairing print and sound, the motivational aspects of the computer, and the fact of actually reading for 25 minutes a day with accurate word feedback for difficult words all probably contributed to the gains made by the trained children in both studies.

The failure to replicate the advantage for segmented feedback could indicate that the advantage was a chance result by the eight children in the subsyllabic condition in the first study. However, it could also be a result of the reduced training and the poorer and more passive use of the system by the second phase students. To clarify this possibility, we have improved our training procedures this year, adding explicit instruction in either a whole word contextual strategy or a segmentation and blending strategy. We have also added two games to provide active practice in the use of the strategies, and one game to improve children's awareness of their word recognition errors.

3.3 Taking Advantage of DECtalk's Flexibility

We are also developing other programs that take advantage of DECtalk's ability to apply phonological generalizations to alphabetic text, to allow children to discover for themselves how these generalizations work. We have used one game as a motivator, where children just type in 40-character lines and hear how the synthesizer pronounces them. Students' continuing positive response to this game has lead us to develop a simple children's talking word processor, where children can hear DECtalk's pronunciations of their changing attempts at a word and can use a spell checker to correct spellings.

In another example that capitalizes on the interactive possibilities of synthetic speech, we are currently testing a spelling program where the computer pronounces a word and asks the child to attempt to spell it (Wise, 1990). During training, the computer gives orthographic feedback (three times per word) concerning the correct choice and placement of the letters. For half the training time, the children receive orthographic feedback, hearing speech only for the whole word being attempted, as one could do with digitized or recorded speech.

For the other half of the time in this study, children can request speech feedback for their intermediate attempts at spelling each word. With this feedback, children can discover for themselves, for instance, that "burth," "berth," and "birth" all sound the same, or that a silent e changes the pronunciation of "pan" to "pane." Our hypothesis is that, for all children, intermediate speech feedback will result in greater benefits to spelling and phonologic coding than orthographic feedback alone, due to its greater engagement and information. We expect even greater benefits for intermediate speech feedback over orthographic only feedback for children with initially low phonologic skills, since the program provides the phonological associations that they presumably cannot.

3.4 Limitations of DECtalk

One limitation in using DECtalk is its incapacity for modifying speech signals beyond its phonemic coding symbols. Thus, even though some subjects confuse DECtalk's pronunciation of isolated /h/ with /p/ or isolated /f/ with /v/, there is no way to program more or less frication or voicing in these phonemes. However, learning rates have been high even in our studies of isolated words, indicating this limitation is not crucial. DECtalk's biggest limitation is cost. Many parents of dyslexics and many adult disabled readers have expressed interest in acquiring our programs for home use. However, DECtalk costs $4,000 to individual users and $1600 for public institutions under a Digital Equipment Corporation Grant Program. We are hoping that a computer speech board becomes available that is as flexible and intelligible as DECtalk, but costs closer to the few hundred dollar range of ECHO and Smoothtalker. Then creative programs can be marketed that help children discover print-to-sound relationships and improve their phonological coding skills, enabling more children to become independent readers.

4. References

Bradely, L. & Bryant, P. (1983). Categorizing sounds and learning to read: A causal connection. *Nature*, 301, 419–421.

Calfee, R., Lindamood, P. & Lindamood, C. (1973). Acoustic-phonetic skills and reading: Kindergarten through twelfth grade. *Journal of Educational Psychology*, 64, 293–298.

Cunningham, A. (1989). Phonemic awareness: The development of early reading competency. *Reading Research Quarterly*, 24, 471–472.

Lundberg, I., Frost, J., & Peterson, O. (1988). Effects of an extensive program for stimulating phonological awareness in preschool children. *Reading Research Quarterly*, 23(3), 263–284.

Lundberg, I. Olofsson, A., & Wall, S. (1980) Reading and spelling skills in the first school years, predicted from phonemic awareness skills in kindergarten. *Scandinavian Journal of Psychology*, 21, 159–173.

Olson, R., Foltz, G., & Wise, B. (1986). Reading instruction and remediation with the aid of computer speech. *Behavior Research Methods, Instruments, and Computers*, 18, 93–99.

Olson, R. K., Wise, B., Conners, F., Rack, J. & Fulker, D. (1989). Specific deficits in component reading and language skills: Genetic and environmental influences. *Journal of Learning Disabilities*, 22, 339–348.

Rack, J.P., Snowling, M.J., & Olson, R.K. (in press). The nonword reading deficit in developmental dyslexia: A review. *Reading Research Quarterly*.

Roth, S. & Beck, I. (1987). Theoretical and instructional implications of the assessment of the two microcomputer word recognition programs. *Reading Research Quarterly*, 22, 197–218.

Snowling, M.J. (1981). Phonemic deficits in developmental dyslexia. *Psychological Research*, 43, 219–234.

Stanovich, K. E. (1986). Cognitive processes and the reading problems of learning disabled children: Evaluating the notion of Specificity. In J. K. Torgeson & B. L. Wong (Eds.) *Psychological and educational perspectives on learning disabilities*, New York: Academic Press.

Williams, J.P. (1980). Teaching decoding with an emphasis on phoneme analysis and phoneme blending. *Journal of Educational Psychology*, 72, 1–15.

Wise, B.W. (1987). Word segmentation in computerized reading instruction. Doctoral dissertation.Dissertation Abstracts. University of Colorado, Boulder.

Wise, B.W. (1990). Improving word recognition and phonological coding with a talking computer system. Paper presented at the annual meeting of the American Educational Researchers Association, Boston.

Wise, B.W. (submitted). Whole words and decoding for short-term learning: Comparisons on a "talking-computer" system.

Wise, B.W., & Olson, R.K. (1991). Remediating reading disabilities. In J.E. Obrzut & G.W. Hynd (Eds.), *Neuropsychological foundations of learning disabilities:* New York: Academic Press, 631–658.

Wise, B., Olson, R.K., Anstett, M., Andrews, L., Terjak, M., Schneider, V., Kostuch, J., & Kriho, L. (1989). Implementing a long-term remedial reading study in the public schools: hardware, software, and real world issues. *Behavior Research Methods and Instrumentation*, 21, 173–180.

Wise, B., Olson, R.K., & Treiman, R. (1990). Subsyllabic units in computerized reading instruction: Onset-rime versus postvowel segmentation. *Journal of Experimental Child Psychology*, 49, 1–19.

Chapter 23

Design of a Hearing Screening Test using Synthetic Speech

Corine Bickley[1] and Gerald Kidd, Jr.[2]

1. Introduction

This section describes some considerations involved in the development of a test which uses synthetic speech to screen children for hearing loss. The test we describe does not exist at present. Here we discuss preliminary work that could lead to the development of such a test (Bickley and Kidd, 1989); we acknowledge at the outset, however, that the process of preparing and validating this type of clinical tool is a significant task, and is beyond the scope of this report. A description of some preliminary experimental work which pertains to our project is being written (Kidd, Bickley, and Stevens, 1992).

Currently, the most widely used method of hearing screening is to measure the audibility of pure-tones presented at a fixed level above standard estimates of normal hearing sensitivity (ASHA, 1985). That technique, particularly when coupled with acoustic immittance measures, appears to be effective in identifying preschool and school-age children with auditory disorders (ASHA, 1990).

An interesting alternative to the standard pure-tone screening test has been developed recently by Gosy and colleagues (Gosy et al., 1987). The test they describe uses speech synthesized in the Hungarian language presented in an open-set format via tape recorder at known sound pressure levels. They

---

[1]Sensimetrics Corporation and Massachusetts Institute of Technology

[2]Boston University

analyze the responses of the subjects with regard to the precisely specified acoustic characteristics of the test items using patterns of errors to estimate the hearing sensitivity in various regions of the spectrum. They report remarkably high correlations between pure-tone audiograms and the audiograms derived from their synthetic-speech screening test. They suggest that such a test may be superior to pure-tone tests with young children because of the inherently more interesting nature of the stimulus, an observation that has been often made about speech tests with children (e.g., Martin, 1987). For children who do not respond well to testing methods that use pure tones, a speech-based test might provide more information on hearing loss than would be indicated by pure-tone responses. Also, for children whose pure-tone results would imply a greater hearing loss than is consistent with their ability to understand speech, a hearing test based on synthesized words may provide useful information.

The alternative we are proposing to using pure tones in hearing screening is to use speech stimuli and to ask the child to identify which word was heard. Although speech is inherently more compelling than tones, particularly for hard-to-test populations, there are potential problems with using speech stimuli. One difficulty with using speech materials, especially naturally-produced speech, is that errors in identification can be difficult to relate to standard, frequency-based methods of describing hearing loss (such as an audiogram). This difficulty is due in part to characteristics of naturally-produced sounds: multiple frequency regions carry information that can be used by listeners to distinguish sounds, and redundancies in acoustic cues result. In synthetic speech on the other hand, the difference between two sounds can often be restricted to a limited region of the spectrum while the intelligibility can be maintained. Thus although transformation from percent correct in word identification to an audiogram is not simple, it is somewhat more straightforward for synthetic speech than for naturally spoken words.

Another potential problem with using speech materials is that the linguistic skills of the listener affect his or her ability to identify words. However, a screening procedure that requires certain other competencies (e.g., linguistic or cognitive) could be an advantage: errors inconsistent with a hearing loss could be used as the basis for referral to speech/language evaluation.

We propose to use synthetic speech stimuli instead of naturally-produced words in order to reduce the first difficulty discussed above. It is now possible to synthesize speech materials that are highly intelligible (Klatt,

1980; Klatt and Klatt, 1990) and also appropriate for a hearing screening test. For the purpose of the test it is necessary that the spectral characteristics of the words are precisely controlled in a way that facilitates the interpretation of identification errors with respect to broad classes of hearing loss.

Our approach is basically to choose pairs of words that differ primarily by a single cue that has energy restricted to a limited region of the spectrum. One example of such a pair is /ɪ/ and /æ/, which differ mostly by the frequency of the first formant: approximately 540 Hz for /ɪ/ and 800 Hz for /æ/. Listeners who exhibit a pattern of failing to distinguish between words such as "slip" and "slap," or "tin" and "tan," might have a hearing loss in a region which includes 540 Hz and 800 Hz. Several pairs of contrasting words will be used to test each frequency range.

As a method of response, we have chosen pointing to a graphic representation of the stimulus word. Pointing to pictures is, for most children, a simple and familiar task (Proctor and Bickley, 1988). Responding non-verbally also separates perception abilities from production abilities. It is, however, a complex task, and linguistic, cognitive, visual, and motor skills could affect the ability to point to the correct picture.

As each stimulus word is presented, four pictures are displayed. The stimulus word is represented by one of the pictures and differs from the words that correspond to the other three pictures by only one or two acoustic characteristics. An example quadruplet is "slip," "slap," "flip," and "flap." The words "slip" and "flip" differ from each other in exactly the same way as do "slap" and "flap." The /s/ in the words "slip" and "slap" has more energy in the frequency region above 3000 Hz than does the /f/ in "flip" and "flap." The vowel in the words "slip" and "flip" differs from the vowel in "slap" and "flap" by the frequency of the first formant (F1). Our assumption is that if a child points to the picture representing a word such as "slip" (which is distinguished by high-frequency energy) as often as he selects the picture for a word such as "flip" which is identical in the low- and mid-frequency ranges) when he is presented with one of them is presented then he or she cannot use spectral information above 3000 Hz to distinguish speech sounds. We plan to present several examples of each contrast and to use the pattern of errors to form the basis for our evaluation.

In this chapter, we describe the choice of word sets for the sort of test we have proposed, explain the process of synthesis of these words, show sample pictures of quadruplets of words, and describe the protocol for presentation of the test materials.

2.   Word sets

Each word set consists of four words that are phonetically similar. The words were selected according to two criteria. The first constraint concerns phonetic structure. Each word differs from two others in the set by only a single phoneme (e.g., "sit" *vs.* "sat" and "sit" *vs.* "fit", or "fat" *vs.* "fit" and "fat" *vs.* "sat"). Similar sets of words are utilized in the FAAF hearing test (Foster and Haggard, 1984; Foster and Haggard, 1986). The second requirement is that the words must be common English words that are easily represented by pictures which are recognizable by young children. Four quadruplets meet these requirements are listed in Table 1, along with the corresponding phoneme contrasts.

Table 1:   Sample word sets and corresponding phoneme contrasts

Set	Words	Phoneme contrasts
1	slip, slap, flap, flip	/ɪ/ vs. /æ/, /s/ vs. /f/
2	many, Benny, bunny, money	/ɛ/ vs. /ʌ/, /m/ vs. /b/
3	tin, tan, pan, pin	/ɪ/ vs. /æ/, /t/ vs. /p/
4	tech, deck, duck, tuck	/ɛ/ vs. /ʌ/, /t/ vs. /d/

The contrasting phonemes listed in Table 1 differ primarily by a single cue that has energy restricted to a limited spectral region. Spectral differences between phonemes in a pair which occur outside of the region of primary interest are minimal. In the ideal case, there would be no differences between the phoneme pairs other than those in one region. However, in order to create natural-sounding synthesized words, minor differences in more than one region were necessary. For the differences which exist outside of the primary regions, the energy is substantially lower that the energy in the region of interest.

The frequency spectrum was divided into four regions for the purpose of word set development. Phoneme pairs were selected for each frequency region. Six pairs of phonemes were used to construct the word sets. These pairs are grouped in Table 2 by the frequency region that contains the salient spectral differences. Phonemes were selected to form a contrasting pair if their spectra differed in the region of interest and were similar outside that range.

Table 2: Sample phoneme contrasts and corresponding spectral differences

Frequency region	Phoneme contrast	Spectral difference
very low (0-300 Hz)	/m/ vs. /b/, /d/ vs. /t/	energy vs. no energy
low (300-1000 Hz)	/ɪ/ vs. /æ/	F1 at 540 vs. 800 Hz
mid (1000-3000 Hz)	/ɛ/ vs. /ʌ/	F2 at 2000 vs. 1400 Hz
high (above 3000 Hz)	/s/ vs. /f/, /t/ vs. /p/	more vs. less energy

3. Synthesis of speech material

In order to illustrate the differences between the phoneme pairs listed in Table 2, spectra of the synthesized phonemes are shown in Figures 1 through 4. The spectra were computed near the middle of each phoneme.

Spectra of the synthesized /m/ and /b/ are shown in the first panel of Figure 1. For the /m/, there is low-frequency energy throughout the interval. The /b/, in contrast, is characterized by having no energy in the interval preceding the onset of the vowel. The transitions of the lowest three formants of both the /m/ and the /b/ into the following vowel rise rapidly, with F1 increasing by 290 Hz in 10 ms in both cases, and F2 and F3 each rising 300 Hz in 20 ms in the /m/ and in 10 ms in the /b/. The /b/ was synthesized with no burst. Thus, the salient difference between the /m/ and the /b/ is the presence or absence of very low-frequency spectral components. The spectra of the synthesized /d/ and /t/ in the second panel of Figure 1 show a similar difference: low-frequency energy throughout the closure interval for the /d/, and silence for the /t/ closure.

Differences in the low-frequency range are apparent in the spectra of the synthesized /ɪ/ and /æ/ (see Figure 2). The most significant difference between these spectra is the frequency of the first formant (F1). The overall gain of the samples has been adjusted so that the levels of the first harmonics are comparable (as would be the case for vowels spoken with approximately equal vocal effort). The frequency of F1 of the synthesized /ɪ/ is 540 Hz, and of the synthesized /æ/ is 800 Hz; that is, the major difference between /ɪ/ and /æ/ is contained in the low-frequency (300-

1000 Hz) region. The frequencies of the second and higher formants are the same in /ɪ/ and /æ/, and are the average values of the corresponding formant frequencies in canonical forms of these vowels. The duration and pitch of the vowels have also been neutralized. These changes do not degrade intelligibility significantly because canonical /ɪ/ and /æ/ vowels are similar in spectral shape (except for the frequency of the first formant), duration, and intrinsic pitch. Neutralization of minor differences facilitates the identification of a single acoustic cue (frequency of the first formant) with the discriminability of /ɪ/ and /æ/.

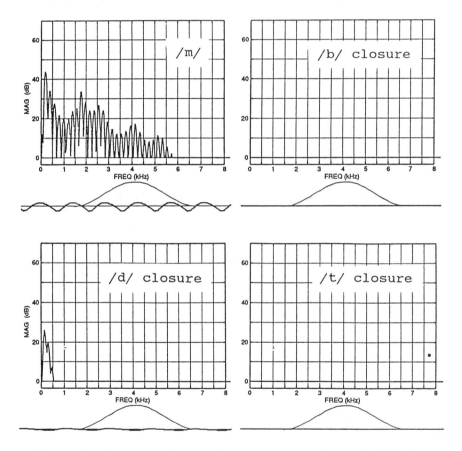

Figure 1: Spectra and waveform segments of sounds differing primarily in the very low-frequency region (0-300 Hz). The upper panels contrast /m/ and the closure interval for /b/. The lower panels contrast the closure intervals for /d/ and /t/.

Spectra of the synthesized /ɛ/ and /ʌ/ are shown in Figure 3. The vowels /ɛ/ and /ʌ/ differ in the mid-frequency region (1000-3000 Hz); ɛ has a second formant frequency (F2) of 2000 Hz while the F2 of /ʌ/ is 1400 Hz. The differences between /ɛ/ and /ʌ/ outside of the mid-frequency range have been neutralized. Thus, the frequencies of the first formant and the third and higher formants are the same in /ɛ/ as in /ʌ/. The duration and pitch were also neutralized.

Two phoneme pairs were chosen for the high-frequency contrast: /s/ vs. /f/ and /t/ vs. /p/. Spectra for the synthesized /s/ and /f/ differ most significantly in the region above 3000 Hz: the level of the spectrum of the /s/ is as much as 25 dB higher than that of the /f/ in this region. The differences between the /s/ and /f/ spectra in the region below 3000 Hz are minimal. The spectra of the alveolar sounds are characterized by a pre-dominance of high-frequency energy, while the labial sounds exhibit (at least in the sample shown) relative predominance of low-frequency energy. The spectra of these four sounds are shown in Figure 4. The formant transitions from the initial consonant into the following vowel and the phoneme durations were neutralized for the /s/ and /f/, and for the /t/ and /p/.

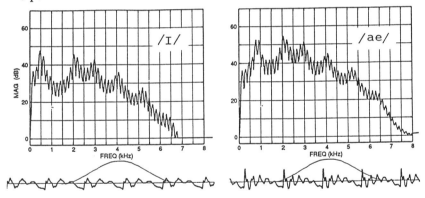

Figure 2: Spectra and waveform segments of sounds differing primarily in the low-frequency region (300-1000 Hz). A spectrum computed near the middle of the vowel /ɪ/ is shown at the left, and that of /æ/ is shown at the right.

All of the synthesized words are identical in acoustic characteristics that do not serve to contrast phonemes. For instance, the fundamental frequency contour of each vowel is the same: an initial value of 196 Hz, followed by a fall of 39 Hz in 105 ms, then a fall of 7 Hz in 45 ms, and a final steady value of 150 Hz for the last 50 ms. Initial and final voiced consonants were synthesized with a steady fundamental frequency equal to the initial and final value of the vowel, respectively.

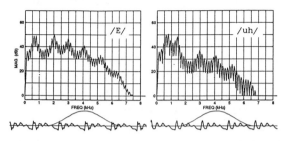

Figure 3: Spectra and waveform segments of sounds that differing primarily in the mid-frequency region of 1000-3000 Hz. A spectrum computed near the middle of the vowel /ɛ/ is shown at the left, and that of /ʌ/ is shown at the right.

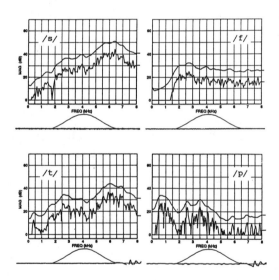

Figure 4: Spectra and waveform segments of sounds differing primarily in the high-frequency region (above 3000 Hz). The upper panels contrast /s/ and /f/. The lower panels contrast the closure intervals for /p/ and /t/. See text for discussion.

Another way in which the words are similar is duration. The length (in ms) of each synthesized phoneme is listed in Table 3. The durations are the average values of the durations of the two phonemes in each contrasting pair. The individual vowel and fricative durations are the values reported by Klatt (in preparation) for the Klattalk synthesizer. For stop and nasal consonants, the durations are the average values of the durations of several repetitions of the phoneme. Because the durations of each phoneme in a contrasting pair are equal, the four words in each quadruplet are identical in total duration.

Table 3: Phoneme durations

Phoneme pair	Duration (in ms)
/ɪ/ and /æ/	200
/ɛ/ and /ʌ/	155
/s/ and /f/	200
/m/ and /b/	80
/t/ and /d/	240
/t/ and /p/	240

Other ways in which the words are similar are sampling rate, frequencies of the higher formants, and formant bandwidths. The sampling rate for all of the words is 15 kHz. The frequencies of the fourth, fifth, and sixth formants are 4060, 5220, and 6830 Hz, respectively. These values were calculated from an estimate of formant spacing, based on an average vocal-tract length for a female talker. The formant bandwidths are listed in Table 4.

Table 4: Formant bandwidths

Formant number	Bandwidth (in Hz)
1	100
2	200
3	300
4	350
5	400
6	600

The synthesized speech materials were evaluated through informal listening tests during the development of the quadruplets. The words were refined until they were easily identified by normally-hearing listeners.

4.   Screening protocol

We propose designing a test with synthesized speech items that are presented auditorily at a fixed sound pressure level. On each trial the child would hear the test word and would see four response alternatives displayed as illustrations on a computer screen. We are assuming that children are sufficiently familiar with the words and pictures to associate each synthesized word with the corresponding picture. An example of a set of pictures is shown in Figure 5. The upper-left corner shows a "slap" and the upper-right sketch represents "slip." The lower panels correspond to the words "flip" and "flap."

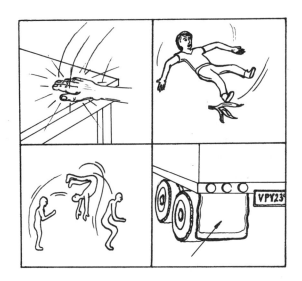

Figure 5:   Graphic representations of the words "slap," "slip," "flip," and "flap."

A second example of pictures of quadruplets is shown in Figure 6. The words are "tin," "pin," "pan," and "tan."

We recognize that validation of such a test is a significant problem, and will require the testing of many children with a large number of synthesized words and computer images. One potential difficulty in this project is to find enough words that fit the constraints of audiometric testing and which are known to children, and also to find associated pictures that are illustrative and are also recognized by the children. Finding words that are in the vocabularies of children, are equally discriminable at some level of presentation, and are equally and highly intelligible given the synthesis scheme will be challenging. In order to find appropriate pictures, we anticipate drawing on resources such as existing picture-based articulation tests. Although these pictures are usually presented in printed form, not *via* a computer screen, the numerous sources of pictures will be a valuable reference in our work.

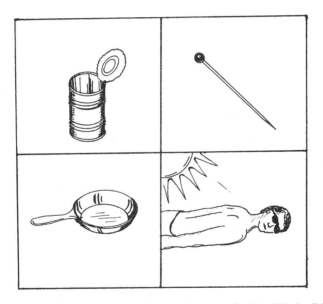

Figure 6: Graphic representations of the words "tin," "pin," "pan," and "tan."

The computer-based mode of presentation and response affords the opportunity for creative reinforcement strategies which may be particularly useful with children who are otherwise difficult to test. The success of recent efforts to include video-game-style computer graphics in psychophysical tests of children (e.g., Allen et al., 1989) would appear encouraging in this regard.

The test strategy requires a sufficient number of items to test different frequency regions with confidence. Not knowing the variability that we will encounter with testing of this sort, we plan initially to use a set of 40 words (we chose this number arbitrarily), which would yield ten estimates in each of four frequency regions. We plan to address the problem of attention span (will children pay attention to 40 words?) and the trade-offs between using a larger set of words (hopefully to decrease the variability) and a smaller set (to increase the ease of administration) during test validation. After locating 40 words and associated pictures that can be reliably identified by normally-hearing children, we will need to pair the images with words and to validate high intelligibility of the words and high recognition of the pictures. Our goal is to estimate the normal variability from testing with a small set of words, and then to develop an adequately comprehensive set of test items.

By using 40 word-picture pairs, we will be able to use statistical methods to establish baseline performance for normally-hearing children and also to determine standard deviations from average performance. These results will form the basis for a pass/fail criterion for hearing-impaired children.

During hearing screening, results would be obtained at two levels: pass/ fail and failure errors. A fail on a test of this sort would most likely be used to indicate simply that the child should be tested further. The proposed test is not anticipated to eliminate the need for further testing. It is hoped though that patterns of failure errors will form a basis for identifying broad classes of hearing loss.

The frequency regions chosen for this test do not map directly to the frequencies tested in a standard audiological test, even a simple screening test. The regions were selected on the basis of characteristics of the speech stimuli. The frequency regions correspond to ranges in which a difference in energy serves to differentiate a pair of sounds in English. Some of the regions (such as the 1000—3000 Hz range and the region above 3000 Hz) cover more than one of the frequencies used in standard pure-tone testing. In contrast, the very low region of 0—300 Hz is often not tested in standard screening methods because high false positive rates tend to result due to low-frequency environmental noise encountered in typical testing situations.

Our test would give a sort of four-point audiogram. The question remains of how to quantify the acoustic energy in each frequency region, and how to compare overall energies in terms of durations and bandwidths. One substantial advantage of our test is the precise control over the temporal and spectral characteristics of the stimuli that is possible with synthesized speech. Thus, it is theoretically possible to determine a true energy function with respect to percent correct responses. A sort of average could be used to determine a threshold performance, with some sort of weighting scheme. We recognize, though, that the results of any psychometric test can be noisy. We might be limited to using simply the pass-fail information in each of the four frequency regions, and might not be able to reduce these numbers to psychometric functions or thresholds. Our results would then indicate only the frequency regions for which a child passed or failed.

5. Summary

We have synthesized words that are distinguished by the energy in a limited region of the spectrum and are highly discriminable. A hearing screening test has been designed using these synthesized stimuli and a test protocol has been worked out.

We plan to relate errors in identification of the synthesized words to hearing loss in one or more of four frequency bands. We are currently investigating the accuracy with which we can predict audiograms from errors in identification of words in the sort of screening test we have described in this chapter.

6. Acknowledgments

This project is based substantially on ideas of Professor Ken Stevens. His contributions are gratefully acknowledged. The sketches were prepared by Kevin Brown, and are greatly appreciated. Portions of this work were supported by grants #R01DC00597 and #IR43NS26979-01 from the National Institute on Deafness and other Communication Disorders.

7. References

Allen P., Wightman, F., Kistler, D. and Dolan, T. (1989). Frequency resolution in children, *J. Sp. Hear. Res.*, 32, 317–322.

American Speech-Language-Hearing Association (1988). Guidelines for identification audiometry, *ASHA*, 27, 49–52.

American Speech-Language-Hearing Association (1990) Guidelines for screening for hearing impairments and middle ear disorders, *ASHA*, Vol. 32, Suppl 2, 17–24.

Bickley, C. and Kidd, G. (1989) Synthetic speech audiometry, *J. Acoust. Soc. Am.*, Suppl. 1, Vol. 86, S49 (Abstract).

Eagles, E. L., Wishik, S. M., Doefler, L. G., Melnick, W. and Levine, H. S. (1973) Hearing sensitivity and related factors in children, *Laryngoscope*, 73 Monograph Suppl.

Foster, J. R. and Haggard, M. P. (1984) *Introduction and Test Manual for FAAF II: The Four Alternative Auditory Feature Test* Nottingham [Great Britain]: MRC Institute for Hearing Research, IHR Internal Report Series B; No. 11–38.

Foster, J. R. and Haggard, M. P. (1986). The Four Alternative Auditory Feature Test—A general-purpose test with multiple special-purpose application and subscores, *Proceedings of the Institute of Acoustics*, Vol. 8, Part 7, 167–174.

Gòsy, M., Olasky, G., Hirschberg, J. and Farkas, Z. (1987). Phonetically based new method for audiometry: The G-O-H measuring system using synthetic speech, *Proceedings of the 11th International Congress of Phonetic Sciences*, Tallinn, Estonia, August 1–7, Volume 3, 185–188.

Kidd, G., Bickley, C. and Stevens, K.N. (1991). Discrimination of synthesized speech in quiet and in filtered noise, in preparation.

Klatt D. (1980). Software for a cascade/parallel formant synthesizer, *J. Acoust. Soc. Am.*, 67, 971–995.

Klatt, D. H. and Klatt, L. C. (1990) Analysis, synthesis and perception of voice quality variations among female and male talkers, *J. Acoust. Soc. Am.*

Klatt, D. H. (in preparation) *Acoustic-Phonetic Characteristics of American English.*

Martin, F. N. (1987). Speech test with preschool children, in *Hearing Disorders in Children*, F. N. Martin, (Ed.) Austin, TX: Pro-Ed.

Pisoni, D. B., Nussbaum, H. C., and Greene, B. G. (1985) Perception of synthetic speech generated by rule, *Proc. IEEE* 73, 1665–1676.

Proctor, A. and Bickley, C. (1988). Elicitation of spontaneous speech production from pre school-age tactile aid users, Journal of Acoustical Society of America, 83, S66. (Abstract)

Chapter 24

Speech Technology in Interactive Instruction

D.G. Bouwhuis
The Institute for Perception Research
IPO Eindhoven, Netherlands

1. Introduction

"If only this thing could speak!" is a frequent lament of beginning users of a complex system. But even without stressing the subtle difference between talking and speaking, a system that could only speak would not seem to be a system that could also talk. Talking implies some sort of conversation, a kind of turn-taking dialogue, and a dialogue implies some common knowledge and mutual understanding (Taylor, Néel and Bouwhuis, 1989). In order to speak in a meaningful way, the complex system should have some understanding and knowledge that it shares with the user, and its knowledge about the user should develop in accordance with the evolving dialogue. In most dialogue systems to date, along with various as yet unsolved problems with real-time speech recognition, context modeling, or answer generation, it is mostly unclear how this common and dynamic knowledge base could be implemented. Fortunately, this problem is significantly less serious in instructional systems for various reasons.

First, in instruction it is natural to assume that the teacher or the instructional system is the holder of knowledge, while the student is to acquire that knowledge. This fact fixes the global intention of the instructional dialogue. Further, the asymmetry in knowledge ordinarily induces a type of dialogue in which the teaching party may give explicit instructions to the learning party, whose intention it is to satisfy those instructions. There is nothing uncommon about this basically asymmetric relationship. It is like, for example, information dialogues in which the information sought may not be entirely available from the information provider, while the information seeker may know many details that the provider will nevertheless communicate (Beun, 1989). The instruction dialogue even seems to contradict a number of generally accepted spoken communication principles known as the Gricean principles (Searle, 1969): be brief, be informative, be relevant, etc. On the contrary, instruction may be very repetitive, singularly uninformative, or may ask questions that are completely independent of the dialogue context.

The upshot of this comparison is that it is much simpler to devise a spoken dialogue system for instruction than for many other purposes, if the dialogue is to be taken seriously by the user. Actually instruction is one of the very few dialogues where it is not strictly necessary that the student replies verbally. A relevant indication of skill acquisition may be sufficient, and may even be preferable to words. Good examples of this are musical performance, sports, games, and motor skills in general.

2. Knowledge versus Skill

Not everything we learn can be termed knowledge. While many fragments of natural languages may be described by formal systems, and so may be called declarative knowledge, by far the greater part of our daily-life language proficiency evolved by overlearning and rote learning, by drill and practice. That is why we know our language by heart[1]; most of it is completely automatized and resists rational explanations of its logic. Sentences just sound good or look right, while a reasoned judgment about them requires time and cognitive effort. It is especially in tasks involving plain skill development, where repeated presentations are necessary, that it is fairly straightforward to design and implement an appealing speech interface for instructional systems.

It is useful to analyze a few properties of spoken instruction that make it preferable to other modes of presentation. By its temporal nature, the speech signal gives evidence of its localized presence in time. By contrast, a screen-displayed verbal instruction appears at one moment in time and stays there. Spoken instruction is delineated much more as a punctuated event, inviting a response or turn-taking reaction, whereas visual instruction may even go unnoticed when the student does not pay attention to its position or appearance. Information dialogues proceed in a very different way when performed by spoken interaction than by keyboard and display

---

1. Knowing something 'by heart' derives in fact from a medieval translation of the French 'par cœur', that was misspelled for 'par chœur'. "Par chœur' (chœur = chorus) referred to chanting or pronouncing collectively expressions to be learned in drill sessions. Unfortunately, the French made the same mistake as the English.

interaction. Specifically, in keyboard-display interactions, waiting times are far longer, corrections of errors are omitted, and partners spend much more time in formulating a considered response. Yet interruptions are frequent, as are sudden topic shifts (Beun, 1989). Speech seems to invite a much more interactive dialogue with close temporal cohesion; in a sense it has a more demanding or inviting character.

A further important advantage of speech over writing, print or graphic display is that not every learner can read. Young children in general are not fluent readers, or may lack the ability altogether. Furthermore, the graphic instructions cannot nearly compensate for absence of verbal instructions due to lack of expressive power and inherent ambiguity.

There is one more subtle argument in favor of auditory *versus* visual instruction. A spoken instruction can, by temporal structure, intonation and accentuation, bring out the intended meaning more clearly and less ambiguously than a visual message. Also tone of voice may be adapted much more flexibly and effectively to the task and to the learner, who may be lacking in initiative. One final advantage is that speech is a very natural component of a multimodal interface. Having, for example, visual items pointed out by other visual items is in general clumsy and causes unwanted visual clutter. By its different modality and expressive power, speech is well suited to act as a message channel in multimodal interfaces. And, unlike most channels of such an interface, speech leaves no trace of its presence once it has been pronounced. It does not sit there obstructing other information sources.

These properties of speech communication may well be less relevant in the acquisition of declarative knowledge, for example, geographical facts and grammatical and morphological rules. There considerable time may be needed for problem solving, calling for a much less interactive, but perhaps much more intelligent interface. Also, students may require a much longer exposure time to learning material in order to consult it repeatedly for full comprehension. Written text seems to have the edge there. The learner can go through the text at his or her own pace, and interrupt or repeat at will. Such flexible access is much harder to realize in listening to spoken text; interruptions are usually unambiguous, but not always easy to implement. Access to arbitrary portions of the spoken text and changes in speech rate are very hard to implement in an unambiguous form to the learner.

While for a number of learning applications the instruction may well be in graphic form, there are many situations in which the actual learning material could be spoken. This is most obvious in language training, where all language material can in principle be in speech form, and it is almost a necessity for tasks involving pronunciation or prosody. Stored or coded speech may function essentially like tape-recorded sound, except that it is far more flexible. Further advantages of employing prestored speech are covered elsewhere in this volume (Schmandt, Chapter 11; Wise and Olson, Chapter 22).

3. Spoken Instruction

In skill training the same material must be presented over and over again. Likewise, corresponding instructions are also of a repetitive nature, and variation in style and content is almost a necessity. When system output takes place by means of short graphic messages, say one or two words, this is seen as a necessary and formal, but nevertheless reliable minimum of information reflecting the limited communicative capability of that system. If output is given in spoken form, so far an almost exclusively human feature, this suggests a far greater communicative capability than actually can be provided. Any shortcomings will be matched against regular human speech communication and become quite conspicuous in comparison. For synthetic or coded speech a number of shortcomings can be distinguished.

3.1 Intelligibility
This is a much-studied variable in speech synthesis. It becomes important in situations where there is little redundancy, and listener action depends critically on speech understanding. Intelligibility is not the ultimate requirement however. Although even human speech is not always intelligible, it is generally understandable. If intelligibility is lower than optimal, much can be improved by increasing message redundancy, or even by making repetition possible.

3.2 Naturalness
This variable has only recently attracted interest, inasmuch as it is harder to establish formal criteria to assess it, and it seems to be rather subjective. Nevertheless it is probably the most important variable, as it relates directly to acceptability. Even if naturalness, or rather unnaturalness, is very easy to identify, it is hard to connect it unambiguously with physical or phonetic properties of the speech signal. The following characteristics may frequently create problems with naturalness.

- Bad temporal structure, both within words and between words

- Speech signal distortion, like buzzing, whistles, noise bursts, and quantization noise

- Inappropriate Phoneme coloring, especially in vowel sounds

- Discontinuities, mostly caused by sudden amplitude changes from one speech segment to another

- Overcontiguity, by which is meant that different synthetic speech sounds can follow each other so fast that they seem to emanate from two or more different speakers

- Incorrect stress

- Incorrect pronunciation

- Breathlessness, which impression arises from the fact that synthetic speech does not need any breathing pauses[2]

3.3 Identical Repetition

No human is able to exactly reproduce a speech utterance; so, whenever a synthetic utterance has any specific phonetic properties, they will gradually become recognized and expected by the listener who will consider this as limited communicative capability. Moreover, one particular utterance will always express the same thing in the same words. This also will not escape the listener and will certainly reduce intrinsic motivation in due time.

If there is any clear recommendation for speech presentation, be it synthetic or coded per sentence, it is that presentations could be short, and never exceed a few sentences, or perhaps even one sentence at a time. Unnaturalness, for example in irregular temporal structure, requires considerable cognitive effort to understand the message, or may be a reason for rejection altogether. In the latter case the listener is not prepared to accept the subjectively suboptimal system as a partner in the interaction.

The acceptability range for synthetic speech varies enormously among individuals. It may be taken for granted that speech researchers have the least difficulty in accepting synthetic speech of whatever quality. Interestingly , children, from say 6-12 years of age, after a short period of habituation, seem not to be particularly bothered by even low-quality speech . In

---

2. It is remarkable that a silent breathing pause, the easiest speech component to synthesize, and that increases naturalness considerably, has not received any serious attention by speech researchers.

general, they are remarkably accepting and prepared to listen intently to even malformed instructions, while at the same time their teachers may find the speech quality definitely unsuitable for children. In trying to introduce equipment with moderately automated speech output into schools or other educational establishments, it may well be found that adults are far more reluctant than children, or even downright opposed to the technology, while their children are happily rehearsing away.

4.   Instruction, Presentation and Feedback

In the following section the use of speech technology for instruction will be illustrated by an example from computer-based reading instruction for initial readers in the first grade. Such a system was developed at the Institute for Perception Research/IPO at Eindhoven in the years 1984-1989 and was called the "Reading Board." A full description can be found in Reitsma (1988), and Spaai and Ellermann (1990).

The instruction points out to the pupil which action should be performed. The action is one which can be performed on the basis of knowledge acquired during the interaction. The instruction may mention an item to be learned, but, in principle, concentrates on the action. In the Reading Board this will always be a pointing action, either by manually touching the screen positions where relevant items are displayed, or by selecting screen positions by means of the mouse. Presentation is the pronunciation of an item to be learned. An example of simple presentation is the situation in which a sentence is displayed and the pupil can point to one word, which is then pronounced by the system. There is no instruction needed, and the pupil can have any word pronounced at will. The word sound production may also be system-initiated, which is a form of self-contained tutoring. Much more often system-initiated presentation will be part of the instruction, for example in the sentence "Now point to the 'm'!", where the carrier segment 'Now point to the' is the action-defining instruction, and the argument 'm' is the presentation. The distinction between instruction and presentation is far from academic; the point is that the instruction is redundant, while the presentation is not. An instruction part can be expanded, varied, shortened, or paraphrased, but will always be expected as a specific, well-known action to be performed, and the action is always similar within an exercise. It is in principle, however, impossible to expand on the item to be learned, and it is also one of many possible items in the exercise. This strong difference in redundancy relates directly to intelligibility requirements. In general, intelligibility enforces increased memory size for sound production which may be impossible or difficult in the application. But also, increased memory usage will slow down operating speed and limit the rate of interactivity. Ultimately, it may even lead to unwanted gaps in speech sound production.

Feedback, finally, relates to the spoken information telling the pupil whether or not the action was correct. Like instruction, feedback may also encompass presentation. Take the example where a child has pointed at the letter 'b' on the screen. As soon as the child selects that position by clicking the mouse, a rectangle is drawn around it in order to show immediate graphic feedback as acknowledgment. The spoken feedback that follows then might say: "No, that is incorrect. This is the 'b'." (The rectangle around the 'b' now disappears and reappears around the letter 'm.') "This is correct. This is the 'm'!" Here there are two presentations, that could be considered system-initiated tutoring. Again, the carrier sentences can be redundant, while the learning items pronounced are not. Yet they should be highly intelligible when the child has shown a lack of knowledge concerning two items.

5. Speech Storage and Production

Speech sound production can proceed by employing two different methods: pre-stored speech (coded in some way) or speech synthesis. In each of the main categories various methods may be employed, each with its specific advantages and disadvantages. For instructional training systems important requirements are:

- speed of response
- controllable intelligibility
- pre-established temporal structure
- prosodic continuity
- limited on-line memory
- real time operation
- reliability
- upgrades and modifications.

Each of these requirements will be discussed below in connection with particular speech production methods.

5.1 Speed of Response

System response speed should fully reflect interactivity to the learner. A response by the system that is felt by the user to be 'immediate' should follow a learner's physical action by approximately 200 ms. Longer latencies lead the subject to believe that his or her action was not registered properly, causing the learner to perform the action again. In some situations one may get around the problem by giving immediate feedback with graphic information that is followed in due time by the speech sound. Nevertheless, a time lapse exceeding one second gives the impression of a very slow and unresponsive system. Unfortunately, time delay is confounded with type of feedback. If the learner action is wrong, initial absence of feedback may already signal that it will be negative. When, however, the learner action is correct, and positive feedback is not immediate, it may suggest an error, lack of responsivity or even limited system knowledge concerning the task. Tardy response will be especially obtrusive when, in the course of the training, ever more correct actions are performed, but are not matched by a corresponding increase in responsivity of the system. In order to shorten waiting time it may be possible to segment the speech message into two parts, a short informative leader, and a more detailed feedback message that comes after some time needed to fetch it from its memory location, or for speech synthesis.

5.2 Controllable Intelligibility

Controllable intelligibility does not mean that the intelligibility of a spoken message should be adjustable on-line, but rather that the intelligibility level of the potential speech messages should be known beforehand. It is hazardous to compose on-line messages whose intelligibility is not well known or predictable, since unintelligible instructions, presentations or feedback would arrest the instructional dialogue. Nevertheless, it may be attractive to employ redundant and relatively frequent speech messages with less than optimal intelligibility if in this way memory requirements can be reduced.

5.3 Pre-established Temporal Structure

Temporal structure will usually be well preserved in coded speech but may be somewhat unnatural in many kinds of synthesized speech. In general, instructional messages contain many common words—so many, in fact, that it becomes attractive to store the different components and to assemble the different messages from them. This reduces memory requirements to a considerable extent as well as speeds up memory search. In assembling such messages a very strict temporal output control is needed in order to attain a natural flow of speech. As the speech files in such a case are handled sequentially by the operating system that also performs a range of other operations in between, fine tuning is always needed to obtain natural timing. It turns out that hardware upgrades, new operating systems and even new software releases can disastrously affect the temporal structure. So while the extreme memory requirements of high quality coded speech can be reduced significantly by speech message assembly, timing remains a refractory problem. It ought to be possible to control the timing of word production on the basis of a pre-established program. This is a practice not realistically possible in cost-effective systems for instruction.

5.4 Prosodic Continuity

In constructing the separate speech segments that are used in composing the messages in an assembly type of speech production system, special care must be taken in order to preserve prosodic continuity in the assembled sentences. Let us take the following example: A feedback message may be assembled from, say, five segments: (1) "No, that is incorrect," (2) "This is the,"(3) "b." (4) "Here is the," (5) "d." Each of the five segments will have been pronounced by the speaker on separate occasions and not in the same temporal order. That means that in most cases there will not be an exact match between the pitches and amplitudes of any consecutive segments. As a consequence the assembled sentence may sound markedly awkward, some segments being pronounced at an audibly higher or lower pitch. Also speech rate during pronunciation may vary and be noticeably different during portions of the final production. Even tone of voice, implying nervousness, determination, etc., may vary from one set of segments to another and give rise to strange sequences of speech. If for some reason a number of speech segments from one speaker must be re-recorded, many features may change in the process. Usually the reason for the new recordings are communicated to the speaker, who may well react by overcorrection. In this way a slow speech rate may become too fast, or a high pitch unacceptably low. As there are usually quite a number of carrier sentences, as well as item names, it is very complicated to devise a recording management system that guarantees proper continuity of all conceivable messages. The use of professional speakers is currently the best way to minimize problems of this kind.

5.5 Limited On-line Memory

Despite its linearly decreasing price over the years (with occasional hiccups), memory remains one of the most capital-intensive parts of a learning system. It is not uncommon to find that memory size practically dictates the method of speech production, in the sense that when memory is limited, economically coded speech must be used. This entails almost invariably some kind of LPC coding which, in turn, requires the use of pre-stored speech. But as the number of potential messages goes up, so does the required memory size. In this respect, an interesting variation on LPC coding is the use of diphone synthesis (Elsendoorn, 1984; for a general discussion, see Syrdal, Chapter 3, on text-to-speech synthesis). In this method not entire sentences are coded and stored, but just the set of transitions from the middle of one phoneme to the middle of the next one. Words and sentences are formed by concatinating consecutive diphones. In this way the only speech material that has to be stored is the set of diphones that covers the phoneme transitions in the language fragment employed. With these building blocks arbitrary messages can be synthesized while having a fixed memory size. Such a system also needs a rule system describing phonological rules for converting text to speech, or rather graphemes to phonemes. In addition, an exception vocabulary must be added for cases that do not conform to standard rules; proper names and foreign words are clear examples of items in an exception vocabulary. In order to produce natural sounding speech, sentence intonation and temporal structure must be provided by prosody grammars that currently exist for a few languages, notably Dutch, British English and German, as used by the IPO diphone synthesis system (Hart, Cohen & Collier, 1991). Empirical evaluation trials show that the prosodic structure obtained in this way is quite acceptable for single sentences at least (Terken & Collier, 1989; Deliege et al., 1989). Despite the considerable progress made in the field of diphone synthesis, the overall speech quality is not as high as might be desirable in many instructional situations, while sometimes intelligibility on the word level may be a limiting factor.

A very attractive way of substantially increasing on-line memory is the use of CD-memory like CD-ROM or, more recently, CD-Interactive, or CD-I for short (Preston, 1988). Total memory size amounts to some 600 Mbytes. For CD-I the default speech capacity is about one hour of hi-fi stereo speech. By using both channels for mono speech signals, capacity can effectively be doubled, and additional increases can be obtained by reducing the sampling bandwidth of the recorded speech, yielding a total duration of 16 hours. Even at the lowest sampling rate, speech quality is noticeably better than the best obtainable synthesized speech, even if it sounds clearly band-limited.

5.6   Real-time Operation

Real-time operation is of course closely related to response speed, but it is not the same thing. Even when real-time operation cannot be attained, the response of the system to a user action can still be instantaneous, although perhaps not complete pending search and computation time. In my experience, speech synthesis systems almost always require noticeable waiting times even for the synthesis of short utterances, and the corresponding delay may reduce perceived interactivity considerably. When using PCM coded speech residing on magnetic memory, search time may take unpredictable idle times. The biggest and cheapest memory system, the CD-I, has an on-line throughput of 170 kbytes per second, which is in fact a stereo audio bandwidth, so that information can only be loaded at a limited speed. While information residing on tracks neighboring the current one may be accessible almost instantaneously, information further away may take waiting times of the order of a second or more before it can be produced. Theoretically the maximum waiting time due to electromechanical operations is 1.5 seconds. These waiting times essentially form a random distribution, albeit with a guaranteed maximum, and so are very difficult to anticipate or to control in the interface management system. With the CD-I system, however, it is possible to buffer contiguous speech segments in advance, so that they are cocatenated seamlessly at production time. Onset of the speech string is then slightly delayed because of the buffering.

Another interesting way around the undesirable waiting time is to mimic more or less human conversation. Beun (1989) found that in face-to-face spoken dialogues humans generally try to avoid silent periods, unlike dialogues with keyboard and display. Frequently humans intersperse these periods with vapid remarks such as "Well," "ehh," or "okay," announcing an utterance coming up. As these are always short words, they could easily be produced on-line in an interactive speaking system with some memory space exclusively dedicated for short interjections. The moments at which these utterances should be produced is a matter of empirical research. This issue points also to the need for close temporal tracking of both learner actions and system response, which should be essentially independent of the overhead involved with the running application.

5.7   Reliability

Reliability is a solved problem from the manufacturer's point of view, but not from the teachers' and learners' point of view. In a sense an instructional system will always put the learner in a more dependent position than most other applications. Frequently the learner also knows less about the instructional system than a professional user about his software application and computer platform. Hang-ups and bugs will therefore have a rather negative effect on the learner's attitude towards the system. Since learners are usually not at all restricted to computer-based instructional systems, unreliability has a devastating impact on acceptance. Even if learners themselves still accept the system, those involved with system management and faced with maintenance or external repair will tend to withdraw it from use. To make matters worse, during speech output, which involves the transfer of large quantities of data at a high data rate and is therefore prone to all kinds of interference and errors, every irregularity is immediately audible. Speech-output hardware and software are not yet so robust that unsupervised correct operation may be expected for extended periods. In evaluation trials conducted for the Reading Board project at elementary schools, an experiment rarely could be completed without at least one equipment failure or program bug, and even the results of an experiment involving a number of instructional systems operated during several consecutive weeks was entirely lost by as yet undiscovered bugs. Successful introduction of instructional systems with speech output might critically hinge on reliability of operation rather than on other advanced features.

5.8 Upgrades and Modification

Perhaps it should not come as a surprise that as soon as learners and teachers are confronted with natural and flexible speech output in an instruction application the desire arises to add other speech messages or remove some of the existing ones. It would go too far here to describe all the technical details involved, but invariably any addition of speech material runs into the kinds of problems that have been alluded to above. Interestingly, similar remarks concerning the modifiability of books are never heard. Although teachers may be able to produce their own reading material or graphics as they see fit, they seldom do. For example, standard commercial versions of simple teaching aids, like flash cards or letter boards are generally used. Putting these issues aside, the need for modifications of the course and improvements in speech quality calls for a software platform that is sufficiently flexible and maintainable to tolerate them at no great expense of programming cost. In this respect instructional systems do not behave differently from other complex software applications, but they are certainly no better.

6. References

Beun, R.J. (1989). The Recognition of Declarative Questions. Doctoral thesis, University of Tilburg.

Deliege, R.J.H., Speth-Lemmens, I.M.A.F. and Waterham, R.P. (1989). Development and preliminary evaluation of two speech communication aids. *Journal of Medical Engineering and Technology*, 13, 18–22.

Elsendoorn, B.A.G. (1984). Heading for a diphone speech synthesis system for Dutch. *IPO Annual Progress Report*, 19, 32–35.

't Hart, J., Cohen, A., and Collier, R. (1991). *A perceptual study of intonation.* Cambridge: Cambridge University Press.

Preston, J.M. (1988). *Compact Disc-Interactive: A Designer's Overview*, Deventer: Kluwer Technical Books.

Reitsma, P. (1988). Reading practice for beginners: Effects of guided reading, reading while listening, and independent reading with computer-based speech feedback. *Reading Speech Quarterly*, 23, 219–235.

Searle, J.R. (1969). *Speech Acts*, Cambridge: Cambridge University Press.

Spaai, G.W.G. and Ellermann, H.H. (1990). Learning to read with speech feedback: An evaluation of computerized reading exercises for initial readers, In J.M. Pieters, P.R.J. Simons and L. de Leeuw (Eds.) *Research on computer-based instruction*, Amsterdam/Lisse: Swets & Zeitlinger BV.

Taylor, M.M., Nél, F. and Bouwhuis, D.G. (1989). *The structure of Multimodal Dialogue*, Amsterdam: North Holland.

Terken, J.M.B. and Collier, R. (1989). Automatic synthesis of natural-sounding intonation for text-to-speech conversation in Dutch. In J.P. Tubach and J.J. Mariani (Eds.) *Proceedings of the European Conference on Speech Communication and Technology*, Paris: September 1989. Vol. II, 108–111.

Index

A

Accentuation, 609, see also Computer-based speech training; Toys

Acceptability, see also Intelligibility
  computer-based speech training, 576
  interactive instruction, 610
  testing methods, 209–213

Access points, 558, see also Text-to-speech, communication aids

Accuracy, see also Errors
  automatic speech recognition evaluation, 364–367
  letter-to-sound rules, 105–106
  recognition systems
    assessment vs. testing conditions, 153-154
    comprehension and perception, 252, 255, 256, 258, 261, 262
    industrial environment, 474–475
    information reduction, 54
    performance and success relation, 152–153
    response time relation, 159
    spoken language interface design, 421–425
    vocabulary, 353
    word monitoring tests, 266, 267
  text-to-speech systems, 107–108

Acoustic coupling, 456

Acoustic theory, 10–15, see also Speech, description

Acoustic tube model, 13, 14, 73

Acoustic utterances, 415–416, see also Utterances

Acoustics
  characteristics of speech, 22–27
  cognitive engineering for speaker-dependent system training, 128, 134–138, 141, 144–145, see also Speaker-dependent systems
  computer-based speech training, 572
  environment in recognition cellular telephones, 447
  perceptual assessment of impaired speakers, 527–531, 534–539, see also Hearing-impaired talkers
  phonetic processing
    perception and comprehension, 270, 271
    intelligibility of speech, 201
    sheep/goat performance, 173

speech coding in recognizer systems, 349
user training in recognition systems, 168–169

Acronyms, 396, see also Voiced mail

Action cues, 439, 612, see also Driving instruction; Interactive instruction

Active filters, see Filters, active

A/D converters, see Analog-to-digital converters

Adam's apple, 4, see also Speech, description

Adaptation, speaker, 85, 143, 145, 171-172

Adaptive delta modulation (ADM), 64

Adaptive differential pulse code modulation (ADPCM), 64–65, see also Pulse code modulation
  embedded/fixed, 460–462
  speech recognition cellular telephone, 448, 450

Adaptive predictive coders (APC), 65, 66

Adaptive-quantizer pulse-code modulation (APCM), 58, see also Waveform

Additive rules, see Rules, additive

Add-on board, 323, see also Analog-to-digital converters

Address, specialized, 101–102

ADM, see Adaptive delta modulation

ADPCM, see Adaptive differential pulse code modulation

ADS, see Audio Distribution System

Affixes, 20, see also Syllables

Affricates, 7, 8, see also Speech, description

AI, see Articulation Index

Air flow, 4, 5, see also Speech, description

Air pressure, 3, 4, 7, see also Speech, description

Alias frequencies, 342, see also Frequency

Aliasing, 67, 324, 326, 328

Allophones, 16, 19, 548, see also Phonemes

All-parallel approach, 82

All-pole assumption, 84, see also Linear predictive coding

All-pole filters, see Filters, all-pole

Alphabet characters, 2

Alphadigit vocabulary, 86, see also Vocabulary

Alveolar articulation, 6, 8, see also Speech, description

Alveolar ridge, 5, see also Speech, description

Ambiguity, 103, see also Text-to-speech systems

Amplifiers, 338

G